A Time of Distance

A Time of Distance

The COVID-19 Visual Project

edited by
Arianna Rinaldo

Gallerie d'Italia | Skira

Gallerie d'Italia | Skira

Gallerie d'Italia
is the Intesa Sanpaolo Project
on art and culture

Skira editore S.p.A.

Massimo Vitta Zelman
Chairman

INTESA SANPAOLO

Giovanni Bazoli
Chairman Emeritus

Gian Maria Gros-Pietro
Chairman

Carlo Messina
*Managing Director
and CEO*

Paolo M. Grandi
Chief Governance Officer

Michele Coppola
Art, Culture and Historical
Heritage
Executive Director
Gallerie d'Italia
Director

Intesa Sanpaolo's unwavering focus on the great issues of our time translates, in the context of the bank's *Progetto Cultura* (Culture Project), into a solid commitment towards the promotion of photography as the principal form of expression of our contemporary moment. It is against this backdrop that the bank is collaborating with the "Cortona On The Move" International Photography Festival, with which we launched – during the lockdown of spring 2020 – an original initiative, in the form of a digital archive called *The COVID-19 Visual Project: A Time of Distance*, which brings together the works of leading photographers from around the world, who were called upon to encapsulate emotions, situations and consequences associated with the challenging period of the pandemic.
Two of these images – the shot taken in Novara by Alex Majoli, and the Gallerie d'Italia in Milan, photographed behind closed doors by Gabriele Galimberti and Paolo Woods – were ranked amongst the 54 most iconic shots of 2020, selected out of 1.7 million entries by *National Geographic International*. The archive has been gradually enriched, and now constitutes an extraordinary set of photographs that makes it possible to survey the present with greater awareness and that, one shot at a time, is building up a wealth of images which, once handed down to the future, may be leveraged to develop a more in-depth understanding of the complex historical moment that we have just lived through. Highly talented, creative exponents of contemporary photography – such as Paolo Pellegrin, Nanna Heitmann, Simon Norfolk and Gideon Mendel – have succeeded in transposing the drama of the pandemic into engaging, beautiful works of art. Today, a selection of these images has become a book published by Gallerie d'Italia | Skira, affording a new opportunity to share the project that we created with the Cortona festival.
Underpinning it all, there is the same idea of photography as a tool for social investigation that infuses the initiatives of Intesa Sanpaolo's new Gallerie d'Italia. The bank's fourth museum, recently inaugurated in Turin's Piazza San Carlo, is dedicated – in synch with the role of the city – to photography, the digital world and the culture of the image.
The new exhibitions on display here will be the result of a programme of projects entrusted to the greatest Italian and international photographers and concerned with current issues – from the climate crisis to the technological revolution – on which to base discussions, workshops and explorations. It is a place where the power of images, like those we can admire in this book, arouses a sense of wonder and gives rise to understanding, reflection and change.

Michele Coppola
Executive Director Art, Culture and Historical Heritage
Intesa Sanpaolo

Contents

04. The Economic Effects

05. A Wounded Society

06. A New Normal

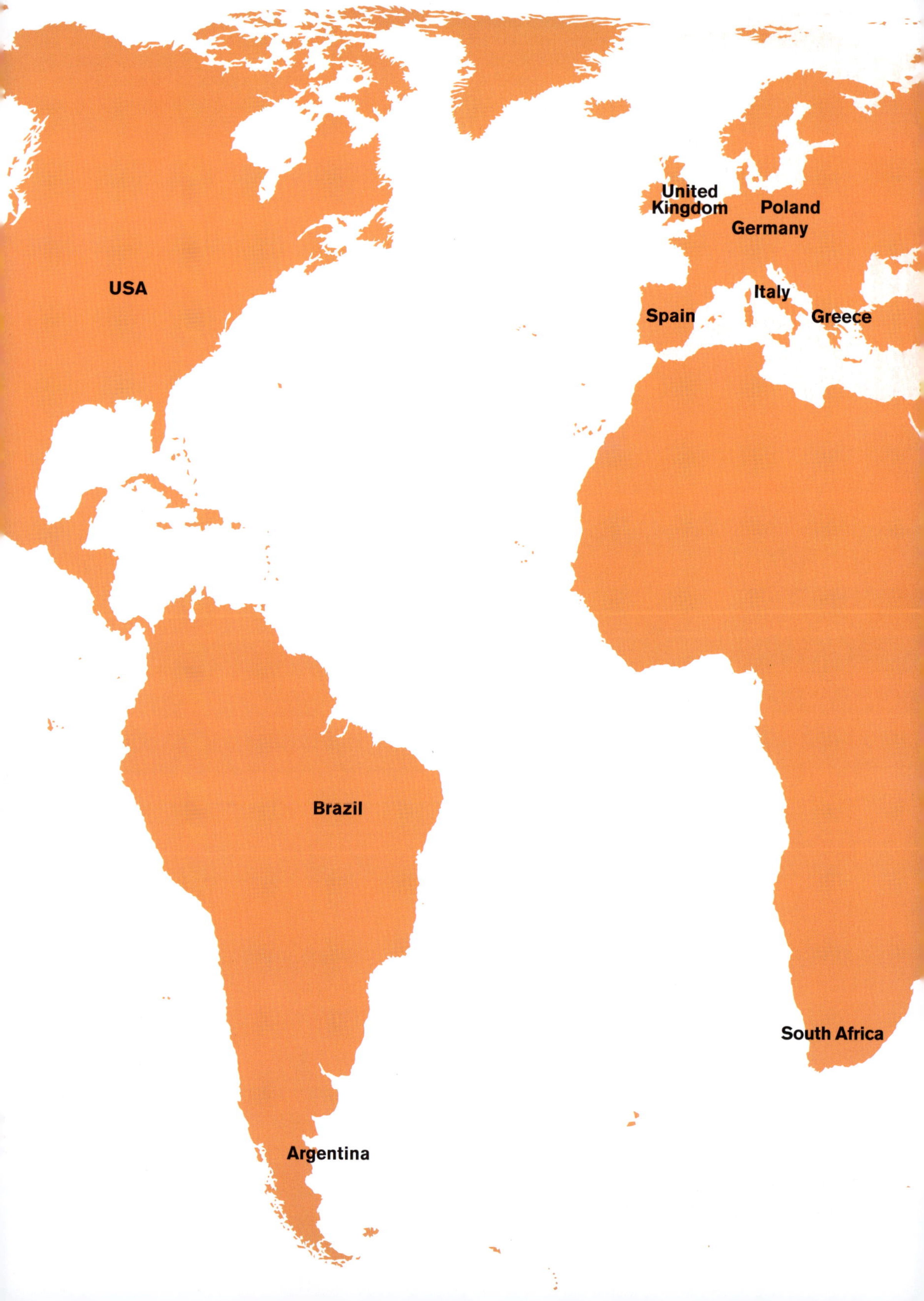
United Kingdom
Poland
Germany
USA
Italy
Spain
Greece
Brazil
South Africa
Argentina

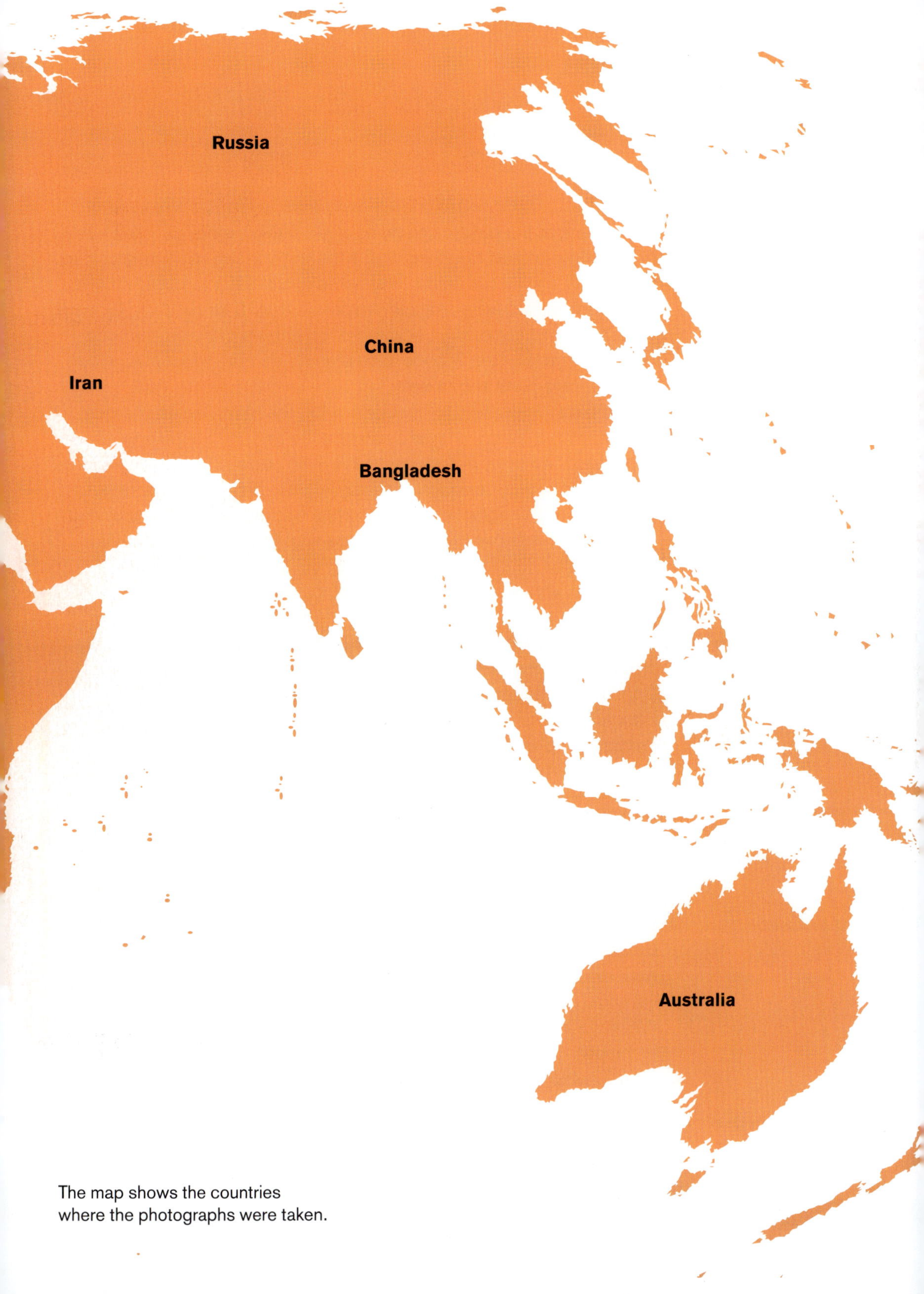

The map shows the countries
where the photographs were taken.

Time and Distance

Arianna Rinaldo
Curator, *The COVID-19 Visual Project*
Artistic director, Cortona On The Move (2012-2021)

When the pandemic began nobody really knew what to do. We were all taken aback by the sudden spreading of this "new coronavirus", as it was continuously referred to in the media in the first alarming news reports (was there an old one? when? most of us asked ourselves). We looked far away to the East and still felt safe in our Western homes. Then suddenly, for many of us, it touched home. Italy became the first hotspot of the virus outside of China, or at least the first one to be severely hit. After a few days, a few hours, it crept closer and closer.

Nobody really knew what to do. Cortona On The Move, the international festival of visual narrative I was curating at the time, got temporarily suspended, like many public events. We really had no clue what was going on. However, those who did know what to do, and always seem to know, are the photographers and reporters who immediately felt the need to go out and document what was happening. That is their job. That is what they do.

I remember very well when Antonio Carloni, founder of the festival, together with the Cultural association ONTHEMOVE, and its director from 2011 to 2021 (the person with whom I have created the programming, the exhibitions and the special projects that have made Cortona On The Move a reference in the world of photography at an international level) called me with a powerful, yet urgent idea: to commission photographers around the world and document this unique historical moment we were living.

With the festival team and partners, we quickly decided to continue being a "place" to share stories about the world: an online project rapidly took shape. We understood we had to be active and proactive in a general moment of suspension. That is how the *The COVID-19 Visual Project. A Time of Distance* was born. It was a necessity for us to continue to spread and produce visual content for a large audience. And we did it because documentary photographers were ready to go around the world, were available to go out there and shoot, risking a disease we still did not know much about.

When we forged the thematic structure of the project we tried to consider all the possible scenarios and collateral effects of the urgent pandemic, many of which we did not yet have a clear idea of. A primary concern was to mirror a global reality: we would start by focusing on Italy as that was the hotspot at the moment and also the physical home of Cortona On The Move. We also aimed to reach different corners of the world. We were treading on unknown waters not sure how lives would shape in the near future.

The result is the multi-disciplinary online platform, covid19visualproject.org, hosting more than 80 photographic stories focusing on a series of interconnected themes that weave the sanitary crisis with economic and social effects. The content is not meant to be exhaustive but aims to touch on issues and matters that were experienced worldwide, albeit with different levels of harshness and gravity.
More than 30 stories were commissioned in the first stage of the production process. Later, an international open call was launched to continue collecting works from other parts of the world. In addition to this curated selection, we also received donations: photographers who felt the need to deposit their work on this platform, to make it available, permanently, as a historical witness of the pandemic crisis.
The first chapter, "A Visual Overview", begins with Alex Majoli's peregrinations around Italy, from South to North, putting on stage the gestures characterising the first weeks of the spreading of the virus. Each place has a name, each person has a story. A year later, the last chapter, "A New Normal", ends with Paolo Pellegrin's uncertain views of the masses and faces trying to find their shape and their place again, in the streets and *piazzas* of the Italian peninsula.
In between, we travel from Patagonia to Bangladesh, from Germany to South Africa, from Brazil to Russia, from Australia to Greece witnessing emergency measures, lockdown desperation, empathy, depression, resilience and hope. Thanks to this collection of visual essays we can look back at how we coped with the interruption of education, the tragedy of the nursing homes, the emptiness of the cities, the silence of the streets and the deaths of our fellow humans. We recall how we rediscovered time and beauty in the little things, how we found connection in the distance, and we felt closer and somehow more united.
Our ultimate goal in creating *The COVID-19 Visual Project* was to offer a stable space for all this to sediment, a place to gather meaningful material we can all return to in an attempt to understand what happened, how and why; and to remember a time when humanity as a whole was forced to press "pause", together. *The COVID-19 Visual Project* thus represents a collective historical memory to help us to not forget the time of distance we all had to experience and endure. Each in our own way, we lived through an incredibly dramatic time in the history of humanity which will shape our future in still unpredictable ways.
This book, *A Time of Distance*, offers a curated selection of the stories collected in the online platform. Thirty-seven visual narratives that witness the struggles and emotions that have accompanied this long and difficult journey: the wish is that we can all look at these images and find a bit of ourselves, a time of distance that we experienced and, hopefully, has passed.

A Sentimental Chronology of the Pandemic

2020, COVID-19. 2021, the vaccine. 2022, a society to rebuild. A collective diary that looks ahead, without nostalgia

Giuseppe Smorto
Journalist
Director of repubblica.it
(2003-2016)
Deputy director
of *la Repubblica*
(2016-2019)

Confined to our homes, concerned only with the borders of the red zone, we have inevitably come to terms with the value of journalism and good information. During the months in which we have been nowhere, our eye on the world has been that of the correspondents, photojournalists, and video-makers. And *The COVID-19 Visual Project* has become our heart and image in the world's media.

Each of us has a mental diary about the pandemic — a burning story, maybe the loss of a dear one. Looking back, there was a time when the Italian government sent a plane to retrieve a student who was in his fourth year of high school in Wuhan. It seemed, in those February 2020 days, that the virus was *their* thing, the Chinese thing. But it didn't take long to get here. We put flags on our balconies, brought out guitars and loudspeakers, to at least get our heads out of the lockdown.

There was a time when masks and sanitizers were nowhere to be found, when the motorway service stations which were always open — even on Christmas Day — were empty. There was a time when the only people around were the pizza delivery heroes, the riders: a job that has become globalised. And, even on the beaches, the police would intervene to punish citizens in deckchairs: the seashore was closed. Children's playgrounds were padlocked, tell me, when will they be back?, when winter is over.

Lonely men gave a sense of history: President Mattarella at the Altar of the Fatherland, and the Pope praying at Saint Peter's in the rain, both accompanied only by silence. Bergoglio walked through Saint Peter's square, a late March dusk had fallen, his breath was audible: "We have realised that we are in the same boat, all of us fragile and disoriented, but at the same time all important and needed, all of us called to row together".

Citizens have been less distracted when it comes to political decisions, which happens every time there is a crisis: it should be a habit that remains with us, that makes us aware. We have been disciplined, by a large majority, we have learnt what PNRR[1] means, and dozens of other acronyms. It is now up to politics to restore a vision. Because, in the meantime, society has become more vertical.

They have been two woeful years, and it is understandable that there is a desire to forget them. Young people have suffered, the virus has stolen the best years from them, DAD[2] has caged them. The folksinger Giovanna Marini, from the top of her outstanding 85 years of age, said it with simplicity: "I never thought I would worry about meeting someone". The newspapers and the news continued to talk about Covid, a long stream that sometimes obscured the certainty of tragedy, too many words.

Since the day the vaccine arrived, everything has changed. 2021 was the year of the jab: me Astrazeneca, you Moderna, them Pfizer. Thousands have been saved, while others have questioned the authenticity of the photos of the military trucks carrying coffins in Bergamo. Every day the count of the infected and the victims has been a fixed encounter with the news: a figure that, in the long run, has become superficial, seen from the right or the left, seen by pro-vax, no-vax and agnostics. The truth came from the hospitals, from the stories of those who were inside those masks and overalls: the medical staff, the doctors who died at work, the distraught nurses who posted angry selfies on Instagram.

In these two years, everyone has been looking for a way to feel alive, like the Borussia Mönchengladbach fans who put up their cardboard silhouettes in the stadium. Theatres and TV programmes invented their audience. In South Africa, where Omicron was born, the police cracked down hard on the protests: how desperate those long queues were to get two bits of social grant. In Brazil, the pandemic has widened the already outrageous gap between rich and poor. In India, a multitude of migrants embarked on a journey on foot to return to their native countries, without protection or services. Not all of them arrived. Large areas of the world, such as Africa, have been neglected. And the idea of a patent-free vaccine found the powerful distracted.

In our own small way, it was also a way of testing new forms of closeness (the distance was obvious). Without being able to hug each other — parents with their children, grandparents with their grandchildren, the sick with the healthy — without the business meetings, the birthday parties. Zoom and Meet have become a kind of bar. And nothing will be the same as before in the world of work: many companies have signed smart-working agreements, with some satisfaction. Many happy employees, but let's not forget how many great ideas and love stories were born in front of the coffee machine. The skyscrapers were empty, there has been a (relative) fall in prices in the metropolises, big cities have lost their appeal, and someone has even signed their resignation letter on Tik-Tok. There has been a return to the countryside and its products, Italians have seen on TV that it is possible to live well even in abandoned villages. Nature has taken its revenge.

And so, we have discovered the centrality of science, not only because of the opinions of virologists: biodiversity researchers have explained in a whisper that these two years have been good for the world, anthropic impact has decreased, hidden species have regained their territory. Chandra Candiani wrote that while this virus kills humans, it saves the Earth, makes animals leap and shine and lets trees peacefully muse on flowers and leaves.

And the video of another poet, Mariangela Gualtieri, played on our smartphones along with that of dolphins whirling in ports without ferries: "we all felt that our pace was too fast and furious".
The European Space Agency showed the traffic of large ships in Venice, comparing two satellite photos, one showing its ancient beauty. Epidemiologists have established a definite correlation between pollution and the spread of the pandemic, the greater pulmonary fragility of those who live in industrial areas. But more topical than all the research, more precise than all the statistics, has been our everyday life, the impact of citizens on health care, both good and bad, neighbourhood welfare also proving useful when it is more efficient than hospitals. Today, the pandemic reinstates our obligation to never leave anyone behind, to build projects against loneliness. To protect the health, education, and cultural systems. And no, we will not be nostalgic for these years.

[1] Piano Nazionale di Ripresa e Resilienza (National Recovery and Resilience Plan).
[2] Didattica a Distanza (Distance Learning).

Beyond COVID-19: A Scenario of Hope and Recovery

Linda Gobbi and
Francesco Morace,
Future Concept Lab

Few people remember that on 21 December 2012 the planet went into a tizzy over the Mayan Prophecy announcing the End of the World on that date. Entire communities of doomsayers in various parts of the world prepared for the Final Event. Something similar happened in December 1999 with the Millennium Bug that announced a dramatic blackout of the entire computer network, which had become a vital infrastructure for the entire human community: in both cases, however, nothing happened.
The great events of history almost always catch us unawares. Think of world wars, the fall of the Berlin Wall, 9/11 in New York: the COVID-19 pandemic is no exception. However plausible and probable it may have been after the appearance of SARS CoV-1 in China in 2002, the pandemic caught a large part of the world unprepared health-wise, socially, and above all psychologically.
The fatigue we still feel is above all *conceptual*. Had we been told that it would last two years or more, we would never have believed it. We had to put up with a level of insecurity to which we were no longer accustomed, manage a personal and family fragility that we thought we had definitively left behind as a painful memory of previous generations, and take on social and civil responsibilities that had disappeared from our existential horizon. For those who have grown up in the age of prosperity, to accept fragility and uncertainty is an almost impossible task; this is a type of sensitivity that has never been taught, either in the family or at school. The world of communication and the media have merely mirrored this same inability, reacting in a disjointed manner, demonstrating the same unpreparedness and inadequacy: after the initial reaction of widespread solidarity, they have entered a phase of asphyxiation and they still seem short of breath, two years after February 2020, when everything fell apart. Lack of breath and forward thinking.
It is not so much a question of infodemic, on which too much emphasis has been placed, as the media were accused of only ever talking about the virus. But what else should have been covered in such an epoch-making event?
Rather, the problem has been the inability to make a qualitative leap, to change pace and broaden the view from the current needs to those of the future, avoiding sterile discussions and taking the bull by the horns instead. What kind of normality do we wish for afterwards? What personal contribution are we willing to make? What personal attitudes are we prepared to question? The entire world of corporate culture must also question itself and find a new meaning, new objectives, and new values on which to base itself.

Knowing that the moment is still challenging, the responsibility of designing a new life, with or without COVID-19, or in different and more acceptable shades of its presence, becomes urgent. We need the courage to get out of the mental cage that still surrounds us, retracing the past, to accelerate the process of Reparation of open wounds and finally close them, for an honest, fair, solidarity-based healing. Citizens, nations, the world of work and culture demand it. And every protagonist, initiative, organisation, company, enterprise, which aims to achieve these objectives, is a creator of the common good. In order not to forget, or rather to treasure the memory of what has been experienced, and to move forward. Memory has the capacity to heal, to provide a stimulus for new benefits generated by adversity.
It curbs the risk of repeating the same mistakes, avoids shortness of breath, timid steps, and short-lived goals, and makes it possible to restore meaning to what has happened in a vision that goes beyond adapting to the day-to-day. These two years of continually alternating openings and closures, relief and fears, vital impulses, and inner tensions, forced solitude and unexpected conviviality, sacrifices and emergency funds, are impressed in everyone's memory. Reliving them, transported in images and organised in the various chapters that bring together the visual testimony of the various authors who took part in *The COVID-19 Visual Project* — conceived by the international festival of visual narrative Cortona On The Move — is like giving strength to hope, if it is a memory of the future.
To go beyond a still uncertain present with the right awareness of the past, which has colours and chiaroscuro shades, feelings and plurality of perceptions, places and people so far away and so close, and much more enclosed in a shot. Art, in our case photographic and visual art, has an incredible mnemonic power, capable of stimulating connections that would otherwise fall into oblivion or be deliberately forgotten. The seven chapters, bringing together the various artistic expressions translated into photography, form an extraordinary contribution to capturing reality and the feelings we have experienced, structuring them into a system: in this way they will live on in us with greater practical and symbolic power. A collective memory that becomes everyone's self-awareness, for a new consciousness, common and supportive, that involves us and sees us as protagonists: all of us. This is the great challenge: feeling involved, remembering the past and creating a new, regenerated perspective, prepared to face new uncertainties. Above all from the point of view of communication, which is fundamental in this time and in this game, with so much at stake even in the digital world.
On 21 December 2021 — reshuffling the same numbers nine years after that December 2012 — we therefore find ourselves at a symbolic transition that was not just imaginary, but also real. And so, in this new year and after two years of dealing with Covid, we must not prophesy, but *propitiate*, that is, as the Italian Treccani dictionary puts it: *to gain favour*, to make the context in which we live favourable. We need antidotes and vaccines to defend ourselves, but above all we need replenishments to get going again.

Hope becomes the replenishing agent in this fragile condition and the premise for building more favourable times. Hope implies not only that a desired result is achievable, but above all that it functions — in terms of motivation — as a compensation for uncertainty. It therefore does not coincide with optimism (everything will be all right!), but with awareness: it combines the strong desire for a positive outcome with the feeling that this might not happen. Hope appears as an anticipatory pleasure (joy before joy, wrote Aristotle), which is played out in the future and in desire. Its relationship with time plays the same role with respect to future events that memory plays with respect to the past and that sensation plays with respect to the present. Hope is therefore memory of the future, and only in this way can it become propitiatory. Hope shares the status of every fragile reality requiring care: it needs to be nurtured, caressed, cultivated, and encouraged to grow. Like love, hope can be learned — with a daily training that becomes a virtuous habit — and it can happen where, while feeding on its own uncertainty, it resists the impossible, becoming a generative reality.

Utopia, Cure, Regeneration and Uncertainty: the four principles of hope indicated by Edgar Morin, who at the age of 100 gave us his post-pandemic therapy: *Changeons de voie. Les leçons du coronavirus* (*Changing paths: lessons from the coronavirus*). This is the challenge that awaits us and in the next few years we will have to prepare ourselves to meet it. The culture that characterises contemporary society (politics, business, bodies and institutions, art) has never seriously developed a *vision of hope*, and if it has, it has considered it a luxury, the icing on a cake whose ingredients are mainly economic: today the icing must be mixed with the yeast of the cake, to be raised and baked. And then the pieces must be distributed fairly to all diners.

Over the past two years, we have experienced uncertainty and the unexpected in their most dramatic form: the dark side of uncertainty and resilience. Today we are experiencing that there is also a vital side to uncertainty (challenge, courage, vision) which the world of culture, communication, economics, social and personal development can and must intercept. The main responses during the pandemic were protection, resistance, and resilience. Such a phase has ended, and we are witnessing a counterforce that needs to be interpreted. There are, in fact, advantages in facing the uncertainty of the present, which are not limited to resilience as an antidote to fragility, but include, for example: an open mind that helps us to accept the unpredictable; an awareness of how much everything can change for the worse but also for the better; a willingness to experiment with the courage of a vision; an idea of the future that gives room for utopia; the importance of Care and Regeneration. All this translates into a social and economic scenario in which certainties become platforms, uncertainties push us to give our all, and passions are shared in conditions of *weak ties* — as defined by sociologist Mark Granovetter, meaning travelling companions, new neighbours, people met at a concert, old friends from high school seen by chance, and so on — in places of great sociality such as cities.

The advantages of uncertainty also include the creative power of surprise and wonder, which is what we have missed most during lockdowns: the surprise that comes from the small worlds of weak ties, from chance encounters, from unplanned conversations, from people different from us met at the bar or the cinema, from that slice of unexpected life that always makes a difference. And it is this that we will want to recapture in the future, reshuffling the cards that certainly cannot be dealt by remaining remotely connected.
We have to distinguish between what saved us (the technology that made the strategy of distancing possible) and what will make us happy again in the future: the extended frequentation of attractive places, the expression of collective passions (sport, music, art) and of ritual consumption.
The experience of a century of life, recounted by Edgar Morin in his latest, small but great, book *Leçons d'un siècle de vie* (*Lessons from a century of life*), provides us with valuable pages for reflecting on the condition of humanity and on a destiny that is perpetually invoked or expected. The great sociologist maintains that, with COVID-19, the human adventure has entered a gigantic crisis in which our destiny is at stake. The odds are in favour of the worst. But, as always, the improbable and the unpredictable are also possible. It reminds us that fortune and misfortune chase each other, nothing is acquired forever, the unexpected and the uncertain are part of the history of the world and that of each of us. There is no perpetuity of the present, no continuity that makes it possible to predict the future with certainty. Many things are unexpected, and the unpredictability of the COVID-19 pandemic is one of the many in the present. Integrating the unexpected into human history is a valuable lesson to be better prepared for the future, and to react more quickly and more effectively by caring for people and Mother Earth. Therefore, memory is as useful for the future as this book, which trains people to hope.
In the paradigmatic fault line of uncertainty, it is thus important to redefine innovative experimentation strategies, shifting the boundary between public and private, indoor and outdoor, on the basis of a renewed social pact, in which generations and social classes are already involved, for a fairer and more inclusive society. This is the time for social innovation. In a phase of redefinition of the Collective Good, such as the one we are currently experiencing, the centrality of a common space-time emerges that goes beyond our perception, and that welcomes a planetary community increasingly aware of its own destiny. It is a matter of carving out regenerated times and spaces, through a New Deal that Luciano Floridi has called Universal Trust: no longer just a Social Contract between humans, but a more ambitious project that recognises the universal bond between human beings, living creatures and living environments. In this dimension, time and space are inextricably connected and subject to global events (pandemics, climate change, natural disasters) that are beyond our control. It is a shared, collective time, also geographically characterised, to be experienced beyond the classic daily perception and to be measured by a countdown that is regulated by the capacity of peoples to make the planet more livable.

We are living in a time in which Reparation seems to be the most correct attitude in a context which continues to be problematic and, in some cases, causes great distress. Reparation as the ability to mend wounds and recompose fractures like in the art known as Kintsugi, beautifully mastered by the Japanese, using pure gold threads. And then: Economy of Reparation in the sense of recognising the economic damage done to the planet, to society, to people, taking decisions that are equally economic, i.e. in the dimension of business, with the courageous intention of giving back and repairing, recognising the errors of the past. But the term Reparation also includes the idea of rediscovering the art of maintenance (e.g. of the motorbike... as Pirsig, author of the cult book dedicated to these themes, put it) and further, of recognising our limits and shortcomings, as when we failed a subject as young students and had to re-sit our exams. With humility and dedication, with patience and commitment. For decades, institutional and, to some extent, corporate communication (both in form and substance) has instead taken the opposite direction: favouring impact to the point of overbearingness, the spasmodic search for provocation and rupture, rather than repair. Without acknowledging their own limits, their own mistakes, their own induced deceptions.
A decisive and courageous change of tone and direction is needed, and the superficial nature of many statements, the emptiness of many promises, the misleading nature of much communication must be recognised. This transition can count on young generations committed to values and disenchanted in perception, masters in unveiling trickery or deception, in deciphering the cognitive bias of digital and algorithms that now represent their essential dimension – which also deserves to be repaired. The latest judgments tending to curb the overwhelming power of Big Tech are beginning to point the way, as is the increasingly serious and in-depth work of many entrepreneurs, top managers and operators who consider the 17 goals of the 2030 Agenda to be an integral part of their company's vision and mission. Companies are therefore called upon to think about inclusion, to defend the dignity of work, to advocate human and civil rights, to fill the gender gap, to propose a broader and more articulated vision of sustainability. It is not a question, then, of prophesying, as happened in 2012, but of propitiating, of making new behaviours possible: nourishing the paradigms of the future which, without fear of contradiction, see sustainability, surprise, and cooperation at the centre of our daily lives.

Bibliographic references
Morin, Edgar, *Leçons d'un siècle de vie* (Paris: Denöel, 2021).
Floridi, Luciano, *Il verde e il blu. Idee ingenue per migliorare la politica* (Milan: Raffaello Cortina Editore, 2020).
Morin, Edgar (with the collaboration of Abuessalam, S.), *Changeons de voie. Les leçons du coronavirus* (Paris: Denöel, 2020).

00.

A Visual Overview

Alex Majoli, Italy
Covid on Scene

Massimo Razzi

They're dark, dark and engraved like our lives in these difficult days. These shots — taken by Alex Majoli on his journey through Italy at the time of the COVID-19 pandemic — tell of, or rather, are materially made of the darkness that is inside and around us. Majoli left towards the end of February. "I was working in Reggio Emilia," he says, "when the epidemic began. So I took my first shots there. Then, I moved to Palermo and, from there, the journey began. Because an event like this cannot be covered only by shooting what you see in a place, you almost have to enter it from the outskirts. I tried to do so, travelling across Italy: from Rome, Milan, Bergamo to the border with Slovenia." The shots, of course, must have been thousands: "In the past — explains Majoli — I would have used 80 rolls of film, 2,500 shots for a story like this. Today, obviously, it doesn't even make sense to count them. In the end, however, there are about eighty images left and about fifty are the final result". The images, all in black and white, are obtained by subtracting light from the outline which becomes almost dark, lighting only what really matters. Someone, speaking of Majoli's work, mentioned a "Caravaggesque" visual inspiration: from the darkness emerges, overwhelmingly, what the photographer wants us to see. But from a conceptual point of view, the keyword is "History". "In the sense — explains Majoli — that we will remember what has happened in these months for the rest of our lives and it will be remembered forever. Like the Plague told by Manzoni, the Spanish Flu or the Great Wars. Events that mark a period that may be short, yet they transport it into the history of mankind. I tried to bear in mind this responsibility as I was shooting."
History, thus, and a lot of pain. But not just tears, also hollow, astonished faces. And maybe, even more, the amazement and tiredness that pervades us when we are worn out by some kind of pain to which we were no longer accustomed. A pain of yesteryear... and so the machines and protective gear used by doctors and nurses reminded us of Chernobyl and the Soviet Union, a crossroads of technology and poverty. In this way, the blessing gesture of the priest in front of a truck loaded with corpses reminds us of an almost "historical" image of the 1970s: the famous picture of a dead boy on a park bench in a large northern city with a priest blessing his corpse. And so, perhaps, we've already been there and Majoli tried to reach the roots of our grief to remind us that we've already seen even worse: from Fascism to the Holocaust; from the world wars to 9/11.

The complete project tells the story of the whole of society in the presence of the virus. There are tired workers on a joyless lunch break in Rome, homeless people being rescued in the streets of Milan, devotees alone on church benches in Bologna, priests wearing masks who seem almost lost as shepherds without flocks. Even animals are bewildered, stray and hungry dogs rummage through the garbage, a circus elephant reminiscent of Fellini and pigeons in a Milanese square surround a rider who seem to be asking for the crumbs of a leftover pizza. There is a sad-looking opera singer singing an aria on her front door. There is isolation in a hospital and isolation in the bedroom of a house that may become a prison, or behind the bars of a gate. There are the faces of frightened and confused children.
Here we find an intense selection of images, incomplete, but harsh, in which, here and there you can see moments of humanity and hope. Wonderful, from this point of view is the image of the woman sitting on her hospital bed, talking. All around her, five "coveralled" figures seem to listen to her almost enchanted. They are probably doctors and nurses. What does the lady say? She might have been telling about how, when and how badly she's been ill, or talk about other quiet moments... or maybe she is talking about her grandson? Whatever the story is, it's wonderful the attention the doctors around her give. Majoli remembers that picture very well: "We walked in, my assistant and I, wearing this sort of space suit... and there, in that room, there was this beautiful scene. That lady, until two days before, was intubated. Now she was talking and explaining, and they were listening carefully. There was one missing, Covid. Because that's the way it is, in this story, the virus is there, it's present, it's everything, but you can't see it…". And Majoli, in fact, makes you see everything. And indeed, one can imagine the virus: an all-encompassing presence and, then, when things go well, an equally pervasive absence.
And the journey ends where the country ends, at the border with Slovenia. Those stones close a world and tell us nothing of what lies beyond. A sign says that Italy is on this side and it doesn't seem possible, even from the lettering, that it is 2020.

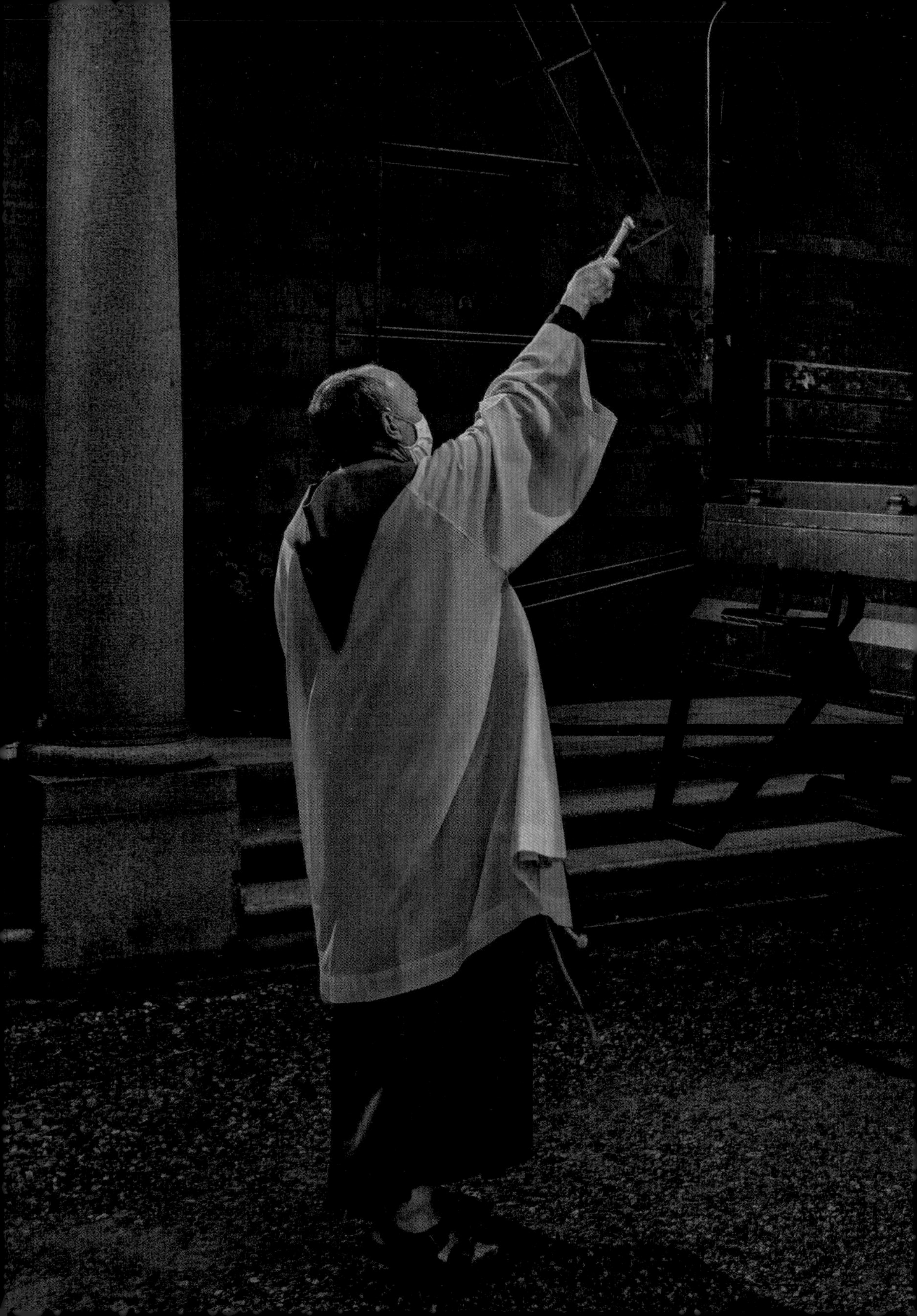

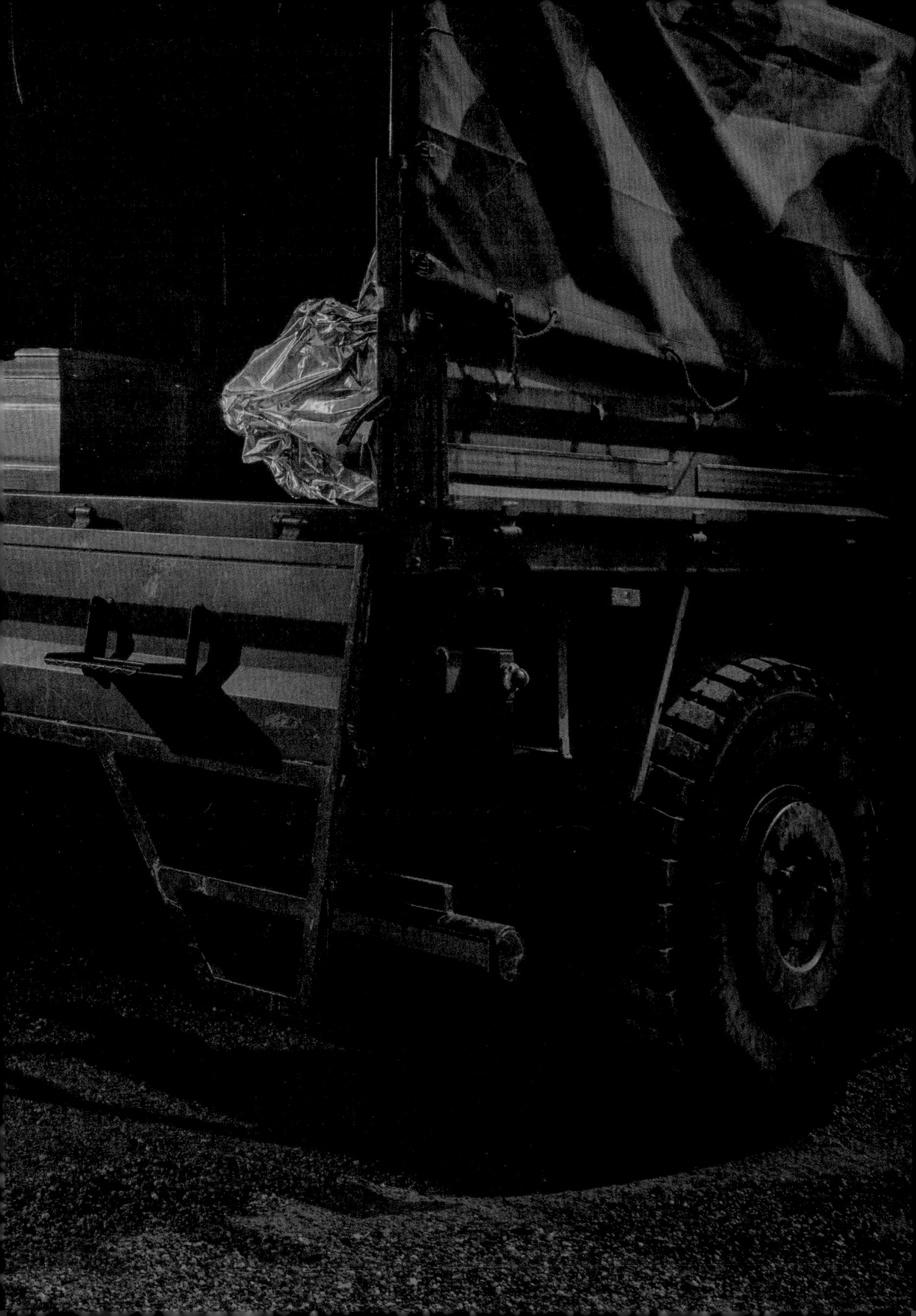

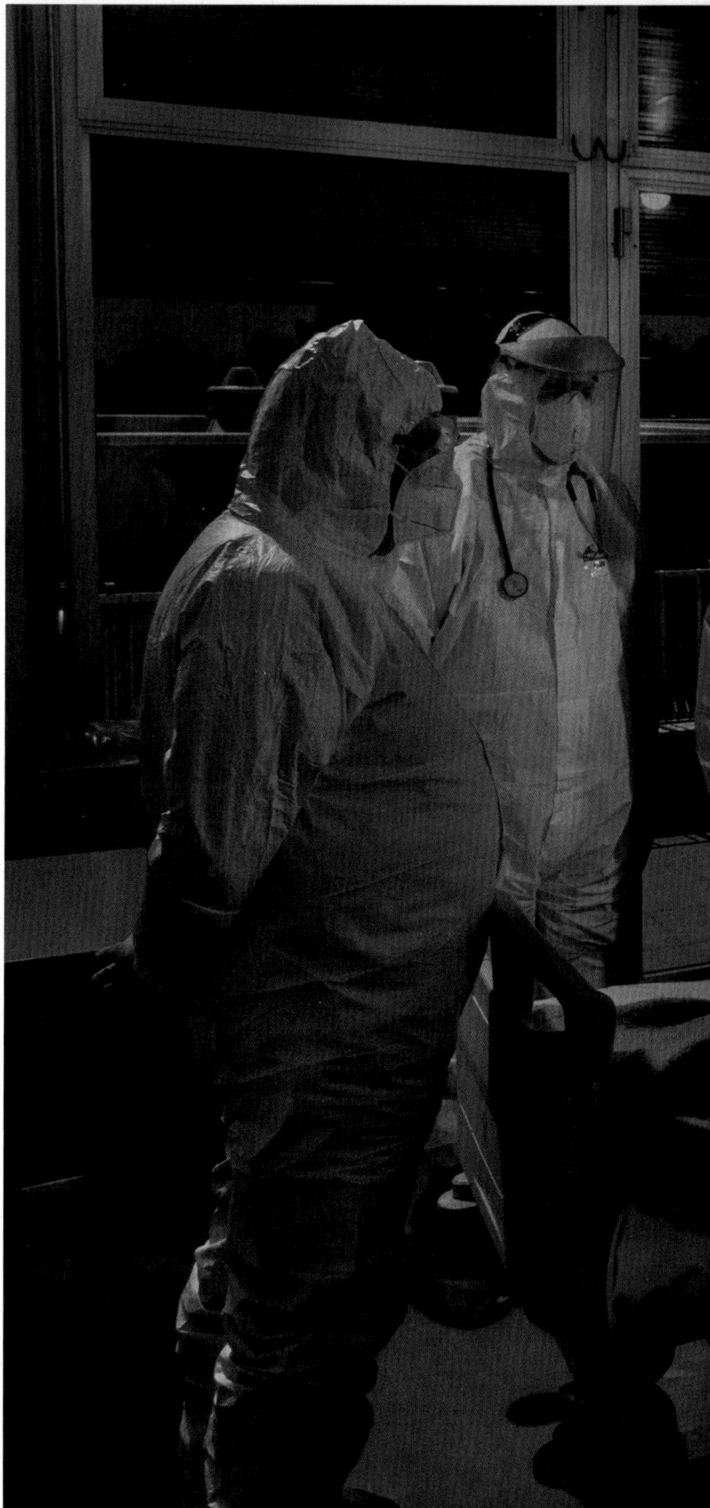

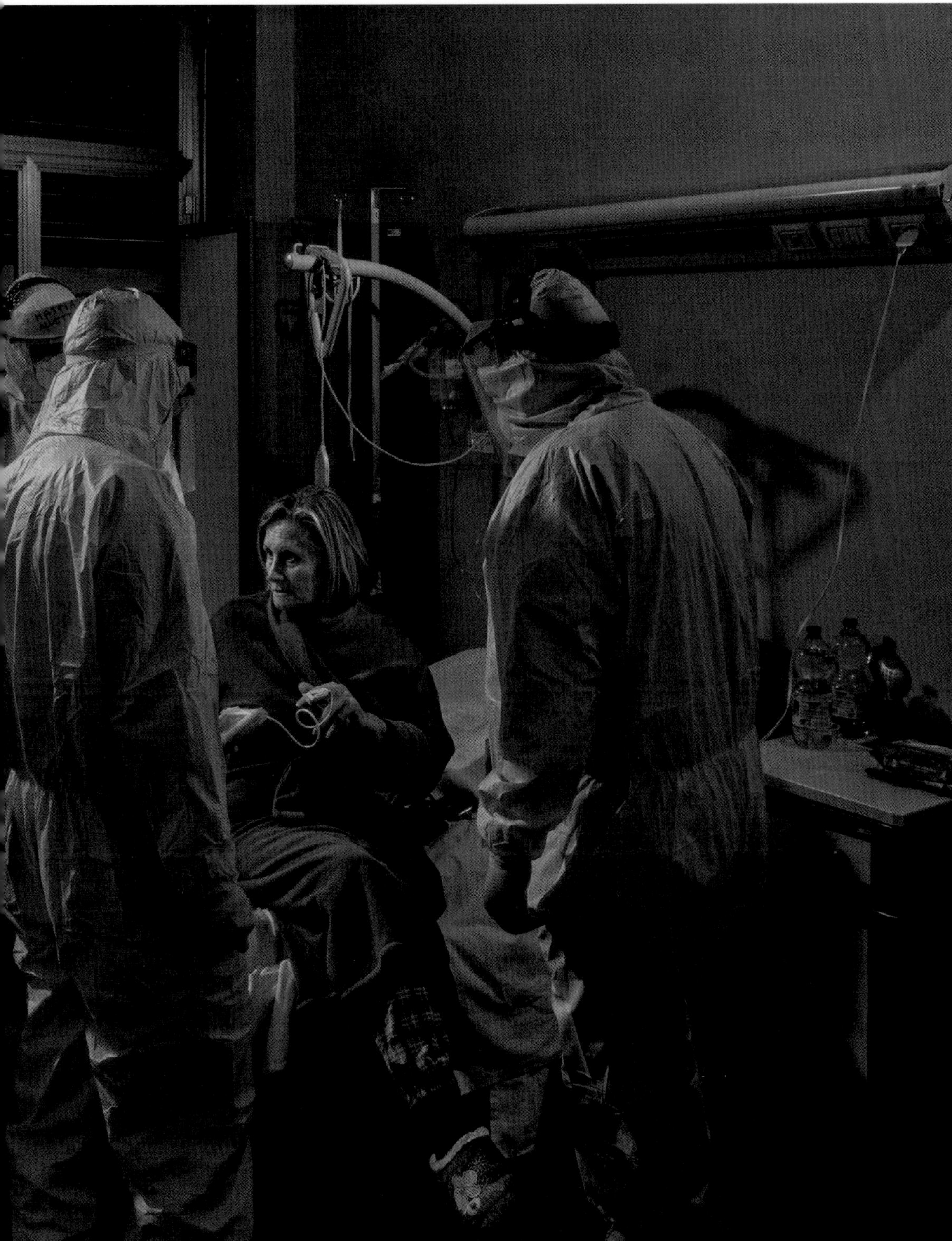

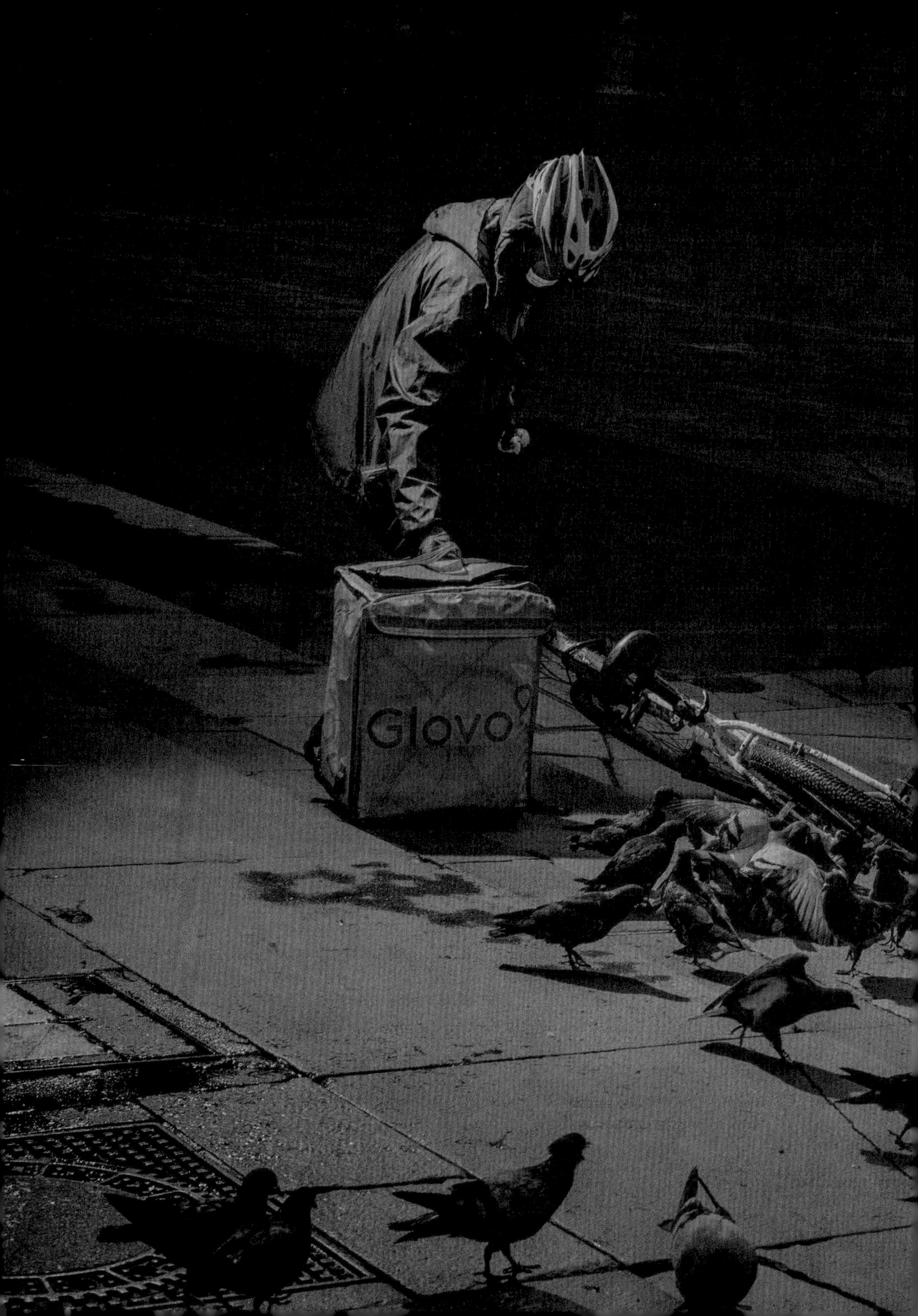
Glovo

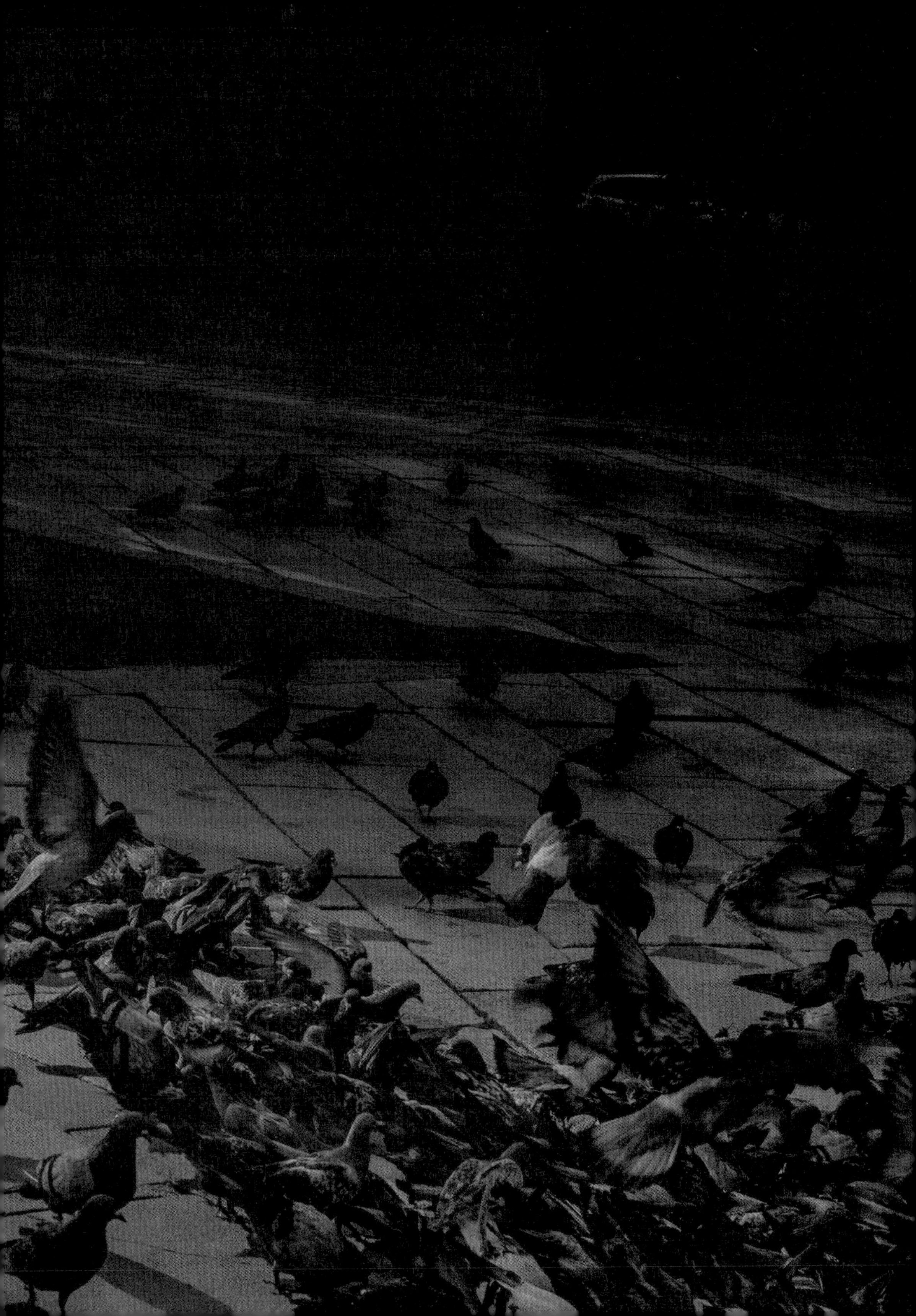

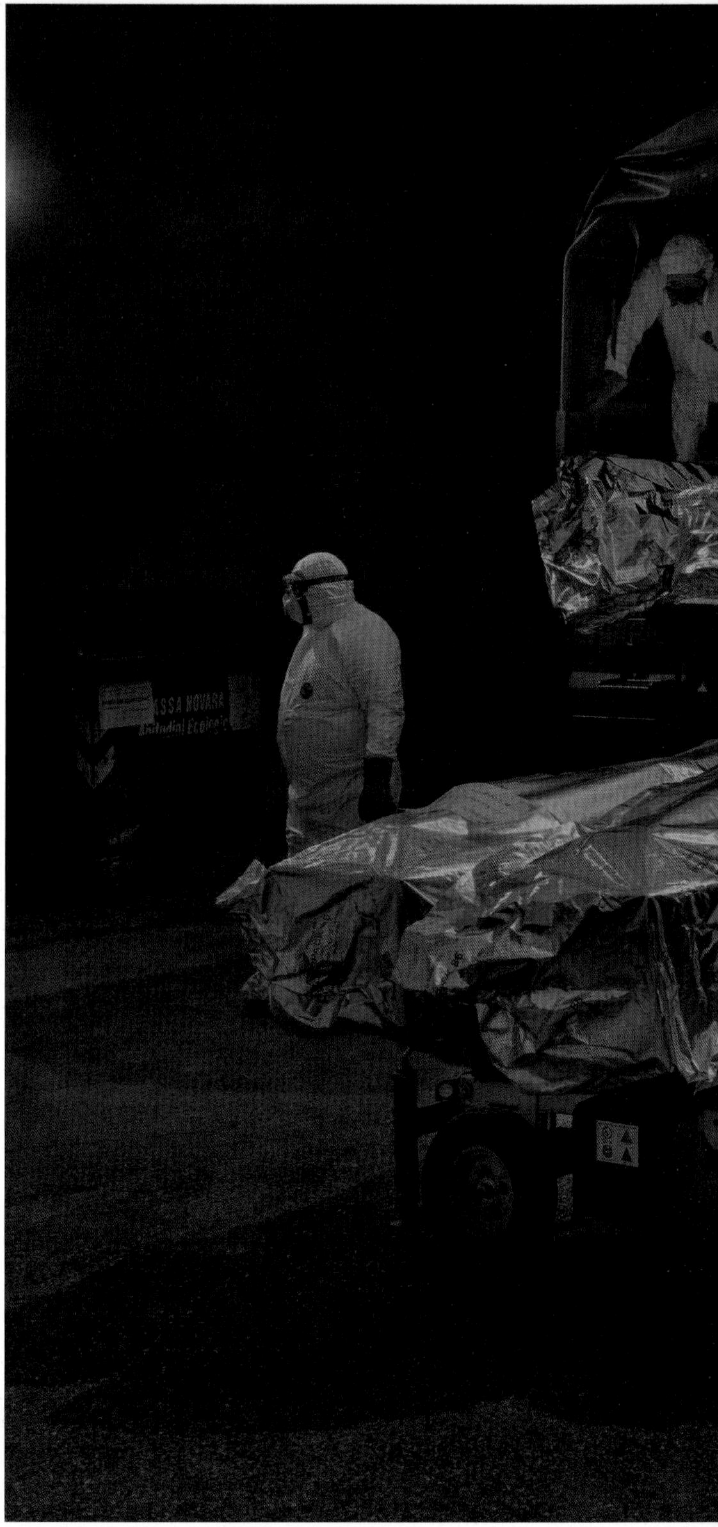

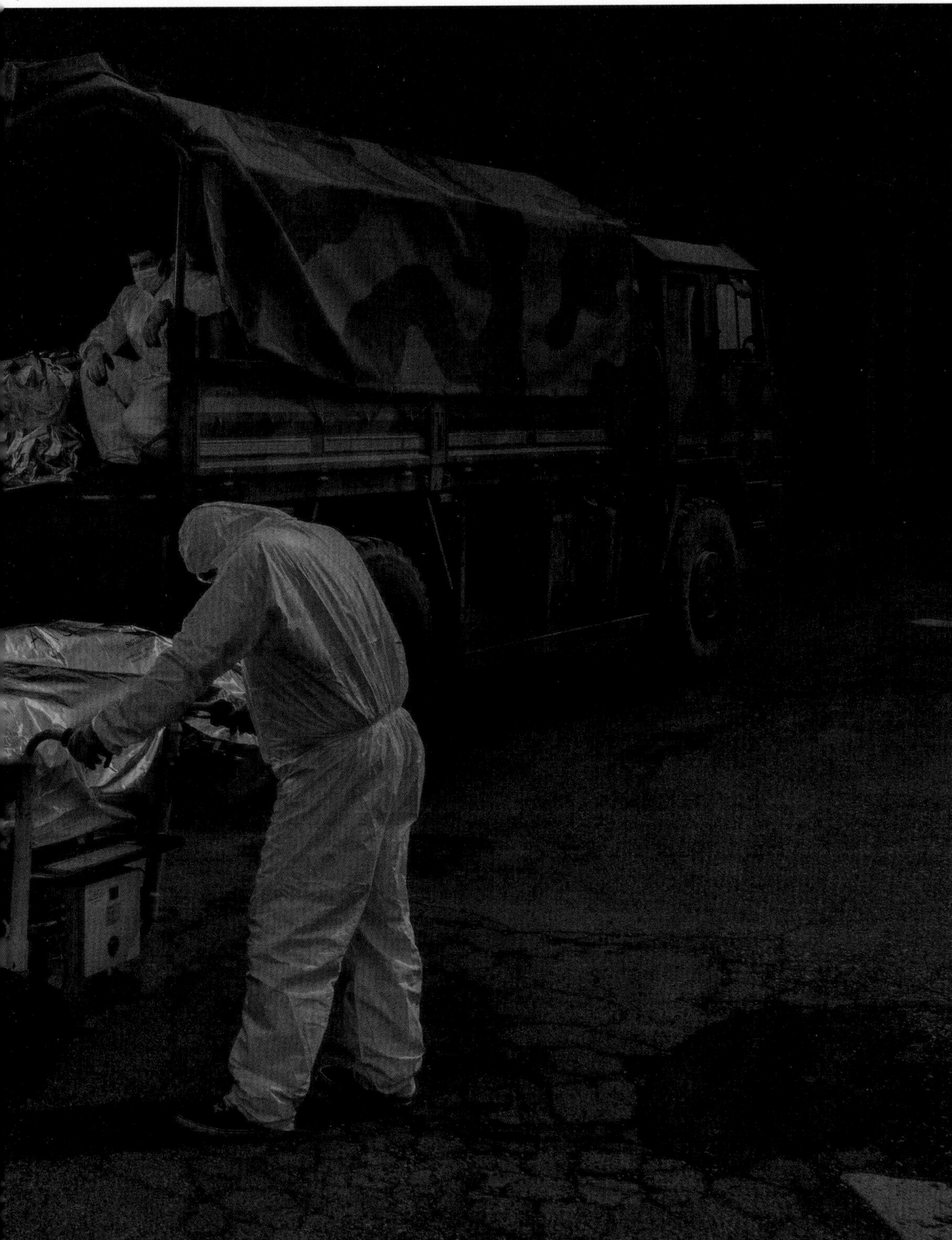

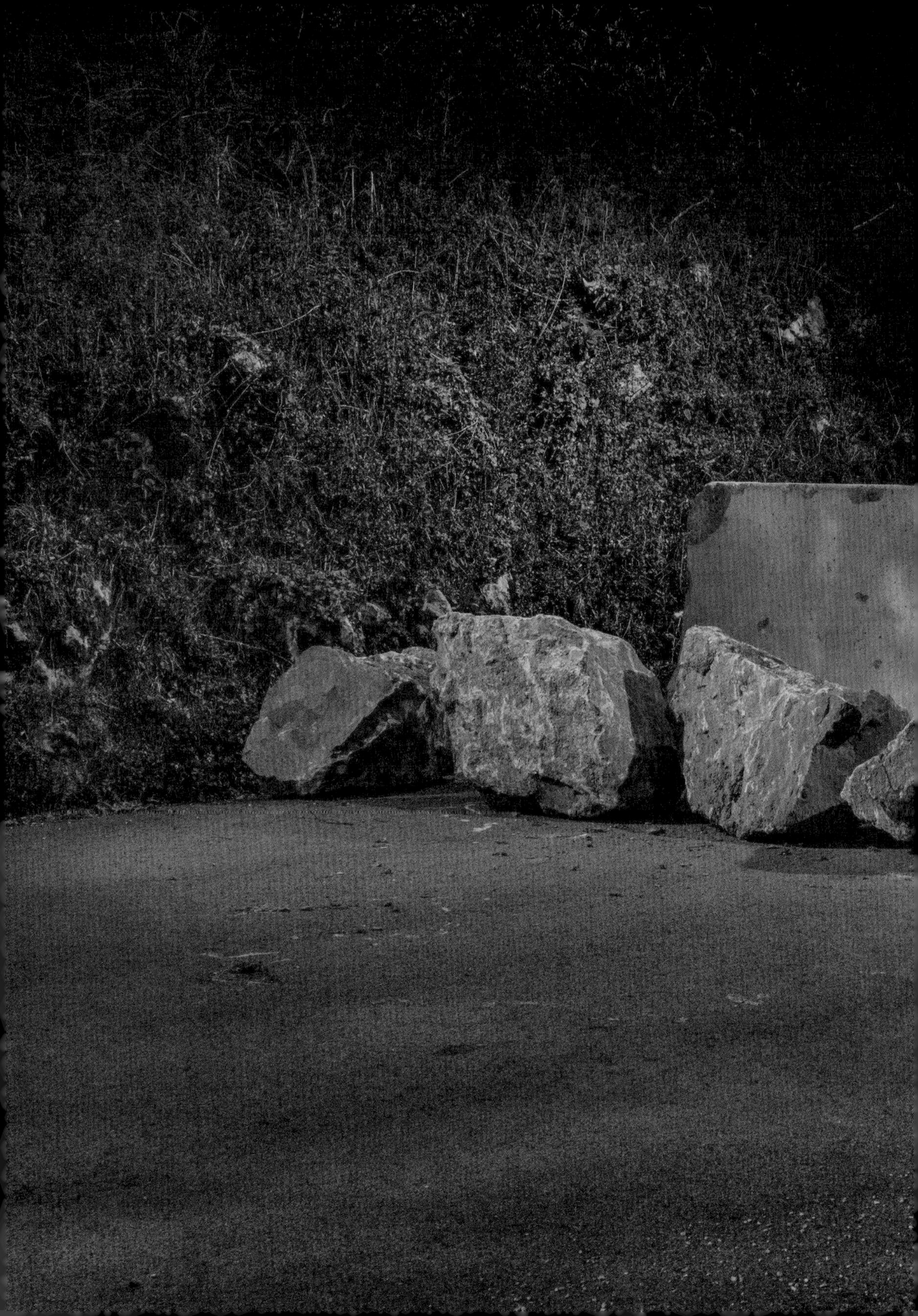

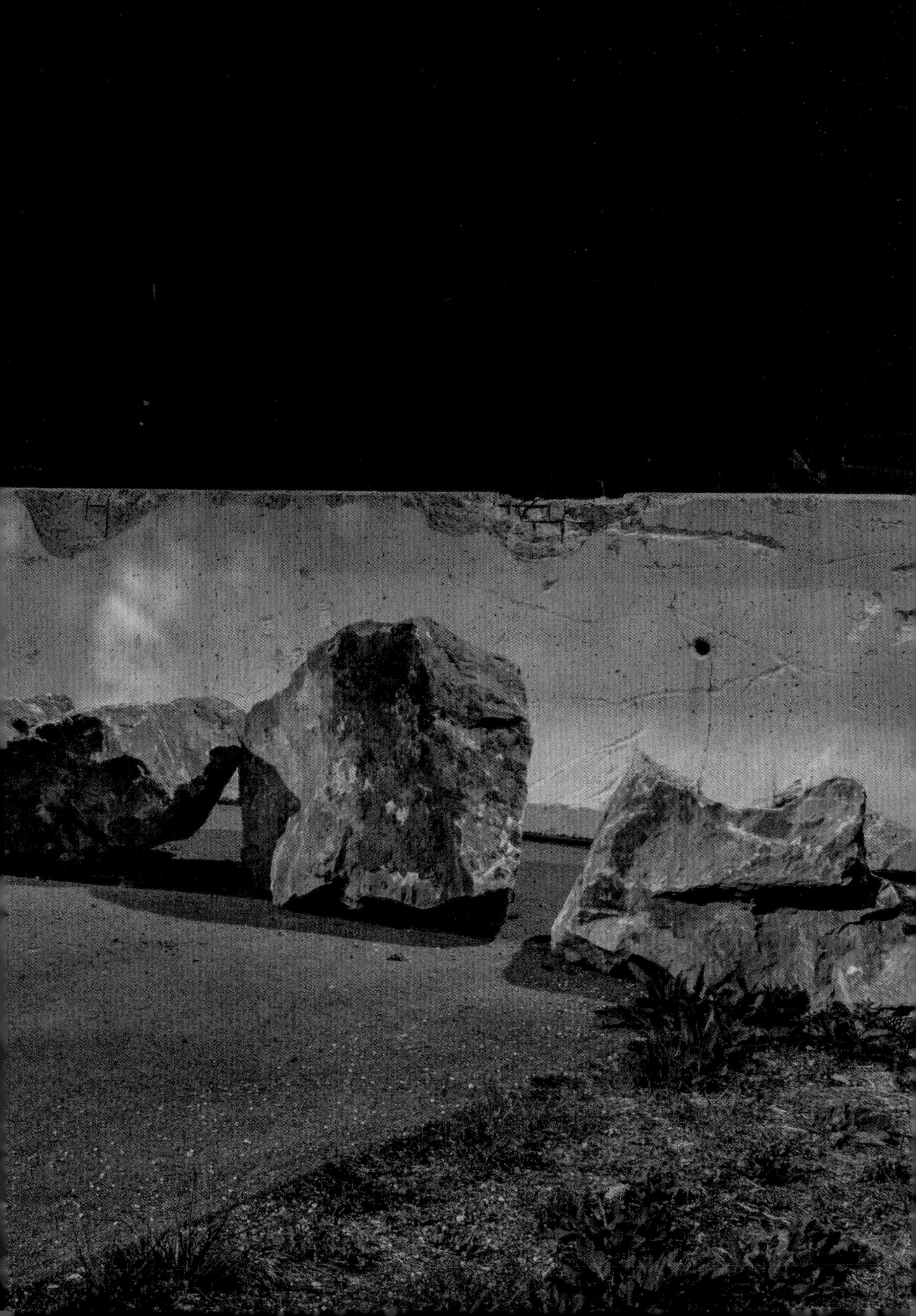

Rafael Heygster & Helena Manhartsberger, Germany
Corona Rhapsody

This project is a contribution to the discussion on the question of what changes in our society will be caused by the pandemic. The work questions how the current situation is presented by the media and perceived by the public and to what extent this corresponds to subjective experiences. But also how the pandemic is possibly being taken advantage for political purposes, and how we will remember the coronavirus crisis in the future.
The outbreak of the coronavirus has changed the world. Like many countries, Germany countered the virus with infrastructural measures, a lockdown lasting several weeks and new rules of social distancing.
Especially at the beginning of the pandemic, the media coverage of the events was often nervous and public uncertainty was great.
Nevertheless, our lives and consciousness are changing due to the pandemic. Even those who do not fall ill are affected: some people are frightened, others are irritated or feel helpless. Some deny health risks and seek responsibility from those in power. Not a few get into economic difficulties. Hugs and physical contacts are no longer a matter of course. Despite the physical distance, people find new ways of being close to each other.
With growing acceptance and adaptation, a feeling of "new normality" has developed.
Often this "new normality" does not feel "normal" to us.
The situation reminded us of a surreal dream.
Based on these subjective impressions we photographed different aspects and scenarios that happened during COVID-19 in Germany. We show governmental measures and the infrastructure behind them. On the one hand, public life is characterised by the need for normality, on the other hand by the desire for change. The people in our pictures move in this field of tension.

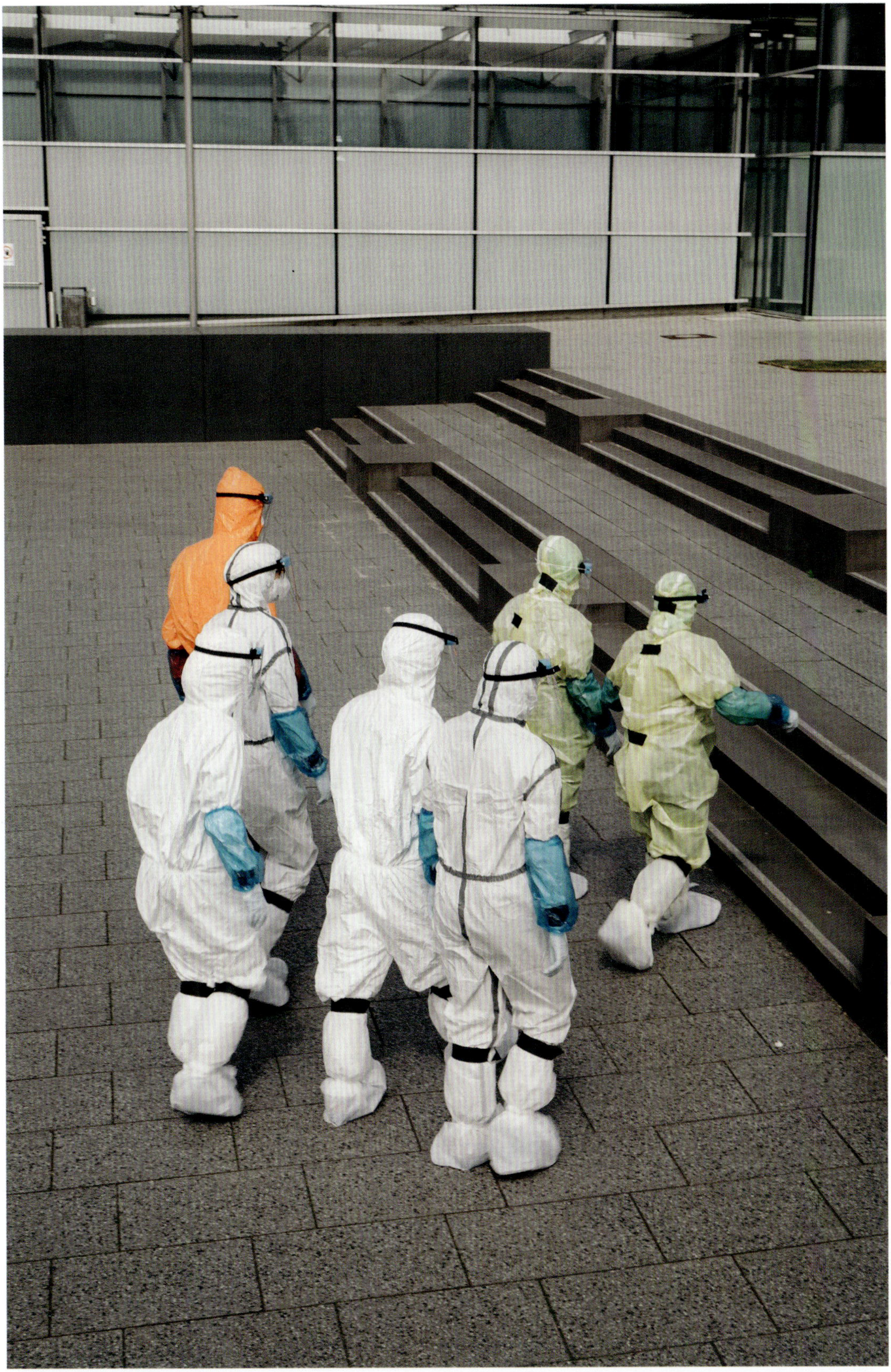

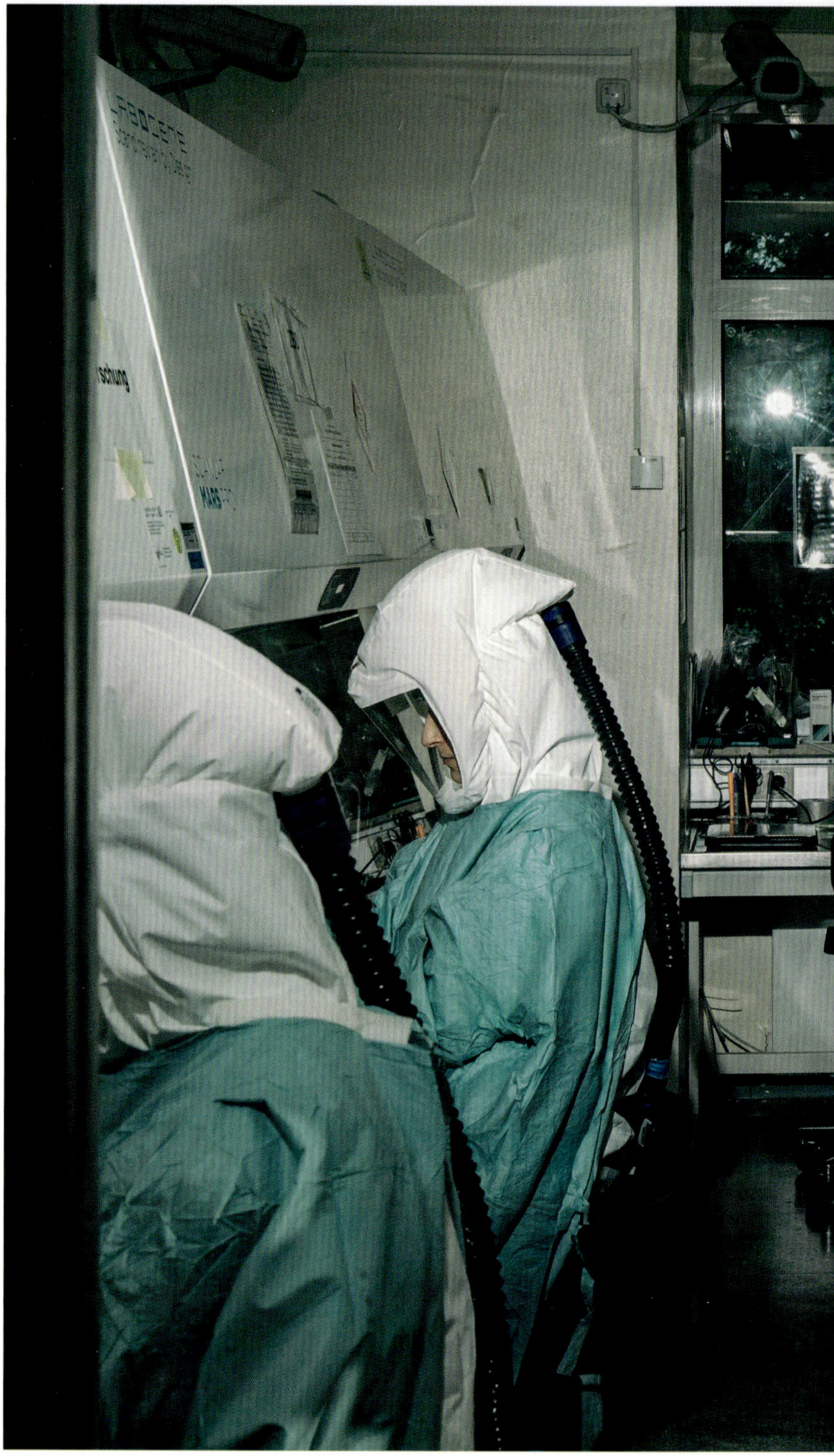

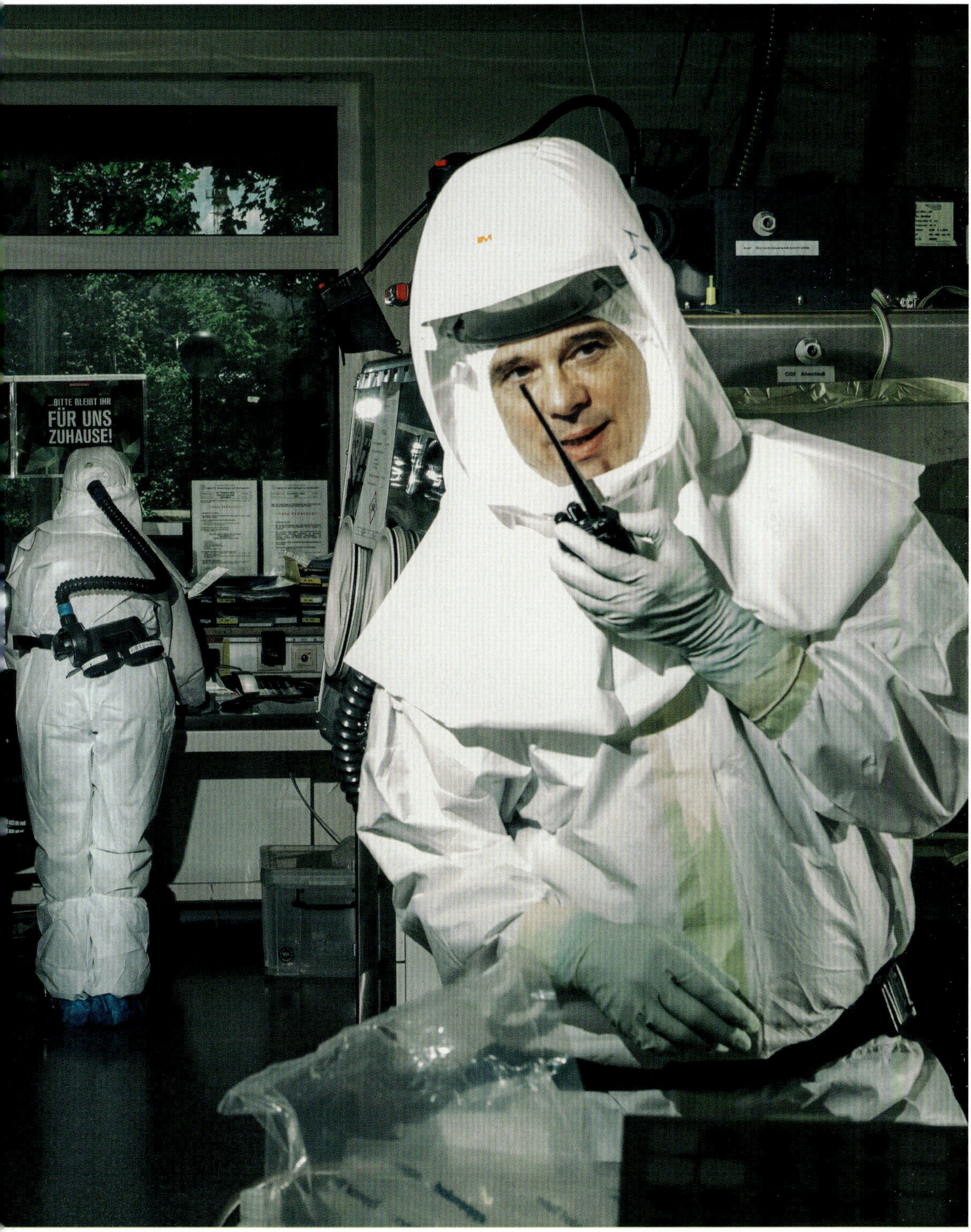
...BITTE BLEIBT IHR
FÜR UNS
ZUHAUSE!

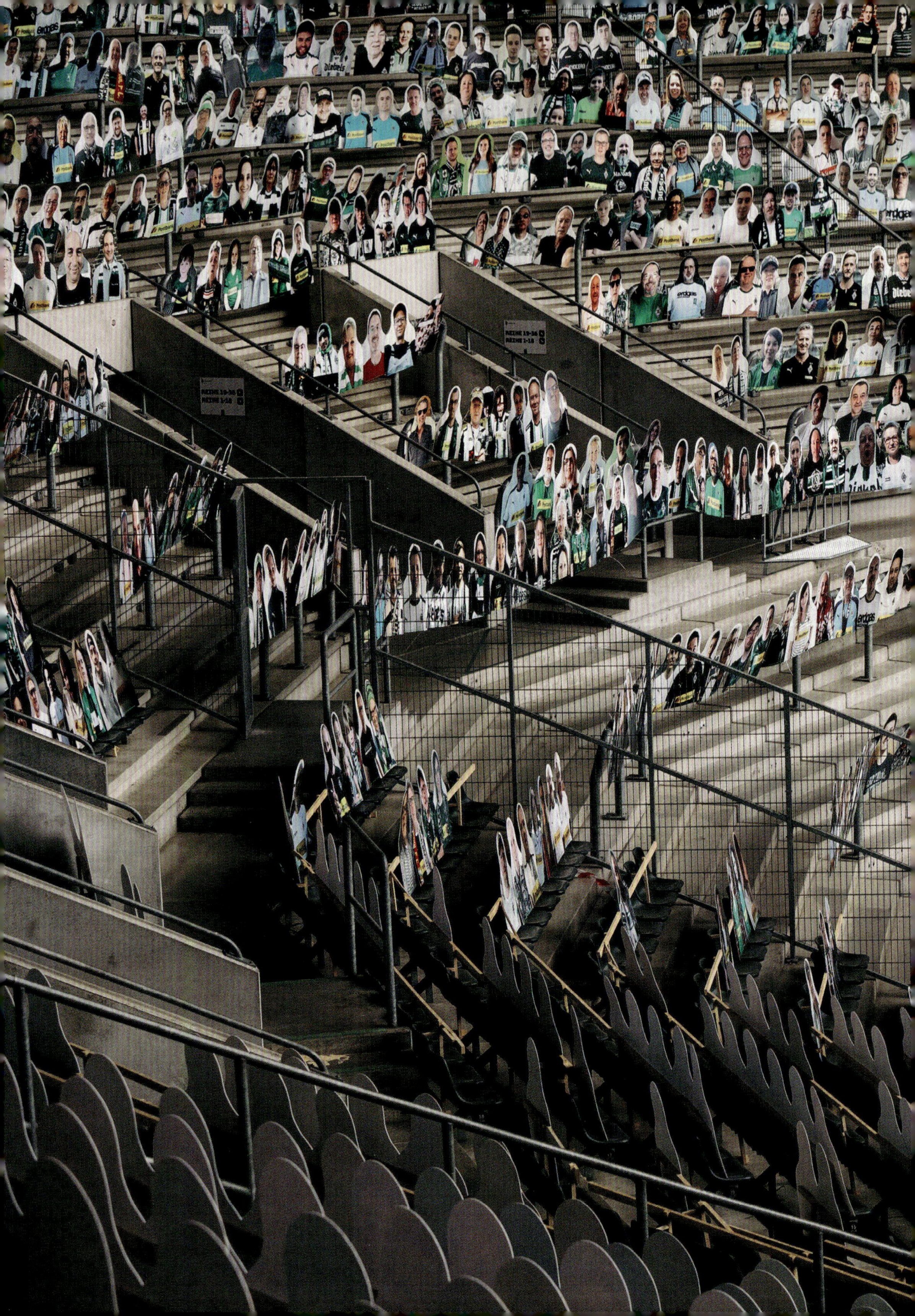

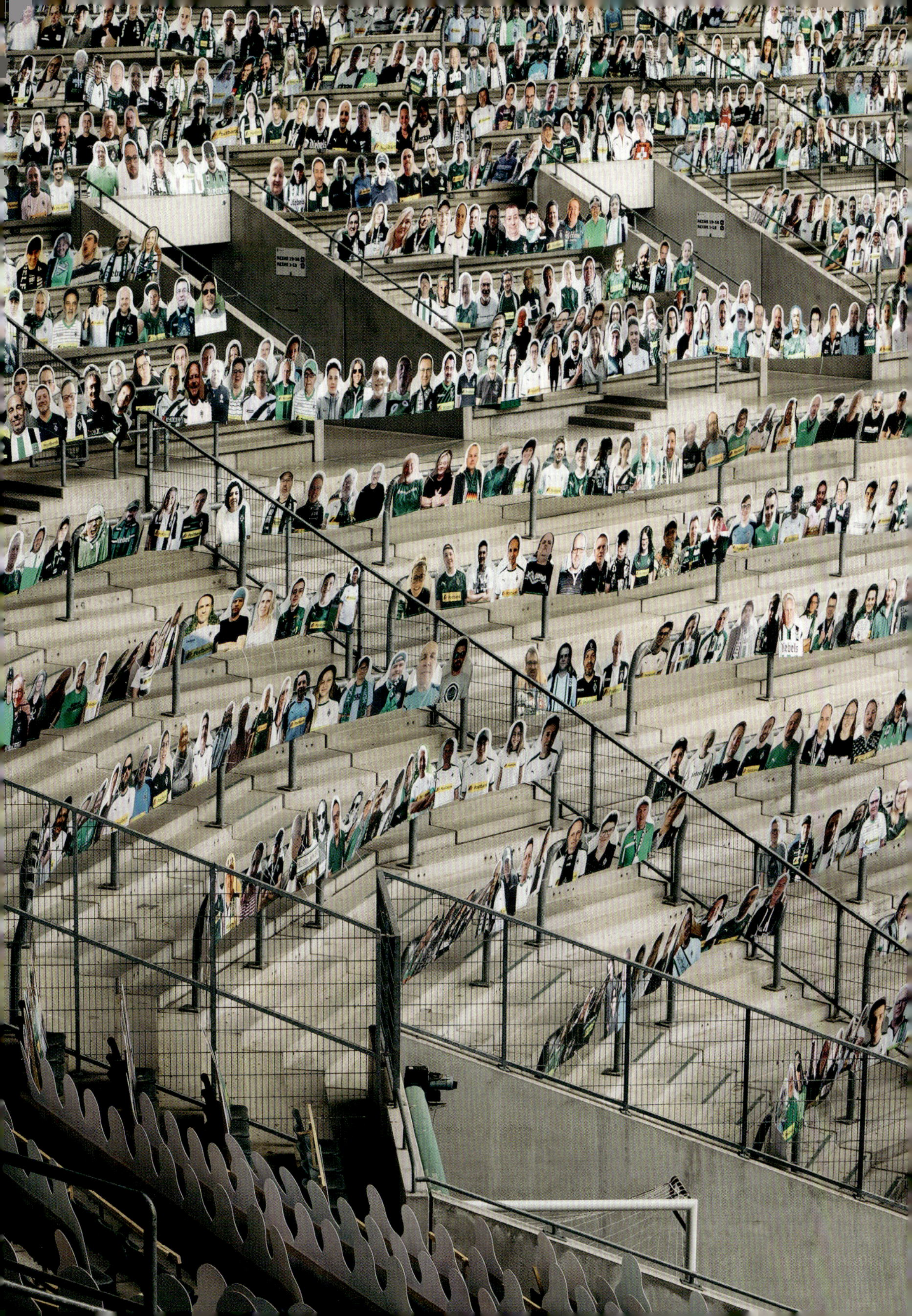

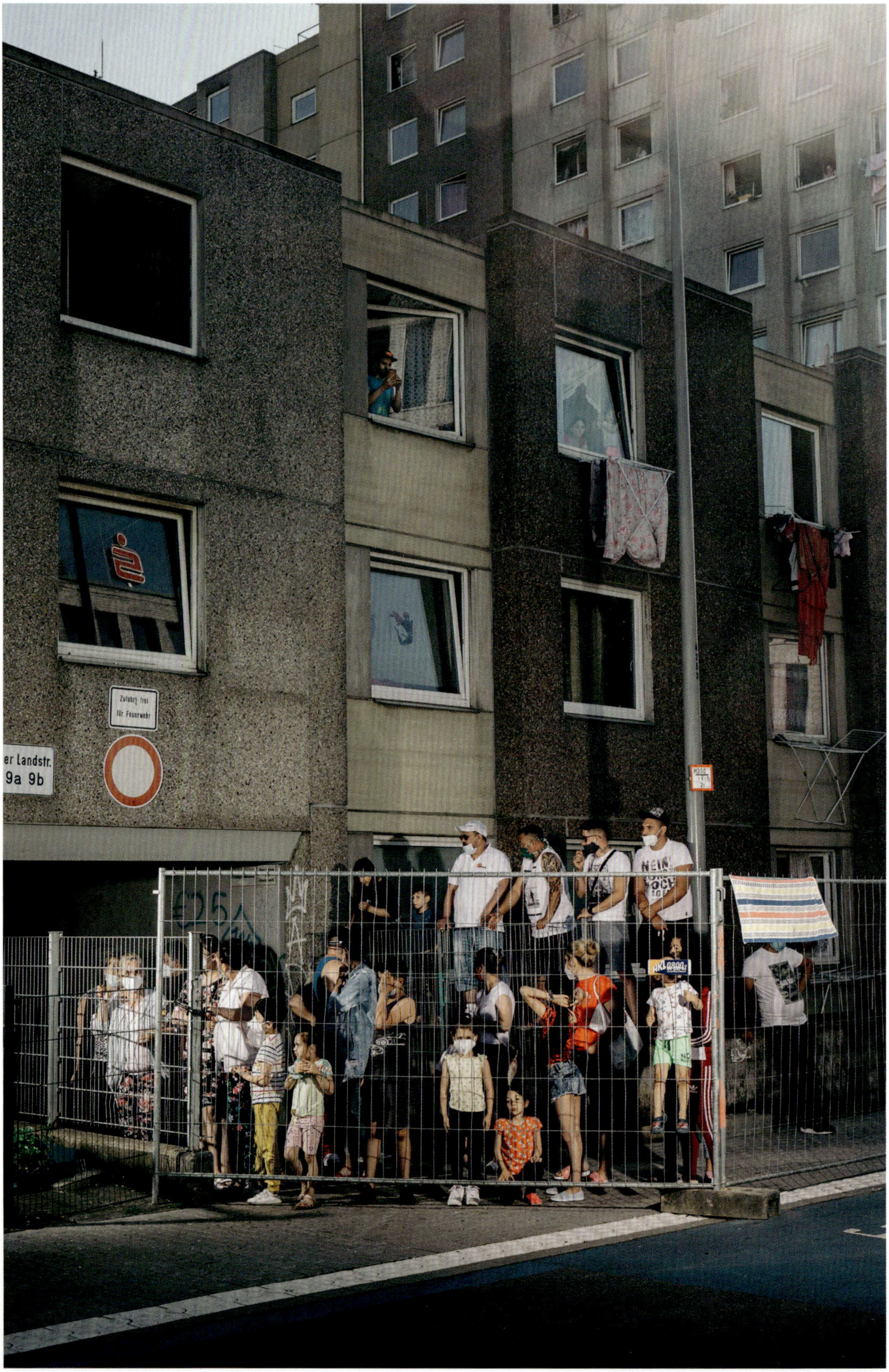
Zufahrt frei
für Feuerwehr
er Landstr.
9a 9b

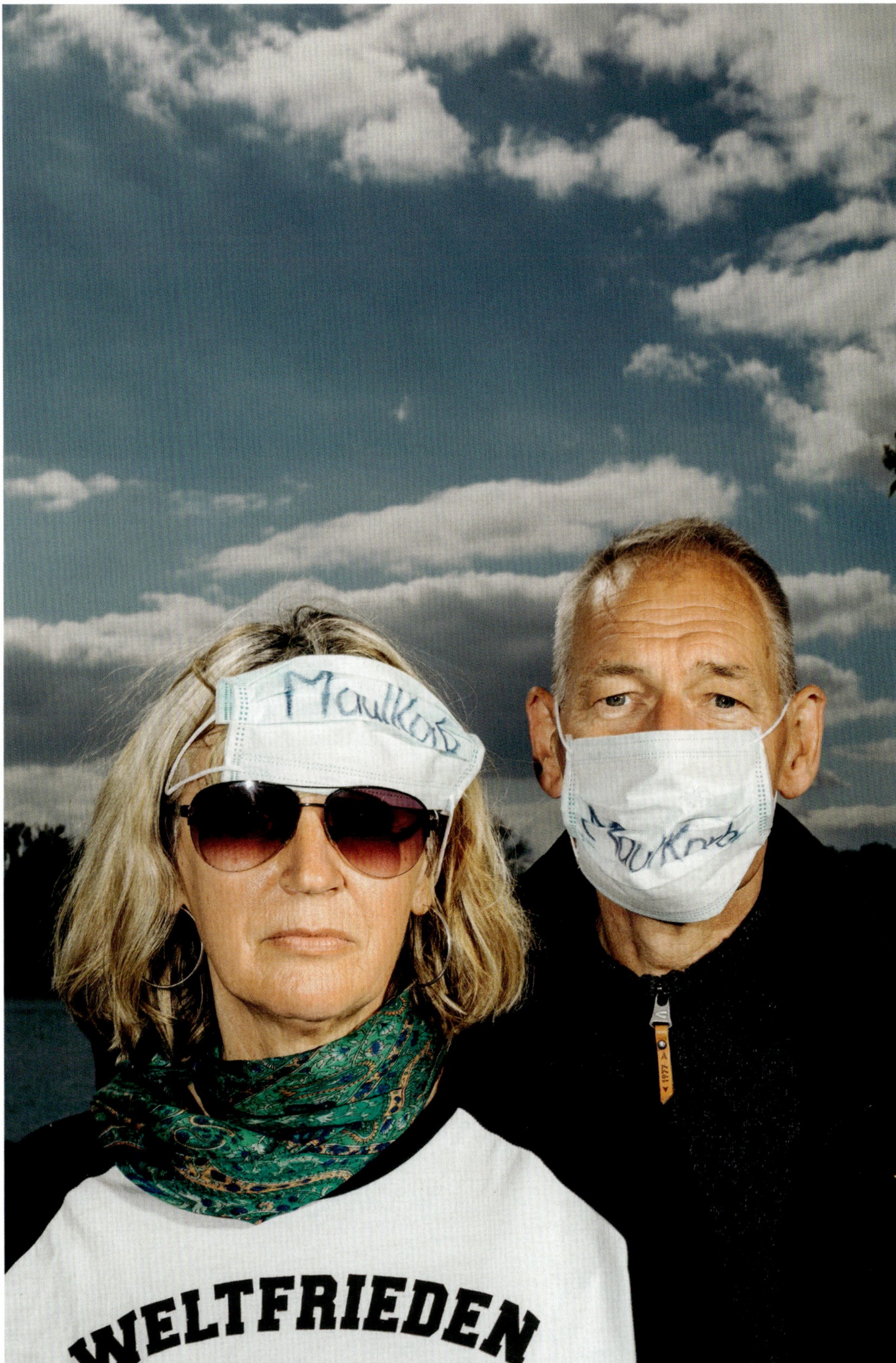
Maulkorb
Maulkorb
WELTFRIEDEN

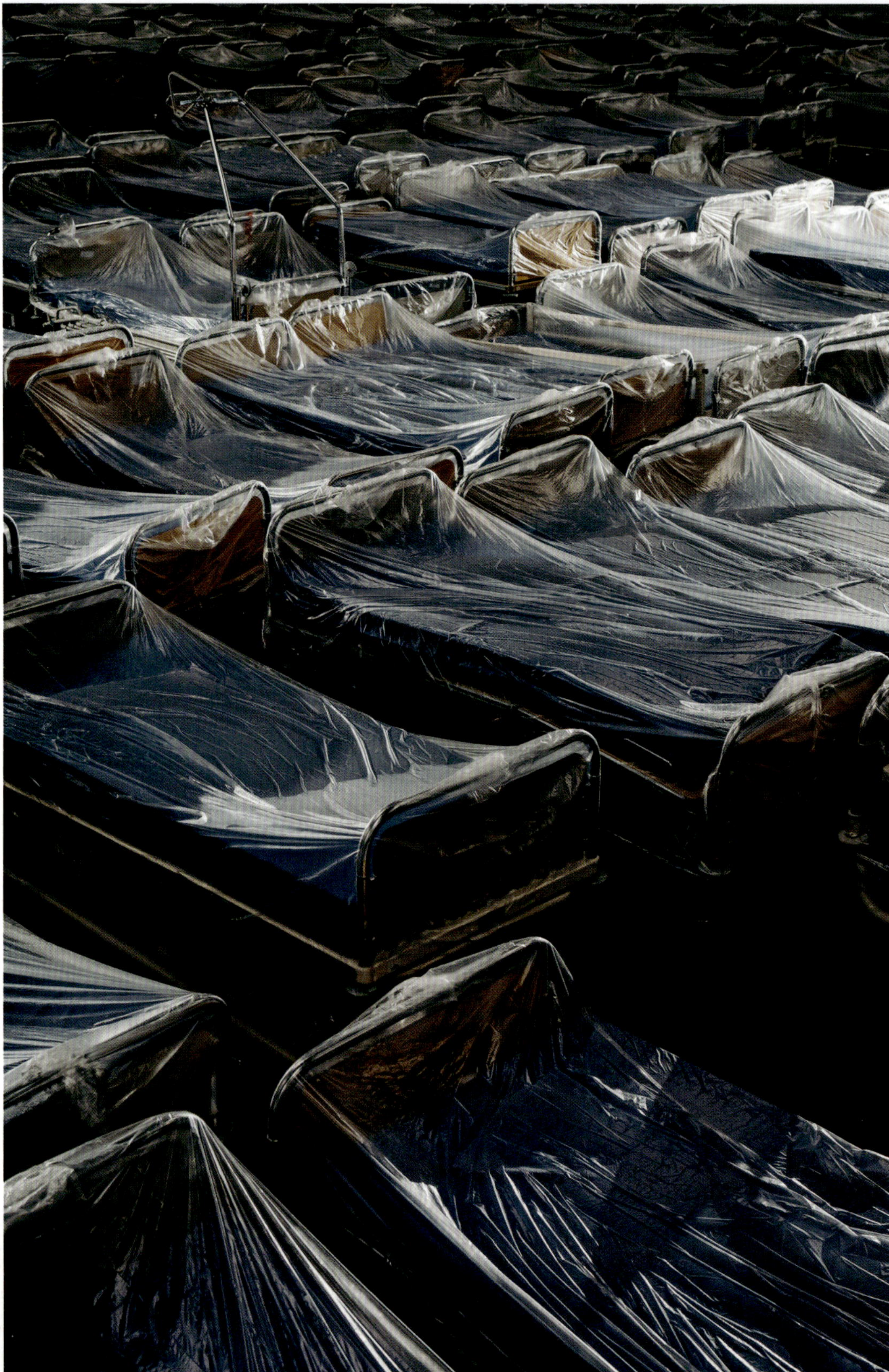

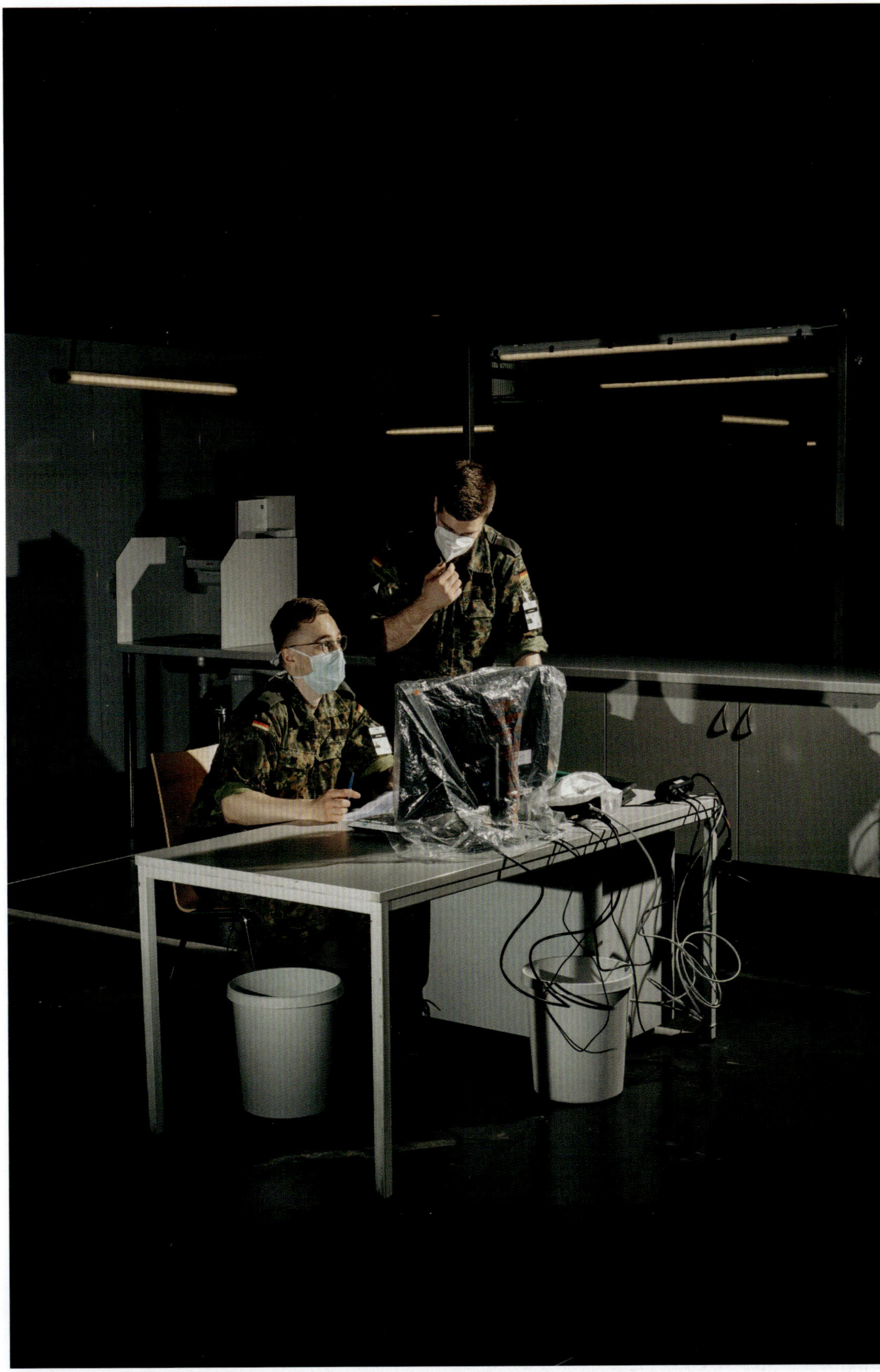

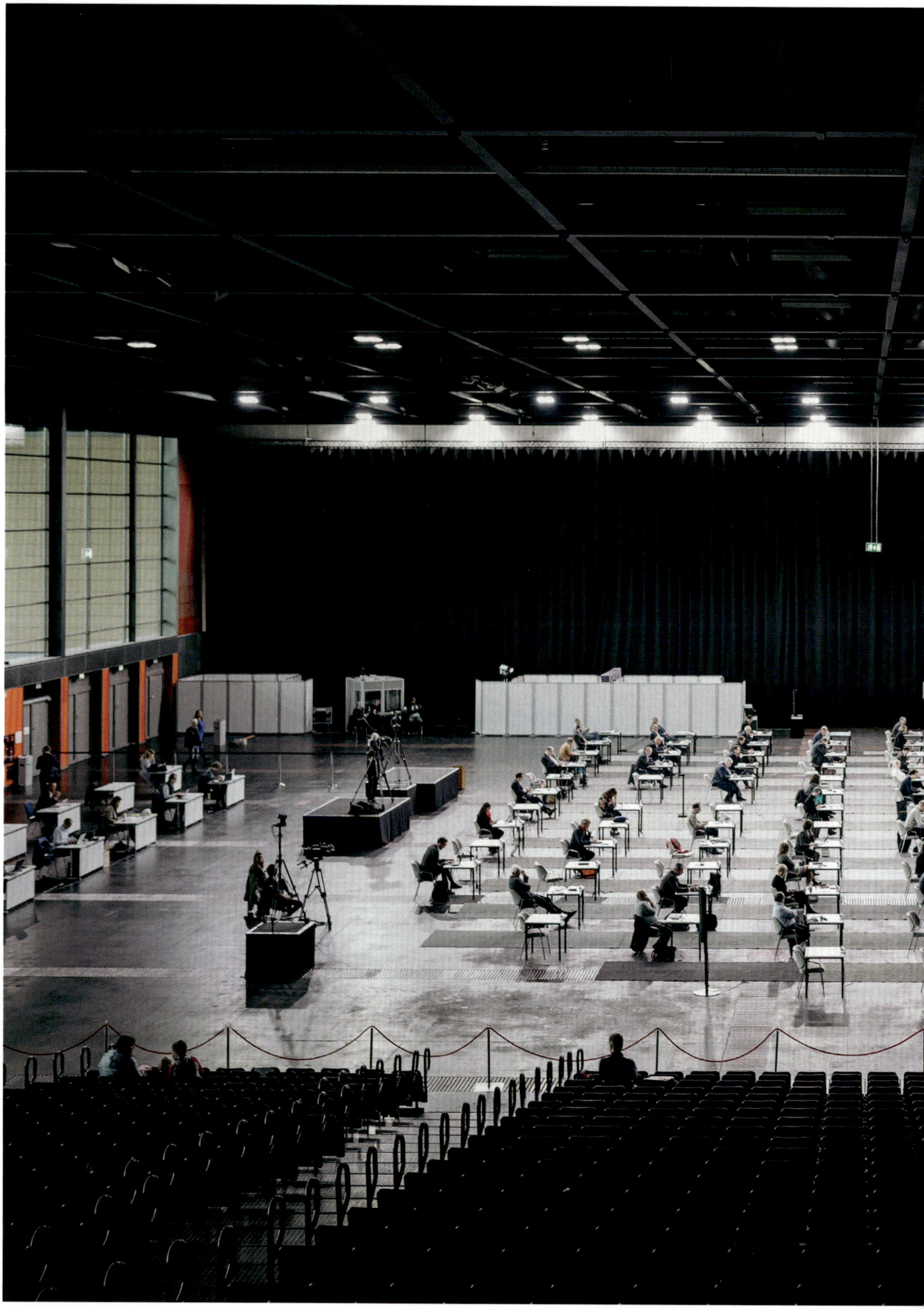

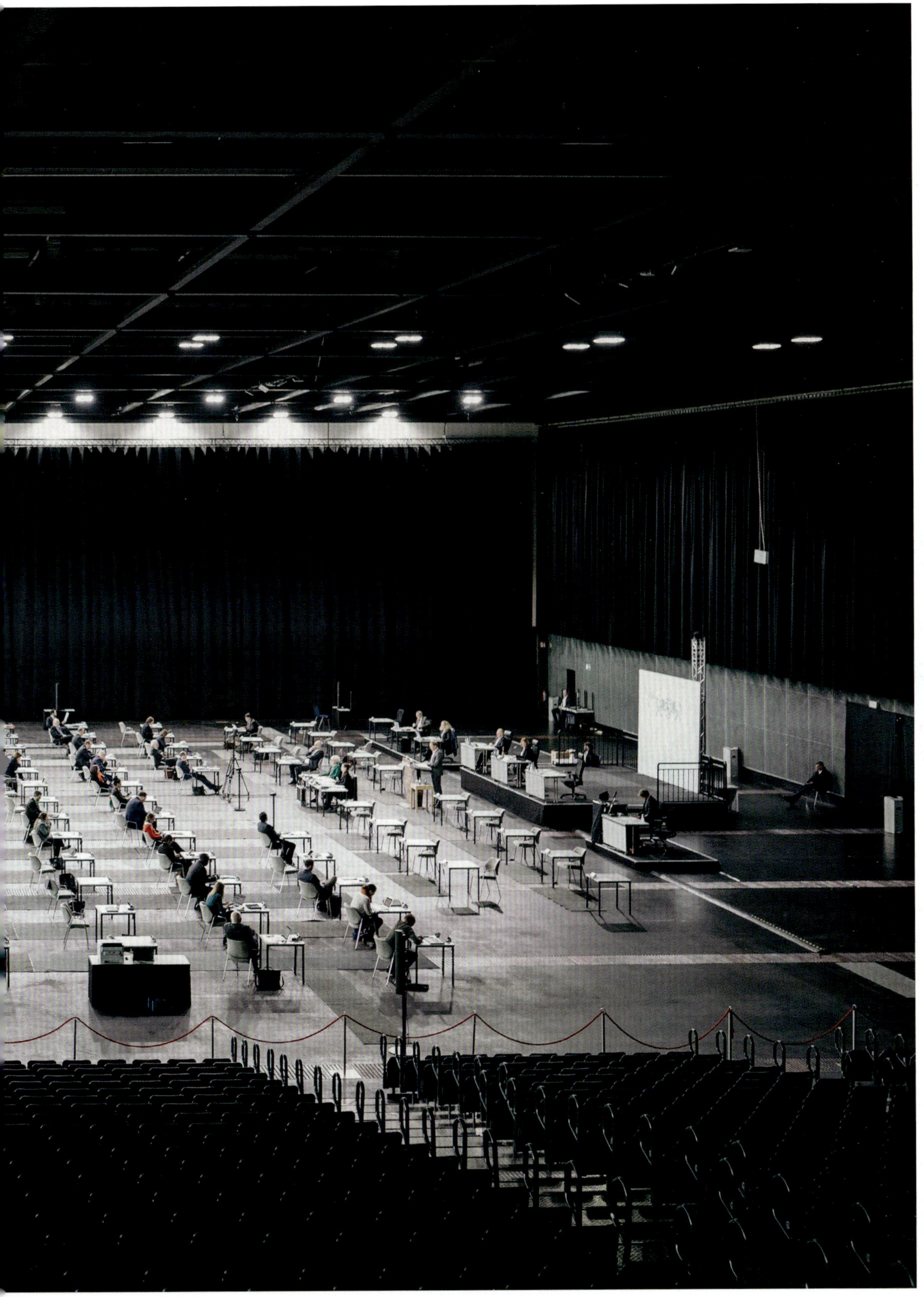

Masoumeh Bahrami, Iran
Inside Living Cells

The coronavirus pandemic, a crisis on this scale, can reorder society in dramatic ways for better or worse.
It can reorder everything in my environment, from my father's face to my city, from the garden next door to the cemetery. On a micro or macro level, a lot of things change their meaning and get a new meaning.
In February 2020, Iran reported its first confirmed cases of SARS-CoV-2 infections. By then coronavirus had spread quickly to other cities. My city, Mazandaran, had become one of the most dangerous and declared a red zone. As a photographer with a lot of fears, I was confronted with a lot of strange and unexpected moments, decisive moments and indecisive moments. I felt like in a tunnel, in a state of transition between life before and after the coronavirus.
Facing mortality, we are all prompted to reevaluate our lives. I observe the reevaluation of life in my environment. A pandemic reevaluation of life in detail. I started taking photos in my house at the scale of my family, then I risked and decided to leave quarantine. Just as personal encounters with mortality can transform a person's life, a societal encounter with mortality has the potential to transform society.
So I want to search for this potential in society. What happened in the transition state outside?
My people have endured a lot of hardship in the last years in Iran, now coronavirus is just like a final blow. What are the action and reaction? How do cities and people deal with it? In the days in which every 10 minutes one person died because of the virus in my country, how are those minutes counted by us? Death becomes the common experience that can make all members of the human race feel their common bonds and common humanity.
Life has meaning in all circumstances, even the most miserable ones.
This means that even when situations seem objectively terrible, there is a higher level of order that involves meaning. This project was the result of my efforts in these situations and the questions that occurred along the way. I've tried to find answers to my questions in all these photos.
For me, though, it was more like a journey between the worlds of images, transformed worlds during the most important crisis of the century.

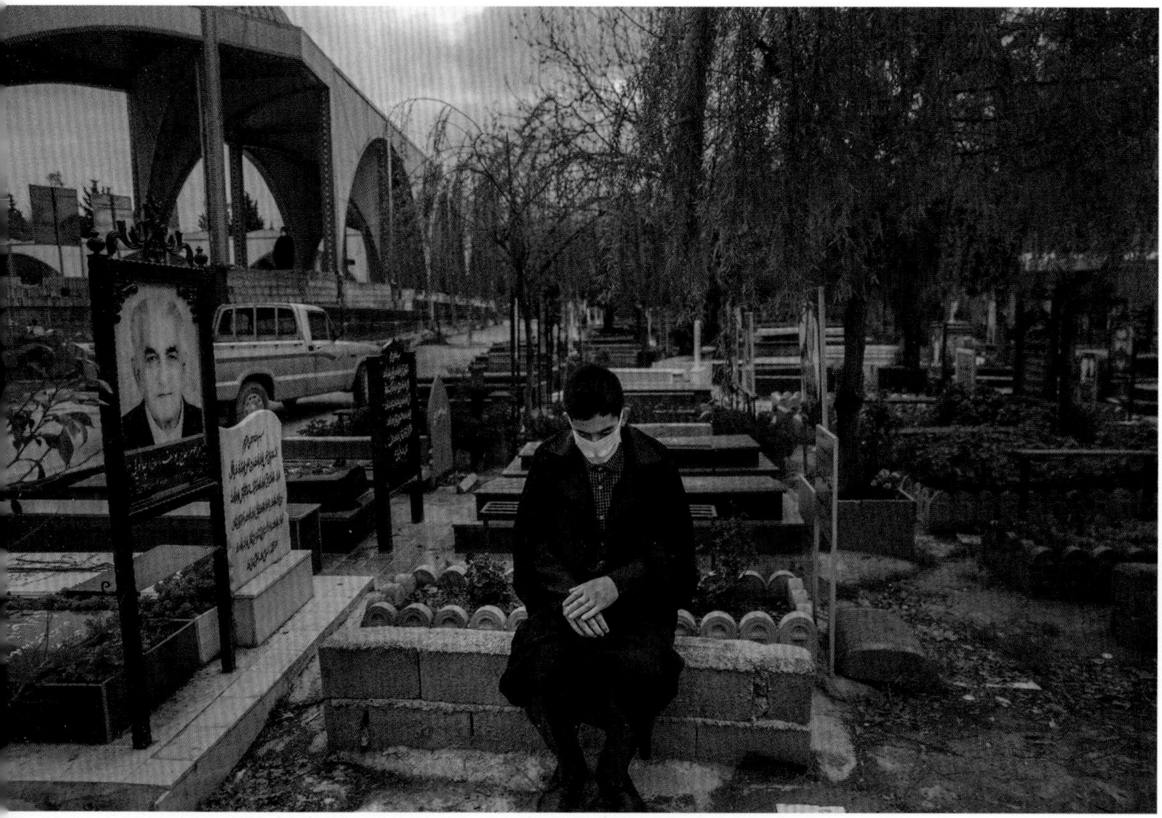

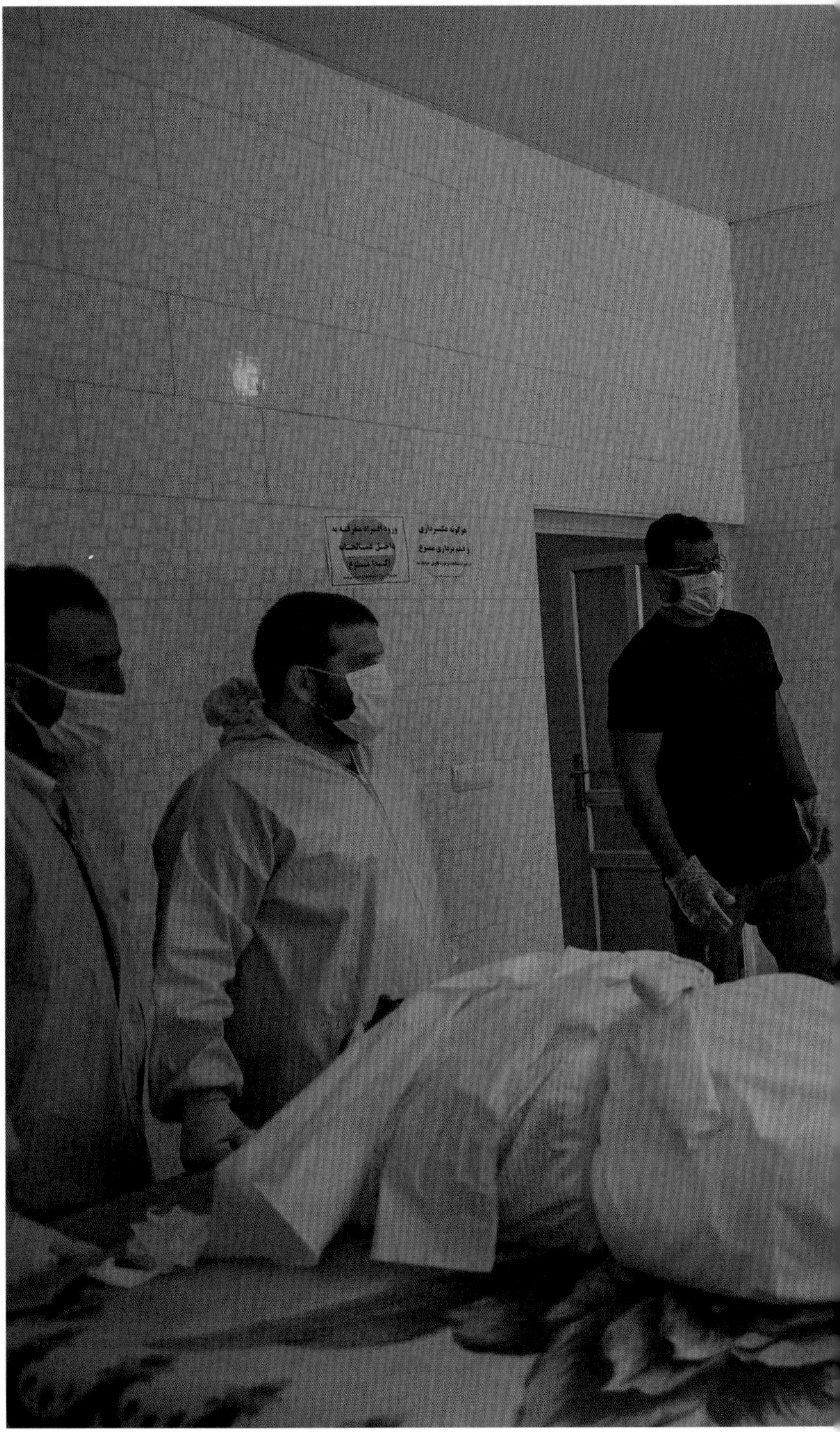
ورود افراد متفرقه به
داخل غسالخانه
اکیدا ممنوع
هرگونه عکسبرداری
و فیلم برداری ممنوع

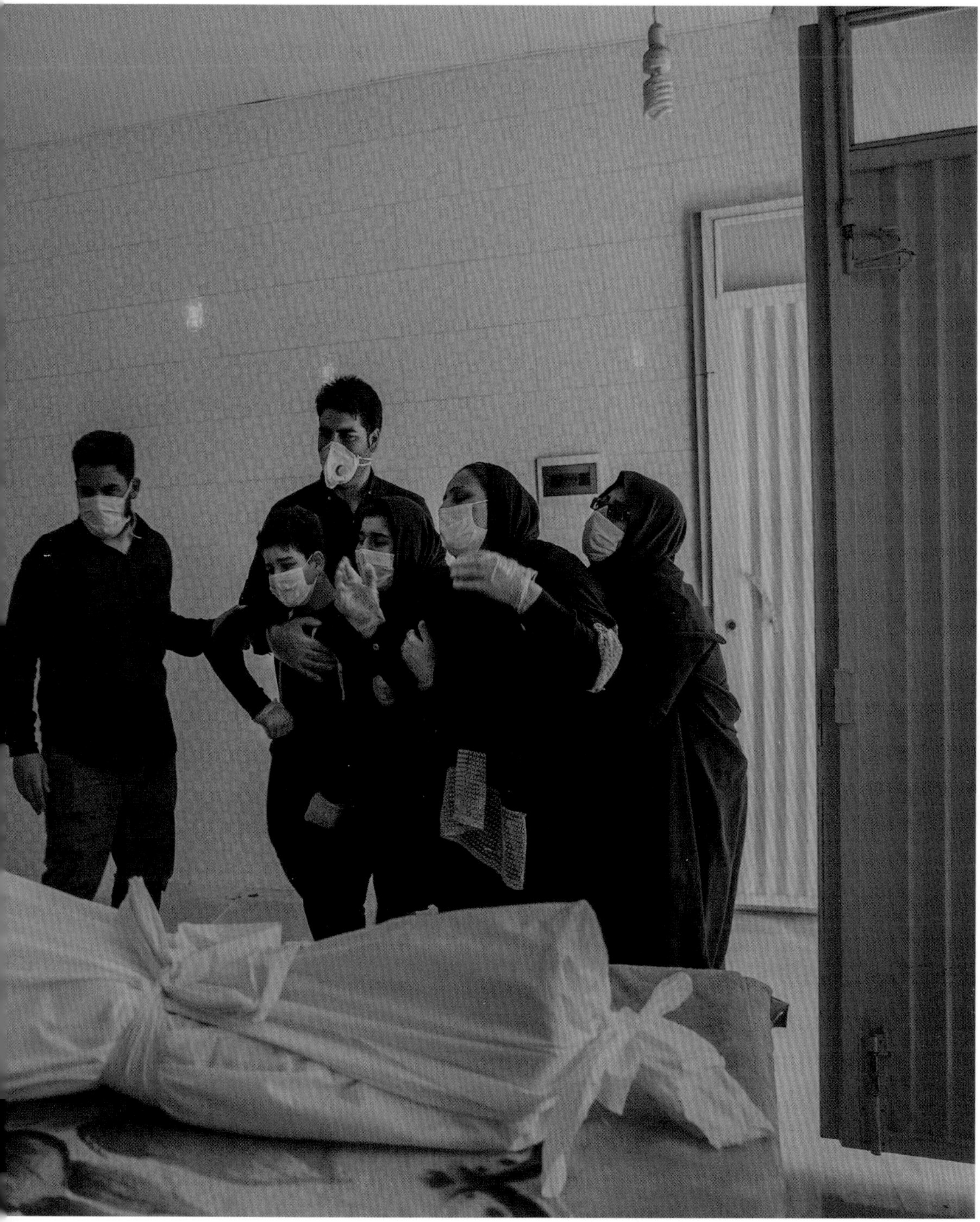

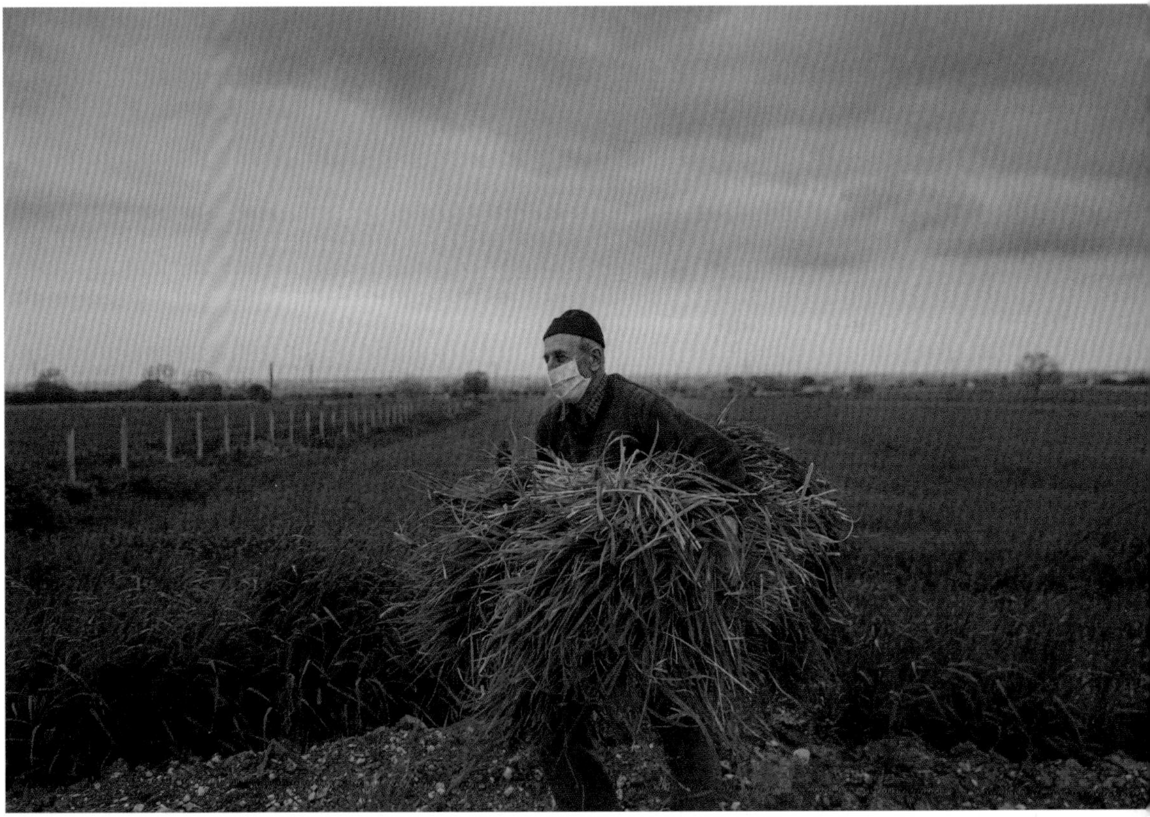

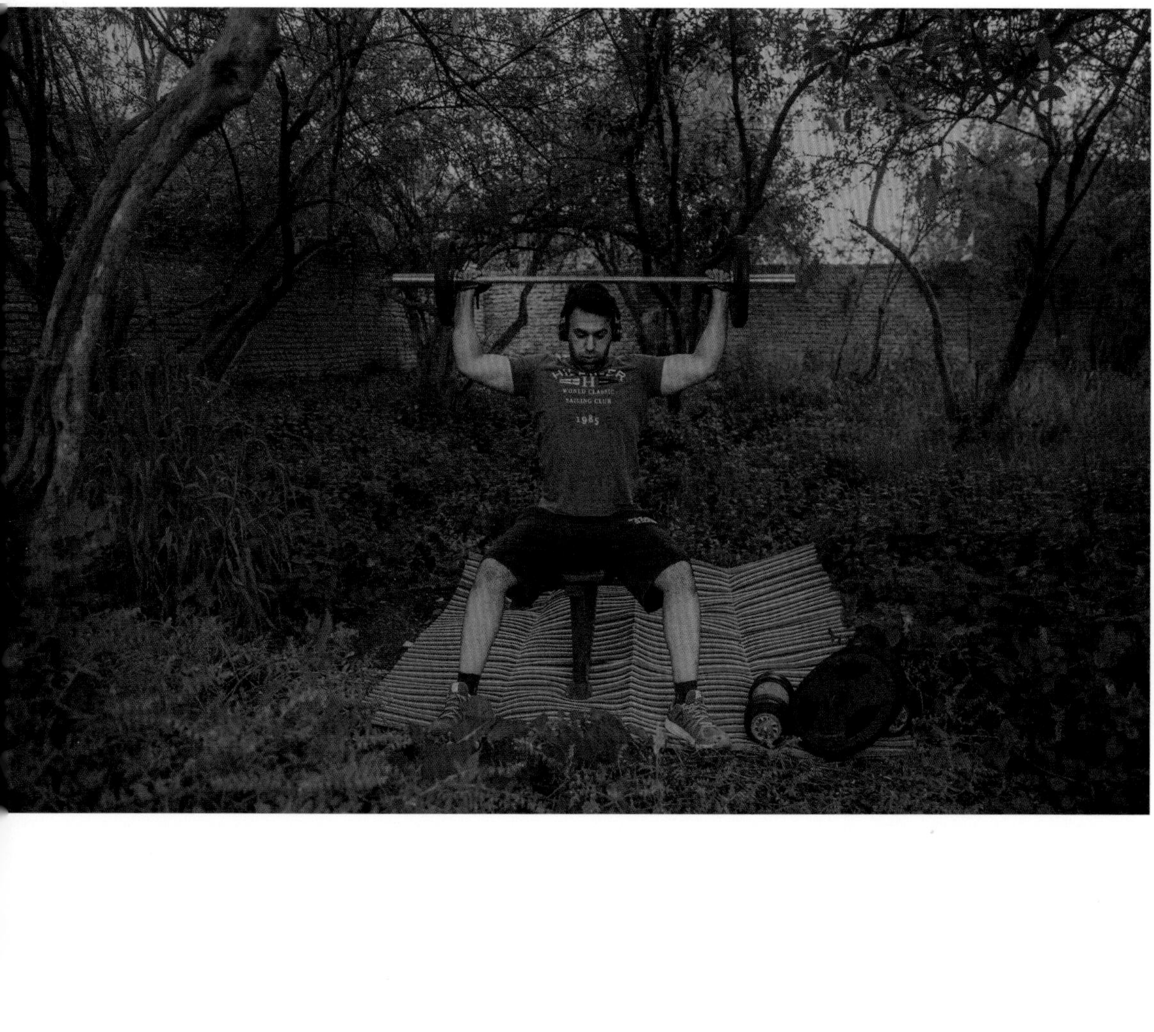
H
1985

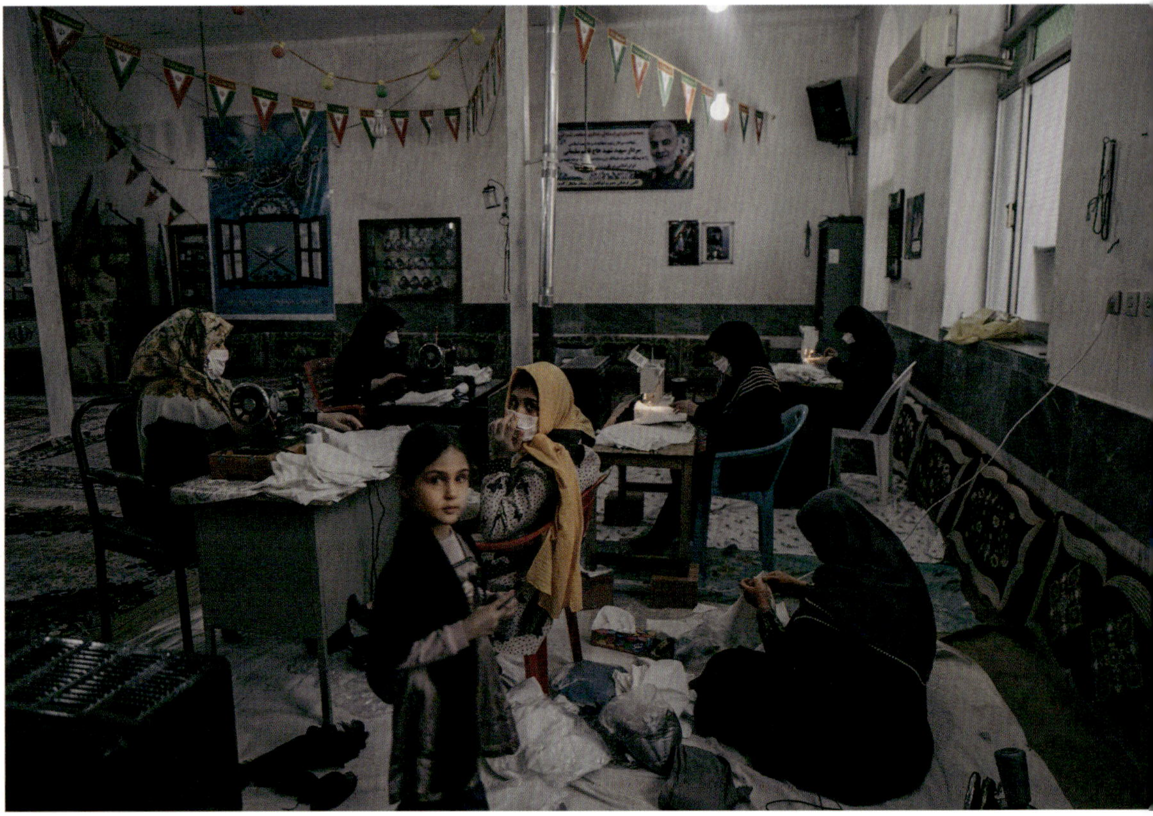

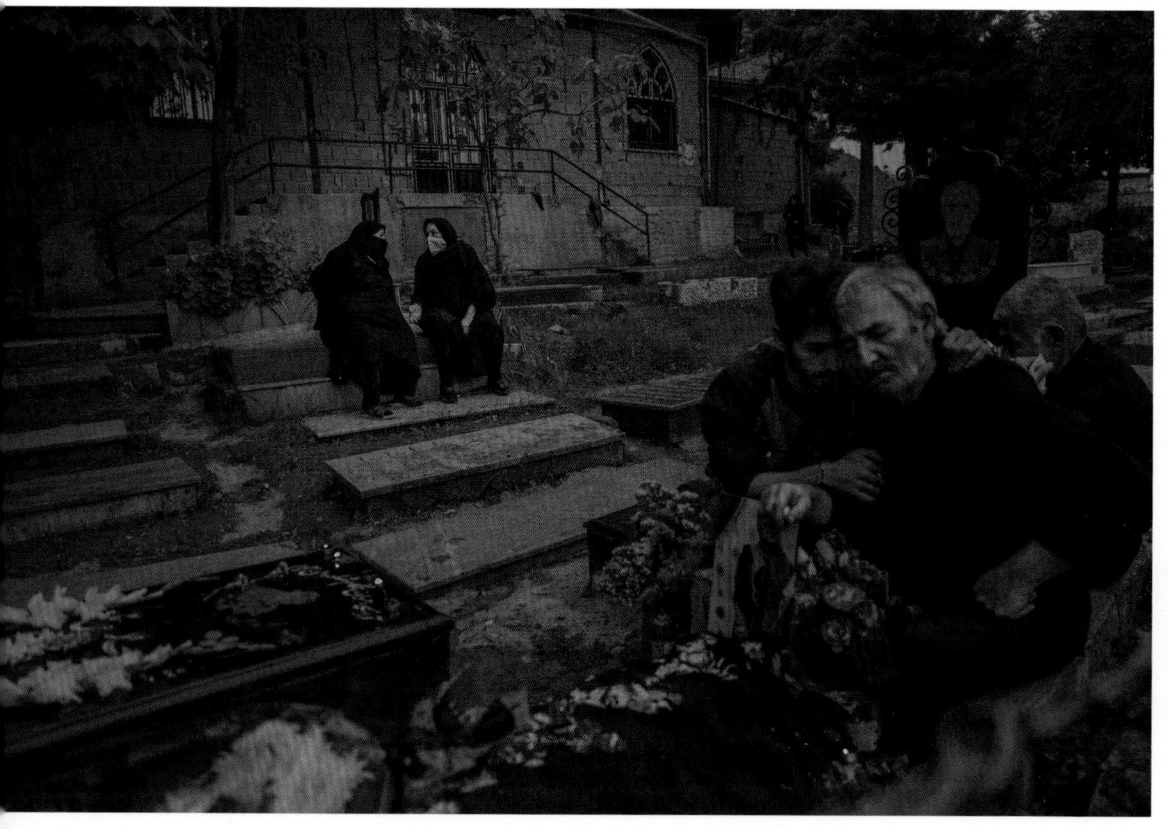

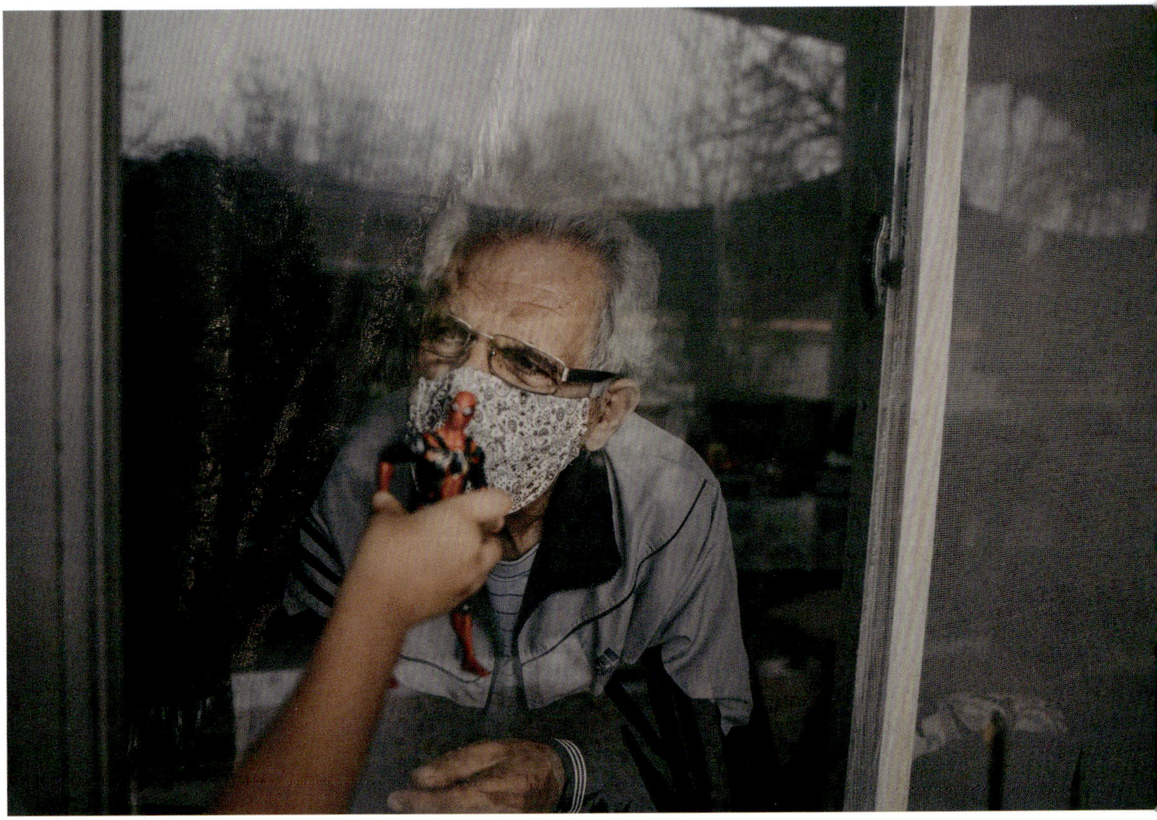

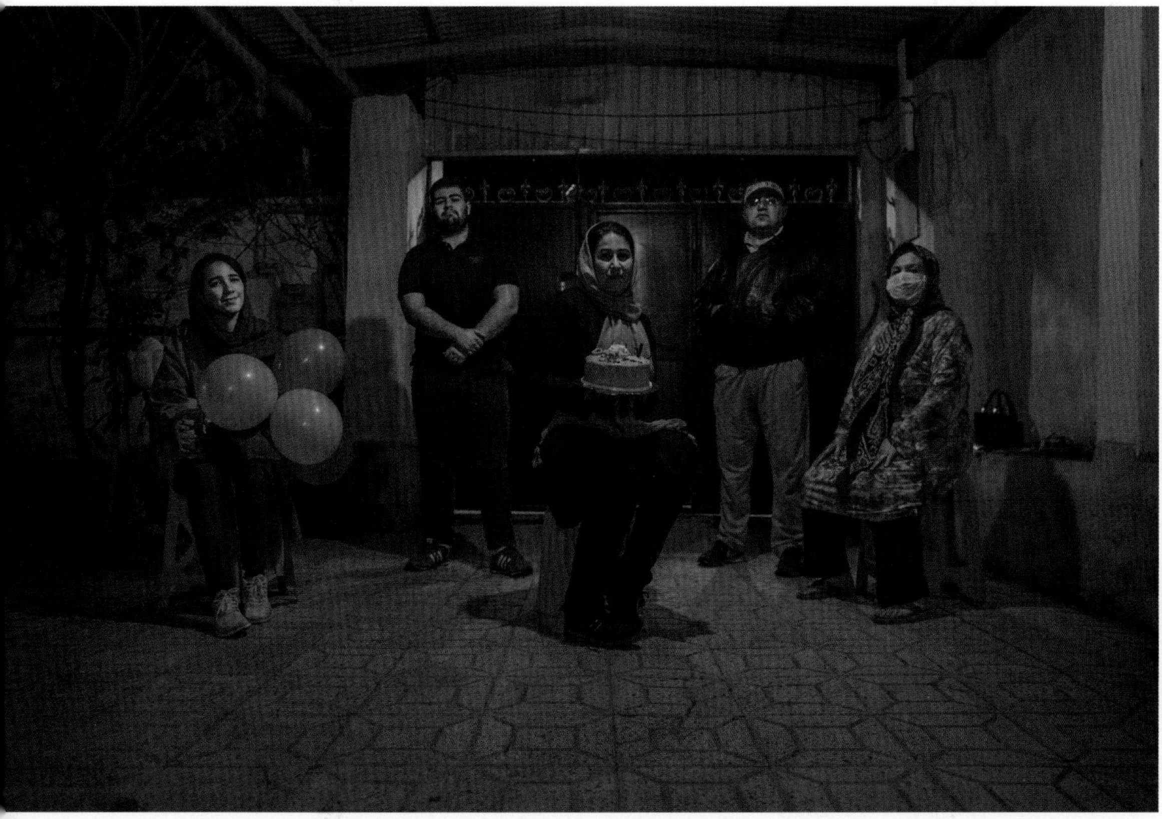

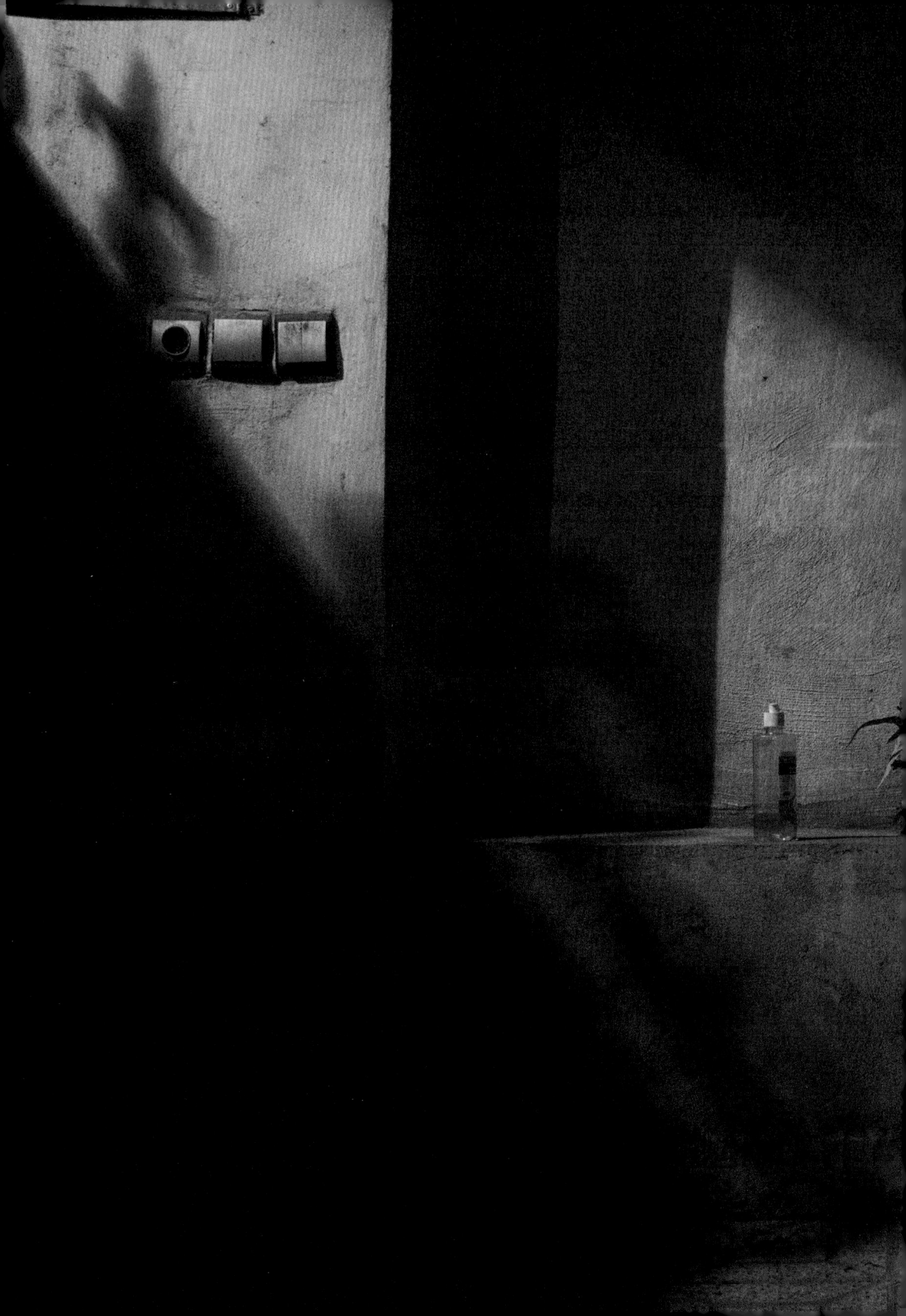

Arek Rataj, China
Wuhan Visual Diary

Coronavirus put more than one-third of the global population under lockdown. The epidemic is believed to have started in November 2019 in Wuhan, China. I arrived there in December and started working at a local university.
One of my students was the first to tell me about a mysterious disease that develops in another district of the city. "It doesn't concern us" — he said calmly. It was about 10–15 km from my university. By that time, there were only a few people in the hospital. There have not been any deaths yet. "It's just some kind of flu or something" — Zhang said with conviction. From then on, I began following reports from various outlets. On January 23, Wuhan City was shut off from the rest of the world and placed under an unprecedented quarantine. Sanitation workers were spraying streets. Staff with biometric devices appeared in Walmart. Coronavirus fears triggered panic buying. Some people threw their pets out of the windows for fear they were carriers. All bridges and tunnels, as well as movement between city districts were blocked. Schools and universities canceled the start of the following semester. In other Chinese provinces, citizens were banned from leaving their homes, with the option of leaving every two days to replenish their food supply. Some people shouted from the balconies "Wuhan Jiayou!" (Be strong, Wuhan!).
Despite the panic, I felt compelled to go out and document the outbreak of the new coronavirus.

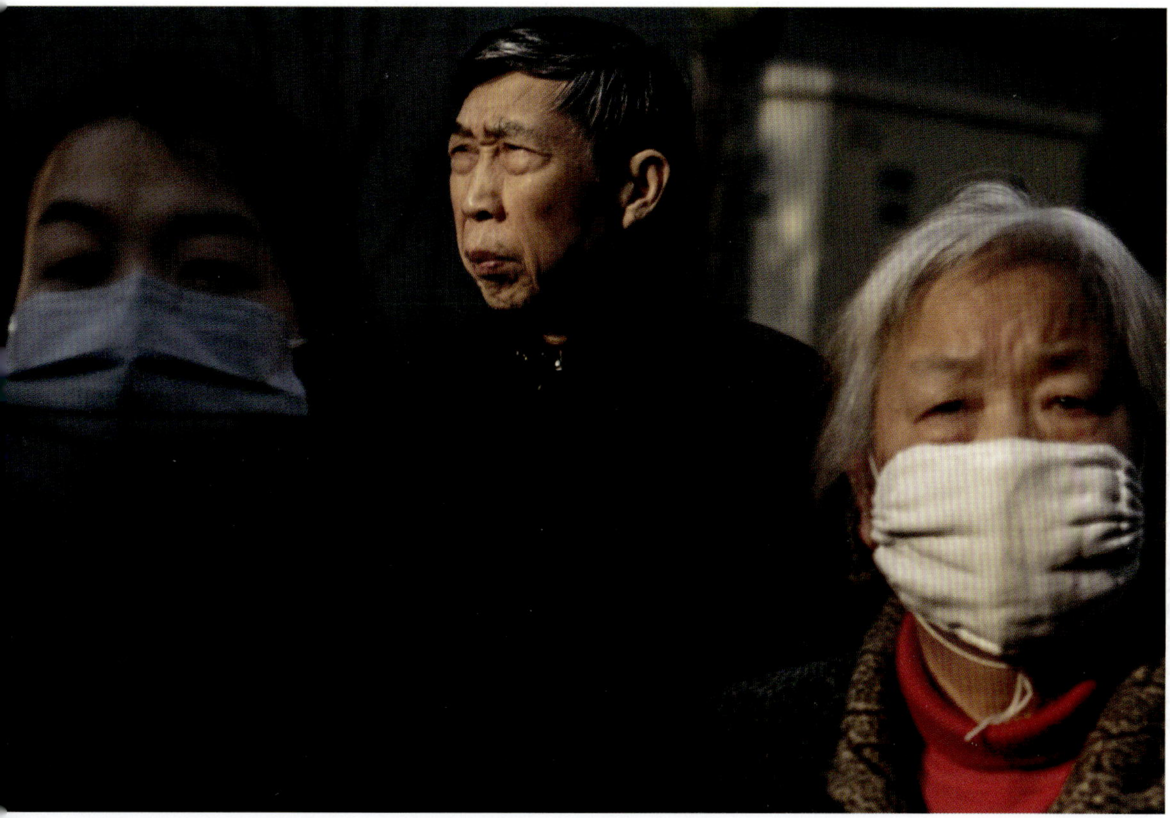

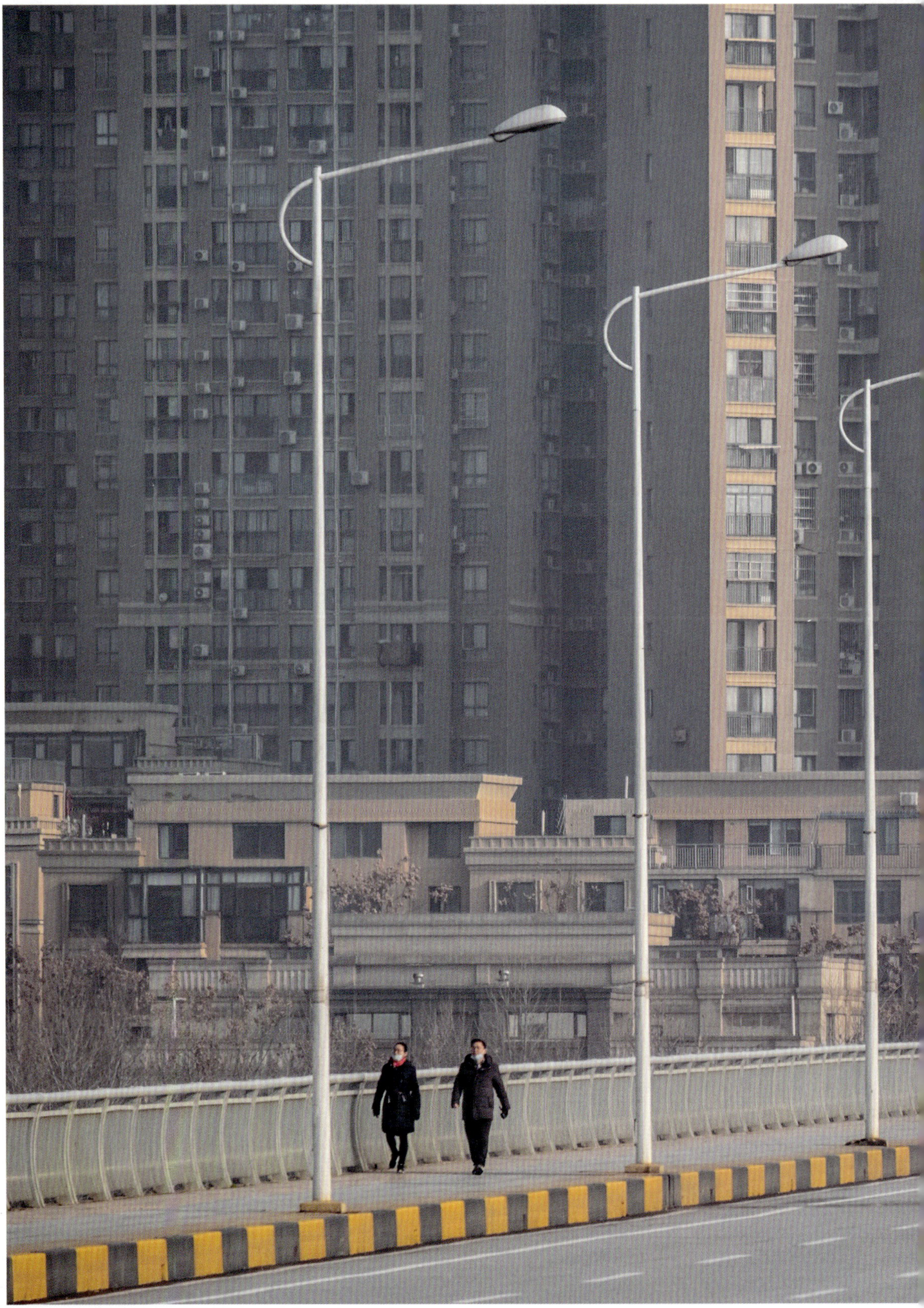

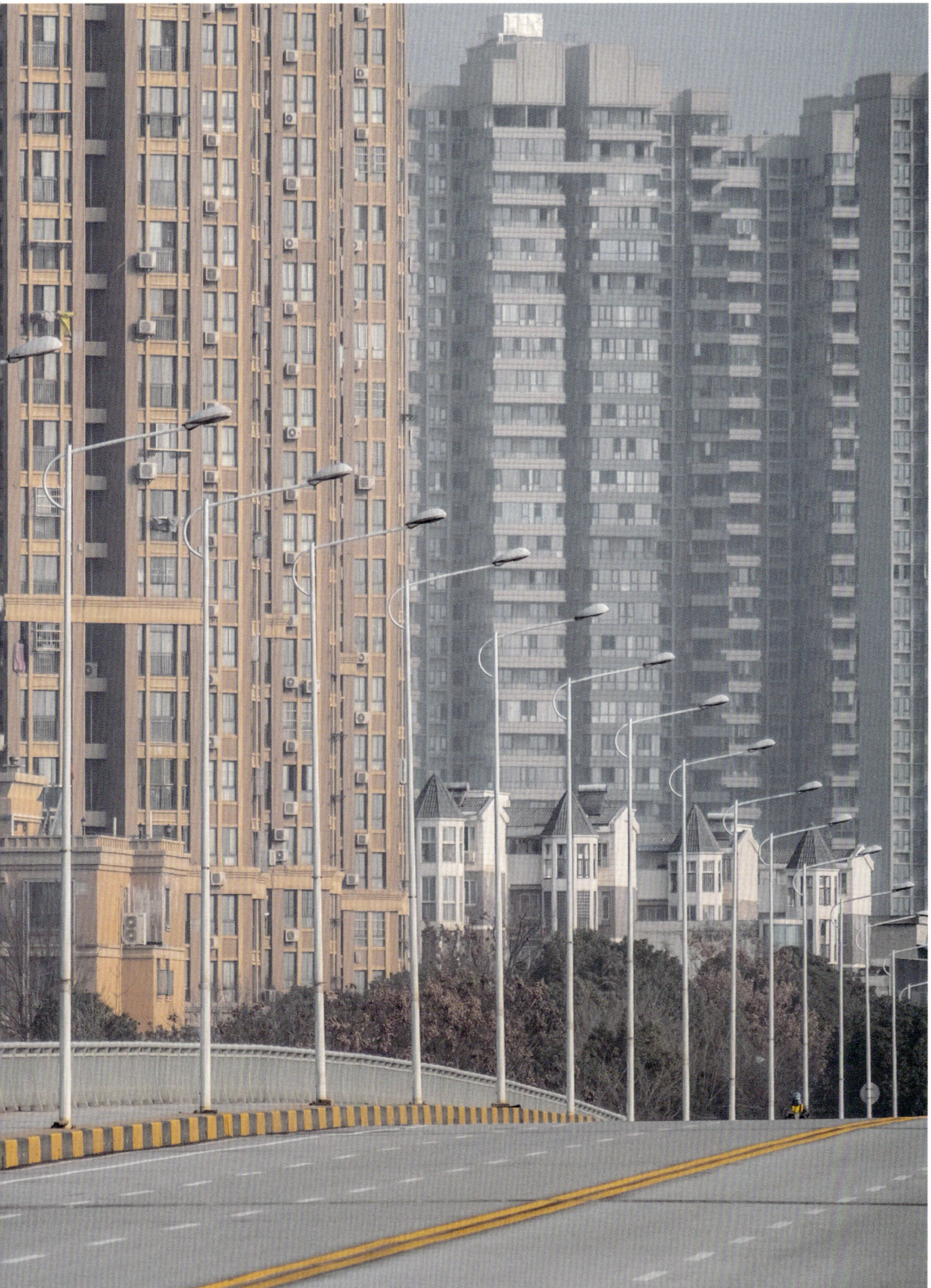

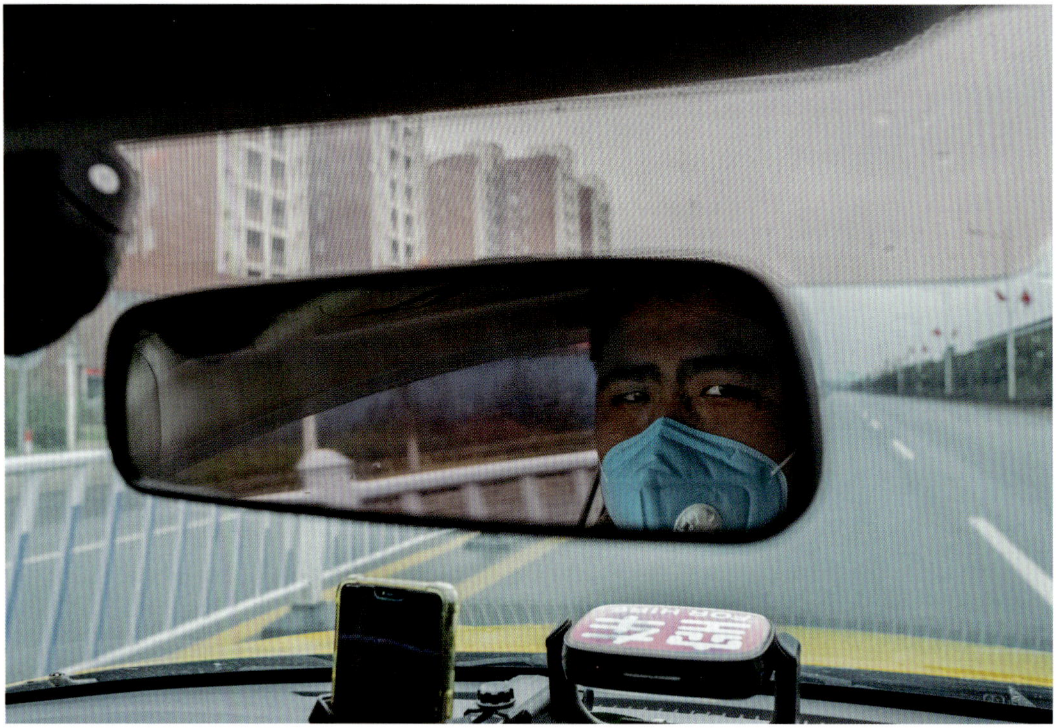

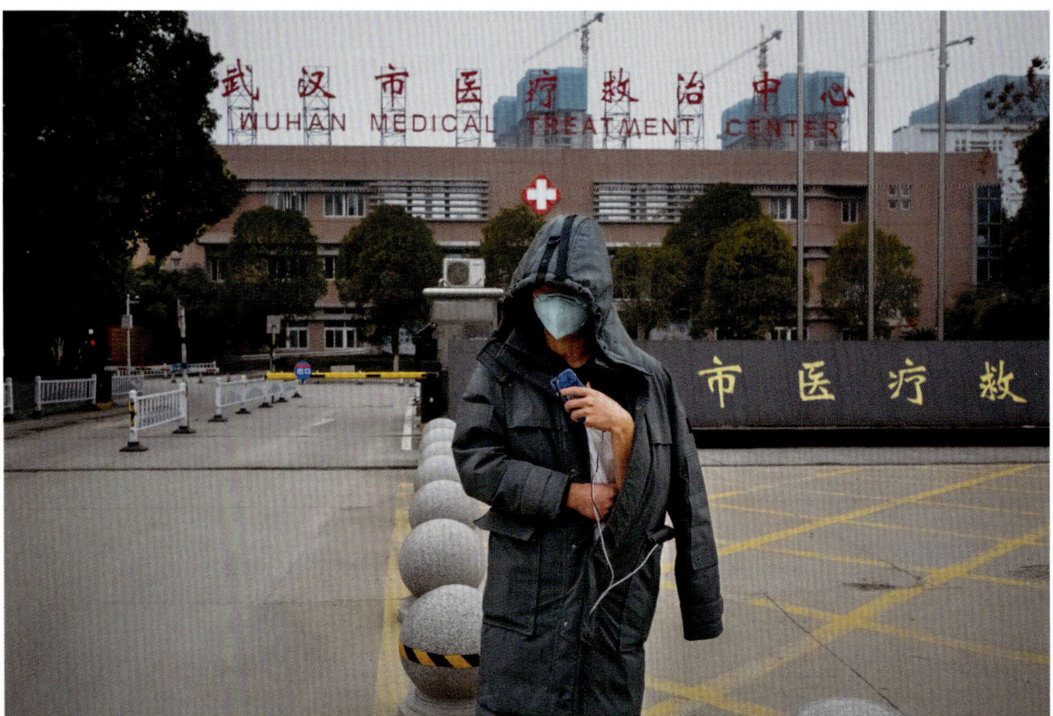
武汉市医疗救治中心
WUHAN MEDICAL TREATMENT CENTER
市医疗救

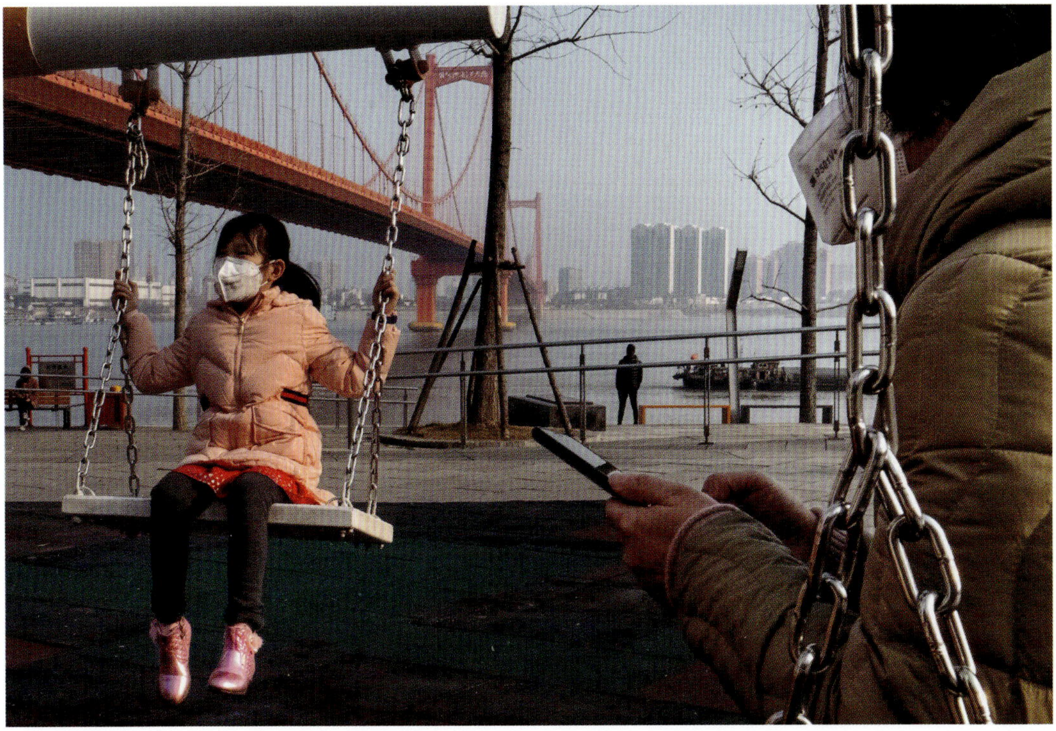

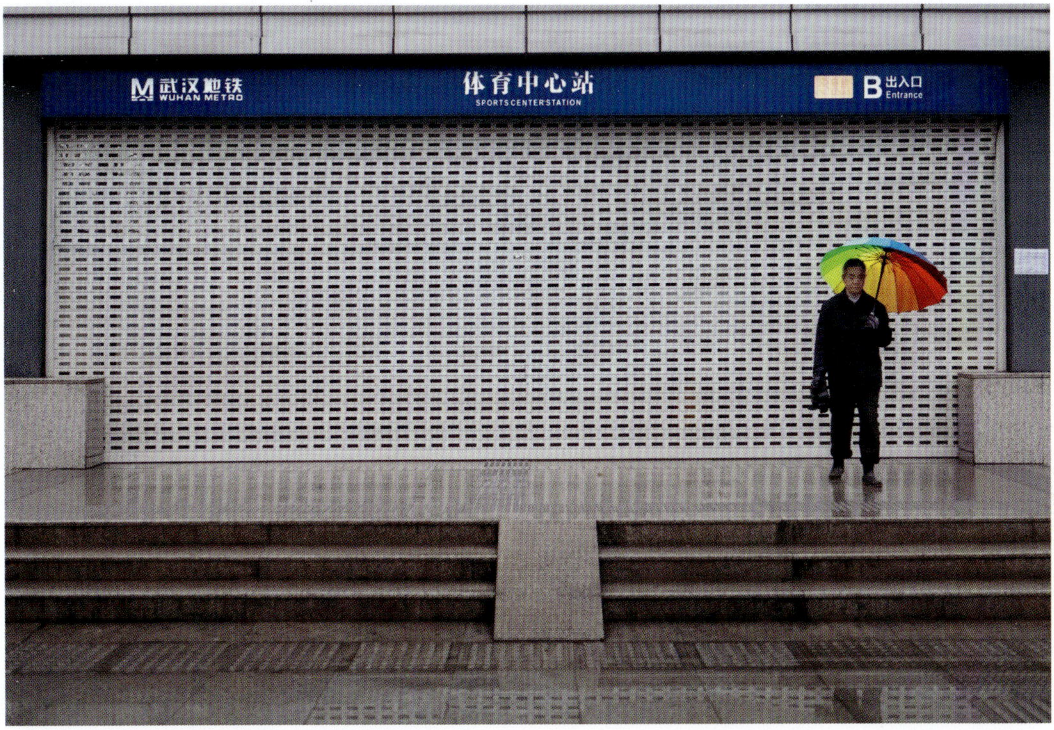
武汉地铁
WUHAN METRO
体育中心站
SPORTS CENTER STATION
B 出入口
Entrance

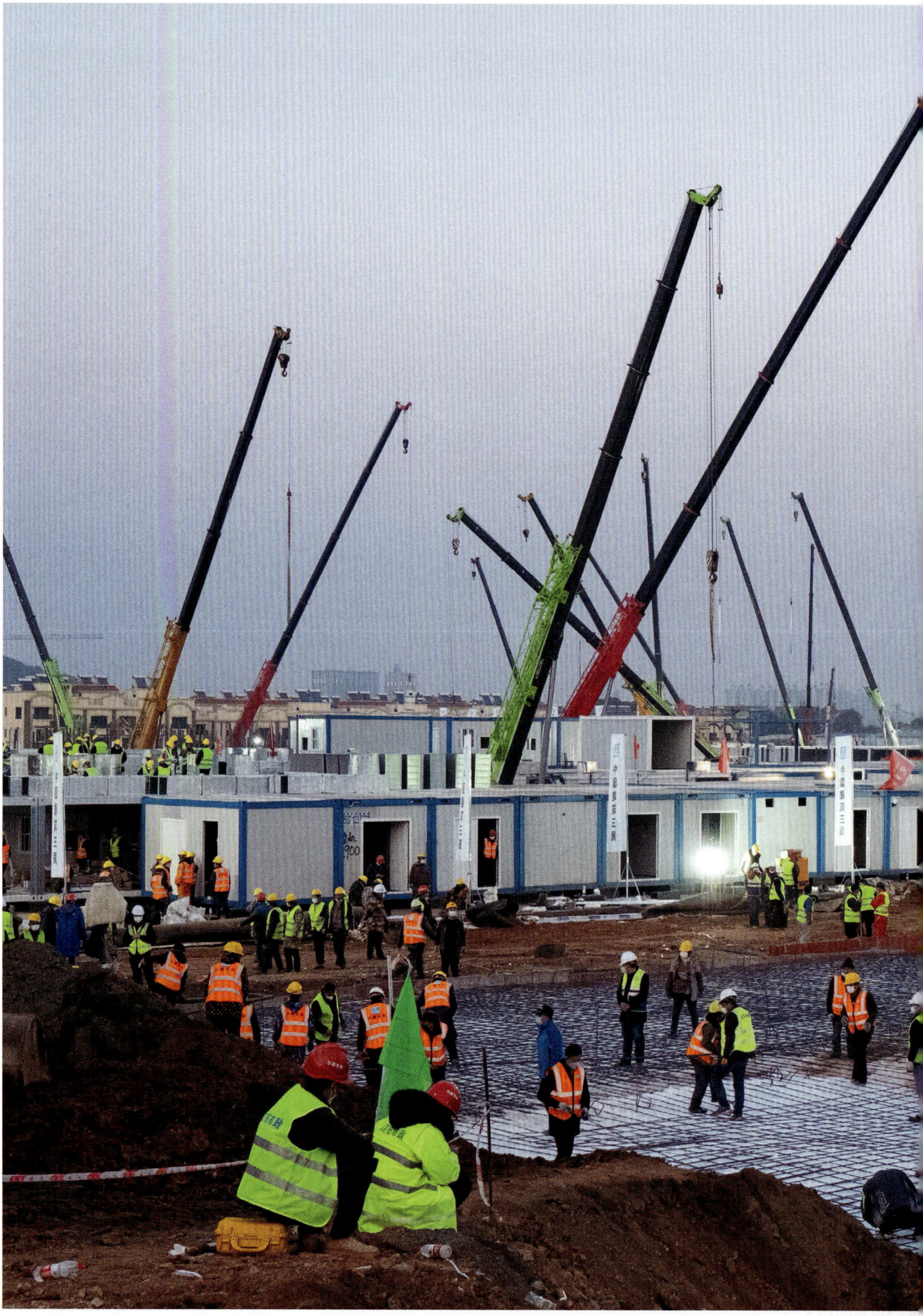

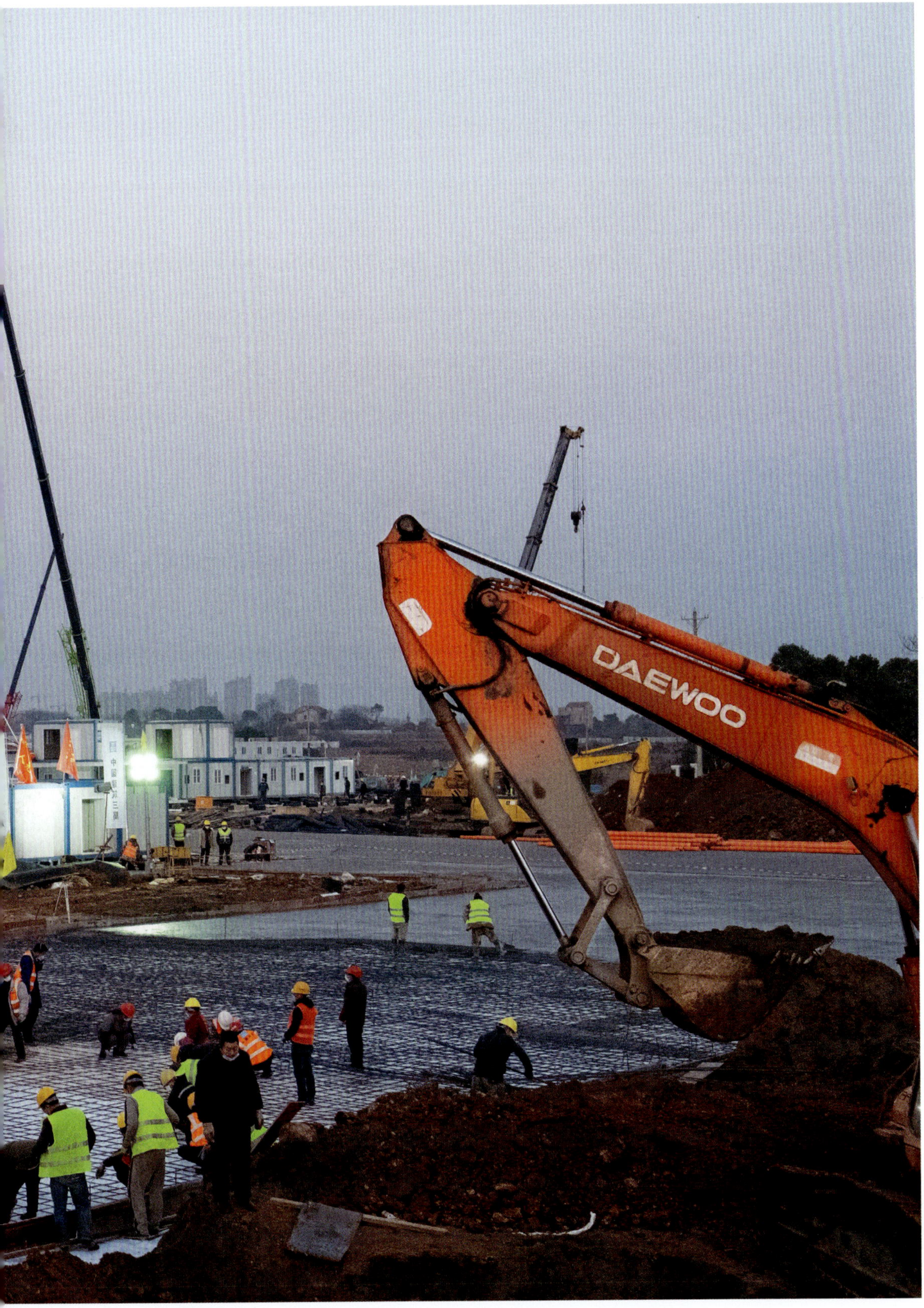
DAEWOO

Tomasz Lazar, Poland
Voids Diary

On the 11th of March 2020, the World Health Organisation announced the COVID-19 virus as a pandemic.
From that moment everyday life in Poland began to change. Firstly, due to the introduction of the epidemic status, restrictions were introduced to protect people from getting infected. Secondly, fear appeared among people. Places, once full of life, became depopulated. In public spaces a noticeable emptiness took over, interpersonal relationships changed. A post-apocalyptic atmosphere and points of view transpired in people's faces like scenes from different movies that they had seen.
With time, the so-called "defrosting" phase of the economy started in Poland. People slowly began to go out into the street, but the feeling of fear remained.
The second wave of the pandemic arrived in the Fall. Finally, humanity faced a new reality that forced them to leave their comfort zone. The individual seemed doomed to total isolation.
In the first phase of the pandemic, according to official data by December 31, 2020, in Poland, over 1,294,878 people fell ill and 28,554 died. Many people believe that this data is heavily underestimated.

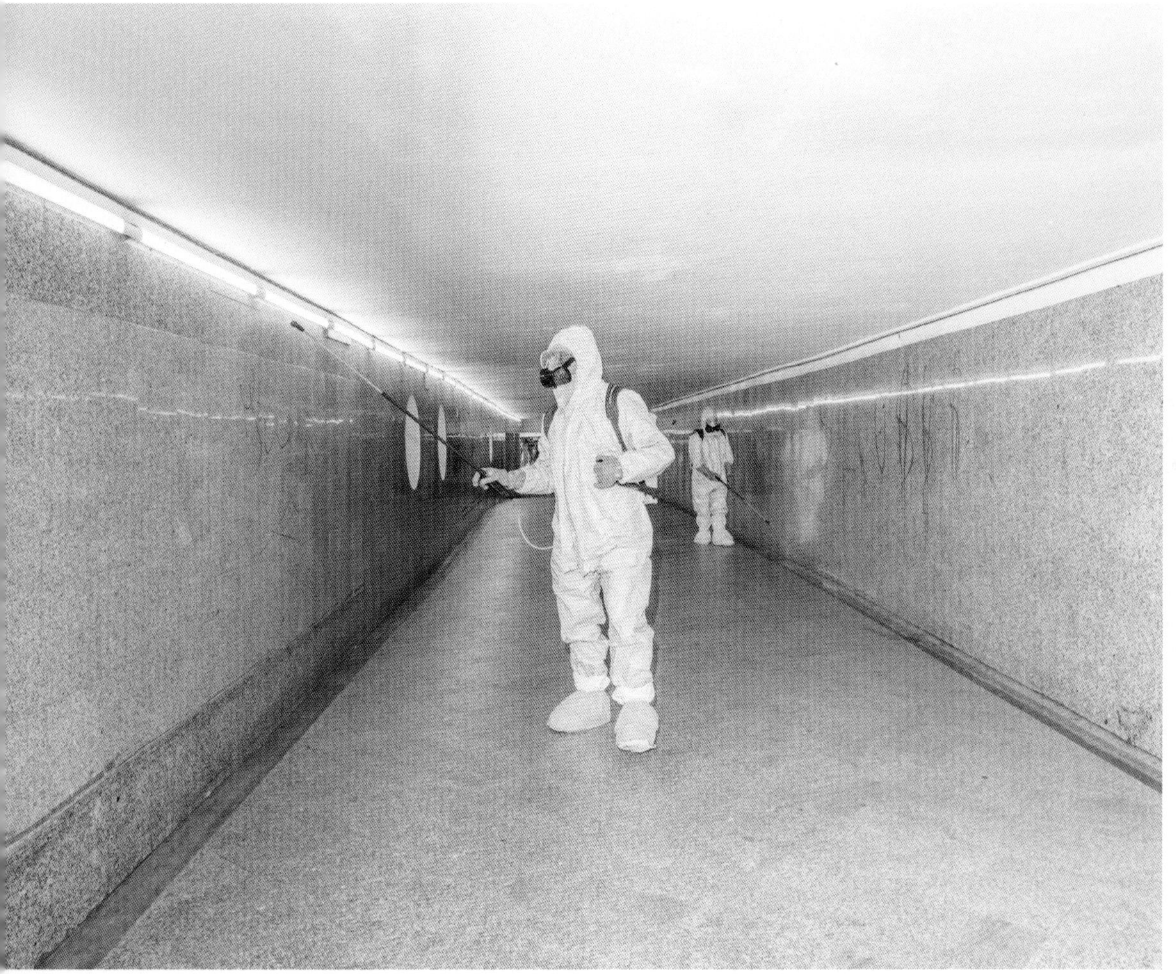

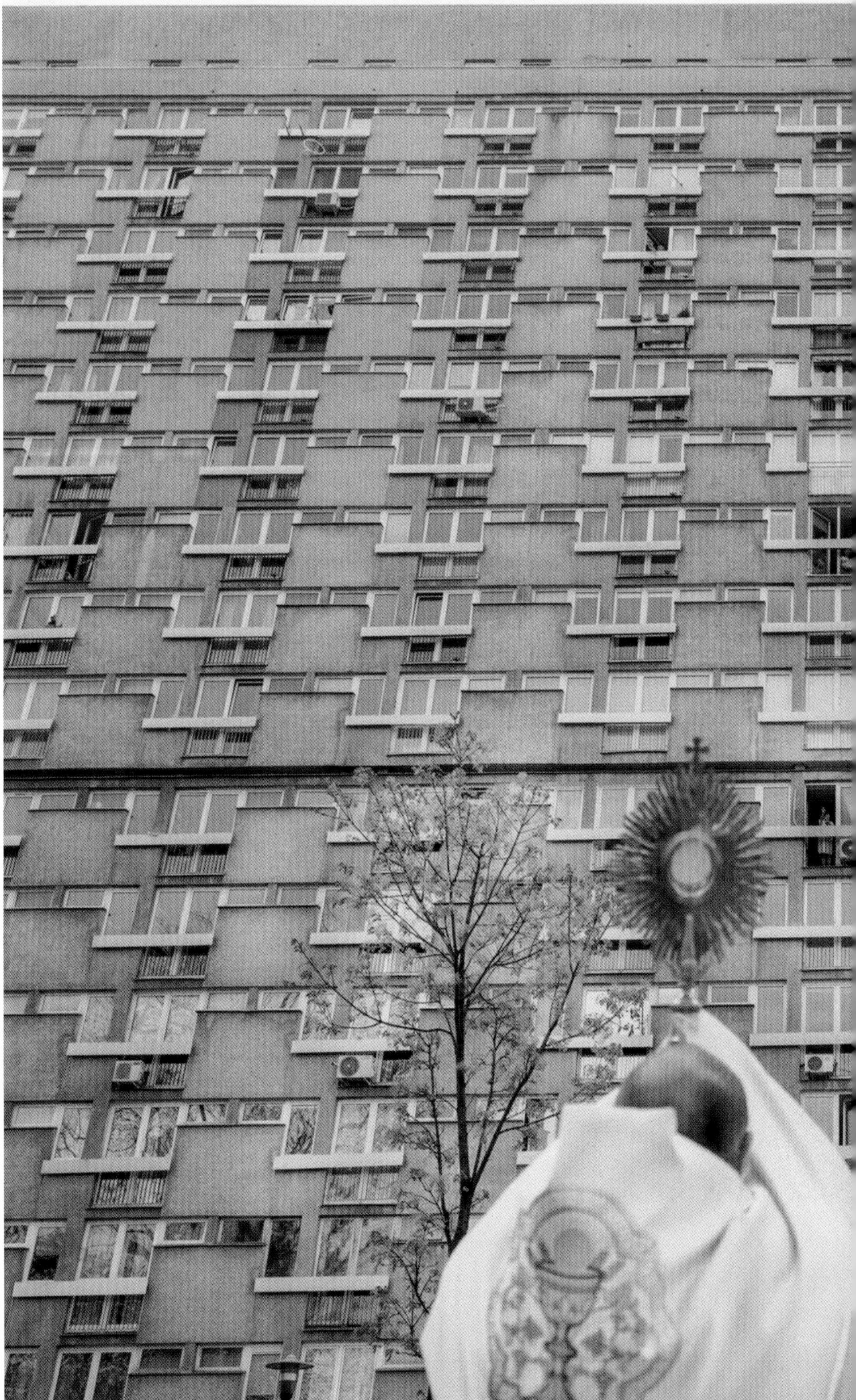

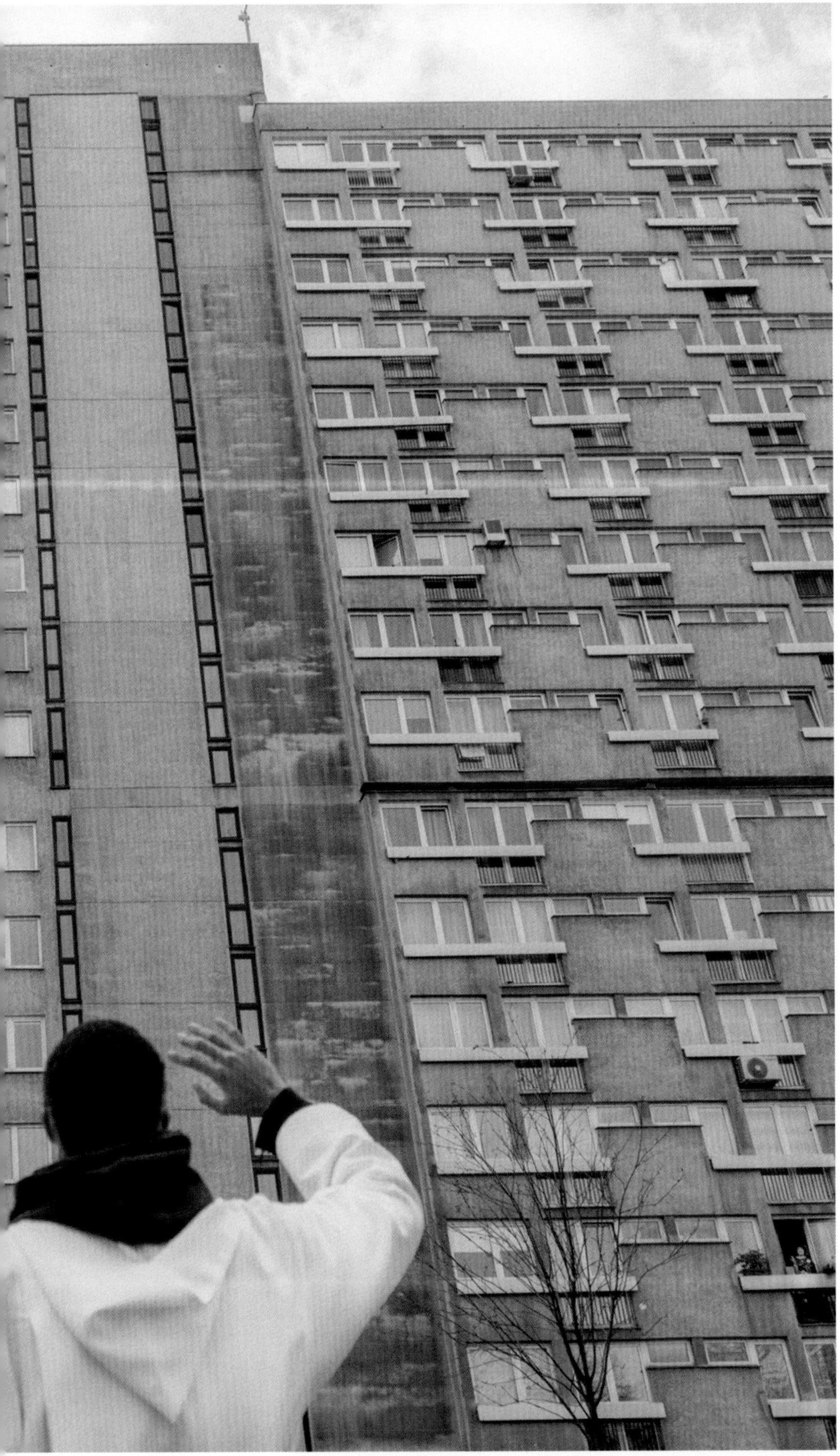

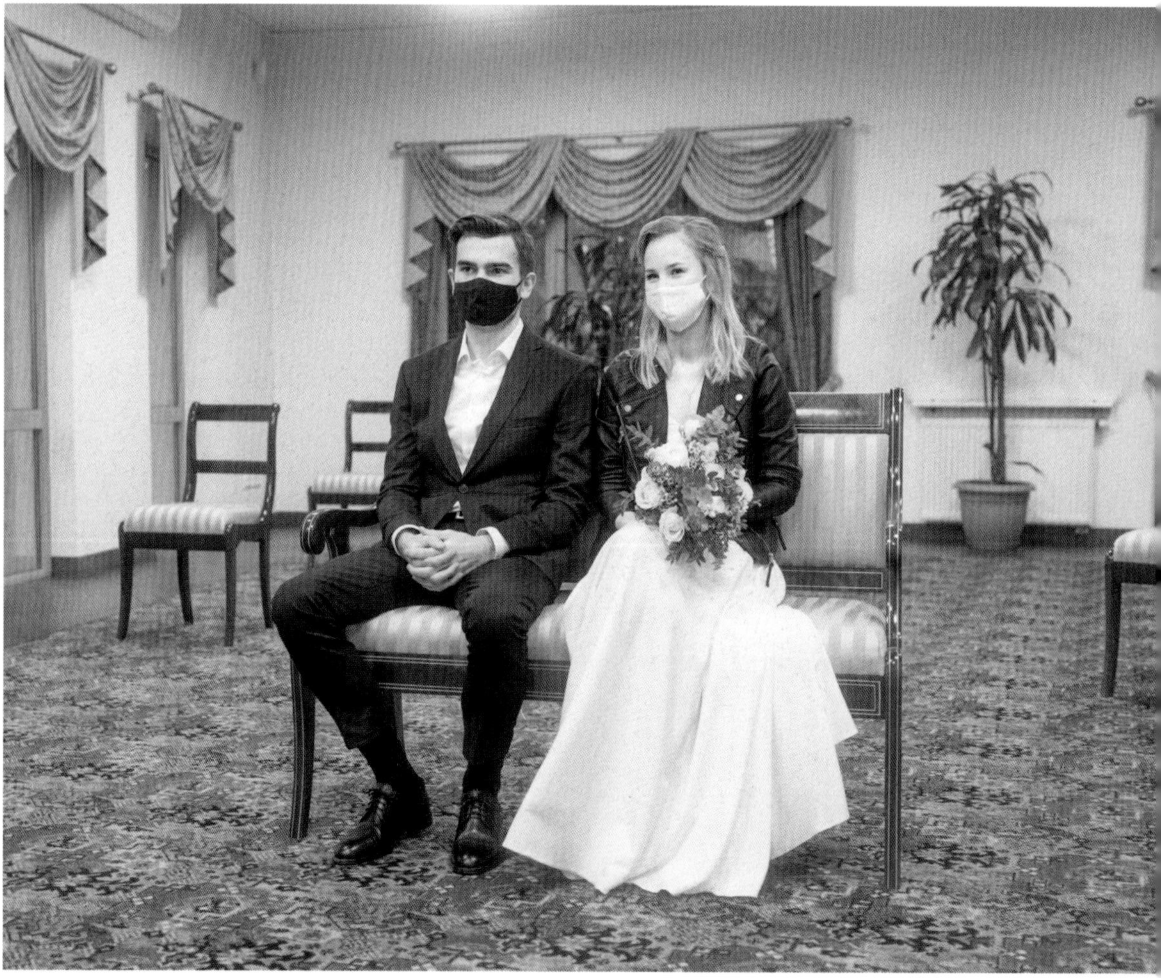

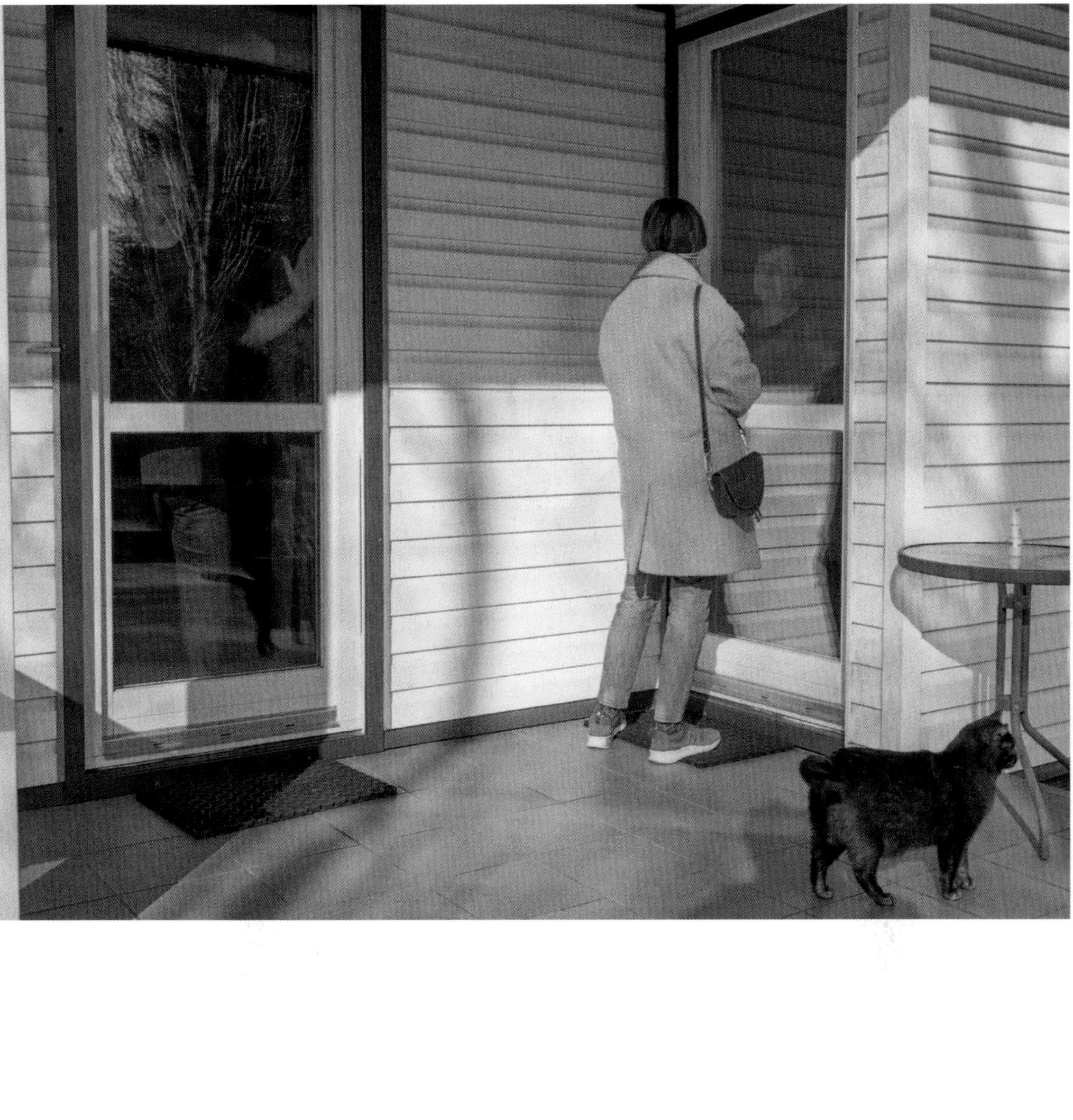

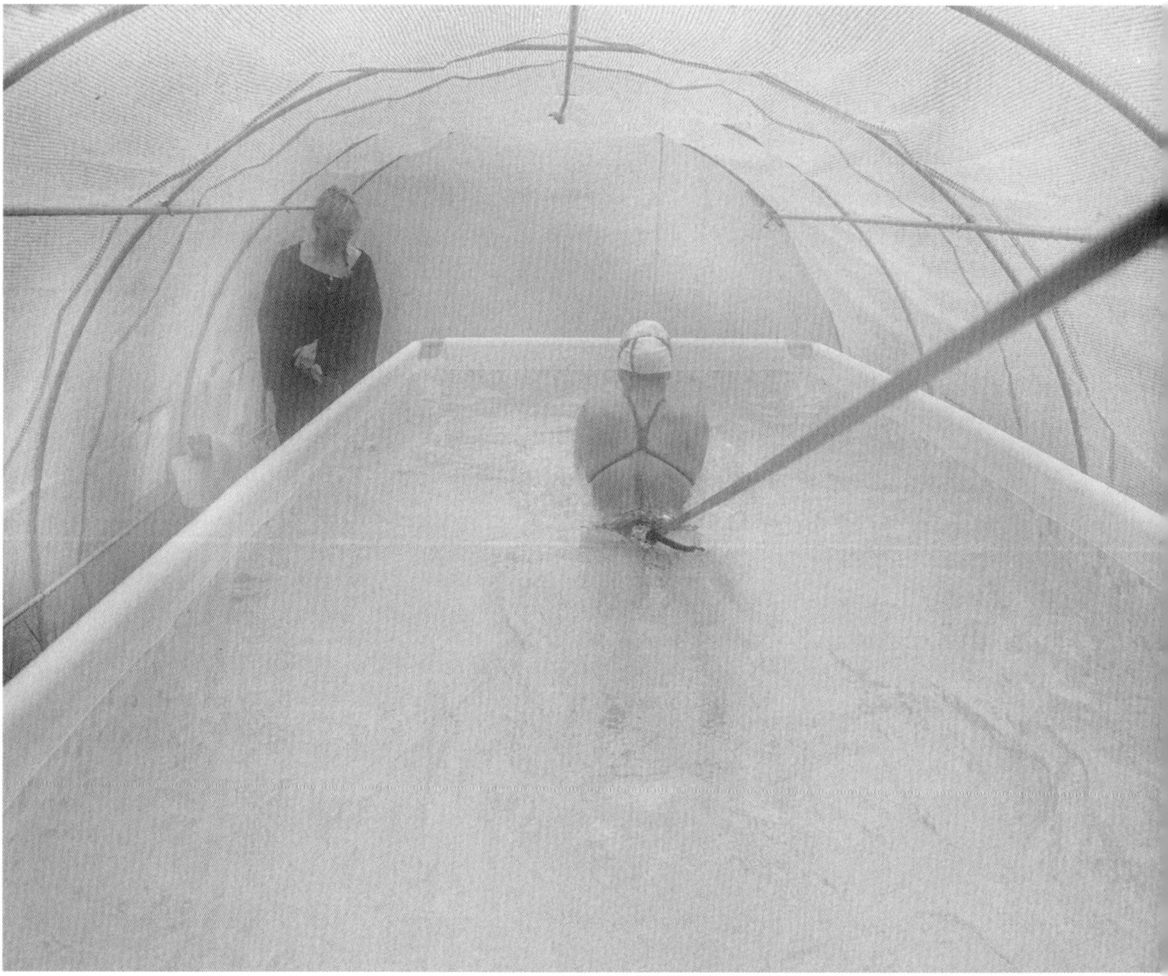

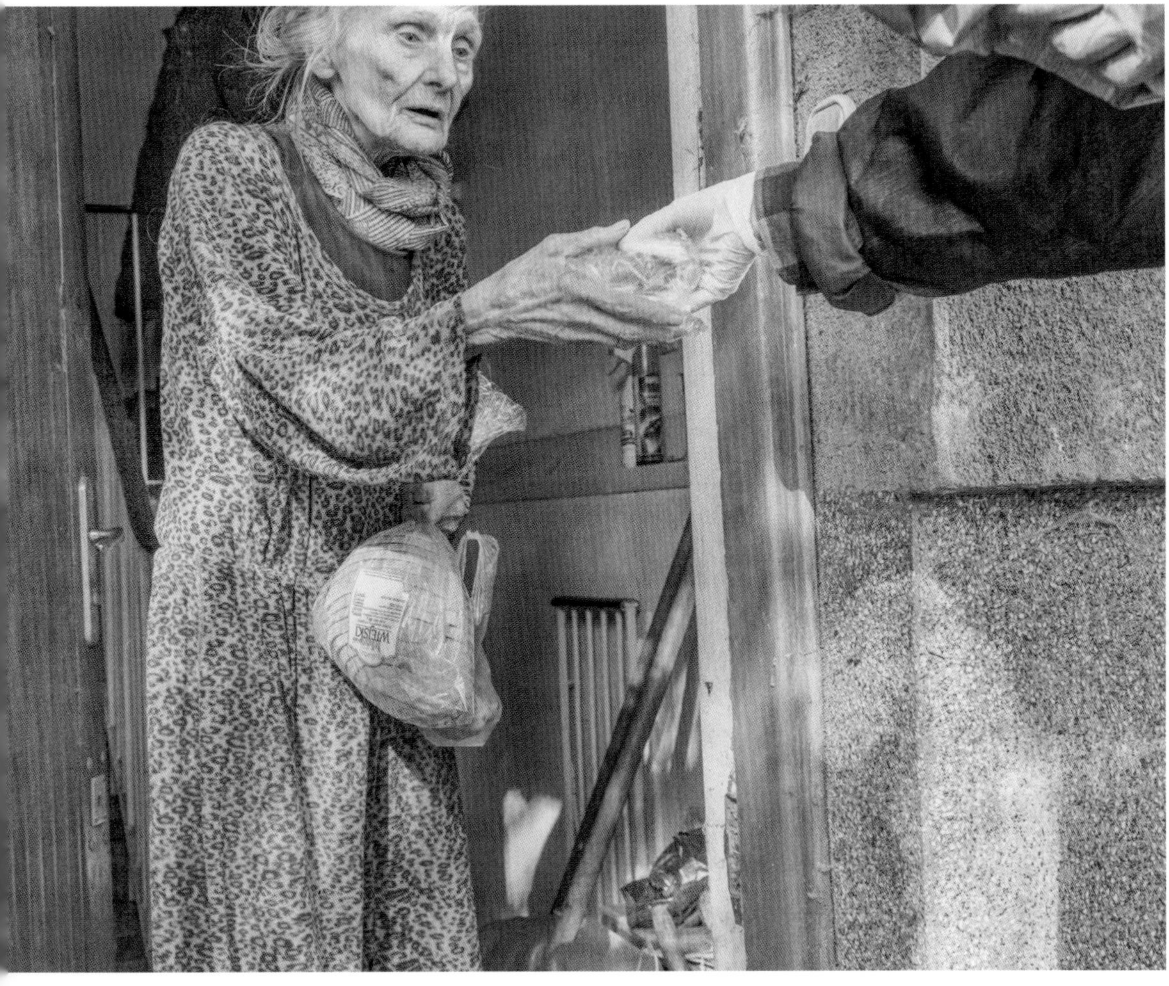

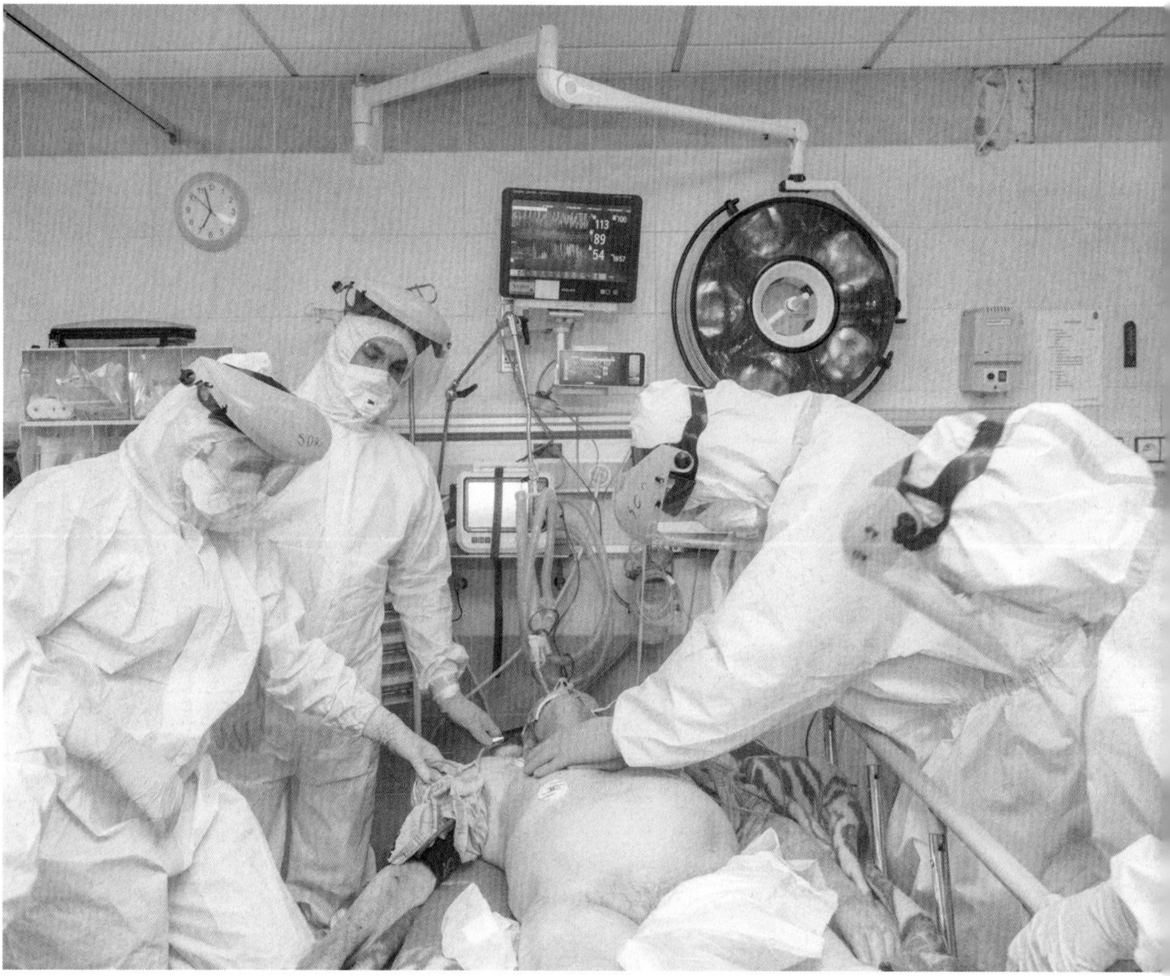
113
89
54

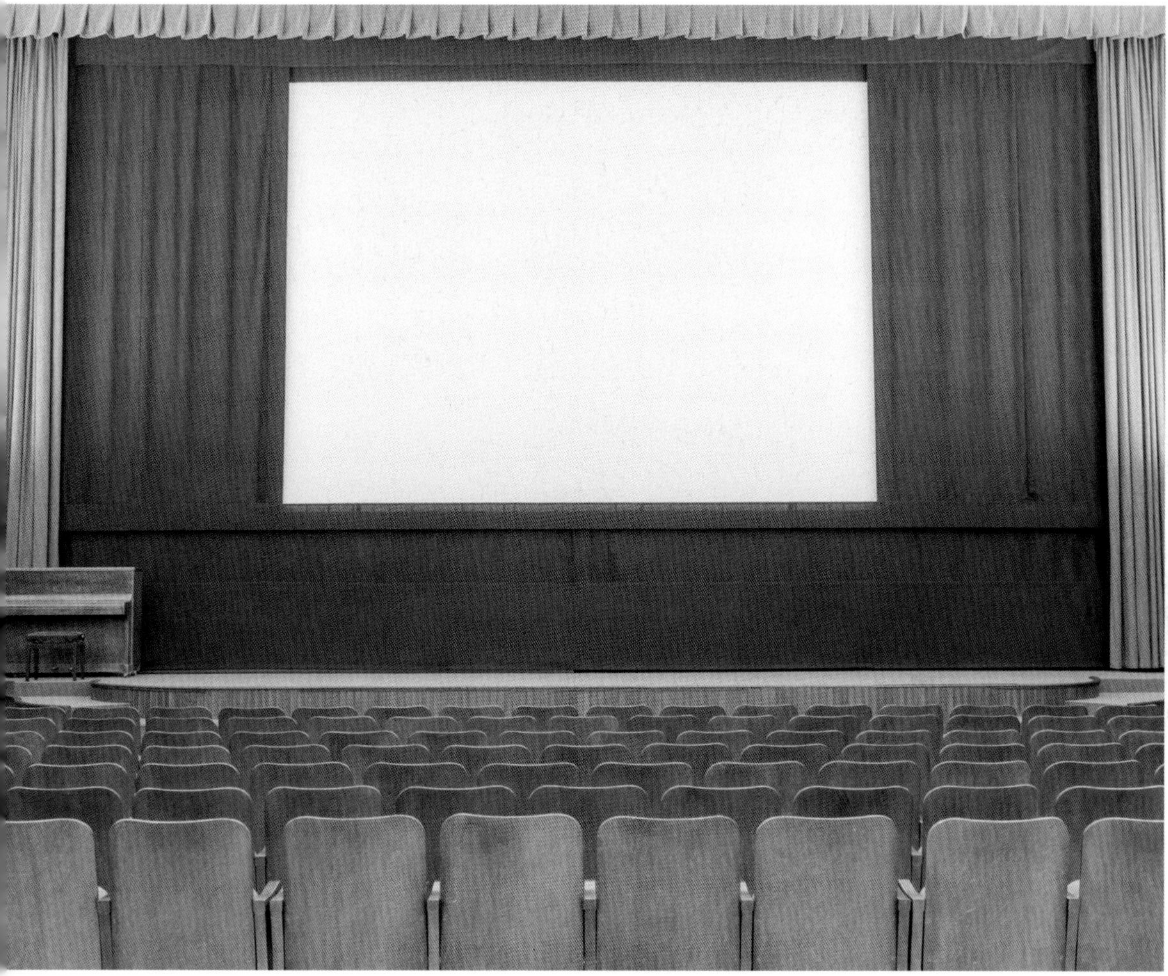

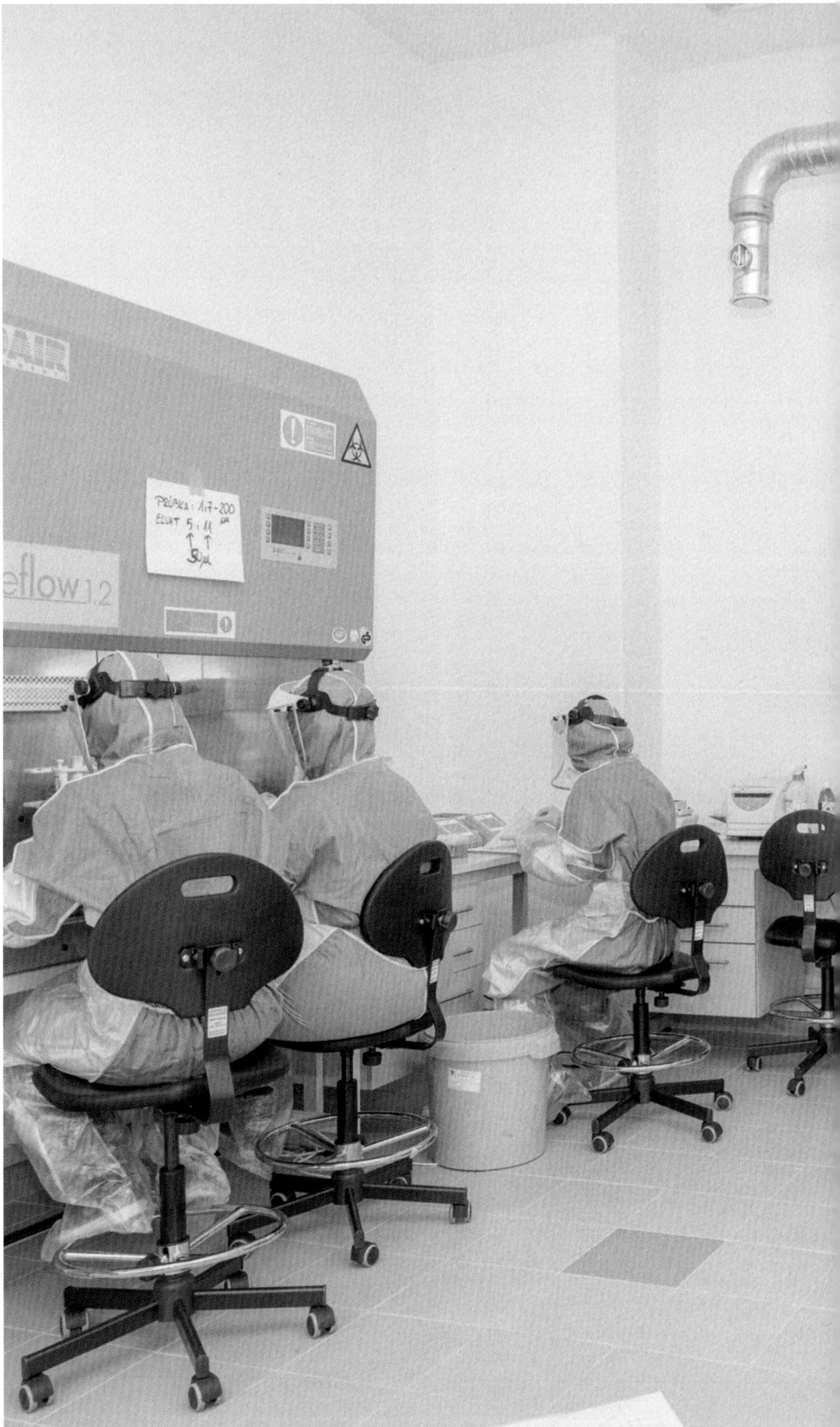
eflow 1.2

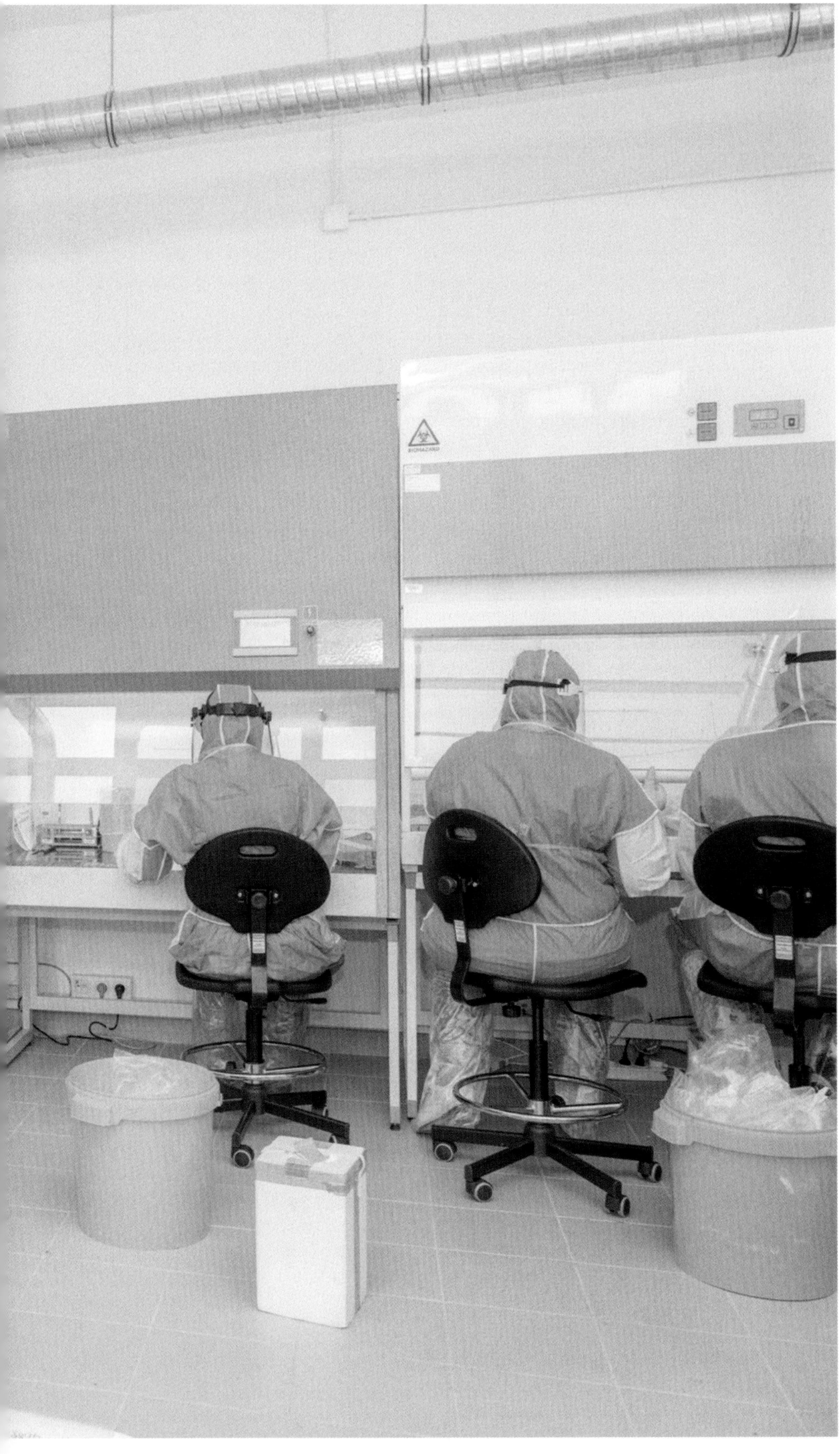

Luján Agusti & Nicolás Deluca, Argentina
The New End of the World

COVID-19 reached the southern end of the planet generating impact even in the most pristine lands. The exact cause of the disease is still unclear, but there is no doubt that it is related to the bad practices that humans exercise over nature. Everything is connected, and straining that balance is dangerous. Nature is our shelter, and our most precious resource.
The New End of the World is born as a hybrid documentary that explores, through photography and video, the traces created by the pandemic in the southernmost city of the world. Between 64 and 70 degrees west longitude of the Greenwich meridian and parallels 52 and 56 of south latitude, the last fragment of South America extends: Tierra del Fuego, the Terra Incognita Australis, open, broken down into islands and endless channels. There are only three cities on the island. Its capital is called Ushuaia, a word that comes from the Yagan language and means "background bay". It is located at the southernmost tip of South America, and it is known as "the end of the world". The end of the world as we know it.
Despite the geographical location, COVID-19 also reached Fuegian territory. Mandatory isolation was decreed and the local government implemented various measures in advance prior to the arrival of the harsh austral winter, such as the creation of a new health centre in a sports stadium.
Since the beginning of history, humans have observed red colour bursting out from their bodies and emerging from the flames that devastated their lands. In Tierra del Fuego, the Yaganes used fire to warn each other of danger. Red has historically meant to our species that something alarming was happening. The pandemic revealed before us that dystopian scenarios are closer than we thought. We forget that our well-being depends on the well-being of the planet we inhabit. Nature is our shelter.

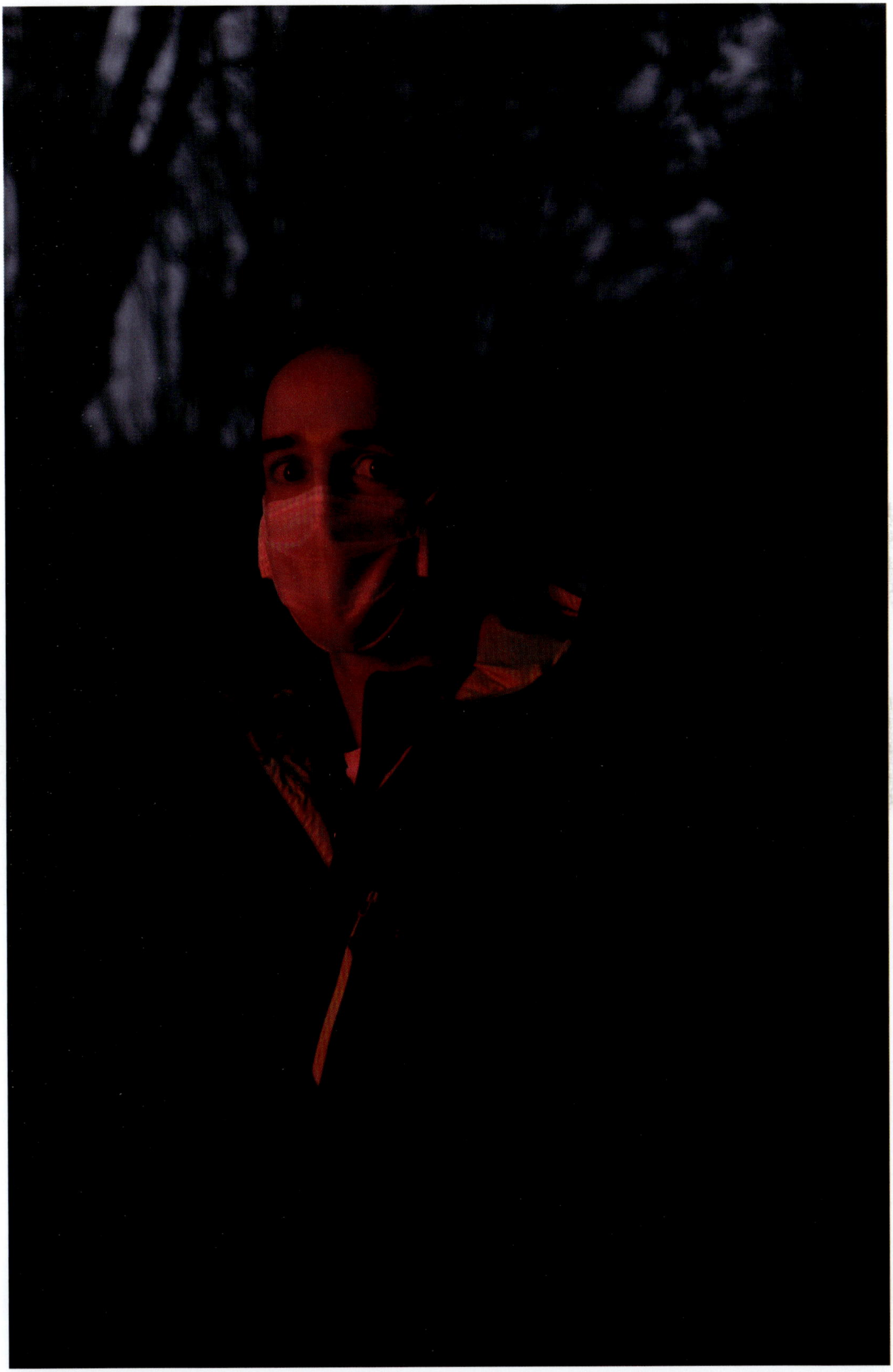

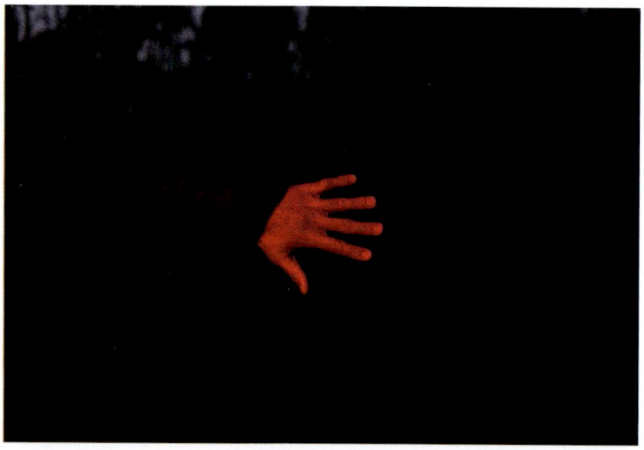

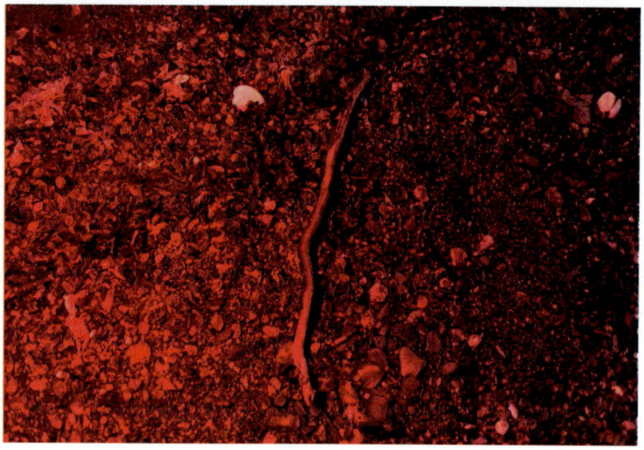

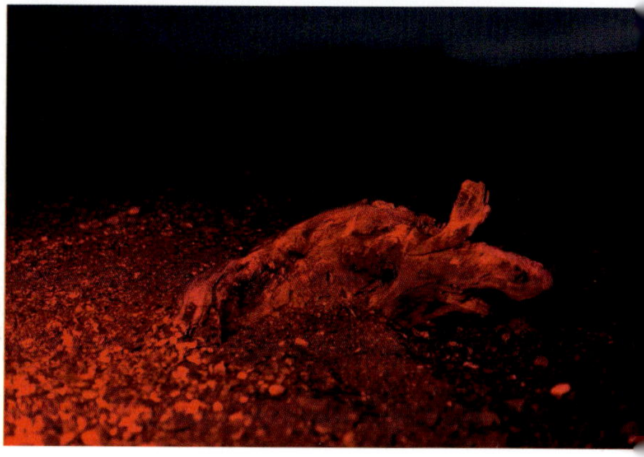

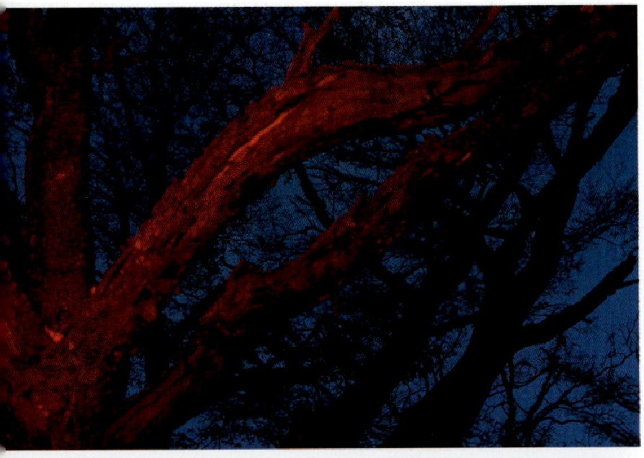

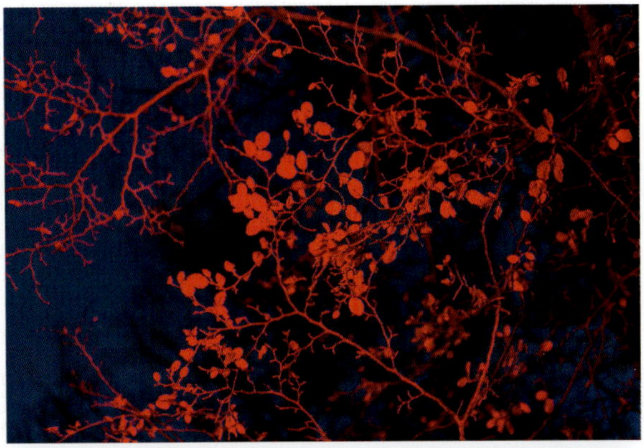

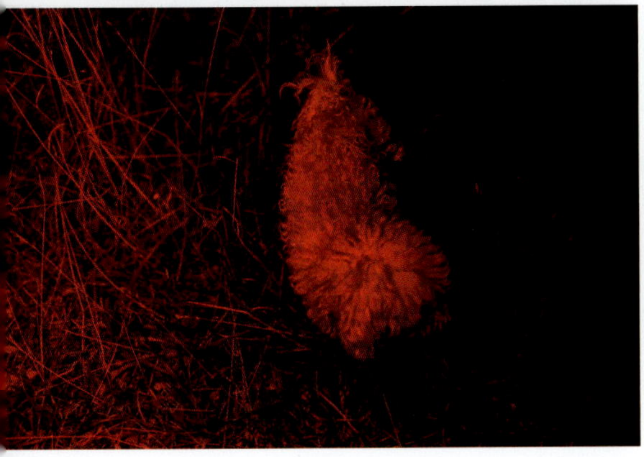

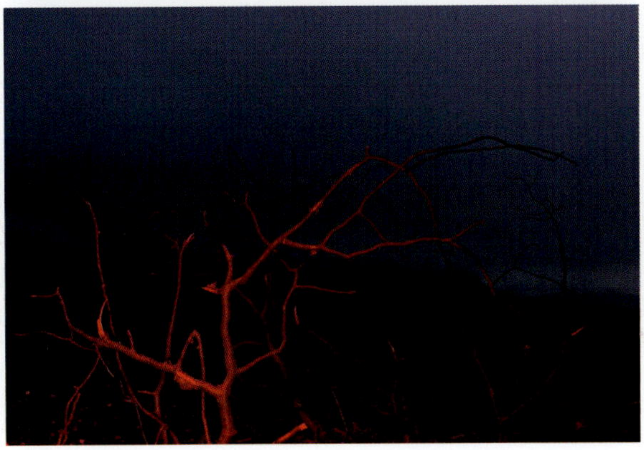

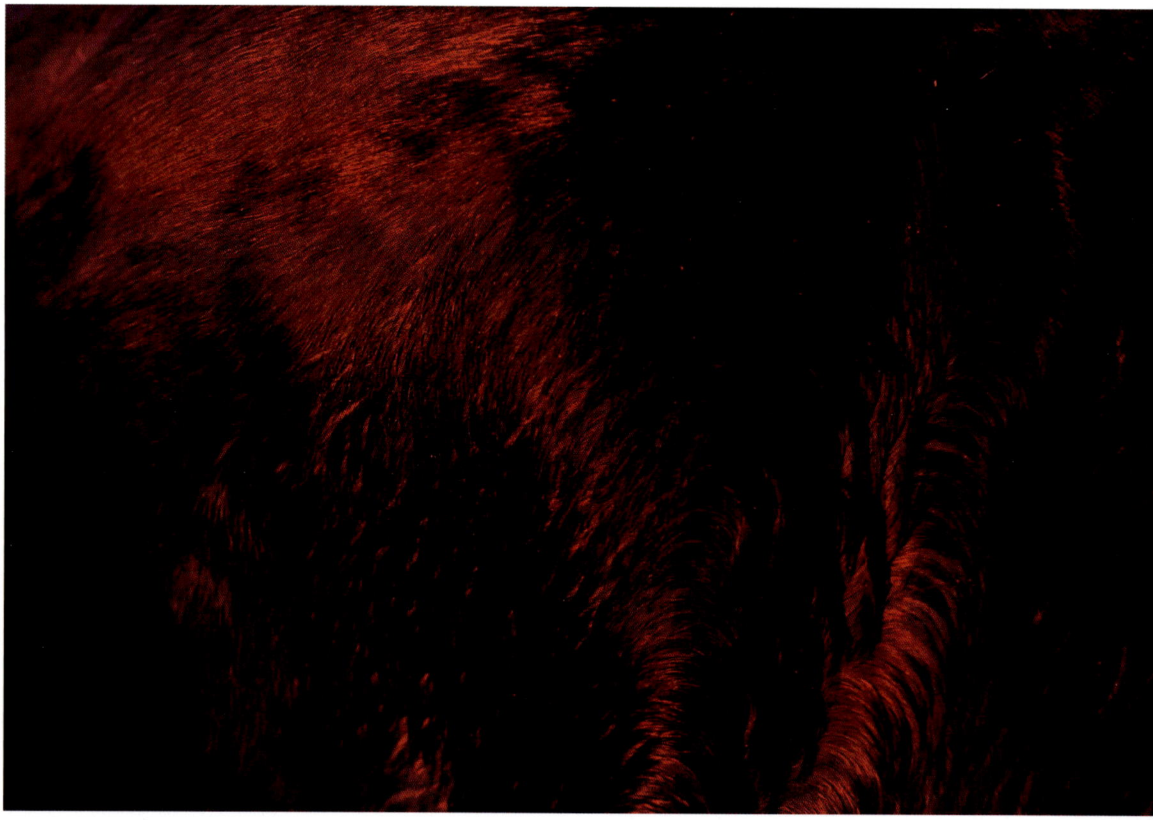

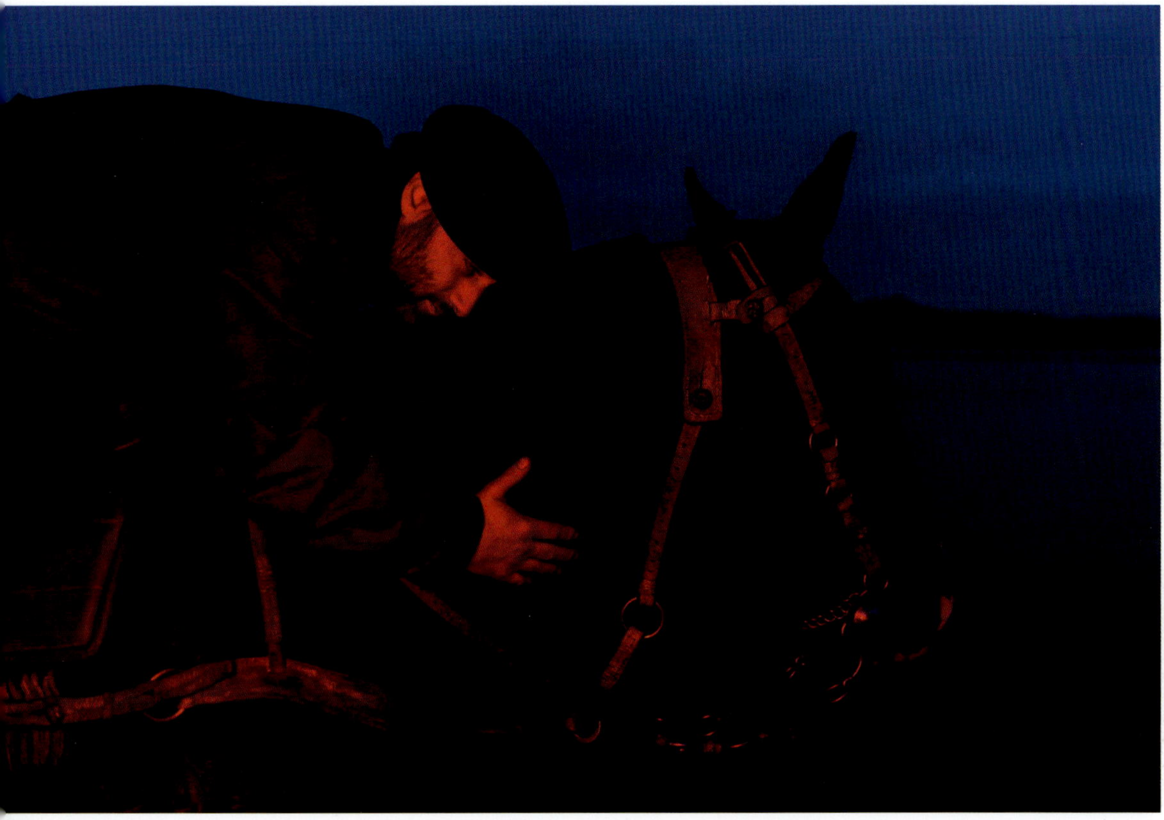

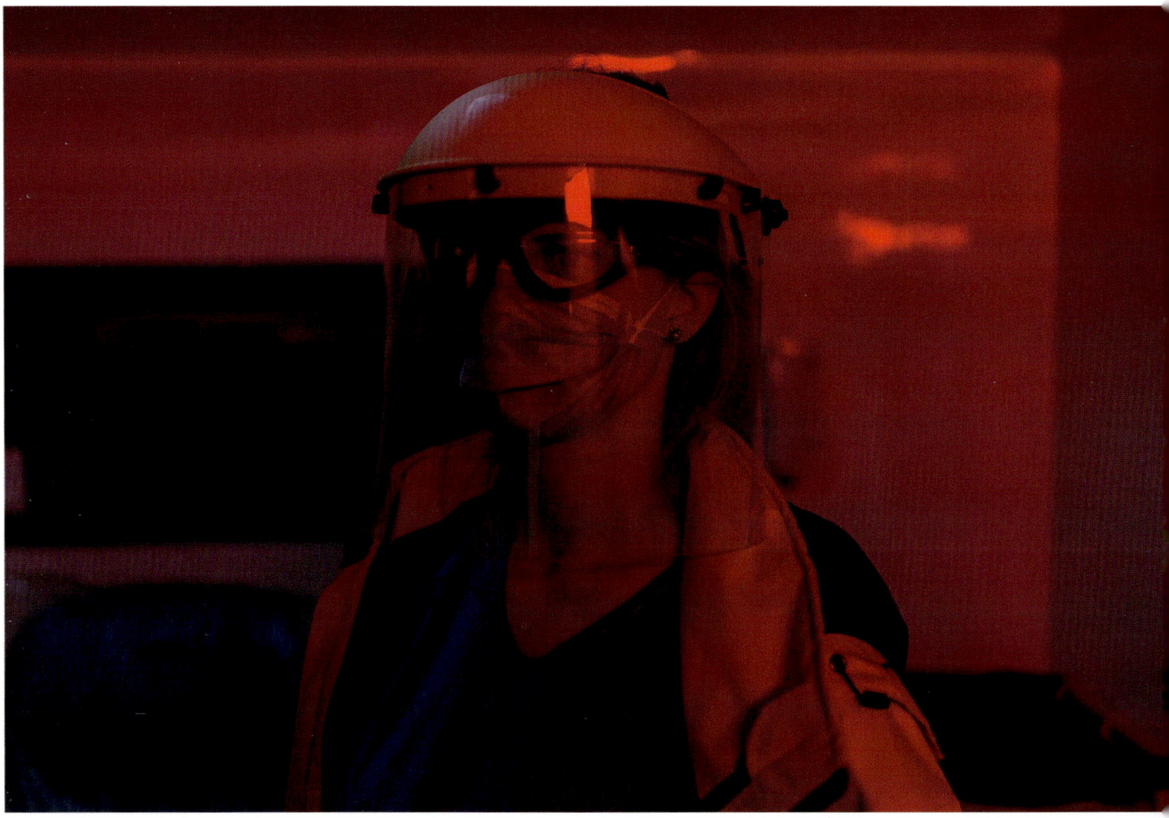

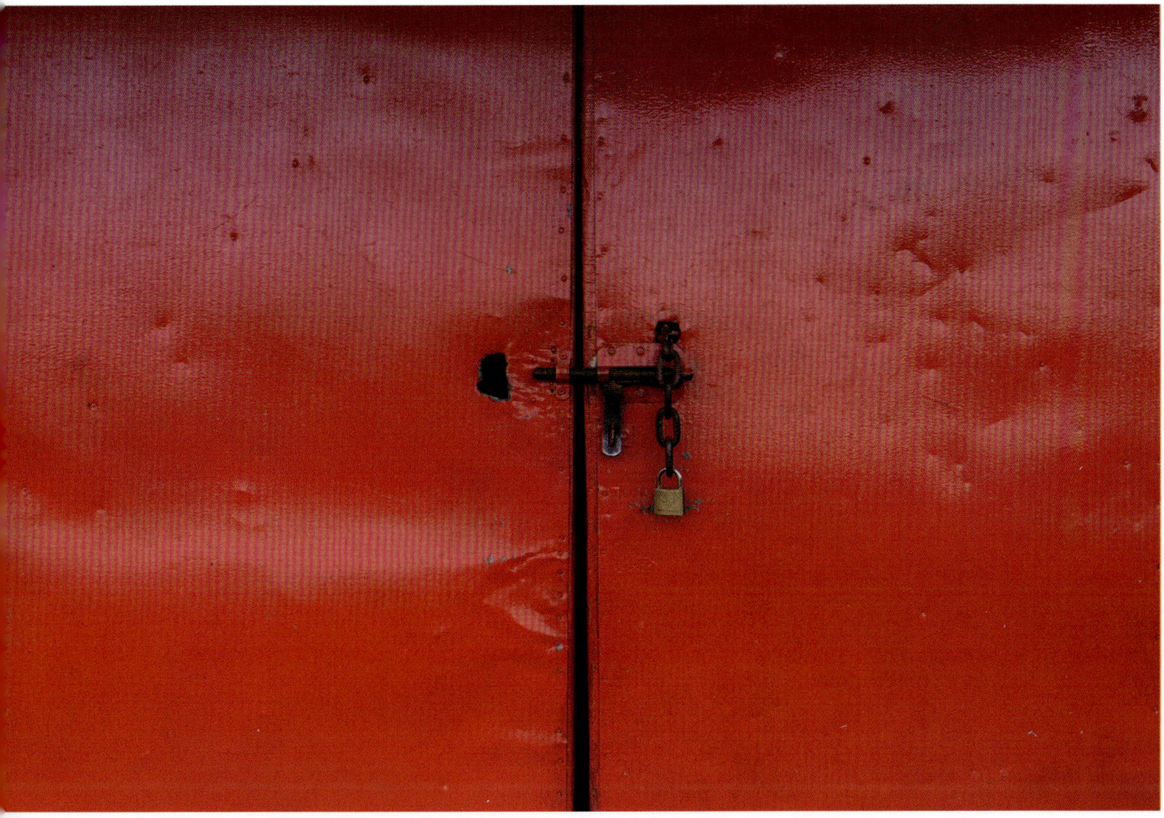

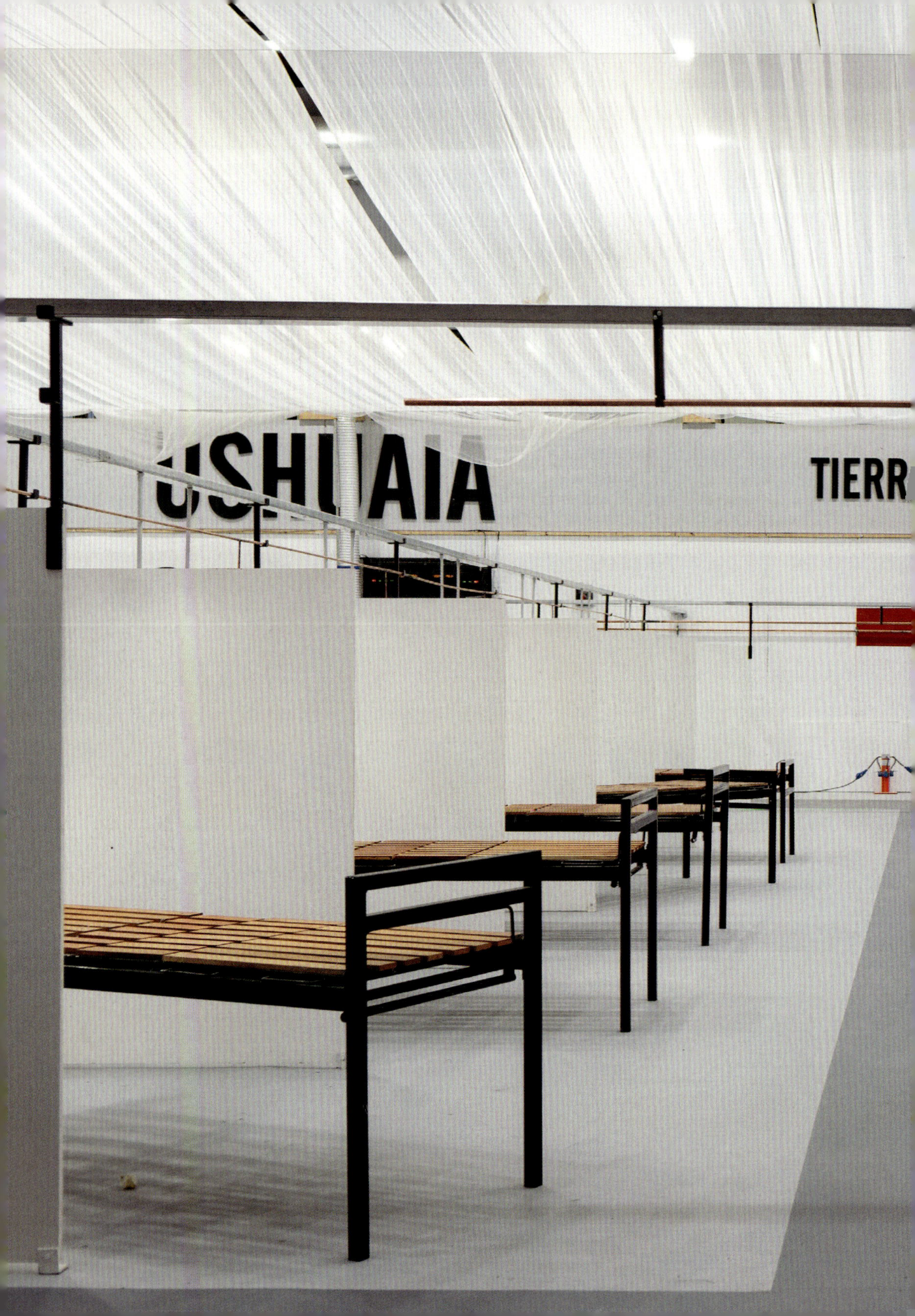
USHUAIA
TIERR

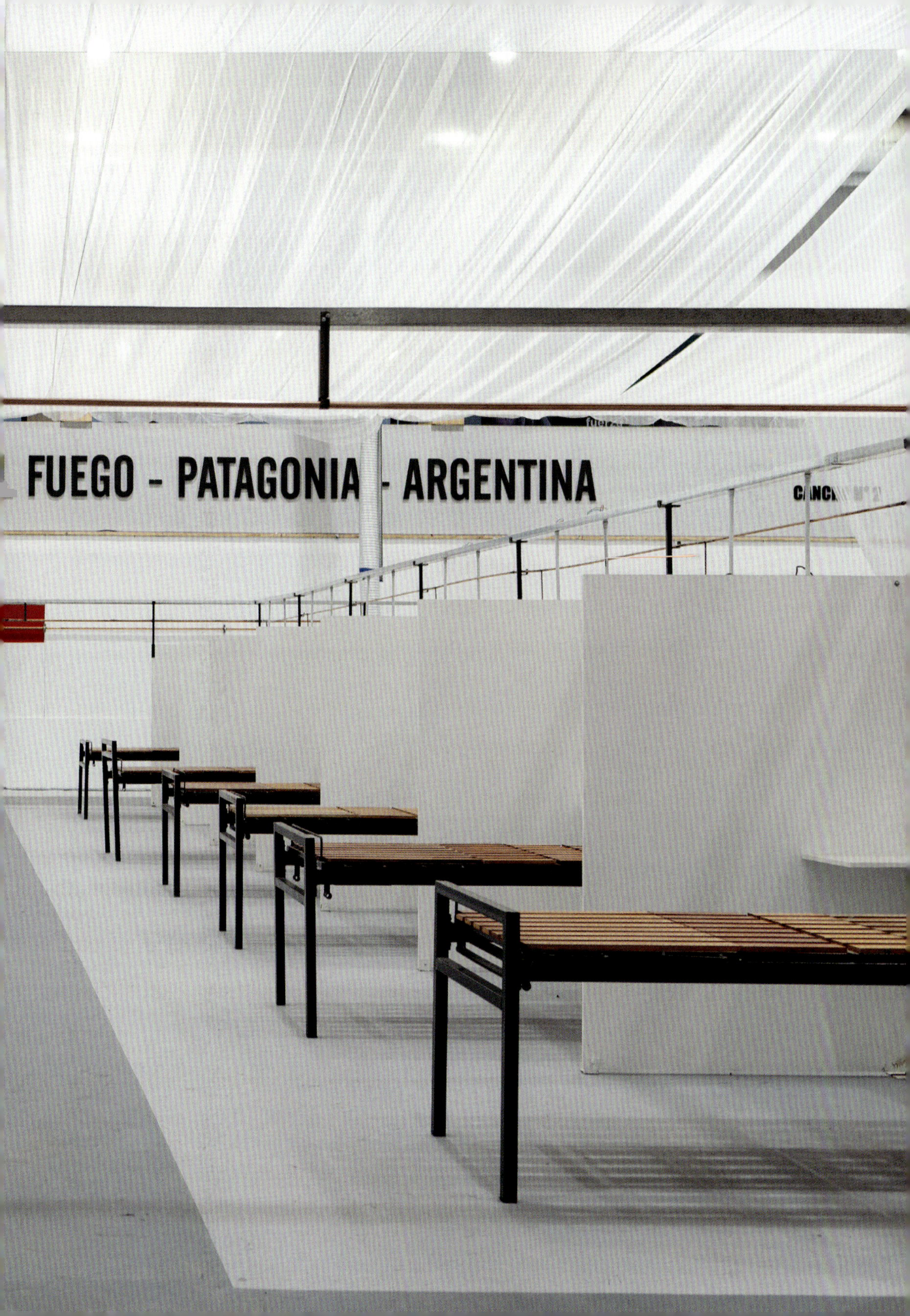
FUEGO - PATAGONIA - ARGENTINA

00. A Visual Overview
Captions

Alex Majoli, Italy

The photographs were taken during lockdown in Italy, between March and April 2020.

SCENE#2756
At the cemetery a priest blessing coffins just arrived from Bergamo. The Italian Army has been brought in to ferry coffins out of Bergamo. Along with other Northern cities mayors, Alessandro Canelli offered support to the city of Bergamo. Novara, Italy, 2020.
(Pages 26-27)

SCENE#1445
Inside the COVID-19 unit, a team of medical staff is checking the condition of one of the patients. Caltagirone, Gravina city Hospital, Italy, 2020.
(Pages 28–29)

SCENE#3569
In Duomo square a food delivery rider is emptying his bag. Since March 9 Italy has been locked down to contain the spread of COVID-19. Towns became ghost city where only delivery riders were the only people seen on empty streets. Milan, Italy, 2020.
(Pages 30–31)

SCENE#2830
At the cemetery coffins are carried out from a military truck. The Italian Army has been brought in to ferry coffins out of Bergamo, amongst Italy's most plagued towns, as its morgue and its crematorium struggle to cope with the surging coronavirus death toll. Novara, Italy, 2020.
(Pages 32–33)

SCENE#3104
For the past 35 years the EU's borderless zone has ensured freedom of movement and residence for persons and goods across its member states. Following the outbreak early this year, on March 17, EU leaders decided that the best course of action was to stop the movement between member nations and re-establish border checks. Even little alley and passes have been blocked by Slovenians as of March 10th. Polava, Italy-Slovenia Border, 2020.
(Pages 34–35)

Rafael Heygster & Helena Manhartsberger, Germany

Soldiers on the way to an exercise at a makeshift hospital in the exhibition halls in Hannover. 14 April 2020.
(Page 37)

The Bundeswehr Institute for Microbiology in Munich specialises in researching and combating biological warfare agents. Research into the SARS-CoV-2 virus plays an important role in the current crisis. The first German COVID-19 case was already diagnosed by the Institute at the end of January 2020. Since then, thousands of SARS-CoV-2 suspected cases have been tested and antibody research is continuously carried out. 27 May 2020.
(Pages 38–39)

In the stadium of the football team Borussia Mönchengladbach, cardboard mates were set up as a backdrop for ghost games. Fans can upload their own photos online, these will be printed on cardboard stands and placed in the stadium. At the time of the photo, about 21,000 soccer fans have participated.
22 May 2020.
(Pages 40–41)

In mid-June, 120 of 700 residents of a prefabricated building are infected with coronavirus. The city bans all residents from leaving the housing complex, imposes a quarantine and puts up fences. 13 June 2020.
(Page 42)

Ilona W. and her husband Andreas demonstrate at a "hygiene demo" in Hannover together with right-wing extremist conspiracy believers against the measures to limit the spread of coronavirus. They have written "muzzle" on their protective masks.
25 April 2020.
(Page 43)

In the Hannover Exhibition Halls, a makeshift hospital has been set up in March. Where usually trade fairs take place in Hannover, treatment facilities were created for 500 COVID-19 patients. Until today it still not necessary to open the new builded infrastructure. 14 April 2020.
(Page 44)

Candidate officers of the German Armed Forces who are studying medicine work out emergency procedures in the makeshift hospital on the Hanover exhibition grounds. 14 April 2020.
(Page 45)

In the improvised parliament in Bremen, all politicians strictly adhere to the valid distance rules in order to set a positive example for the citizens, a member of parliament tells.
As soon as they leave the hall, however, many of them take the distance rules less seriously and stand closely together in groups without a mask. 13 May 2020.
(Pages 46–47)

Masoumeh Bahrami, Iran

17 year-old Hossein Droudy is waiting for the corpse of someone who died because of coronavirus. He is a student in a religious school. After the death of his grandfather, who was also a mullah, he started to take care of his responsibilities (the funeral related works) at the Behshahr cemetery. Although coronavirus has been raised the fatality rate over the past few weeks, he was the only mullah who works in cemetery for months. He said at the first days he was frightened but thinking about the martyrs whom went to war calm him down. They may have been afraid first and worried about their families but they went to war anyways.
(Page 49)

The family and relatives of Yazdan Mortazavi came to the washing house for the last visit. Yazdan Mortazavi, 53-year-old, passed away because of a coronavirus infection in the hospital. Yazdan and his daughter were hospitalised because of coronavirus. The doctor told Yazdan's wife to take the daughter home, since Yazdan was becoming distressed because of his daughter, and his body got weaker. The mother took the daughter home and Yazdan passed away in the hospital. When they entered the washing place, the mother said that he loved his children and he always laughed. "I must keep my children happy now. I will live with his memories. How can I continue without him?"
(Pages 50–51)

Mashti Karim is a 66-year-old vendor who sells potatoes and fruits on the sidewalks. Due to the spread of coronavirus many jobs have faded away. Karim talks about his job, now he can earn less money. "It seems that people do not eat fruit. Maybe they think our fruits are infected with the virus. I take the risk and come out to earn money for my family, but nobody buys. I stay here beside my car without selling anything. I go around the street and collect grass for my cow and my neighbor's cows. I keep myself busy and work for the cows. This way the time passes faster and I do not think about coronavirus."
(Page 52)

My 36-year-old brother, Borzoo, was in a bodybuilding course when the coronavirus pandemic started. He continued his exercises at home during the quarantine. During the first days because of cold weather he exercised inside the house but after a while when the weather got warmer (during the spring) he continued his exercise in the garden. There is a garden next to his house and we played there when we were young. He said, "Doing the exercise in courtyard is weird because it was unbelievable for me to see my bodybuilding equipment in a garden not in a gym. I look at the quarantine as an opportunity, and honestly I think I have no other choice".
(Page 53)

Volunteer women are gathered at the mosques and sewing. Due to the rapid expansion of the coronavirus, the shortage of medical equipment, for example mask and covers, made the situation worse. Somayeh Ahani, the supervisor, suffers from Fibromyalgia. One of the tailor women said that during the war we used to gather at the mosque to help people and this pandemic situation is similar to that.
(Page 54)

It was the 7th day of ritual for Rezvan Hashemi, a 54-year-old woman. She had respiratory disease and she died because of coronavirus. Rezvan was hospitalised in the ICU section of Khatam for one month. After a long course of the disease she died in the hospital. At the end of the ritual, when people left the cemetery, her husband went near the grave and said "now, it is my turn" and started crying at that time and his son-in-law hugged him.
(Page 55)

This is first day of Nowruz (new year), Bahram is wearing a mask at home and watching his grandson, Bardia, who pasted his toy to the window. To follow the social distancing guidelines according to the World Health Organisation, Bardia wants his grandfather to kiss his toy from the other side of the window on his behalf. Because of his pre-existing conditions, Baraham quarantined himself and used a mask even at home. He felt shortness of breath and sometimes coughed. He said it was the strangest Nowruz of his life, even stranger than Nowruz during the war. "I miss my grandchildren and I would like to see them even through a window", he said.
(Page 56)

My brother's wife is sitting in the centre with a cake which she bought for me. It is my birthday, in pandemic days and with social distances. After months, my brothers and their family came in our yard to celebrate my birthday.
(Page 57)

A view from our court during the coronavirus quarantine. In the corner of the room, where there were slippers and disinfectant material. When someone comes from outside, they need to change their shoes with a clean slipper and clean their hands with disinfectant. The eucalyptus leaves are used for eliminating the shortness of breath. My uncle picked them from the nearby plain and put them behind the door.
(Pages 58–59)

Arek Rataj, China

On January 19, 2020, a few days before Chinese New Year, people are queuing up to purchase discounted traditional steamed bread.
(Page 61)

On January 28, a couple wearing face masks walk down an empty street. The normally bustling streets of Wuhan became deserted after implementing restrictions.
(Pages 62–63)

On January 24, a taxi driver drives through the empty street of Wuhan a day after imposing lockdown. A few days later Wuhan officials temporarily abolished taxi services for more than two months.
(Page 64, top)

On January 17, a Chinese man stands in front of the Wuhan Medical Treatment Centre, which hospitalised the very first coronavirus patients.
(Page 64, bottom)

On January 29, a girl wears a face mask as she plays on a swing near the Yingwuzhou Yangtze River Bridge in Wuhan.
(Page 65, top)

The panic began on January 23, when public transport was closed two days before the Chinese New Year. Communication stopped, the metro, buses and the airport were shut down. It was reopened after a 76-day lockdown.
(Page 65, bottom)

On January 30, a 1,000-bed Huoshenshan Hospital in Wuhan, created in response to the COVID-19 pandemic, was built in just 10 days. It has run under the management of the People's Liberation Army.
(Pages 66–67)

Tomasz Lazar, Poland

Ozonation of the underground passage in the city centre. Warsaw, 7 April 2020.
(Page 69)

Father Lech Dorobczyński, priest of the Franciscan reformers parish in Warsaw, while walking around the estate and blessing parishioners who do not leave the homes with the monstrance. Warsaw, 19 April 2020.
(Pages 70–71)

Klaudia and Szymon getting married during the pandemic. According to the Covid regulations in Poland, only the couple, witnesses, photographer and the person celebrating the wedding may be in the wedding hall during the ceremony. Wesola close to Warsaw, 28 November 2020.
(Page 72)

Portrait of a family during the COVID-19 pandemic in Poland. Paula says goodbye to her parents Ewa and Krzysztof, after delivering the shopping to their home. For their safety, she does it through the glass door. Older people are at high risk for this disease. Ewa and Krzysztof made the decision to isolate themselves from everyone until they were vaccinated against COVID-19. Warsaw, 28 March 2020.
(Page 73)

Paulina Cierpiałowska (15-year-old), multiple Polish champion in swimming, during training in the pool constructed by her parents in the garden. As a result of COVID-19, the Olympic Games in Tokyo have been postponed, which means Paulina still has the chance to qualify for the Olympic Games. Malbork, 19 May 2020.
(Page 74)

Jola, who worked as a flight attendant for 30 years, receives food from people from the Senior Aid campaign. This action was organised by the Warsaw Group and every day helps an increasing number of elderly people who stay at home for fear of being infected with COVID-19. Warsaw, 10 April 2020.
(Page 75)

A man undergoing resuscitation in a Hospital Emergency Department. Warsaw, 23 May 2020.
(Page 76)

View of the empty Iluzjon Cinema room. Pursuant to the ordinance of the Minister of Health of March 14, all facilities such as cinemas, museums, libraries, theaters, etc. are closed until further notice. Warsaw, 27 March 2020.
(Page 77)

Technicians doing Covid tests in the Alab lab. Alab is the second-largest private laboratory in Poland. Warsaw, 13 May 2020.
(Pages 78–79)

01.

The Health Challenge

Andrea Frazzetta, Italy
The Life and Death Shift

By the middle of March, Northern Italy had become the epicentre of a global pandemic. The coronavirus had infected tens of thousands of Italians, devastating the country with Europe's oldest population. In the region of Lombardy, where the virus first exploded in the West, a wealthy and advanced health care system had suddenly become a war zone.
Hospitals became the front lines in a gruelling battle. Desperate patients crowded into emergency rooms, sick, dying and afraid. They expanded intensive-care capacity, lined entire wards with ventilators and crowded corridors with oxygen tanks and beds. The doctors, nurses, paramedics and volunteers had little choice but to soldier through day and night with little rest.
Quarantined at home, Italy's citizens took notice. They applauded from their balconies and shared on the web photos of nurses collapsed at a desk or bearing the bruises of tight masks. These are the faces of the men and women who fought to save them.

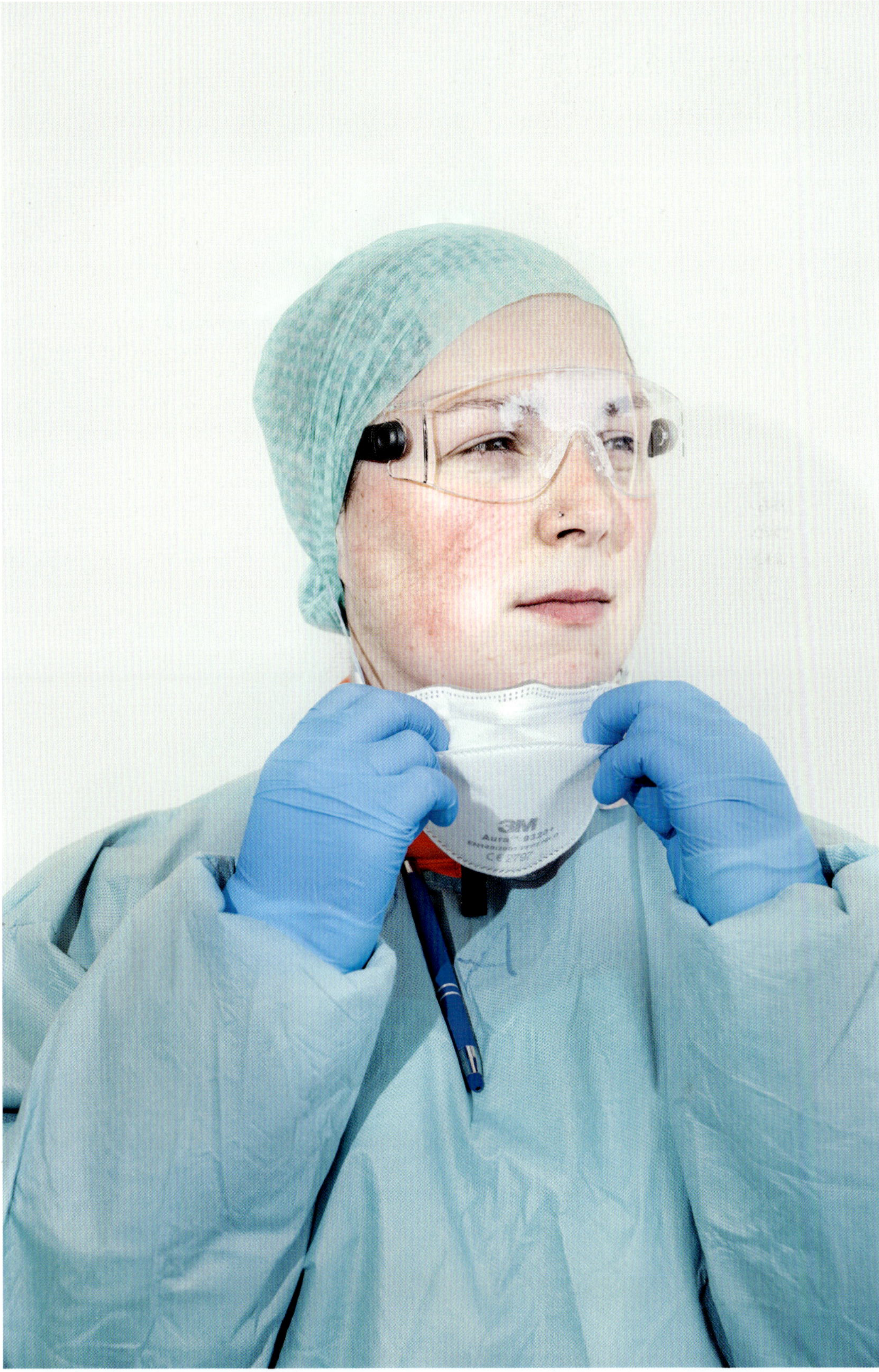
3M
Aura

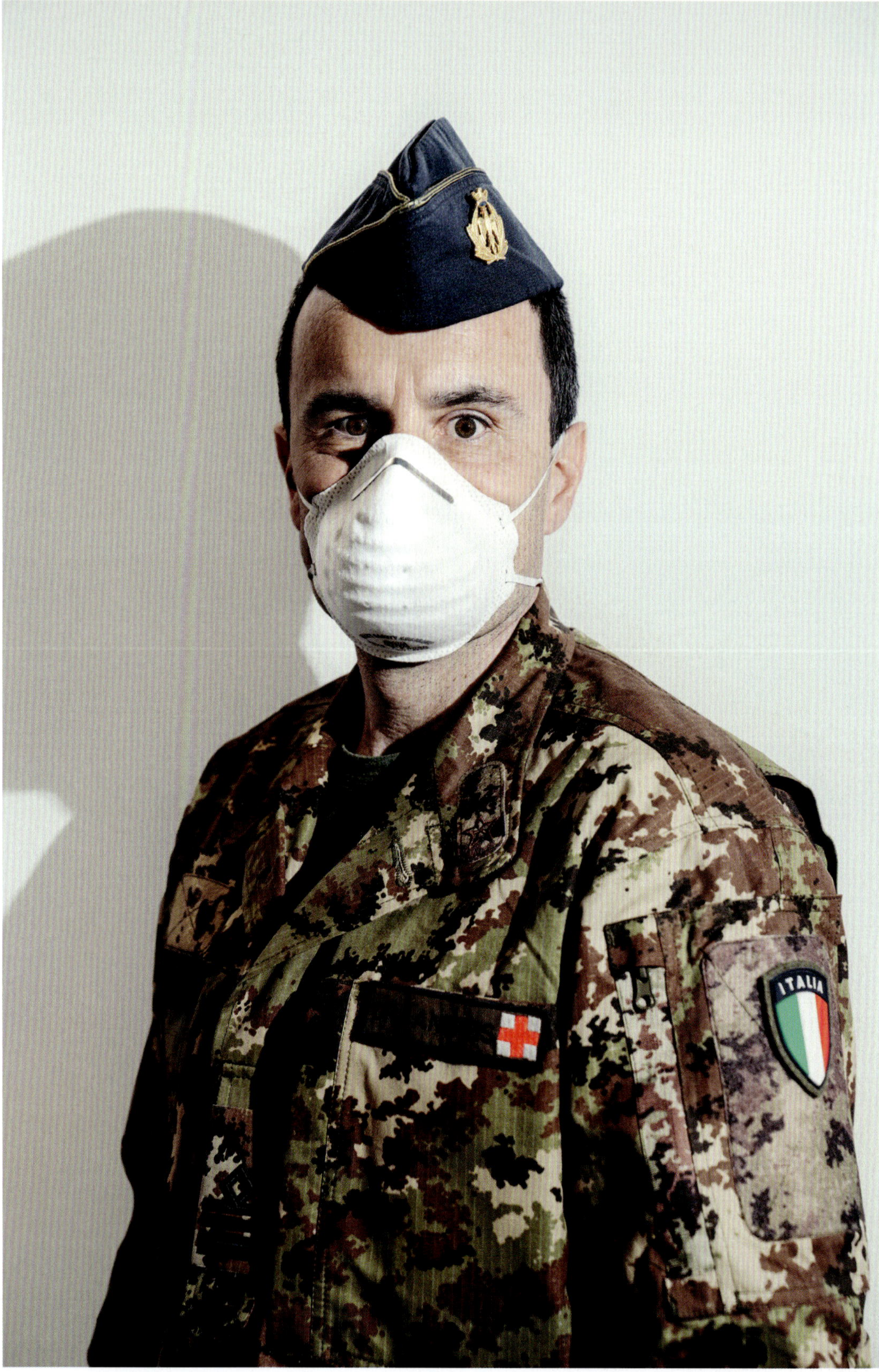
ITALIA

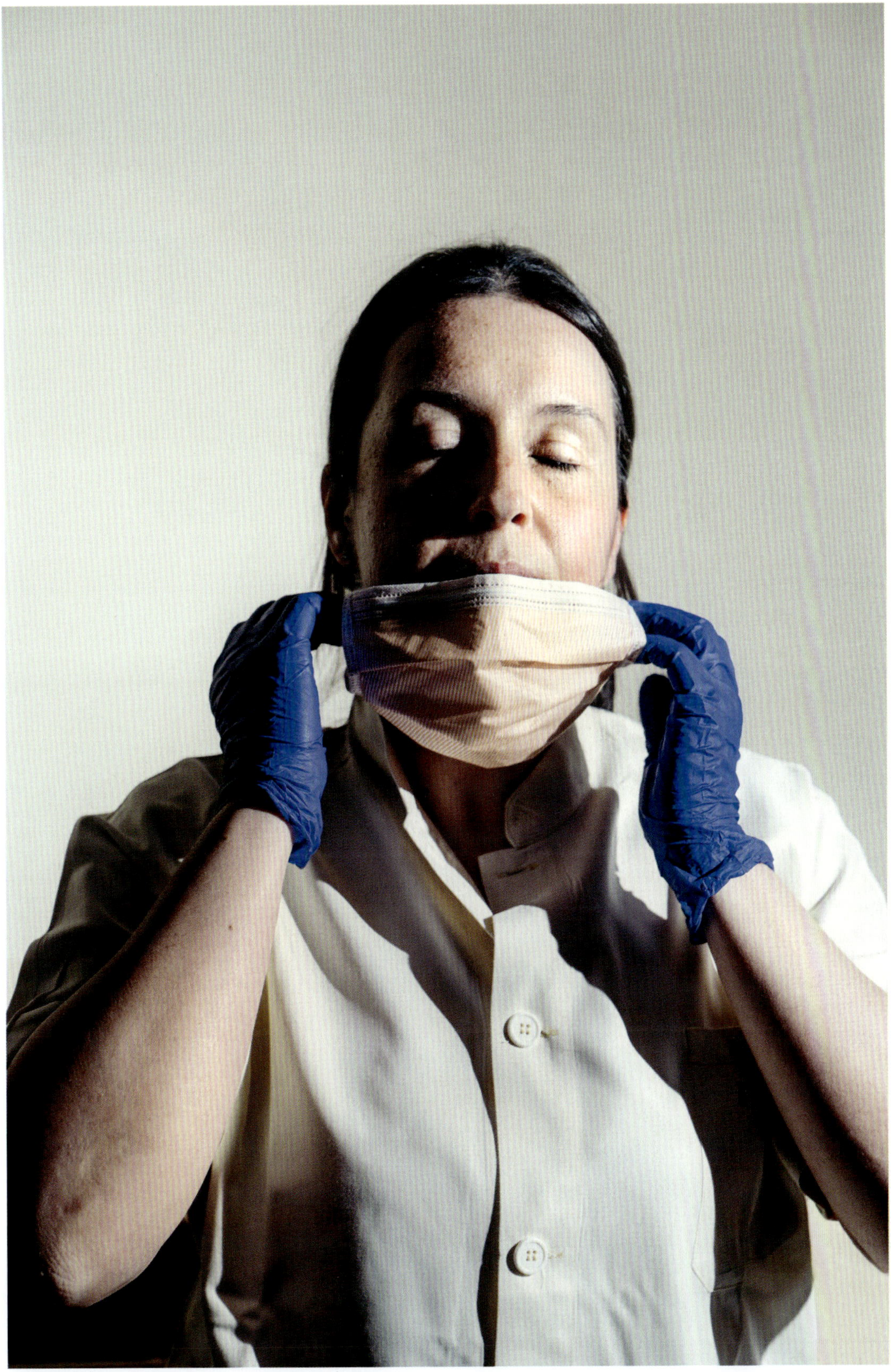

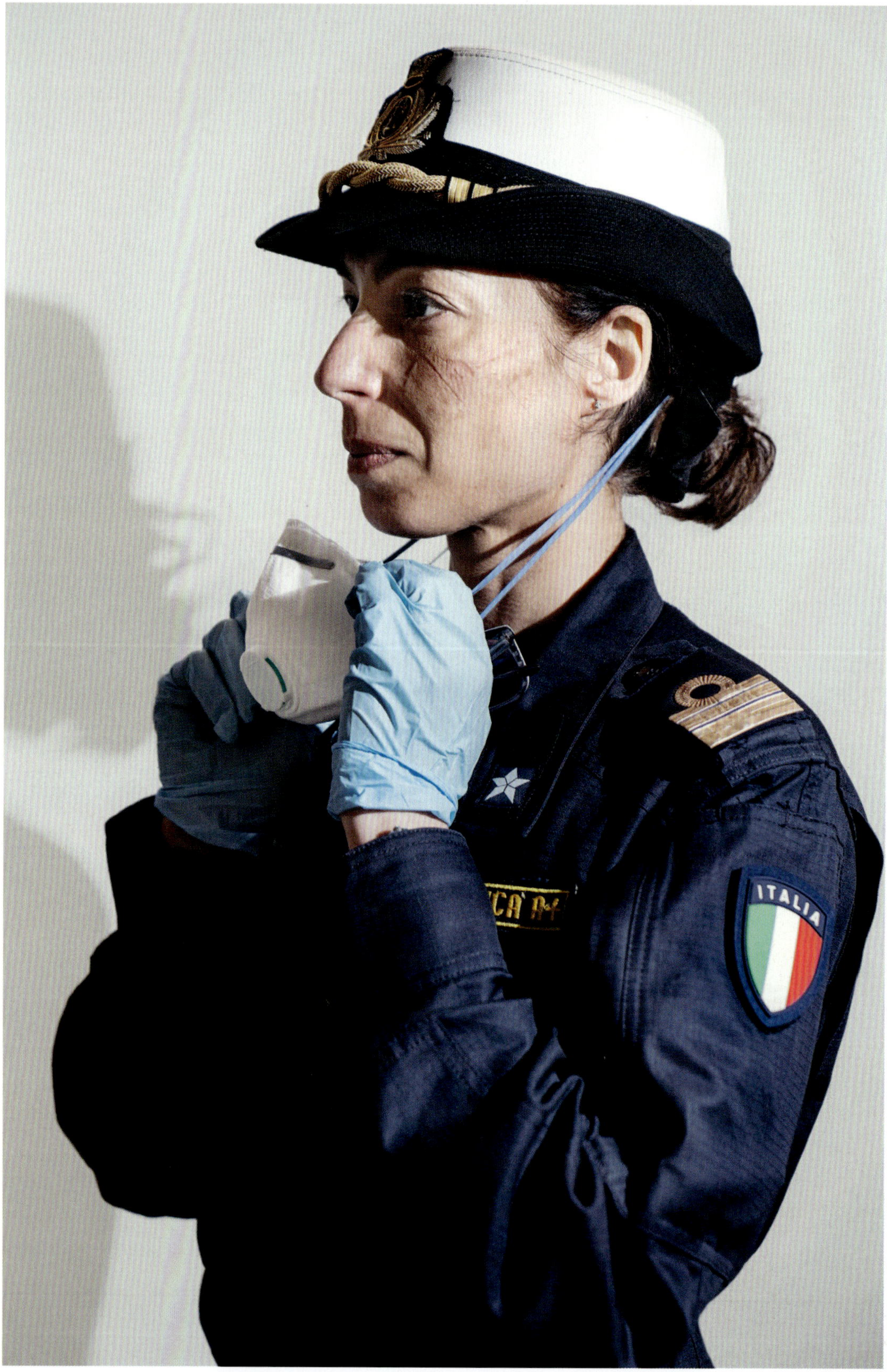
ITALIA

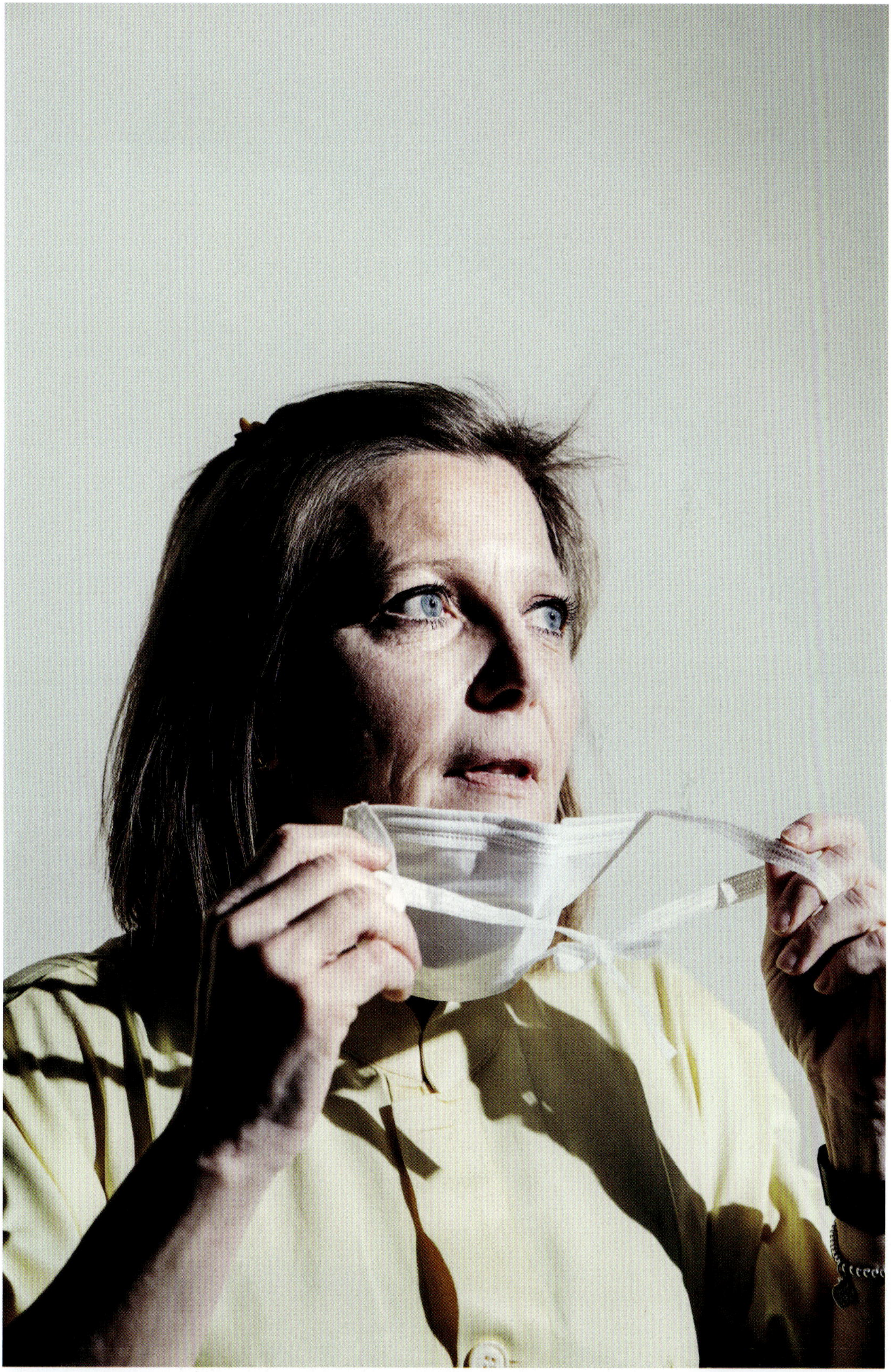

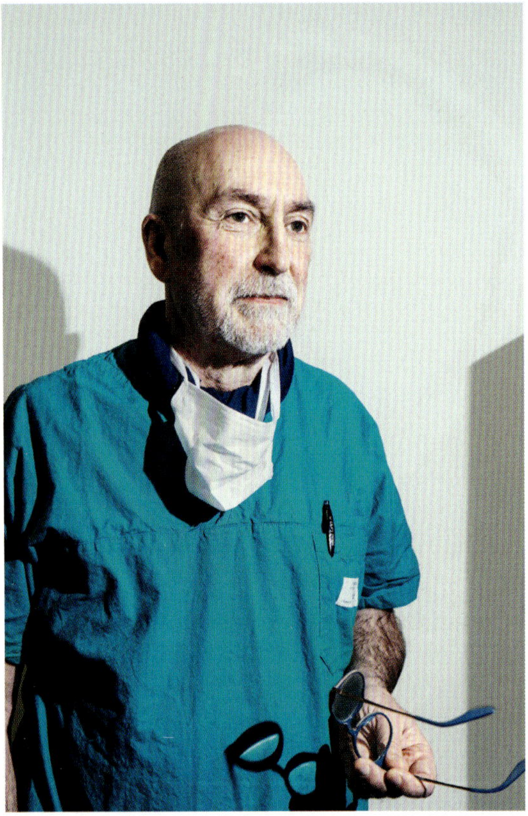

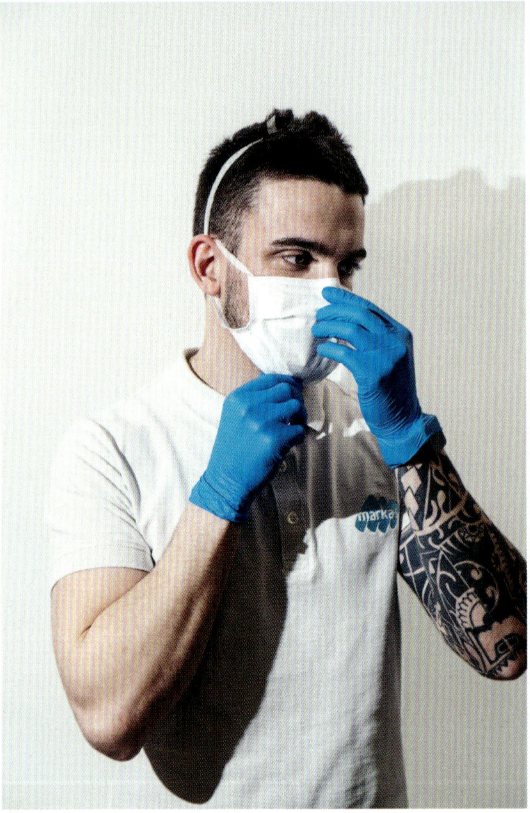

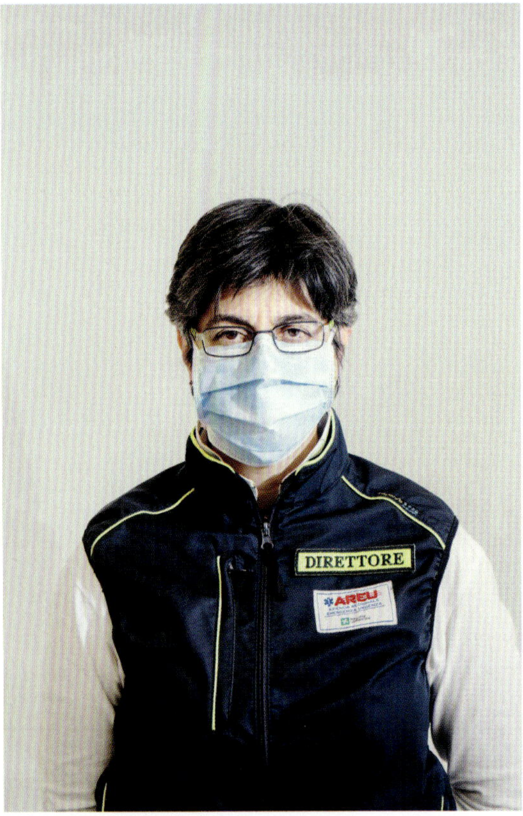
DIRETTORE
AREU

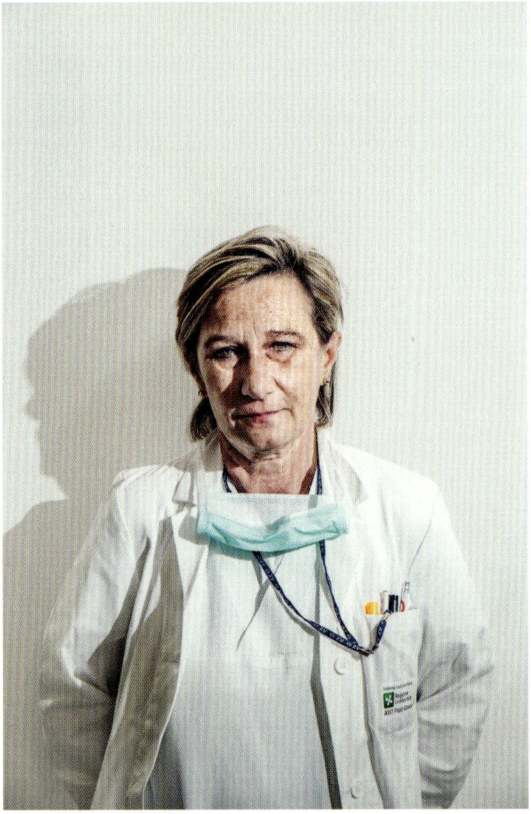

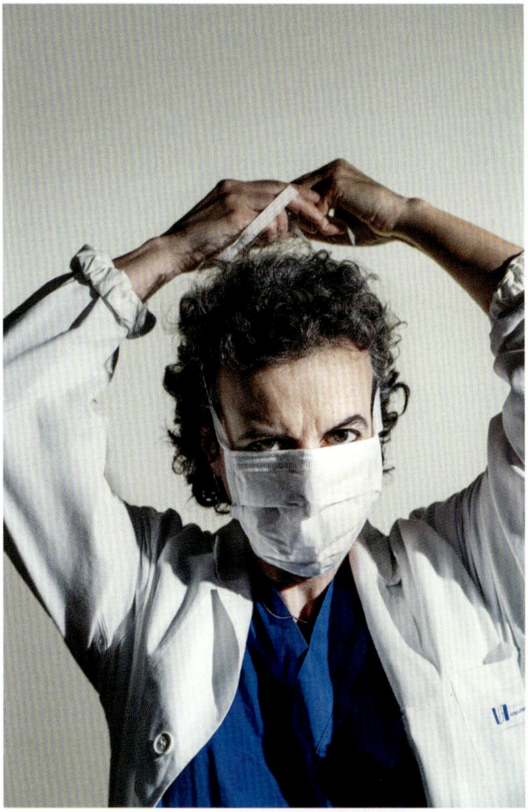

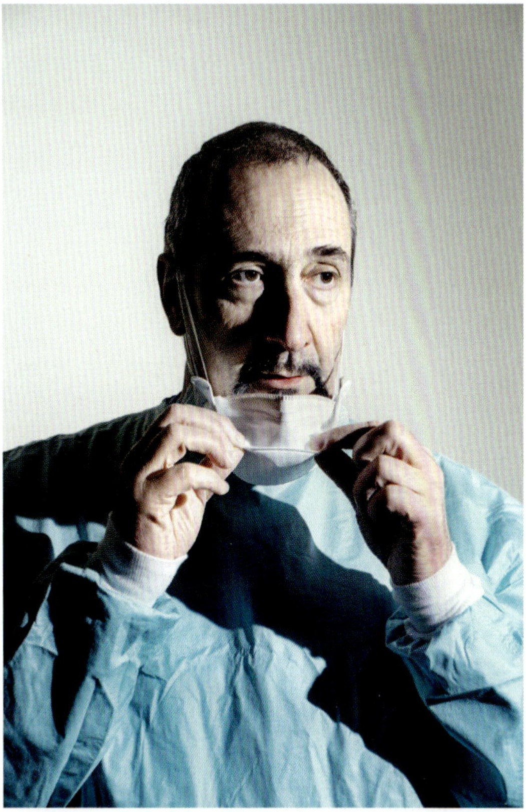

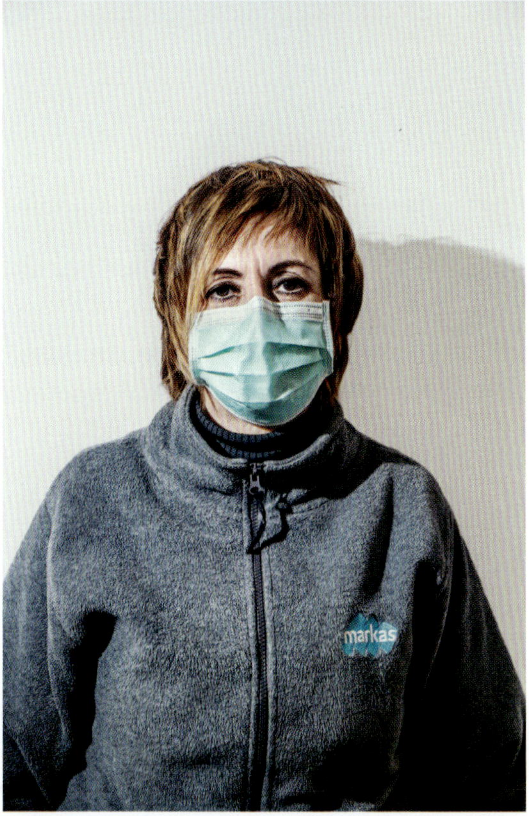
markas

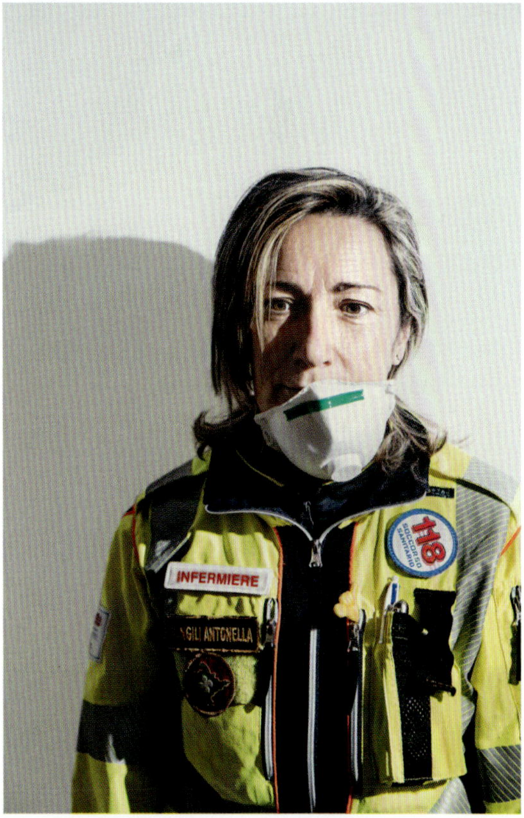
118
INFERMIERE
ANTONELLA

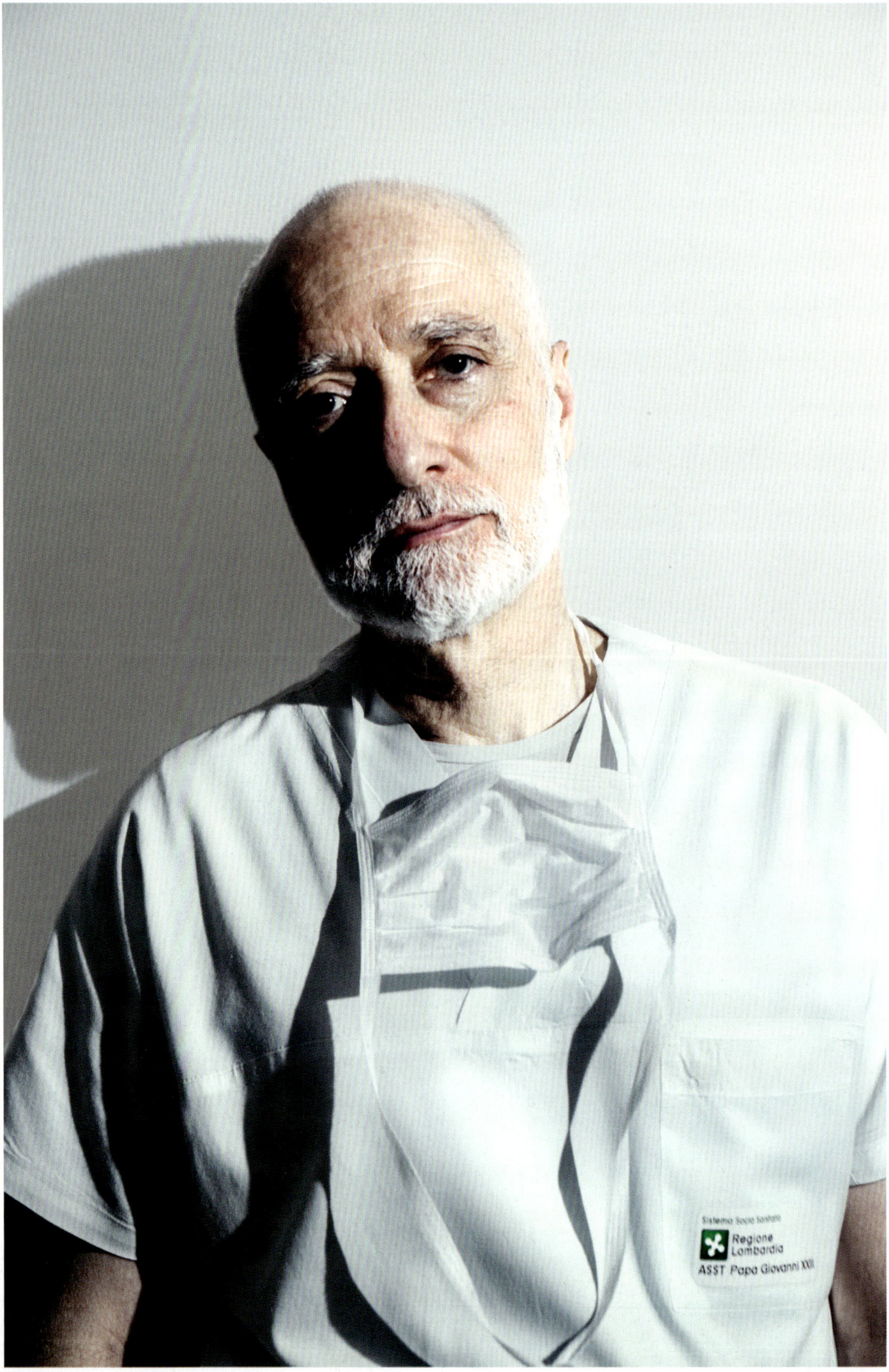
Sistema Socio Sanitario
Regione
Lombardia
ASST Papa Giovanni XXIII

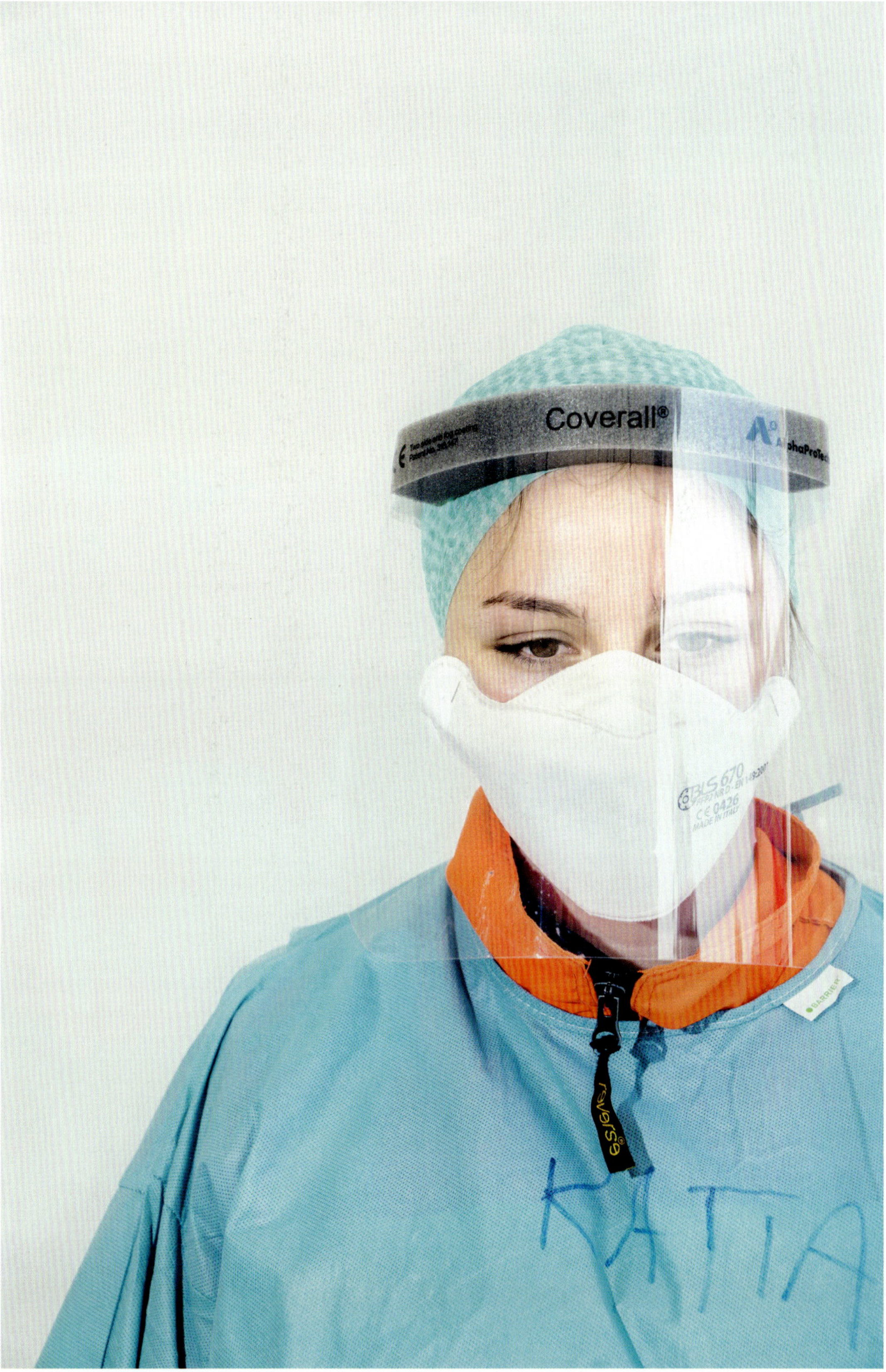
Coverall®
KATIA

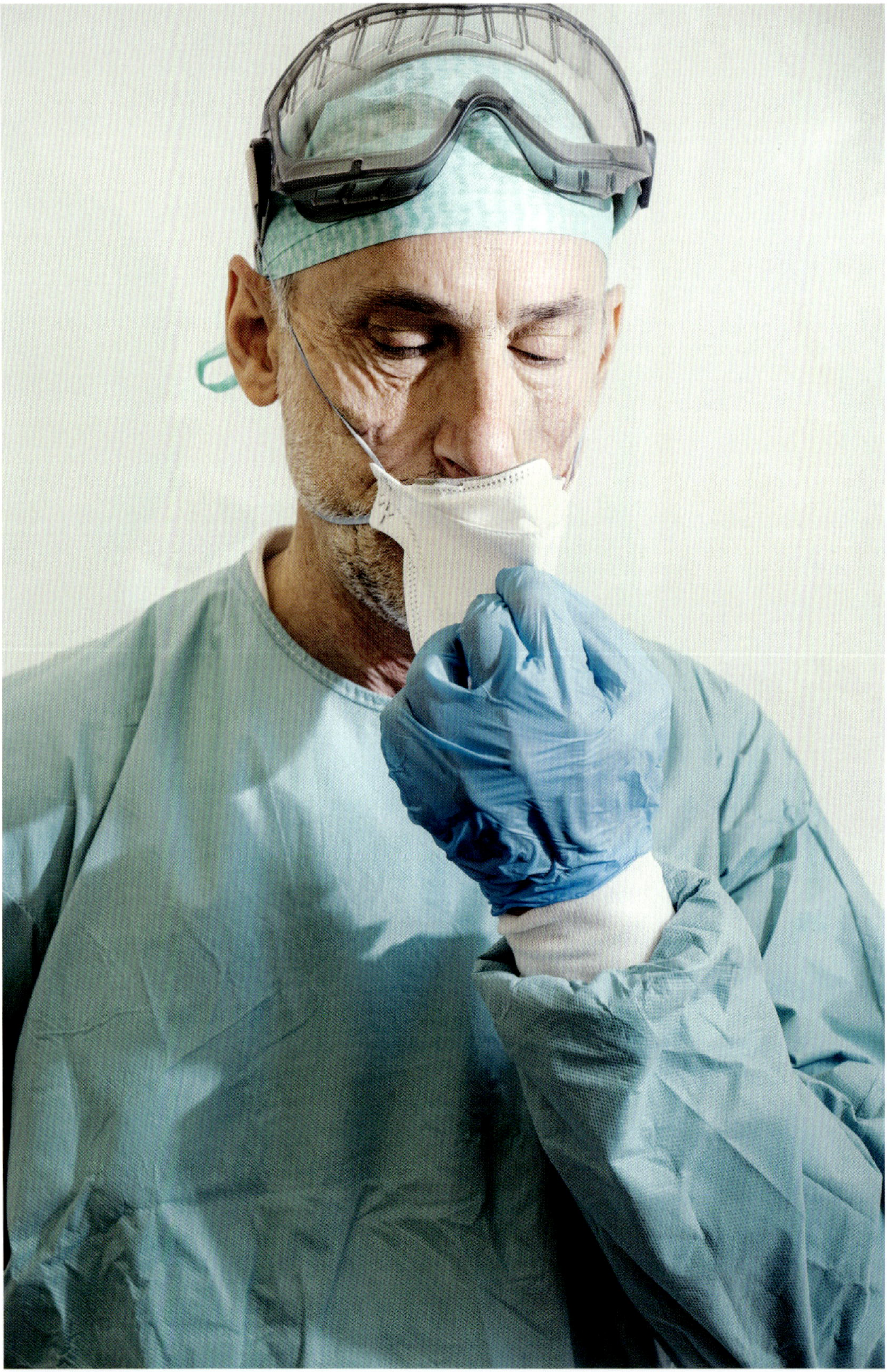

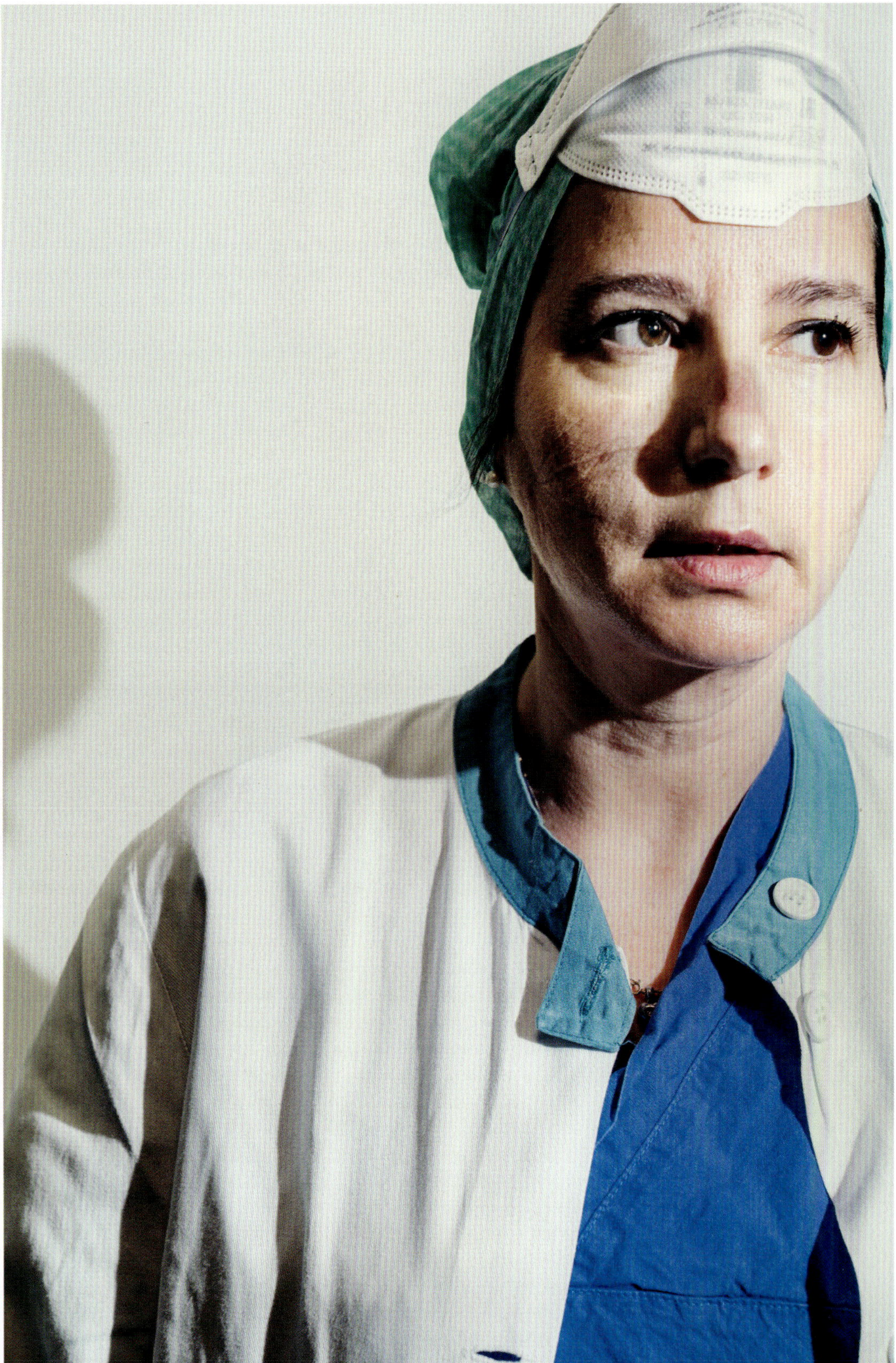

Gaia Squarci, USA
New York's Health Card Diaries

Gaia Squarci is a young Italian photographer living in New York. She is there when her home country is hit by the COVID-19 crisis. In a short while, New York becomes the epicentre of the pandemic in the US. With her heart in Italy, where family and many friends are, and her camera around Manhattan, the Bronx, Queens and Brooklyn, where her life is, she draws a picture of an intensely intimate experience of the health crisis.
Well aware of the complex and weak welfare system in the States, Gaia witnesses first hand how the medical resources are torn, and the fabric of an unequal society takes a toll when confronted with such an emergency. Her images are accompanied by diary notes which draw us closer to the issues and offer us a space for reflection on themes that go beyond the current health crisis.

March 26, 2020
"I'm in deep water...
Two deaths and two new patients.
If I find a moment I'll join the call."
I've been on a Zoom call by myself for more than an hour waiting for him, wondering if I even should, given the situation. While my friend Alessandro is working as a nurse in a chaotic ward in Northern Italy, it feels surreal to be playing music at my desk, typing on the keyboard while seeing myself framed in the corner of the screen, available to an invisible spectator.
He joins at the end of his night shift, calling from a filter zone. "When you were a child did you ever happen to be trying to swim and gag on water? When your eyes are wide open and you can't breathe? People here look at you that way and you could be the last person they see. They're completely alone, relatives can't even come to the hospital to hold their hand, and entire families are dying nonetheless. Tonight's new patient is the daughter of a woman who died here yesterday."
Ale is usually pretty cheerful, but the last two weeks took a toll on him. When I met him a few months ago the fact that he worked as a nurse didn't make him much different than most. Now it means he's one of the relatively few people experiencing on his skin what the rest of the world can only read and speculate about. Something that remains for us, at our desks, a catastrophic abstraction. He tells me about the extremes he's seeing in Italy. Respirators prioritised for the patients with higher chances of survival, doctors volunteering to work for free and others clearing their agenda and driving to their second house in the Alps, shrugging off the role they could play in saving lives. People at the window insult whoever they see on the streets, even if they might be bringing food to older parents. "There are many denunciations of this kind here. People are angry."
I wonder when I'll see home again. My parents are over 60, I canceled my trip to Milan at the beginning of March and now it feels like ages back. I look at my globe. When I saw it for the first time it was sitting on a pile of trash in the Rockaways, after Hurricane Sandy hit in 2012. Old, beautiful and

abandoned, I brought it home with me and for years it's been complicit to my dreams. Ale asks me when I'm going to host him in New York. We talk about his girl in a nearby city, whom he can't see. "I miss physical contact. I miss stroking a woman's hair. I want a hug. Not the one you give when you're greeting someone. I want a long one. It needs to last at least five minutes. Five minutes would be good."

May 13, 2020

Sometimes names that don't mean anything to most people become ubiquitous in the press from a day to another. I couldn't have named a single hospital in Queens before March. Right now Elmhurst Hospital, in the midst of the most ethnically diverse urban area in the entire world, is on endless headlines and nationally known as the epicentre of the COVID-19 epidemic in the United States. People come and go in the yellow light of the early evening. An old man gets out of the entrance with an umbrella and a broken slipper on a sunny day. He asks me if I can throw the slipper in the trash for him, he can't bend. He walks away slowly, wearing only a white sock on his left foot. Right behind him, I see a nurse sitting on a low wall, her face destroyed from exhaustion. Her name is Sonya, and she came from Texas to work in New York during the pandemic. "The second week I was here I lost both of my patients, hours apart. One was expected, the other was not. This is by far the worst thing I've ever seen. Ever." I ask if she's also seeing young patients being strongly affected. "Yes, several. One of them for instance, very young, was doing good sitting on the bed without oxygen, and within a few hours he was intubated. It's as quick as that." I'm glad I sometimes get health workers to speak to me. They're told not to talk to the press by hospital administrations and I received many NOs, as if masks were like gags stopping them from speaking about the enormity they're going through. I follow the low wall around the building to a patch of light where I meet Carlos' eyes. He stands on the sidewalk with the help of a stick, a bouquet of white flowers gifted by the hospital on the other hand. His glance seems tired, worried. I help him call a cab with his phone, awkwardly trying not to get too close. He's an old man at risk, and I find out that his skin cancer is the reason that forces him to come to the hospital despite the epidemic. Chemotherapy. He's afraid to come, he tells me, but there's nothing he can do. If I understood anything about this epidemic is how fear can come from all sides, taking different paths inside every one of us. Everyone is vulnerable in a different way.

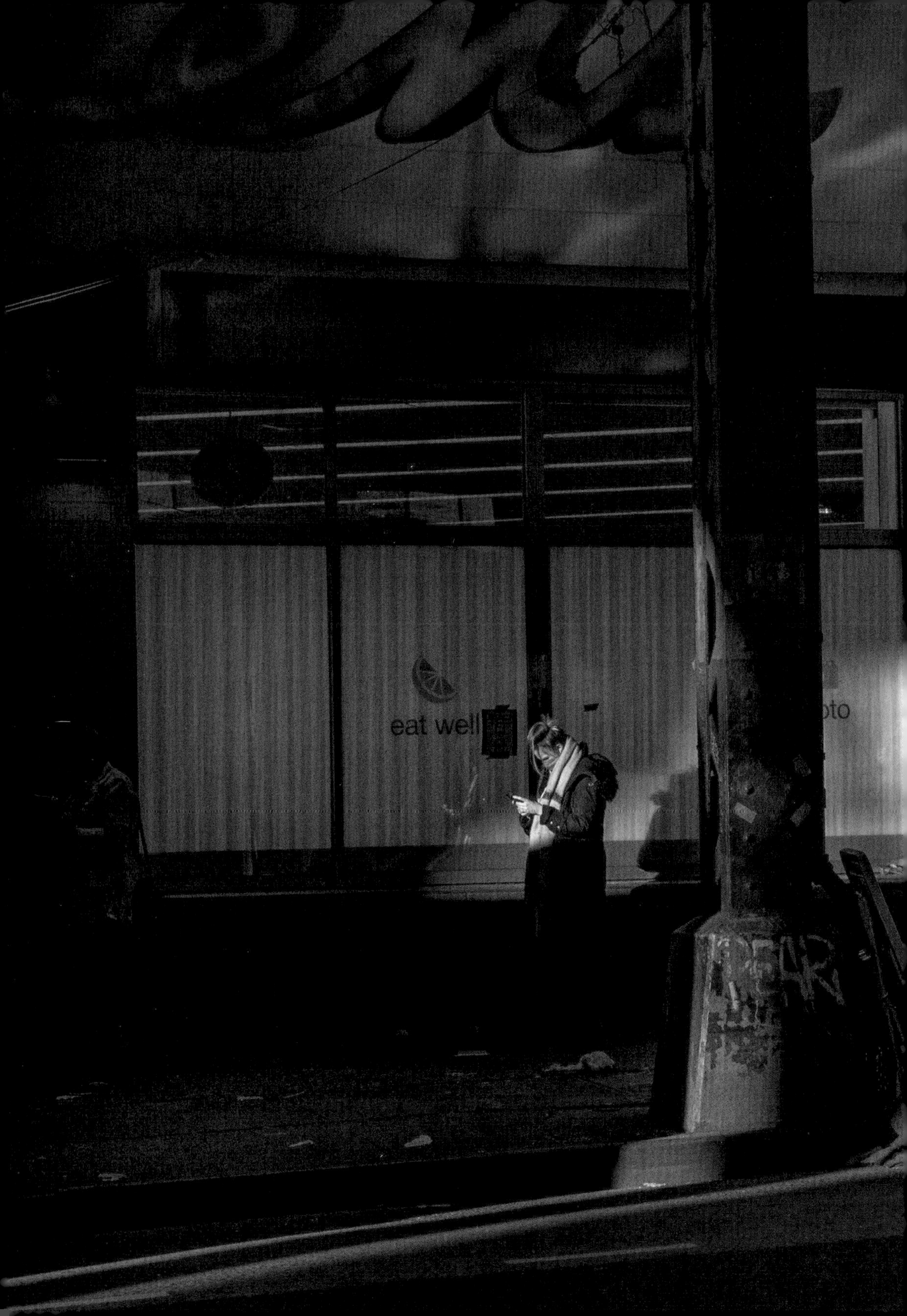
eat well

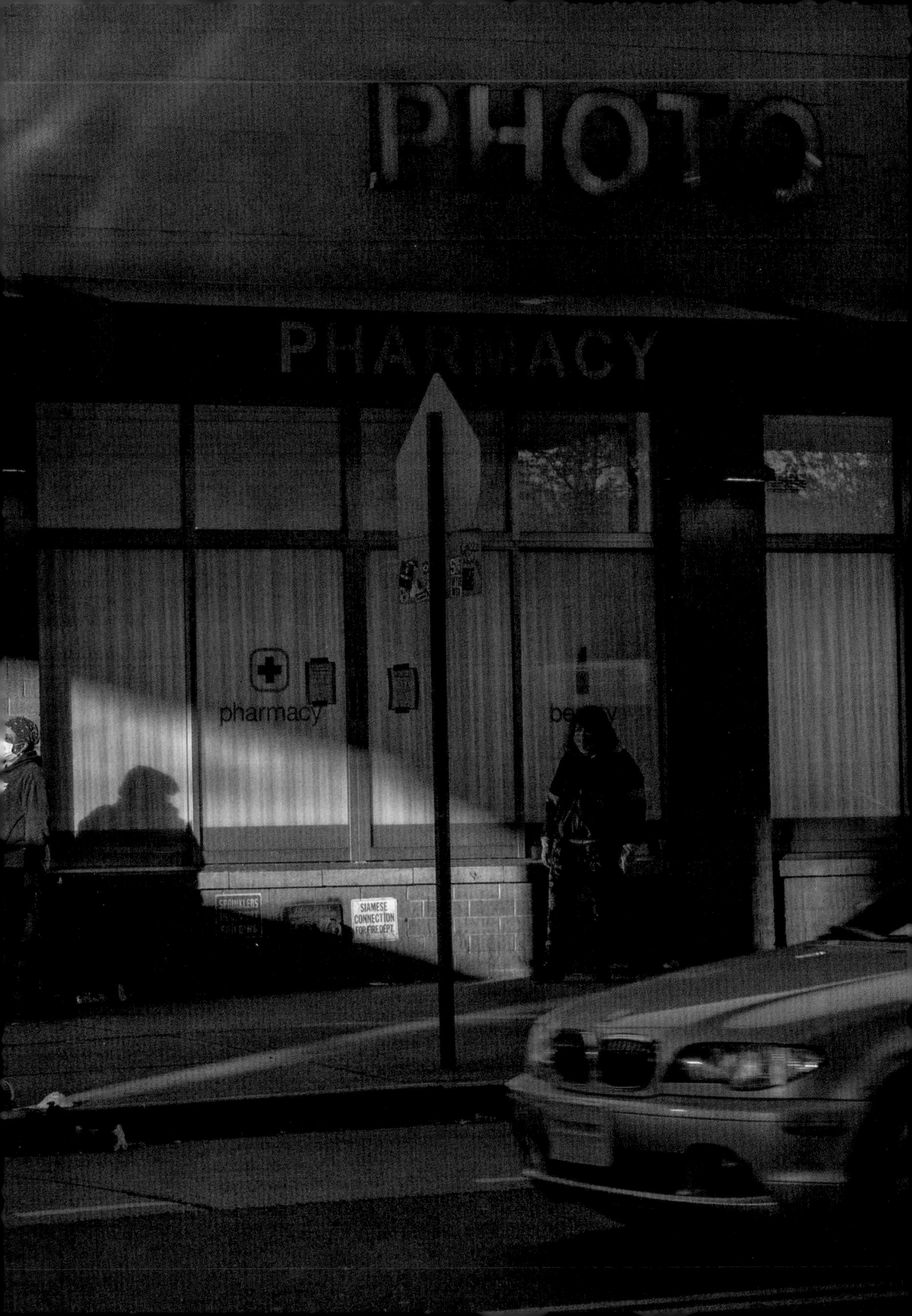
PHOTO
PHARMACY
pharmacy
SIAMESE
CONNECTION
FOR FIRE DEPT.

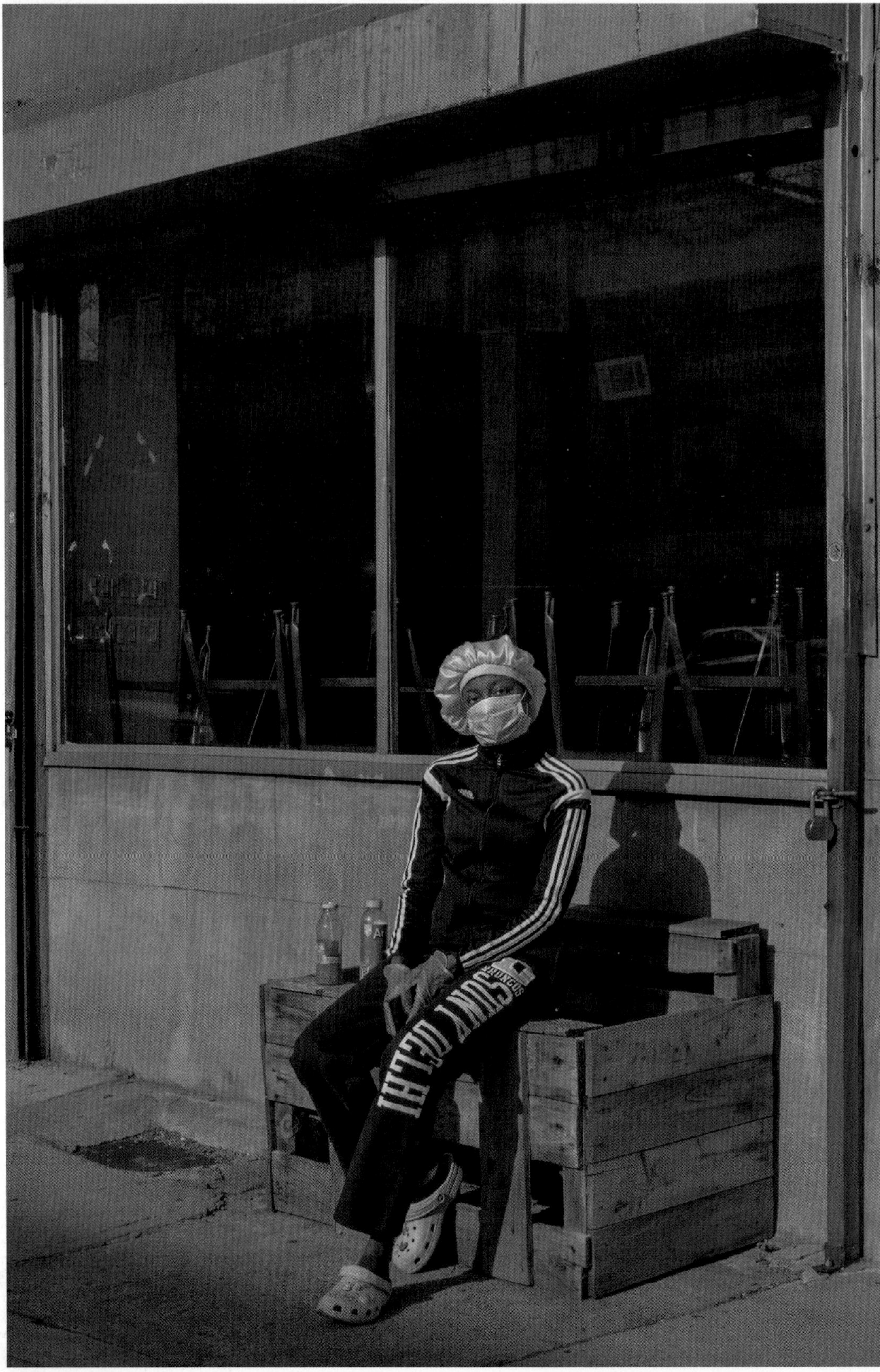
BRONCOS
SUNY DELHI

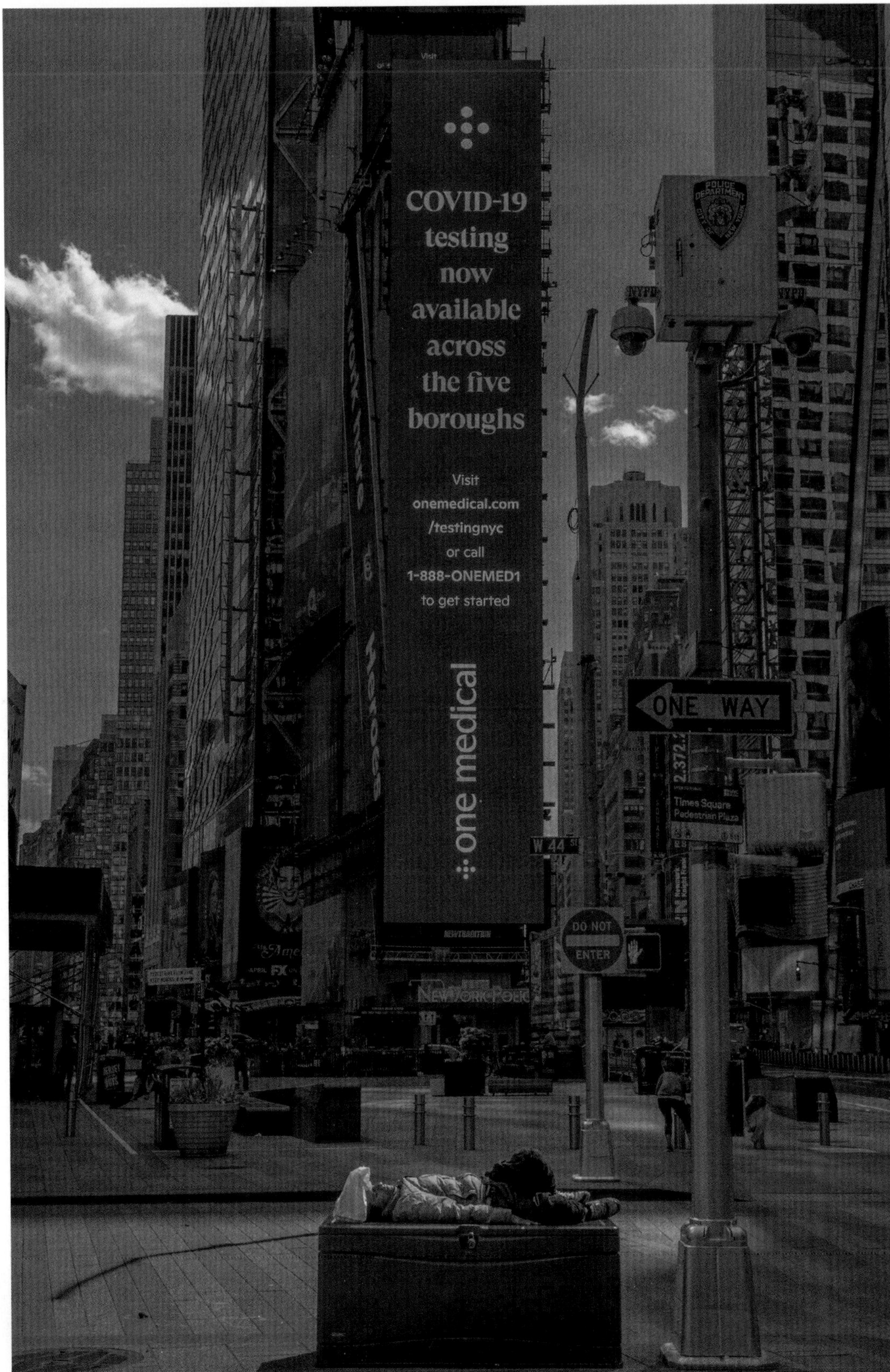
COVID-19
testing
now
available
across
the five
boroughs
Visit
onemedical.com
/testingnyc
or call
1-888-ONEMED1
to get started
one medical
ONE WAY
Times Square
Pedestrian Plaza
W 44 St
DO NOT
ENTER

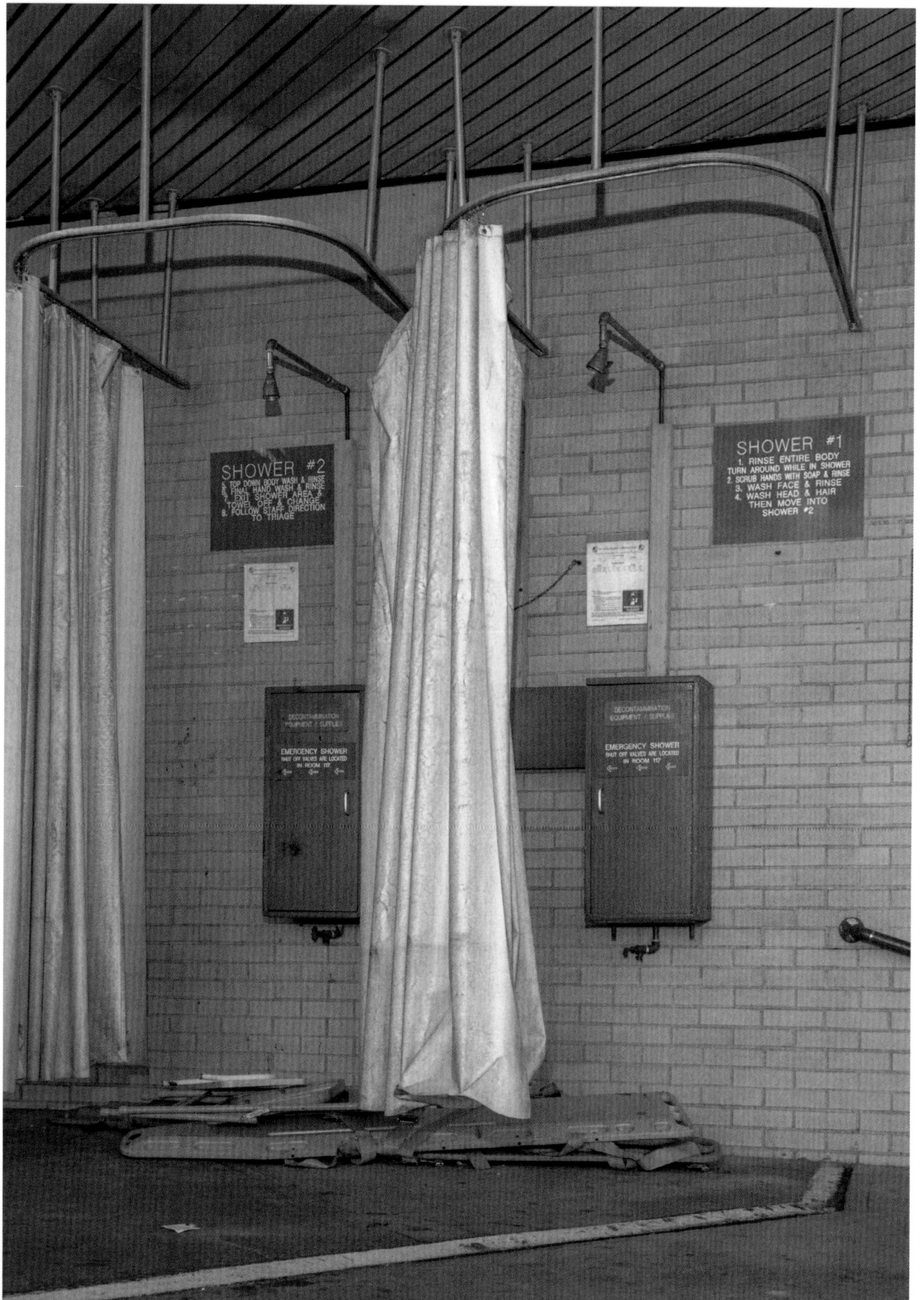
SHOWER #2
5. TOP DOWN BODY WASH & RINSE
6. FINAL HAND WASH & RINSE
7. EXIT SHOWER AREA &
TOWEL OFF & CHANGE
8. FOLLOW STAFF DIRECTION
TO TRIAGE
DECONTAMINATION
EQUIPMENT / SUPPLIES
EMERGENCY SHOWER
SHUT OFF VALVES ARE LOCATED
IN ROOM 117
DECONTAMINATION
EQUIPMENT / SUPPLIES
EMERGENCY SHOWER
SHUT OFF VALVES ARE LOCATED
IN ROOM 117
SHOWER #1
1. RINSE ENTIRE BODY
TURN AROUND WHILE IN SHOWER
2. SCRUB HANDS WITH SOAP & RINSE
3. WASH FACE & RINSE
4. WASH HEAD & HAIR
THEN MOVE INTO
SHOWER #2

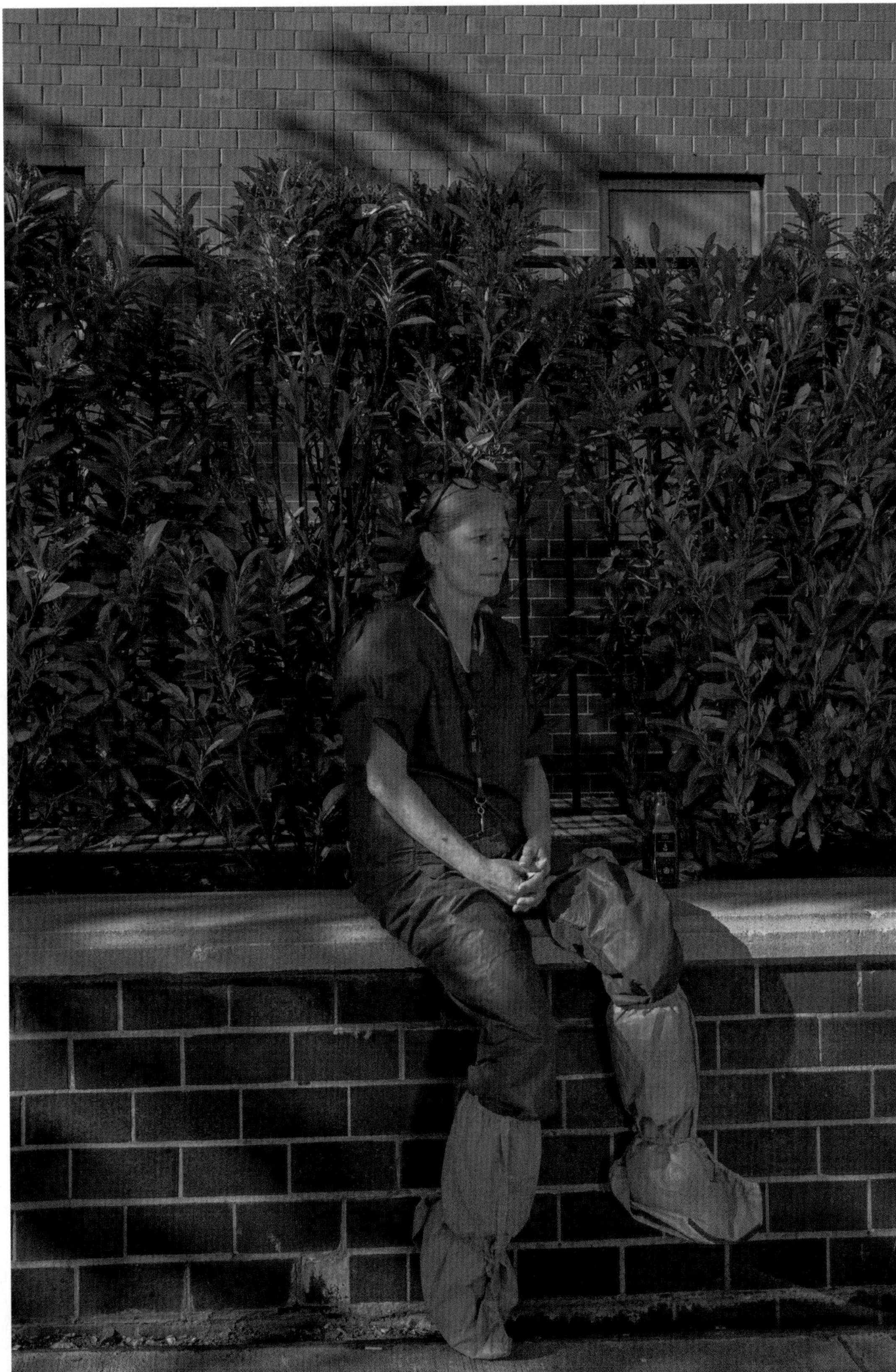

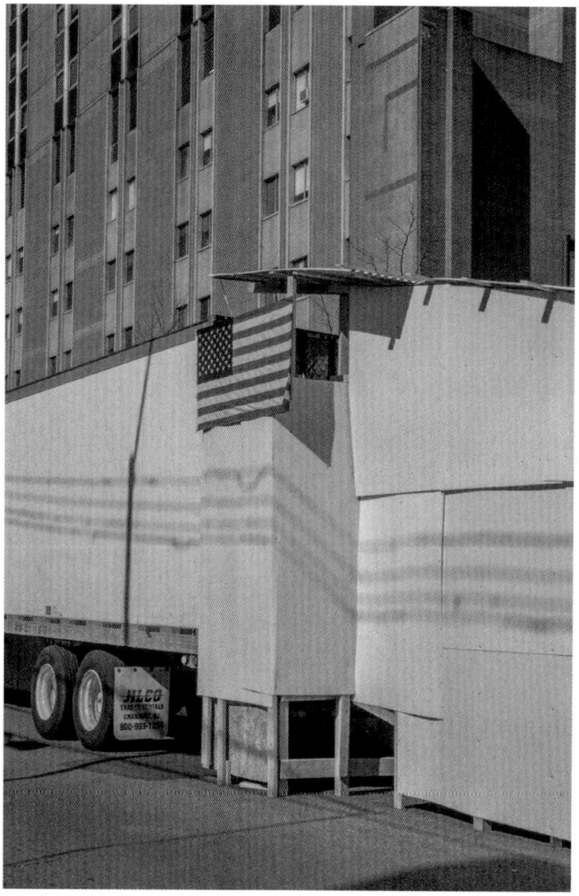

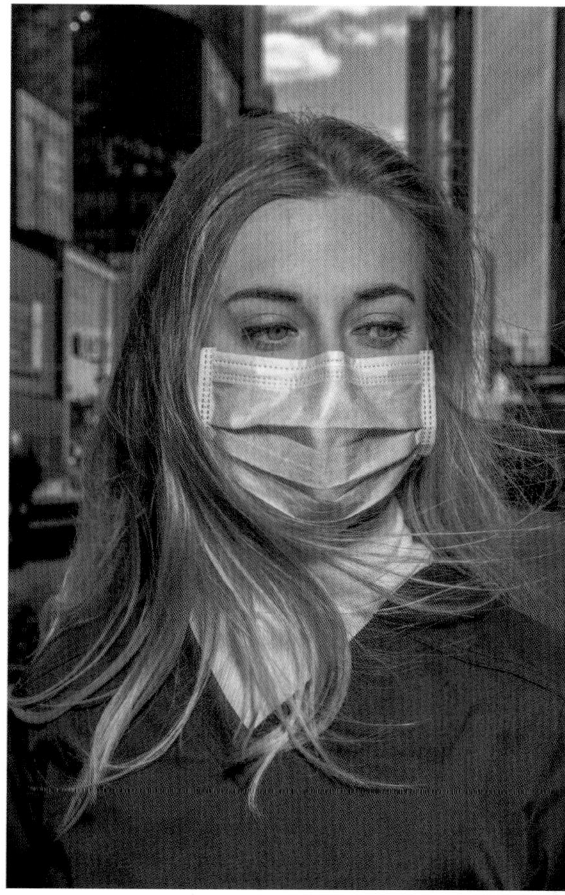

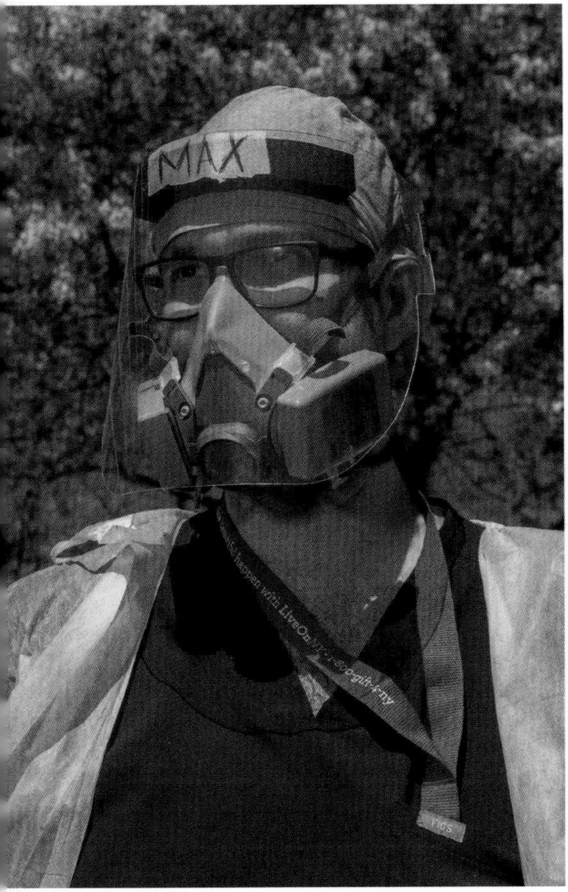
MAX

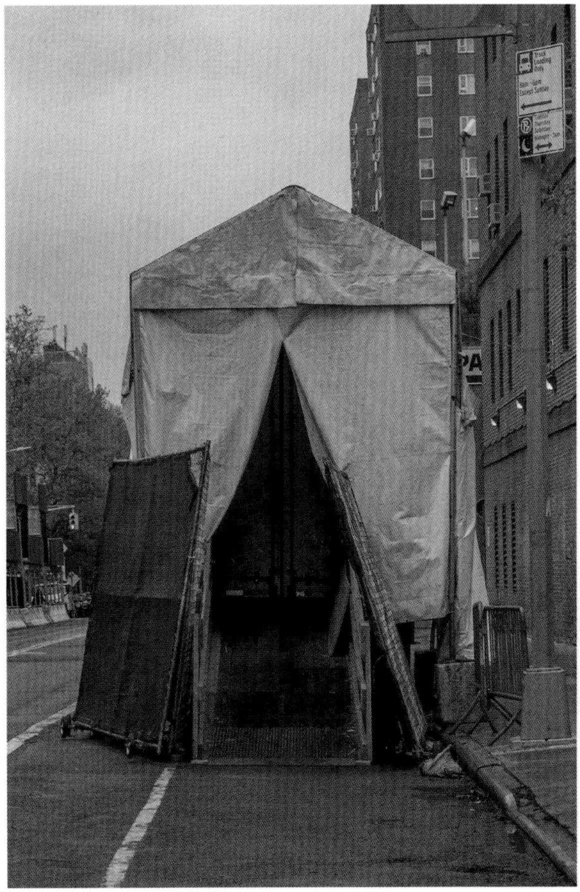

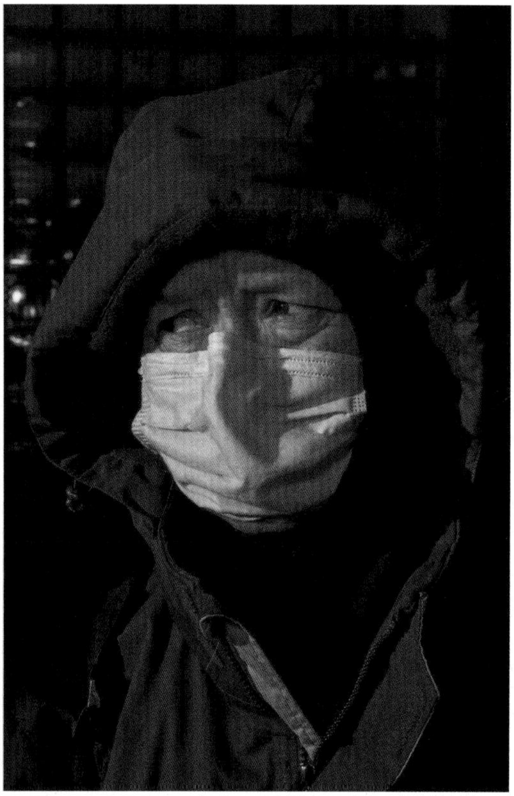
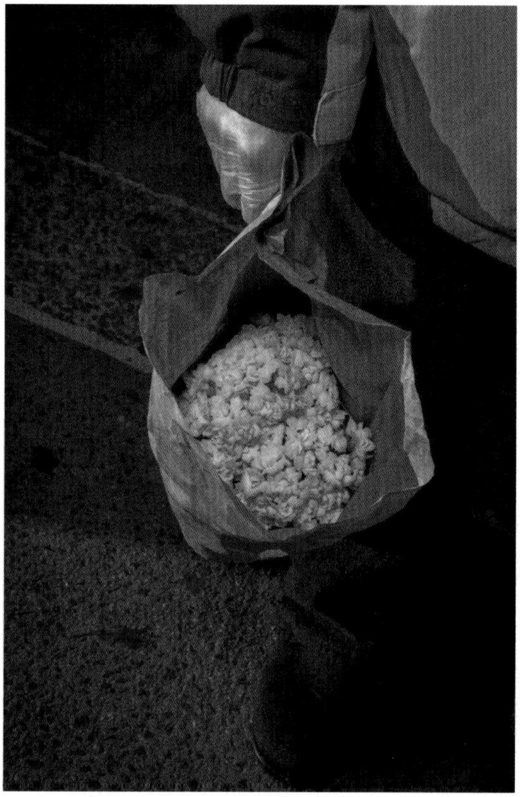

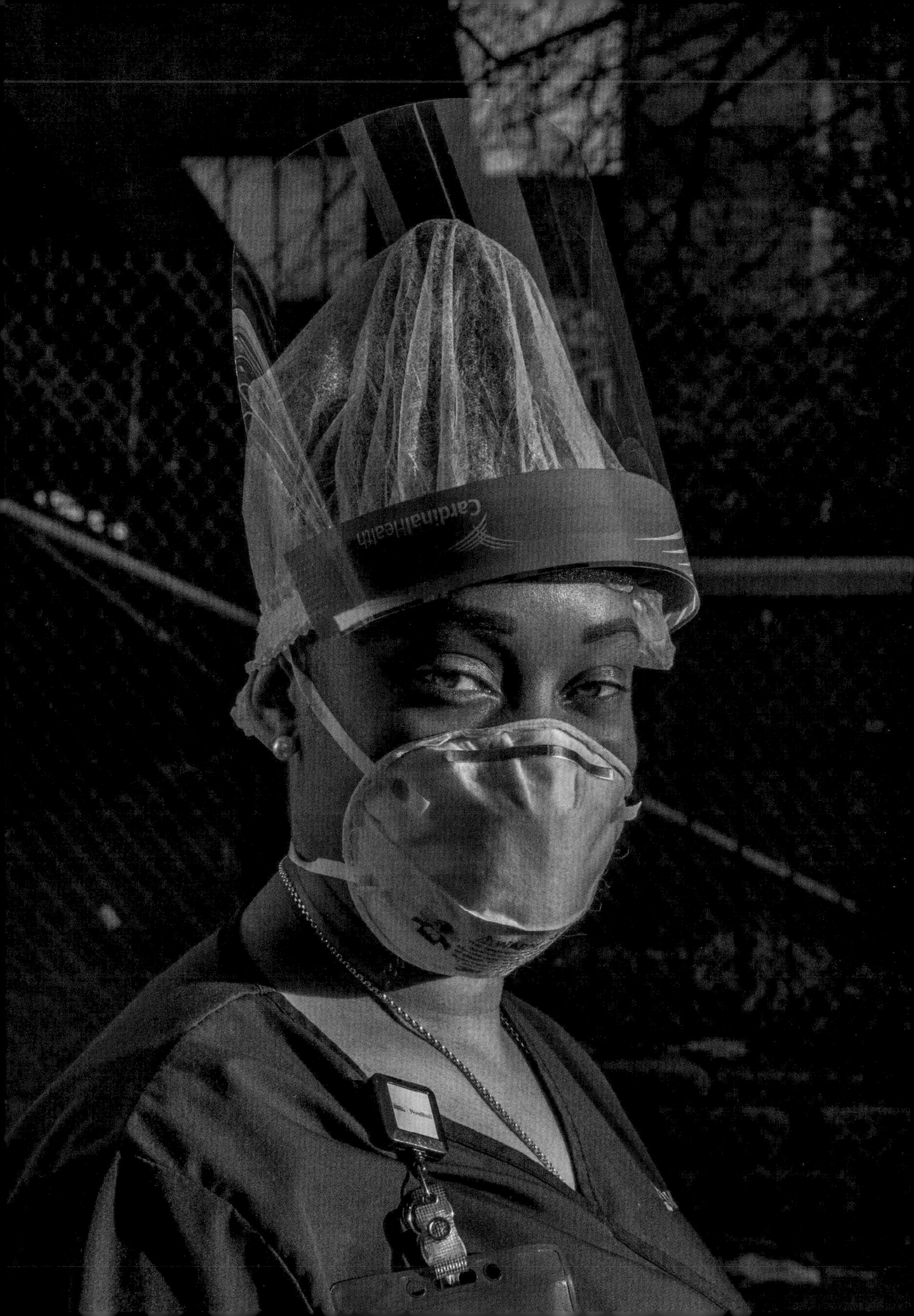
CardinalHealth

Santi Palacios, Spain
Seniors in Solitude

What happens when you are unable to say goodbye? What should you do when that inevitable farewell, death and subsequent funeral comes in such an inconceivable manner? All norms in these scenarios have been wiped out by COVID-19 in a single blow.
Santi Palacios visited nursing homes in Catalonia, Spain, during the state of alarm declared due to the pandemic. Old folks' homes have become one of the tragic focal points in the health crisis caused by the coronavirus in Spain, one of the countries hardest hit by the pandemic. Figures top more than 50,000 deaths in 2020 alone, according to official data. Two-thirds of these deaths correspond to the elderly: more than 25,000 have died of coronavirus, or with symptoms compatible with those of the illness, in Spanish nursing homes in 2020, mostly isolated and unable to say goodbye to their dear ones.
This story takes us into these places the months of March, April and May when the lack of means of protection, misinformation and fear dominated almost everything. The resulting feature gives a true insight into what was happening there while the country was confined.
These photographs evoke the emotions that were experienced inside nursing homes during the worst weeks of the state of emergency caused by COVID-19: loneliness, fear, isolation, fragility, sadness, documenting the most serious consequences of the pandemic: the death of thousands of people. And they do so respecting the privacy of that group that lived through a civil war and the post-war hardships, the Franco regime, the transition to democracy, the arrival of the new century and, now, a pandemic.

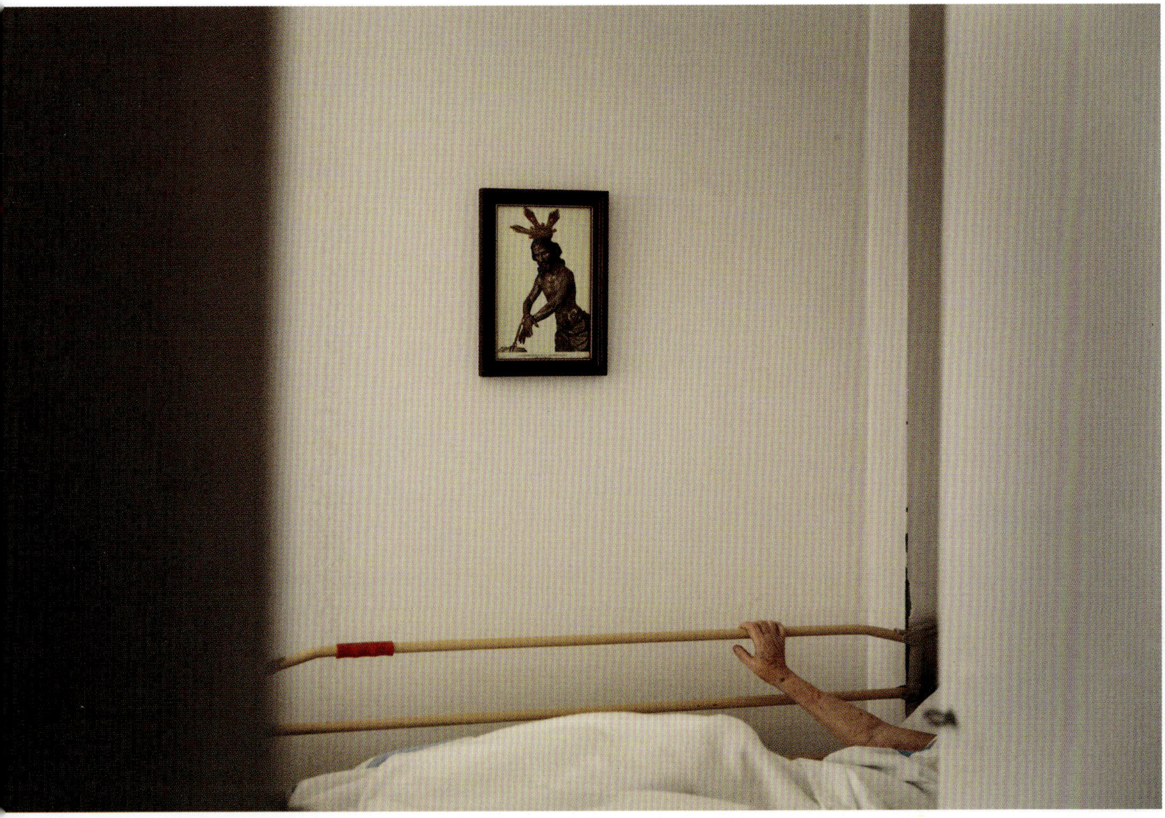

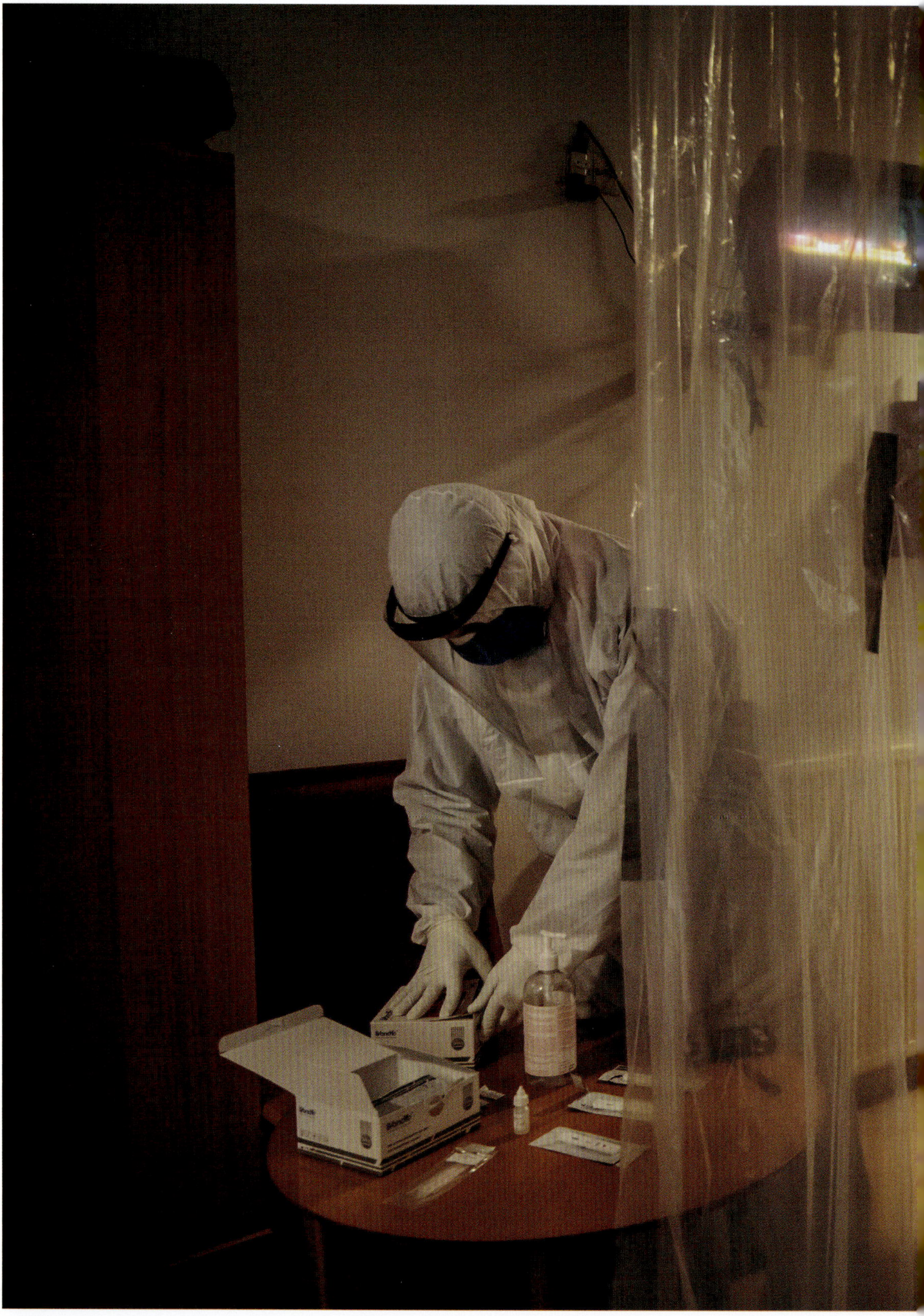

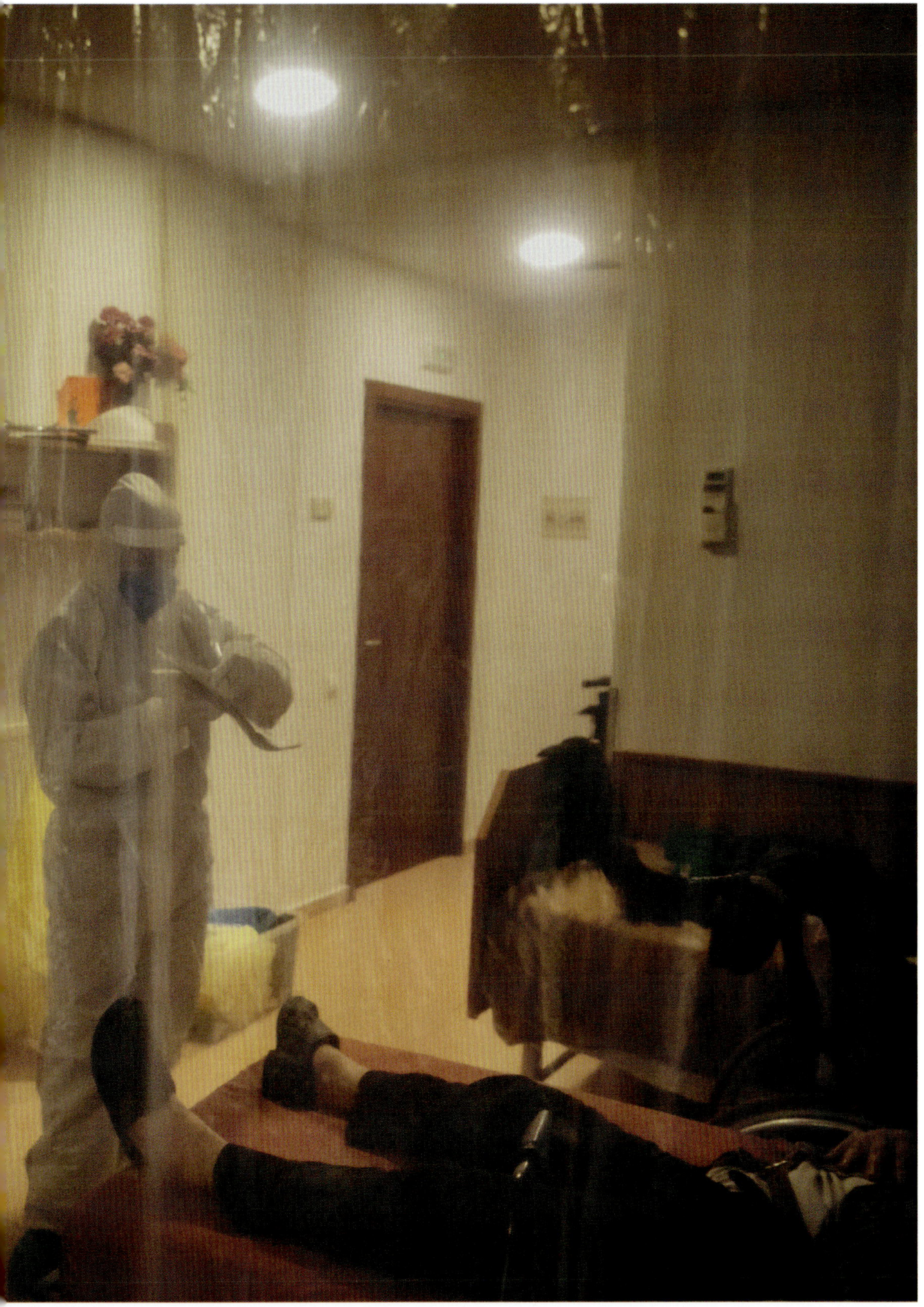

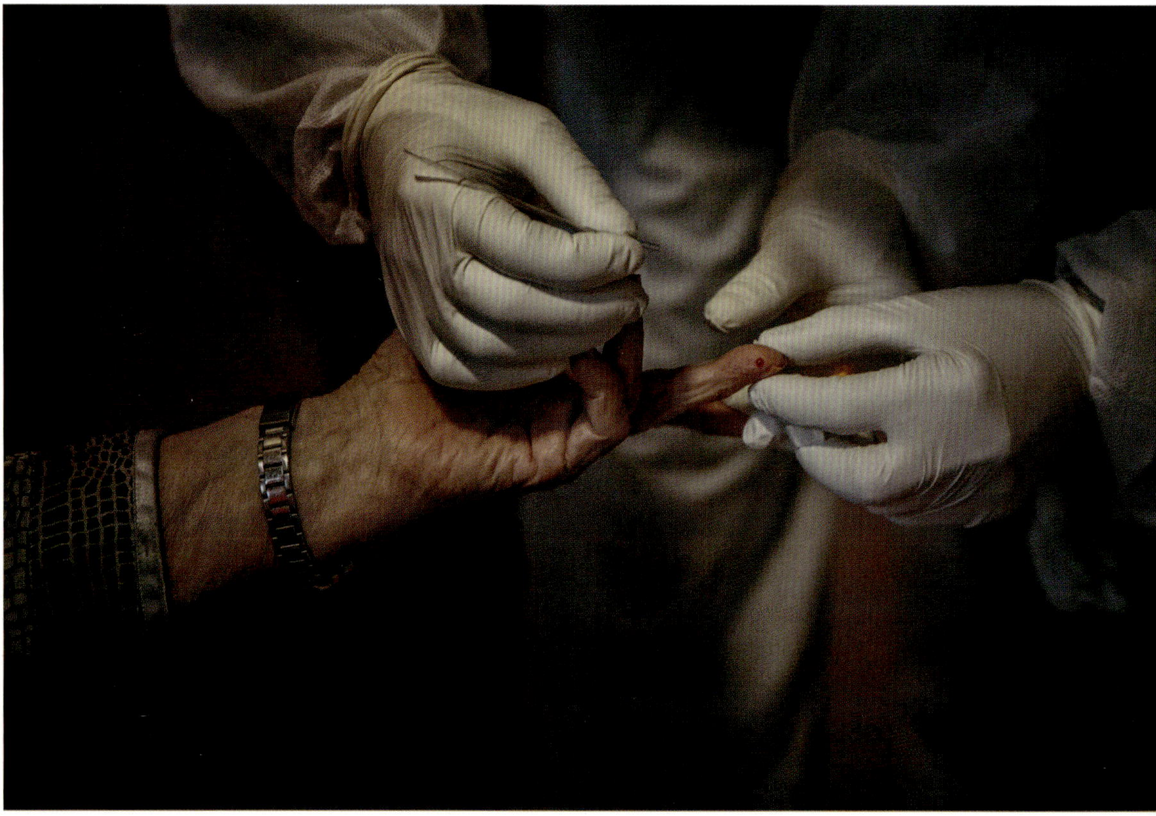

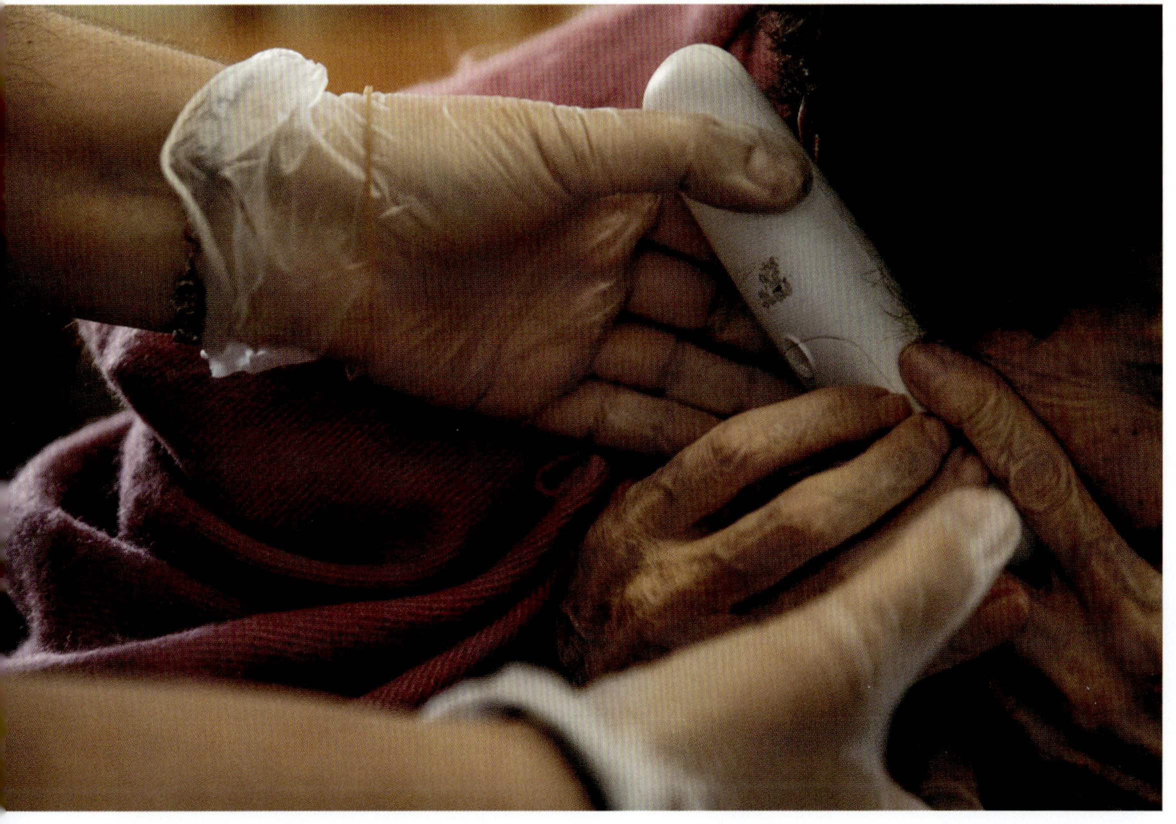

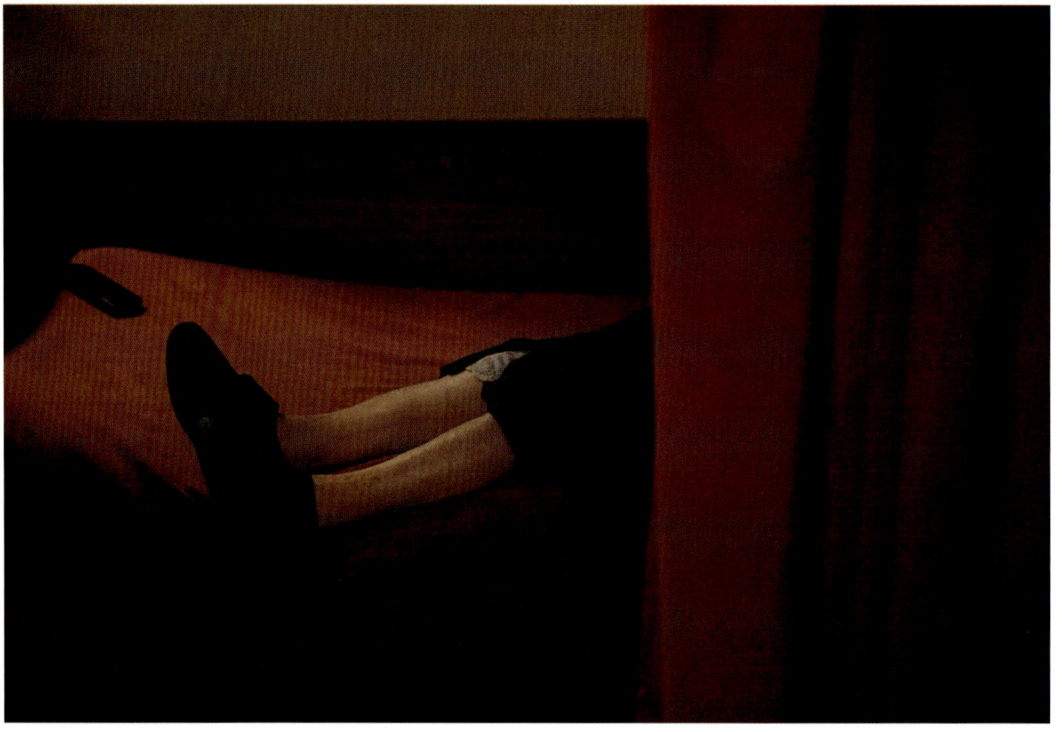

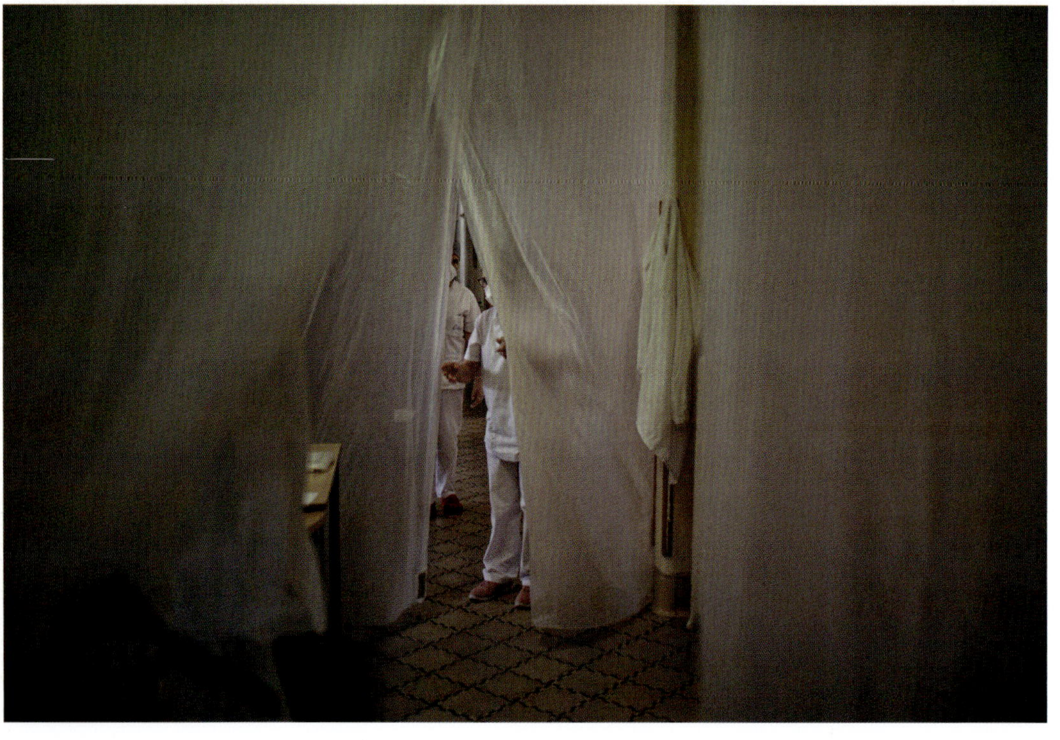

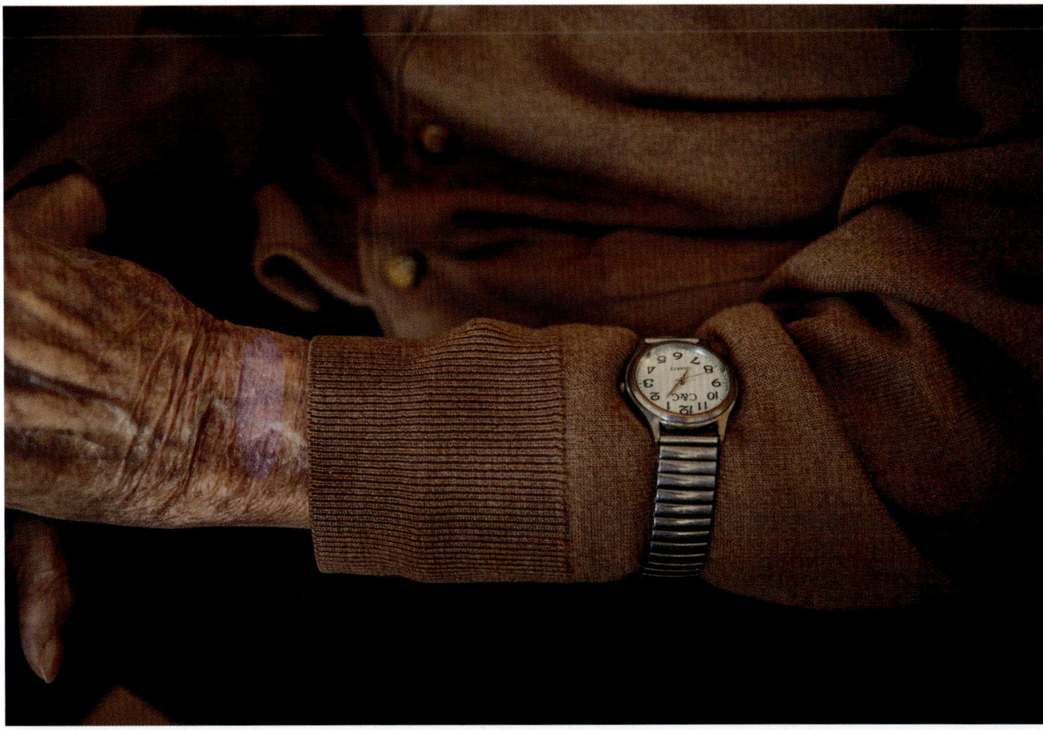
C&C

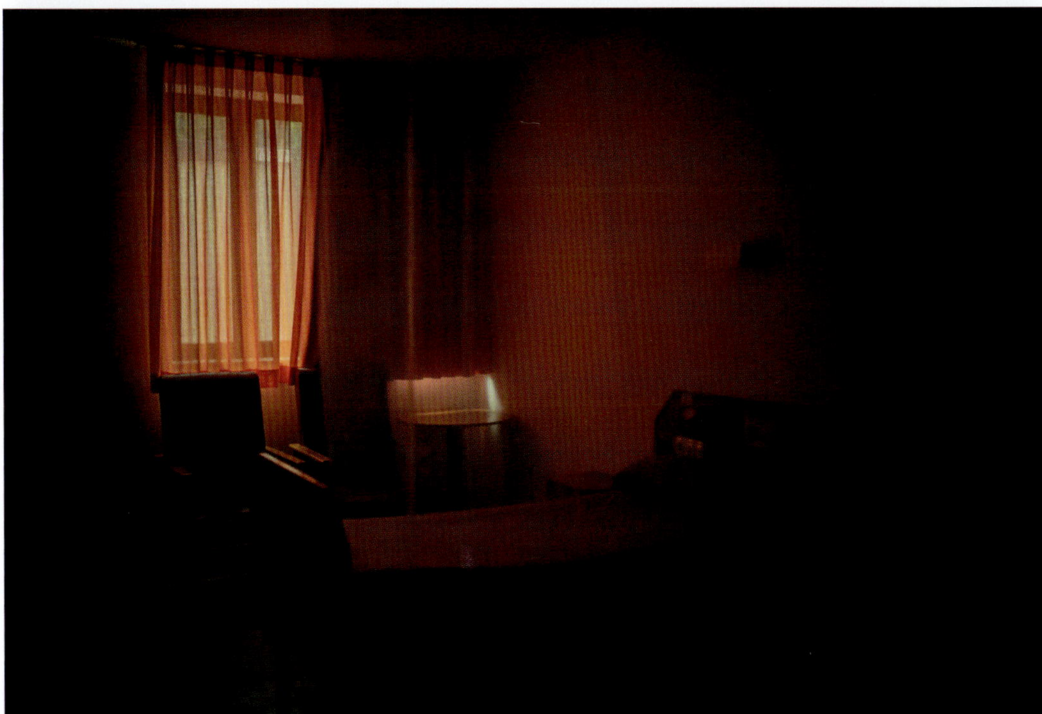

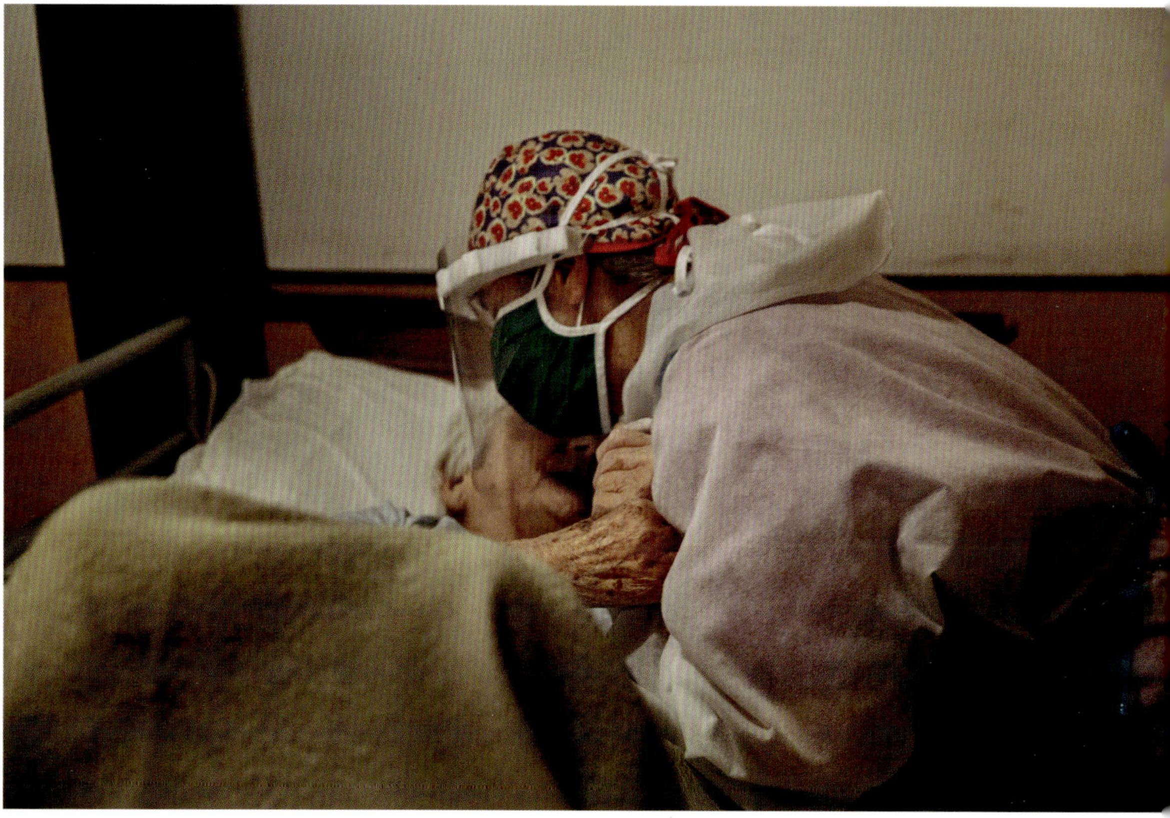

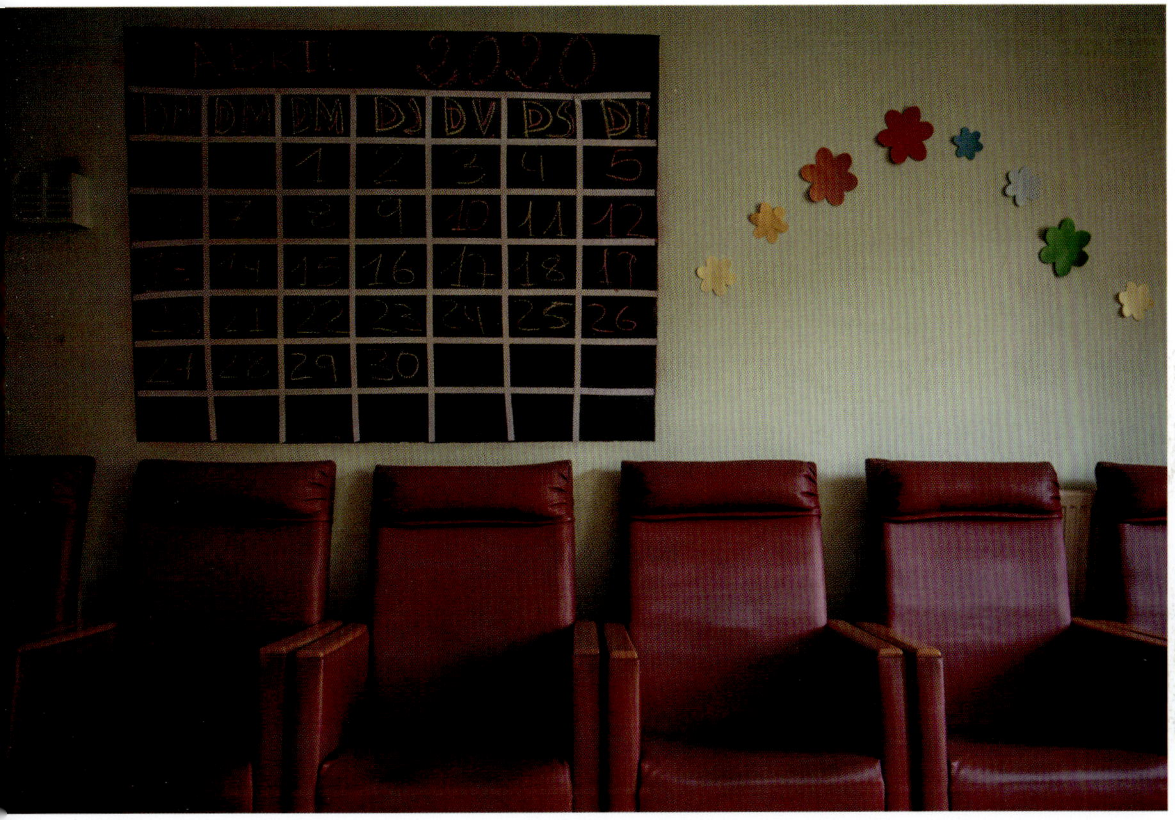
2020
DM DM DJ DV DS
1 2 3 4 5
8 9 10 11 12
15 16 17 18
22 23 24 25 26
29 30

Stefano Schirato, Italy
Awakenings

In Spring 2020, when Italy was coping with the first lockdown due to the COVID-19 emergency, TV programs broadcast images of coffins and funerals with no familiar faces around, of wrecked medical personnel, of a whole country bent on its knees. We all felt so overwhelmed by the situation there was no space in our minds and in our lives but for grief and sorrow.
By the time I started the project, more than 30,000 Italians had died from COVID-19 – the highest death toll in the European Union – but over 100,000 people had recovered. Hospitalisations had been declining since the third week of April. I, therefore, understood that a positive message might have been useful and powerful. So I decided to report on the survivors, on those who made it, who gained a chance of salvation after finding oneself one step from death.
The project tells the story of patients from the Intensive Care Unit and Infectious Diseases Unit at Santo Spirito Hospital in Pescara, my town. Most of them suffered from ARDS (Acute Respiratory Distress Syndrome), which causes a person's respiratory rate to double as the level of oxygen (O_2) in the blood decreases. Often, the only solution is intubation – sometimes for weeks – to let the lungs rest.
Many of them panicked and, afraid of not waking up, made what they feared might be a final call to a loved one. "Unlike others, Covid patients who need to be intubated are lucid and aware. They think about their family members. It is a very touching moment and we take part in that pain every time", said Antonella Frattari, the head of intensive care at the hospital.
They all had been intubated, spent weeks in a coma, then woke up and were finally discharged to go back to their homes and hug their families.
I felt that hugs and returning home are pretty much the same in every country, in every family, and that these local stories could actually speak for all.

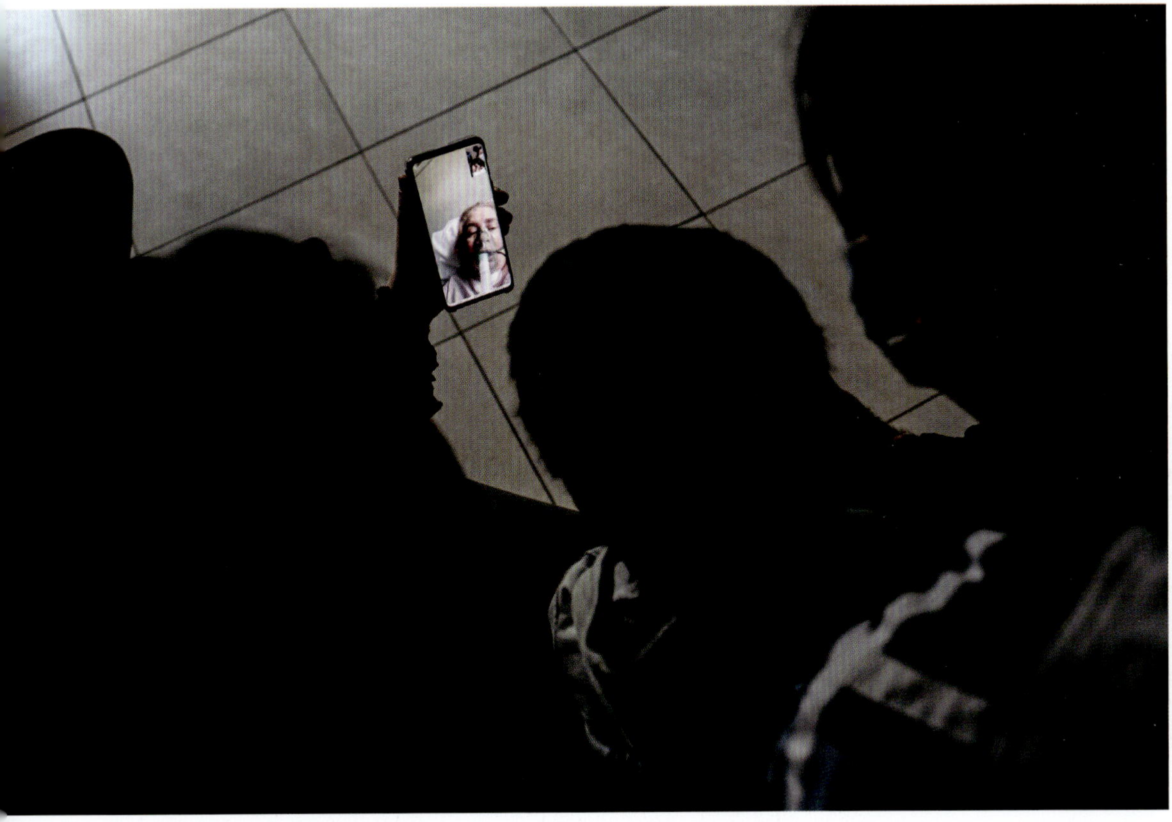

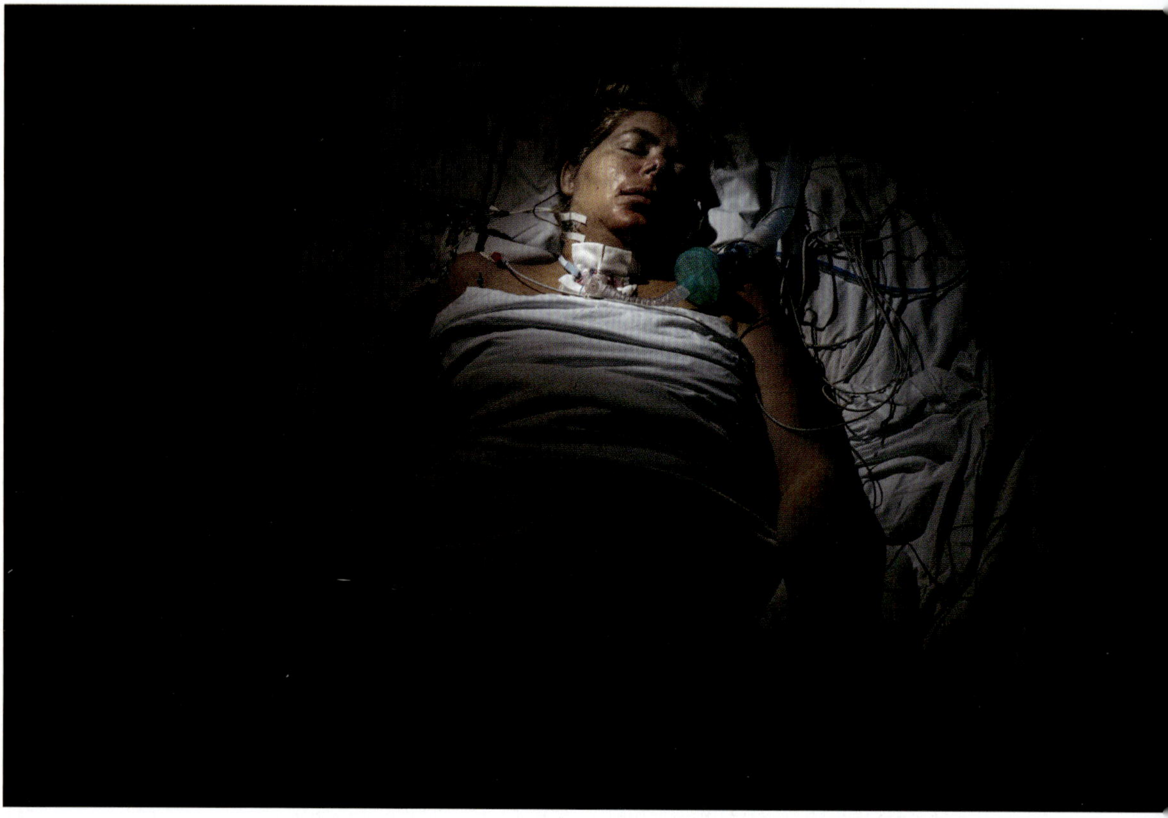

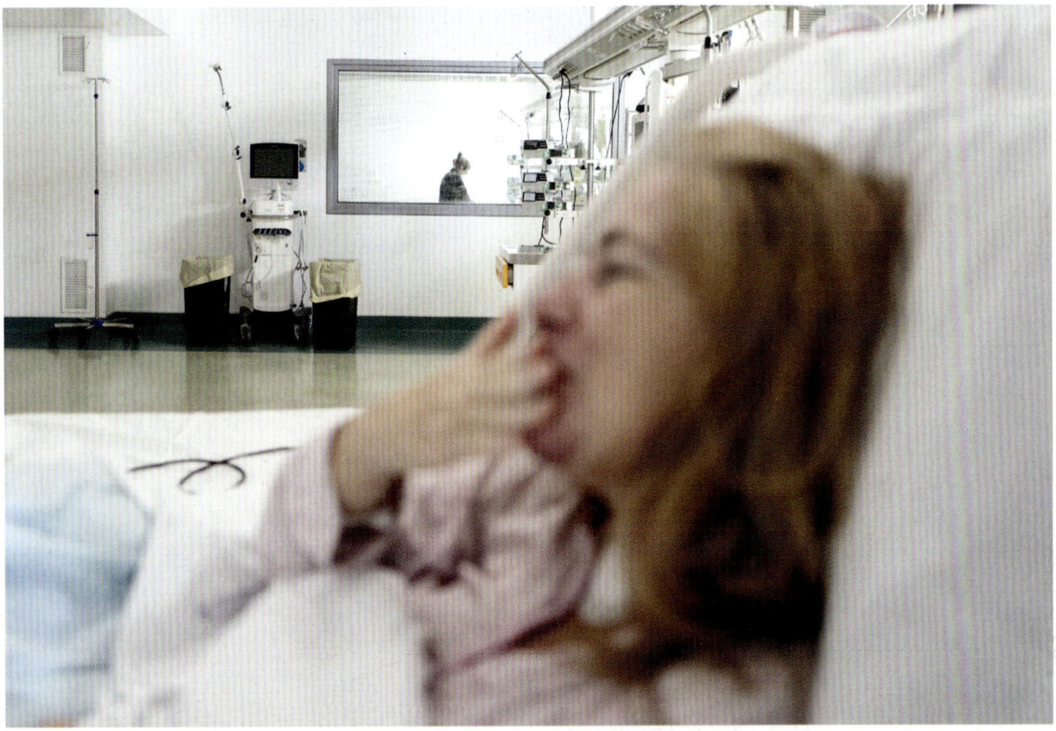

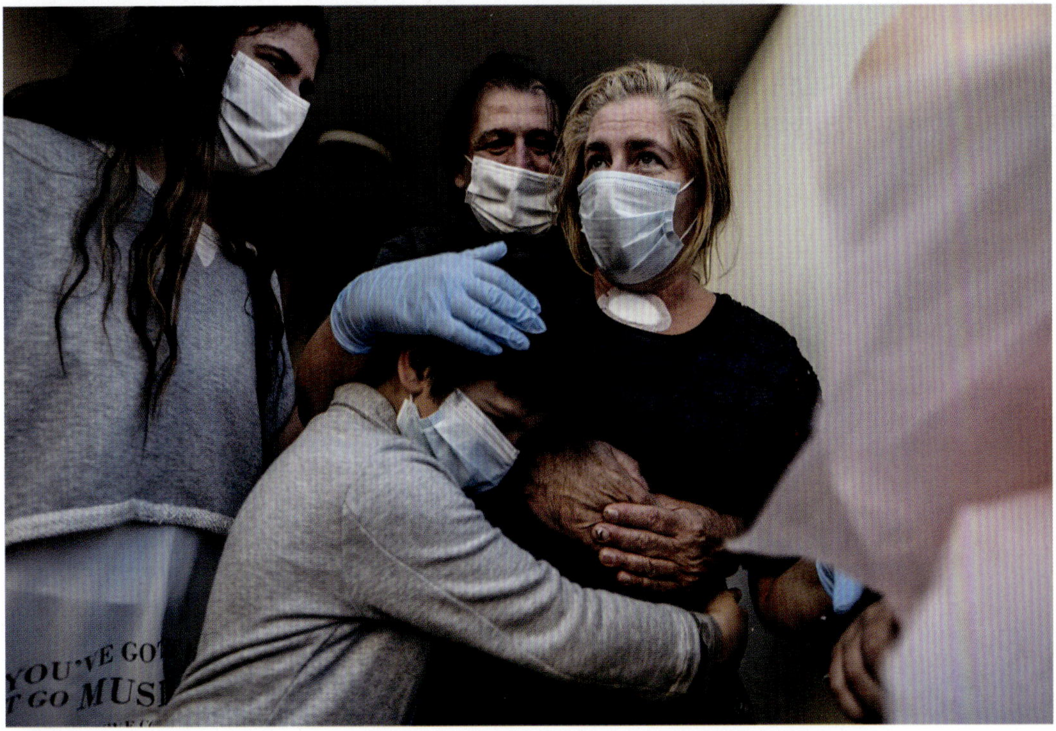
YOU'VE GOT
GO

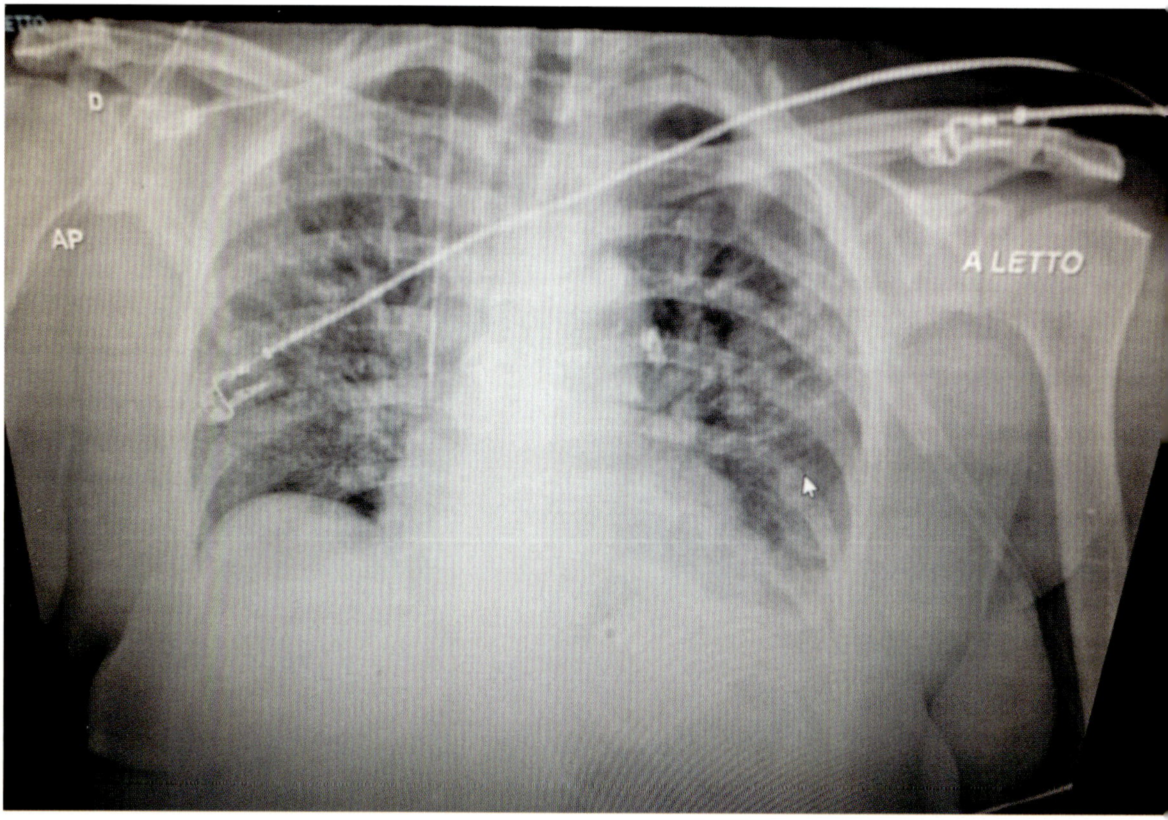
D
AP
A LETTO

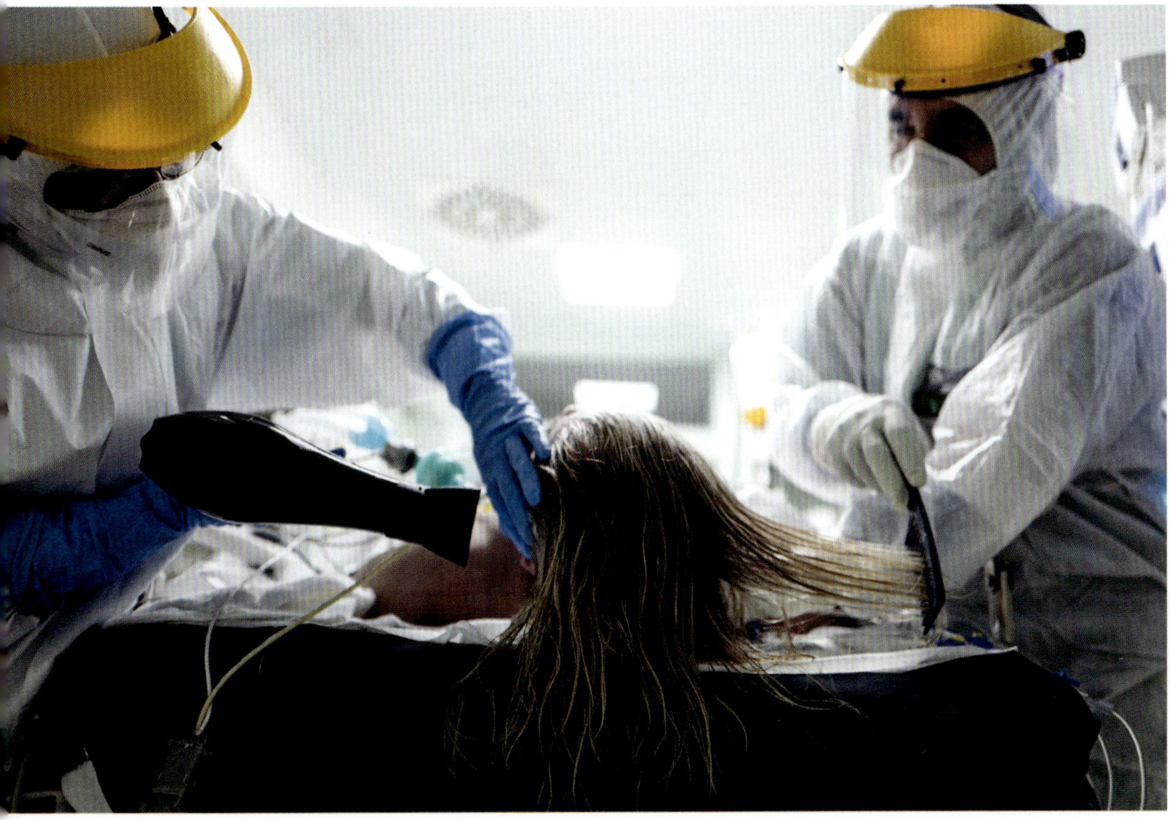

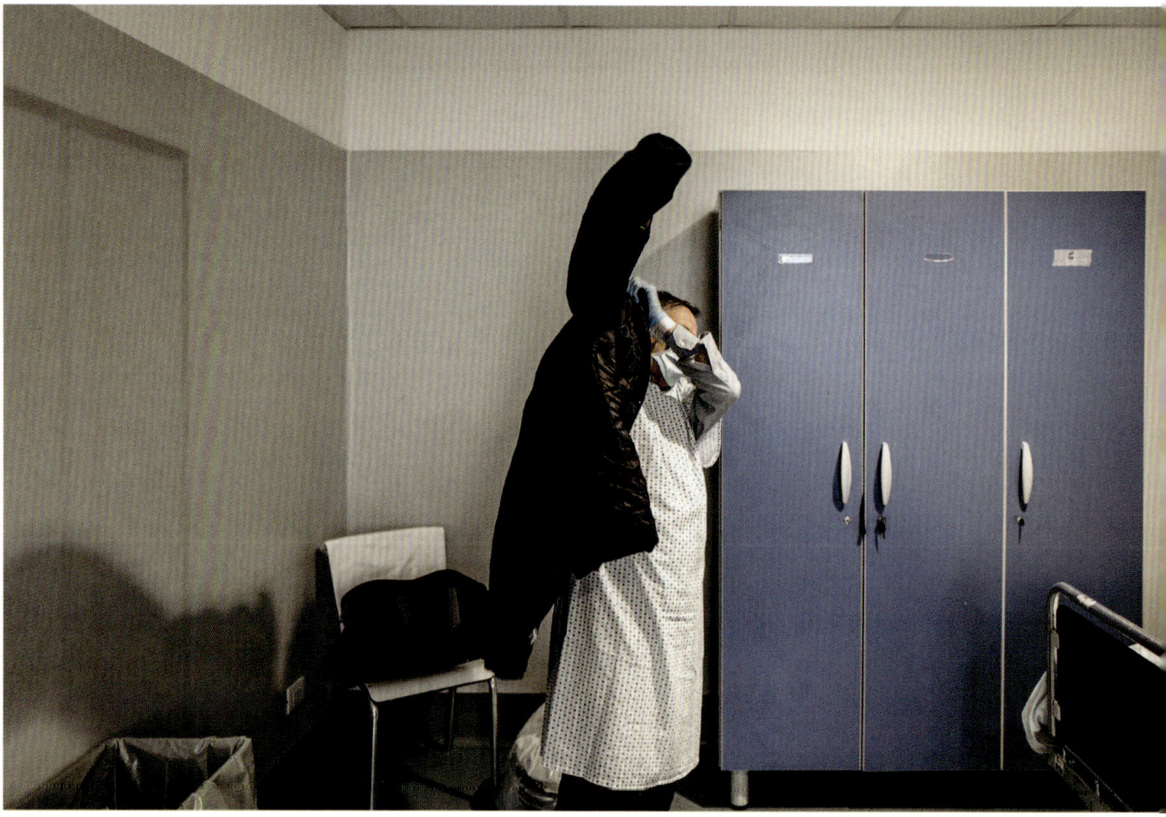

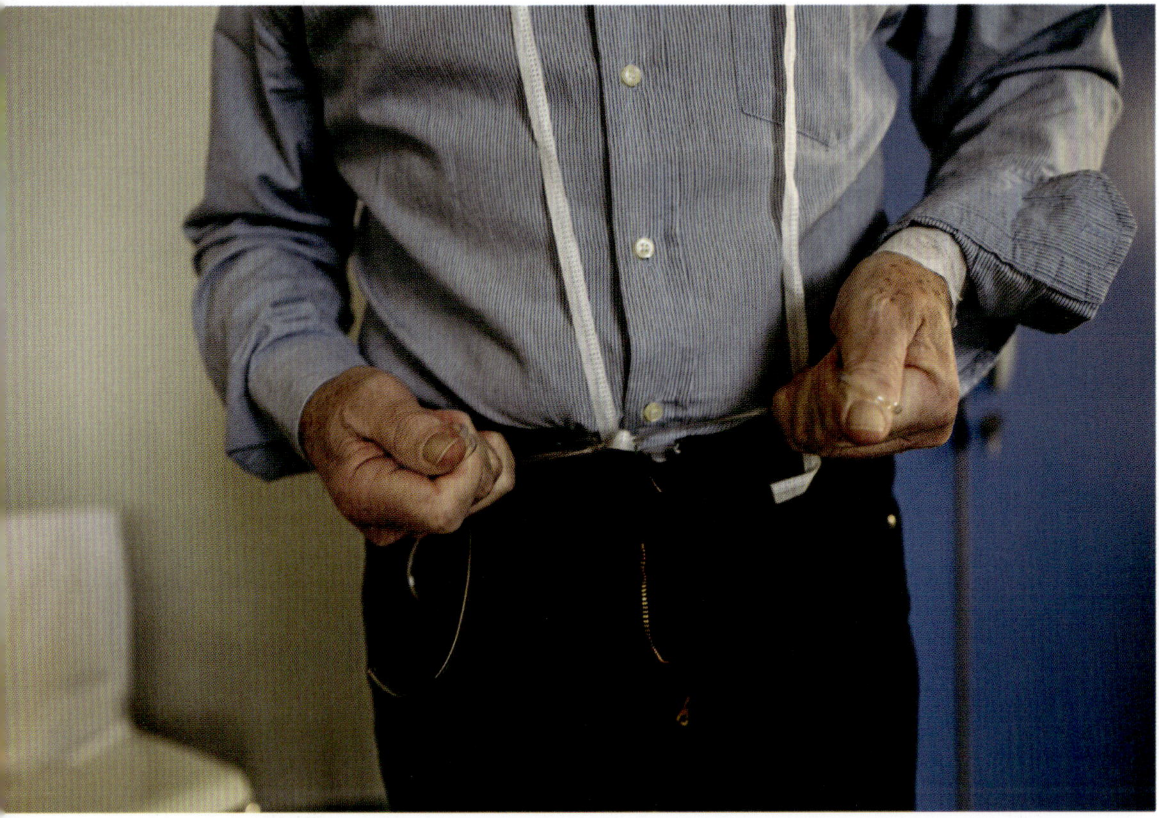

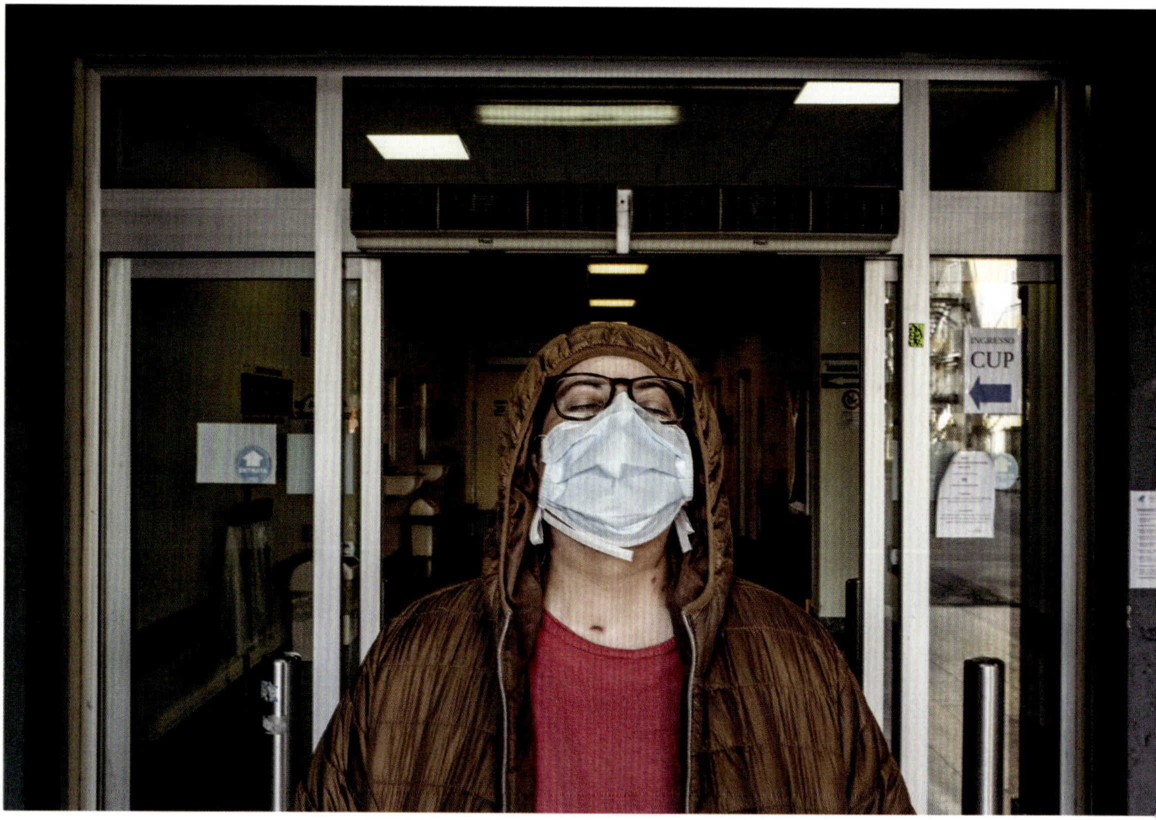
INGRESSO
CUP

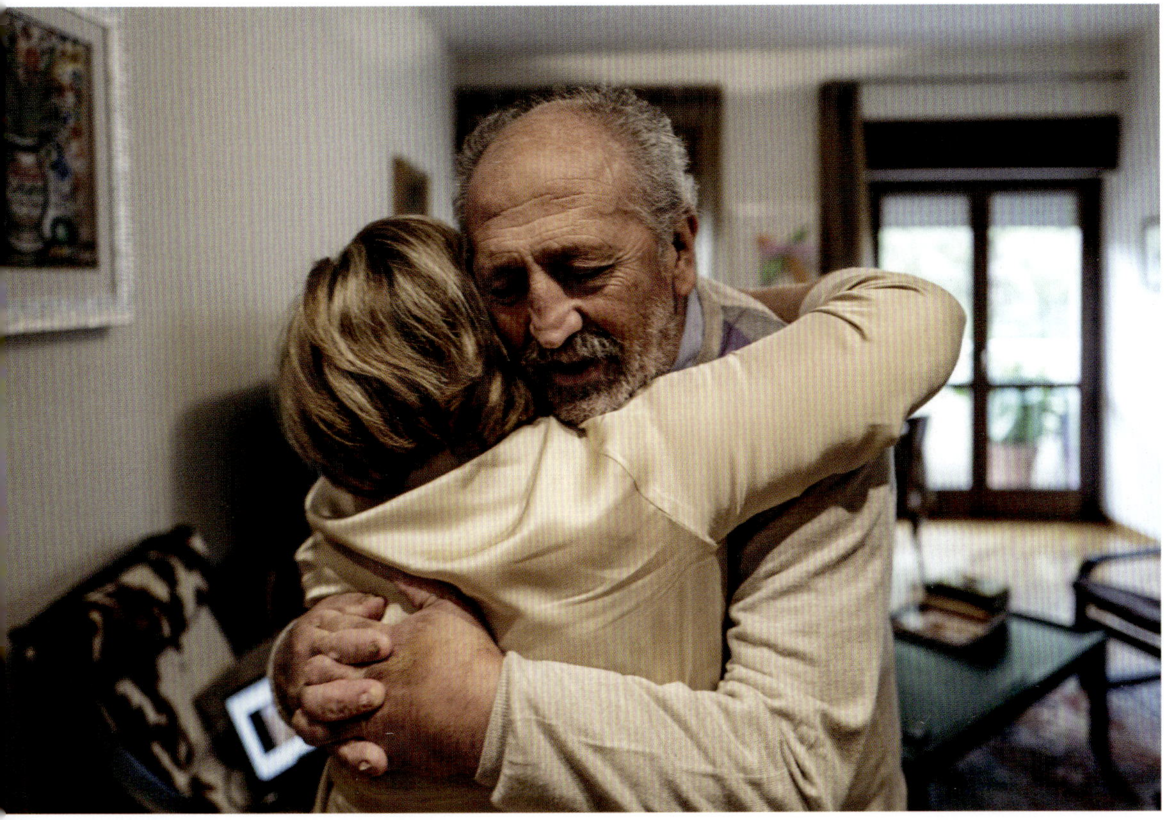

01. The Health Challenge
Captions

Andrea Frazzetta, Italy

The photographs were taken on March 19, 20 and 21, 2020.

Laura Righetti, 30-year-old, volunteer EMT for Croce Blu, Brescia:
"Two months ago, I was teaching elementary school, going out with my friends to get an aperitif after work. Now we are busy all the time. When we go into people's houses, we scare them. They were used to seeing our faces, but now we're all completely covered. It's as if we're aliens".
(Page 97)

Lieutenant colonel Marco Andreis, 44-year-old, physician of the Italian Air Force in help at Papa Giovanni XXIII Hospital in Bergamo:
"The patients are always more or less the same. Any ambiguity is cleared up by listening to the lungs. You hear the friction — like two pieces of paper being crinkled together — in both lungs. You hear it in the bottom of the lungs. And they breathe like a dog. You know how a dog breathes quickly, much faster than a man? A healthy person takes about 12 breaths a minute. This morning, I saw one patient who took 40 breaths in a minute".
(Page 98)

Stefania Ceriani, 38-year-old, nurse at the Infectious Disease Unit at Luigi Sacco Hospital, Milan. As coronavirus tore through Northern Italy, hospitals became the tront lines in a grueling war.
(Page 99)

Commander Giuditta Luca, 43-year-old, pathologist of the Italian Naval Force in help at Papa Giovanni XXIII Hospital in Bergamo:
"There is this sense that the enemy could be anywhere, and in any given moment you can see this in the eyes of the people who live here. They express, without even wanting to, a profound sense of loss. These are scars that stay inside".
(Page 100)

Paola Speri, 53-year-old, head nurse of the Infectious Disease Unit at Luigi Sacco Hospital, Milan:
"The most shocking thing is to see the fear in their eyes, mostly in younger patients. They rely completely on us. Many at night are afraid of falling asleep and never waking up again".
(Page 101)

Gabriele Tomasoni, 65-year-old (and eight children), primary physician at the Intensive Care Unit, Spedali Civili di Brescia, Brescia:
"Every intensive-care procedure must be in proportion to age, to the progress of the disease, to the expectation of life. In normal times, we always try. In these situations, it's not possible. Since the beginning, I have thought of the words of John Paul II: *it is necessary that the heroic becomes daily and that the daily becomes heroic*".
(Page 102, top left)

Marco Scalvini, 25-year-old, cleaner for Markas, the service company for the Papa Giovanni XXIII Hospital in Bergamo:
"The heroism of doctors and nurses has been widely and rightly discussed, but we are there, too. I heard a nurse say that Harvard graduate engineers would be needed to sanitise the environments in this crisis. Maybe that's too much. But securing every corner of an entire hospital is no small responsibility".
(Page 102, top right)

Giovanna Perone, 55-year-old, doctor and director of the Areu AAT 118, the emergency service in Brescia.
(Page 102, bottom left)

Anna Zanotti, 53-year-old, head nurse at Papa Giovanni XXIII Hospital in Bergamo, in charge of finding room for outnumbered patients in other hospitals around Italy:
"No words can give you any idea of what we are living through here. We are devastated".
(Page 102, bottom right)

Annamaria Brambilla, 52-year-old, director of the E.R. unit at Luigi Sacco Hospital, Milan:
"My husband is also a doctor in another hospital, and when I get home, we talk like any two people talking about what happened during the day. We do it calmly, to help each other face things, to share the burden".
(Page 103, top left)

Roberto Rech, 57-year-old, physician and coordinator of a special unit of hospital emergency and pain treatment at Luigi Sacco Hospital in Milan. Roberto had personally ridden in an ambulance down to a small town, Codogno, on the first night of the outbreak. He inspected "Patient 1", who is believed to have significantly spread the virus. Since then, he had worked constantly, trying to understand the invisible enemy.

By the middle of March, Northern Italy had become the epicentre of a global pandemic. Hospitals expanded intensive-care capacity, lined entire wards with ventilators and crowded corridors with oxygen tanks and beds. The doctors, nurses, paramedics and volunteers had little choice but to soldier through day and night with little rest.
(Page 103, top right)

Katia D'Addamo, 45-year-old, cleaning coordinator for Markas, the cleaning service company at Papa Giovanni XXIII Hospital in Bergamo.
(Page 103, bottom left)

Antonella Mangili, 46-year-old, nurse at Areu AAT 118, the emergency service in Bergamo: "The traffic on the streets is down to about 1 or 2 percent of what it was. But we have to keep the siren on anyway. After stabilising the patient, just before loading him in an ambulance, we ask relatives to say goodbye the best they can".
(Page 103, bottom right)

Marco Rizzi, 63-year-old, director of Infectious Disease Unit at Papa Giovanni XXIII Hospital in Bergamo: "To see ambulances in line at the entrance, and not knowing where and how to place the sick, it hurts. All of this will leave a mark".
(Page 104)

Katerina Papeta, 22-year-old, volunteer EMT for Associazione Nazionale Carabinieri, Brescia.
(Page 105)

Alberto Poinelli, 54-year-old, nurse and deputy supervisor of the Areu AAT 118, the emergency service in Brescia.
(Page 106)

Monica Falocchi, 48-year-old, head nurse (supervisor) at the Intensive Care Unit, Spedali Civili di Brescia, Brescia. As coronavirus tore through Northern Italy, hospitals became the front lines in a grueling war.
(Page 107)

Gaia Squarci, USA

The photographs were taken in New York between March and May 2020.

People wait in line to shop at a pharmacy. Brooklyn, NYC.
(Pages 110–111)

Alexis, college student who now follows lessons from home, sits in front of a closed restaurant in Bed-Stuy. Brooklyn, NYC. This photograph has been produced with the support of the ICP, International Centre of Photography
(Page 112)

A man sleeps in Times Square, Manhattan, NYC.
(Page 113)

Emergency showers outside of Brookdale Hospital. Brooklyn, NYC.
(Page 114)

ICU nurse Sonya Hribal, who came to New York to work during the COVID-19 health emergency contracted by FEMA, is photographed in front of Elmhurst Hospital in Queens, NYC.
(Page 115)

A refrigerated truck is used as a morgue for COVID-19 victims outside of Wyckoff Heights Medical Center, Brooklyn, NYC.
(Page 116, left)

Bailey Stephenson, Cardiovascular Intensive Care Unit nurse who came from Georgia to New York City to work during the COVID-19 health emergency, poses for a portrait in Times Square. Stephenson was contracted by an agency. Manhattan, NYC.
(Page 116, right)

Maksim Shmargun, ICU surgeon at Lincoln Hospital. Bronx, NYC.
(Page 117, left)

A refrigerated truck is used as a morgue for COVID-19 victims outside of the Brooklyn Hospital Center. Brooklyn, NYC.
(Page 117, right)

Carlos Rojas, from Ecuador, ill with skin cancer, waits for a car outside of Elmhurst Hospital after one of his chemotherapy sessions. Queens, NYC.
(Page 118, left and right)

Ebony Kinch, who brings food to patients at Woodhull Hospital, poses for a portrait in front of the hospital. Brooklyn, NYC.
(Page 119)

Santi Palacios, Spain

An elderly woman remains confined in her room at a nursing home due to the pandemic, in the province of Barcelona, Spain.
26 April 2020.
(Page 121)

Volunteers of the NGO Open Arms carry out tests to detect the coronavirus to two elders at a nursing home in the province of Barcelona, Spain. 14 April 2020.
(Pages 122–123 and 124)

A worker holds the phone so that an elderly woman can speak with her daughter, at a nursing home, province of Barcelona, Spain.
18 April 2020.
(Page 125)

An elderly woman rests on her bed at a nursing home after a team of volunteers had performed a PCR test for the detection of coronavirus, in the province of Barcelona, Spain. 14 April 2020.
(Page 126, top and bottom)

Carles, born in 1915, three years before the beginning of the pandemic known as the Spanish Flu of 1918, waits to be tested for coronavirus at a nursing home, in the province of Barcelona, Spain. 4 May 2020.
(Page 127, top)

Beds separated by a plastic curtain as a preventive measure against the coronavirus, remain empty in a nursing home during the worst weeks of the health emergency, in the province of Barcelona, Spain. 13 April, 2020.
(Page 127, bottom)

An elderly woman grabs the hand of Isabel, a nurse at a nursing home, and speaks into her ear while Isabel responds spontaneously with the closest thing to a hug she achieves by wearing a face shield, protective suit, gloves, gown and mask, in Barcelona, Spain.
12 May 2020.
(Page 128)

Armchairs remain empty in the living room of a nursing home, during the weeks in which elders had to keep confined to their rooms, in the province of Barcelona, Spain.
14 April 2020.
(Page 129)

Stefano Schirato, Italy

The photographs were taken between April 19 and June 16, 2020.

Montesilvano, Italy. Domenico Pagliara and his children Daniele, Alessandro, Linda and Giada, during a videocall to his wife Marzia Merlin, still in the hospital. Domenico has just come back from hospital where he was admitted because COVID-19 positive, like his wife. While both parents were in hospital, their childen lived two weeks at home alone. Now, they are waiting for Marzia to come back home and get the family back together again.
(Page 131)

Pescara, Italy. Santo Spirito Hospital, Marzia Merlin, 50, was admitted in the Intensive Care Unit and intubated because of respiratory complication. She had to undergo tracheotomy. Her husband Domenico, also suffering from coronavirus, came out of the hospital few days ago. They have four children.
(Page 132)

Pescara, Italy. Santo Spirito Hospital. Marzia Merlin, 50, sending a kiss to the medical staff of the Intensive Care Unit, before being moved to General Medicine Unit. After 18 days in pharmacolgical coma, her lungs finally seems to work well and she is now able to breath by herself. In few days, she'll be discharged and allowed to go back to her husband and her four children.
(Page 133, top)

Montesilvano, Italy. The children of Marzia Merlin, 50, hug their mother after six weeks of hospitalisation for coronavirus. Marzia was in intensive care for 18 days and in a pharmacological coma. Her husband Domenico was also hospitalised in Intensive Care Unit and the four children remained home alone. Finally today the family is reunited.
(Page 133, bottom)

Penne, Italy. San Massimo Hospital. Intensive Care Unit. Lung X-ray of a patient admitted to the ICU due to COVID-19.
(Page 134)

Penne, Italy. Intensive Care Unit at San Massimo Hospital. Nurses are drying Gina's hair after washing it. It's the first time Gina Di Giacobbe, 61, is able to have her hair washed after a long period in the Intensive

Care Unit. Gina was first admitted in Santo Spirito Hospital, in Pescara, and then moved here in Penne due to lack of beds.
(Page 135)

Pescara, Italy. Santo Spirito Hospital. Lino Profeta, 68, from Castilenti. After more than a month in the hospital, he has finally been discharged. He is now getting dressed to go out and come back home.
(Page 136)

Pescara, Italy. Santo Spirito Hospital. Lino Profeta, 68, from Castilenti. He was admitted in the COVID-19 Unit at Santo Spirito Hospital on March 26. He underwent ventilation and, on March 30, he was moved to Intensive Care Unit as his condition was getting worse. He lost 10 kilos during his hospitalisation so now it' s time to go back home, he has asked a nurse for something to tighten his trousers and has been given an infusion tube.
(Page 137)

Pescara, Italy. Santo Spirito Hospital. Emanuela De Nicolo, 44, leaves the hospital after 58 days of hospitalisation for coronavirus. After a few days from hospitalisation she was moved to the Intensive Care Unit because of respiratory failure. Today she finally returns home to her partner and her two English pointer dogs.
(Page 138)

Pescara, Italy. Maurizio Melchiorre, 62, geologist, hugs his wife. Maurizio is finally back home after 33 days in hospital.
(Page 139)

02.

The Urban Void

Simon Norfolk, United Kingdom
Lost Capital

In Gustave Doré's 1873 engraving of *The New Zealander* a lonely traveller, in centuries to come, sits by an overgrown River Thames. Across the water are the lifeless ruins of a future London, the crumbling dome of St Paul's as decayed as the Roman Colosseum is today. New Zealand was imagined by Doré as so remote that it would escape the West's imminent collapse and our Kiwi ponders the ruins of an earlier, collapsed civilisation just as an English noble might have done on his Grand Tour in Rome. One of the things I love about the Grand Romantics was they had the courage to imagine a new society but also the humility to see beyond that, to how the world would be when even their paradise had come and gone. The meme of *The New Zealander* has had a long life. There is a direct line from him to the dystopian cities of J.G. Ballard and Cormac McCarthy, to a thousand zombie movies and he's behind all those computer games that feature the lonely avenger scouring the streets of a post-apocalyptic city.

Constantin-François Volney, who travelled in Egypt and Syria in 1784, wrote in his book *Ruins, or a Survey of the Revolutions of Empires* (*Les Ruines, ou Méditation sur les Révolution des Empires*, Paris: 1791): "What are become of so many productions of the hand of man? Where are those ramparts of Nineveh, those walls of Babylon, those palaces of Persepolis? … Alas! I have beheld nothing but solitude and desertion! Who can assure me that the present desolation will not one day be the lot of our own country? Who knows but that hereafter some traveller like myself will sit down upon the banks of the Seine, the Thames, or the Zuyder Zee, solitary amid silent ruins, and weep a people [extinct], and their greatness changed into an empty name?"

The Romantics thought our society would collapse from the emptiness of its values or the inequalities in our economies. Even the imaginations of Shelley or Byron couldn't factor in a virus from a pangolin in the wet market of a provincial Chinese city.

In photographing Coronavirus London I was astonished that by removing from the streets the daily dross of life (cars, trucks, people) suddenly the architecture shone forth. Buildings look like the architect's plans of them; unblotted, sharp. I'm reminded of the paintings of Giorgio de Chirico, their linear clarity and brilliantly lit dreamscapes. I never noticed how London is a grand imperial chessboard with all the architectural pieces laid out awaiting the cavalcade.

I thought of the city as "lost" because a) this London was lost beneath the cacophony, b) I often got lost down side-streets I thought I knew intimately and c) we're all a little lost, at sixes and sevens right now.

I felt much like I did when I was in a bombed Afghanistan at the beginning of my career searching a shattered battlefield absent of soldiers; a stage without actors and me, the New Zealander, scratching for clues. Empty London is a *memento mori* or a *vanitas* painting; it shows that this microscopic virus has made proud fools of us all. It has shown us to be ultimately powerless and our investments misguided and empty. All our dreams and schemes and the protections that insulate us from the world were found to be as tough as wet cardboard. Even the most comfortable of us is scrambling around the internet for toilet roll and PPE (Personal Protective Equipment). *Omnia vanitas.*

The only people I meet on my dawn trips are the bronze statues of the grandees of the British Empire ("Good morning, Your Grace") who stand slightly-disappointed, looking down on the mess we've made of their inheritance. They resemble Easter Island's Moai left guarding the sacred groves of a religion no one follows. Everyone's gone to the Rapture. London looks magnificent whilst looking as if it has been hit by a neutron bomb. I never imagined the Apocalypse would be so quiet one would hear in Piccadilly the song of a blackbird.

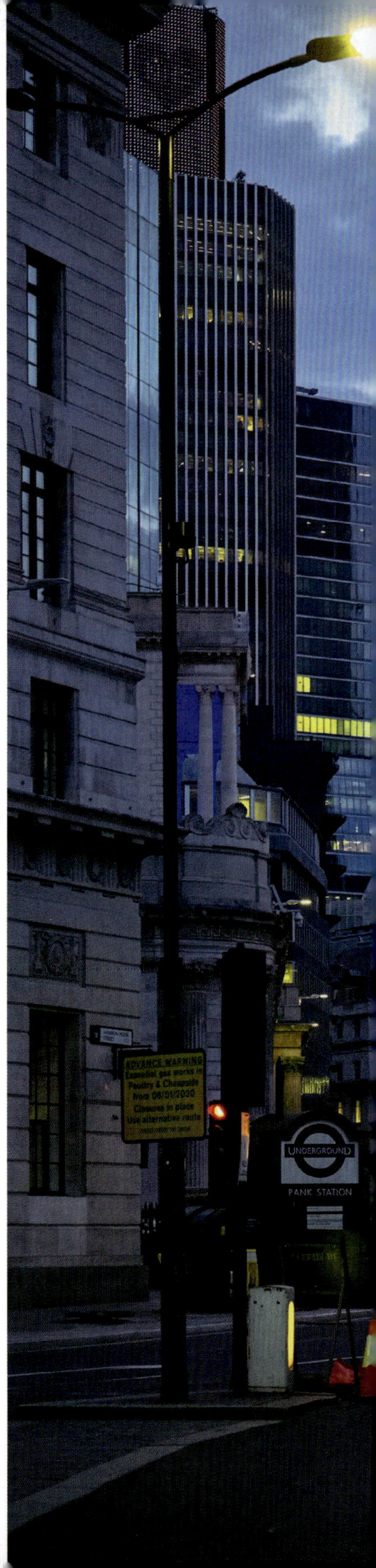
ADVANCE WARNING
Essential gas works in
Poultry & Cheapside
from 06/01/2020
Closures in place
Use alternative route
UNDERGROUND
PANK STATION

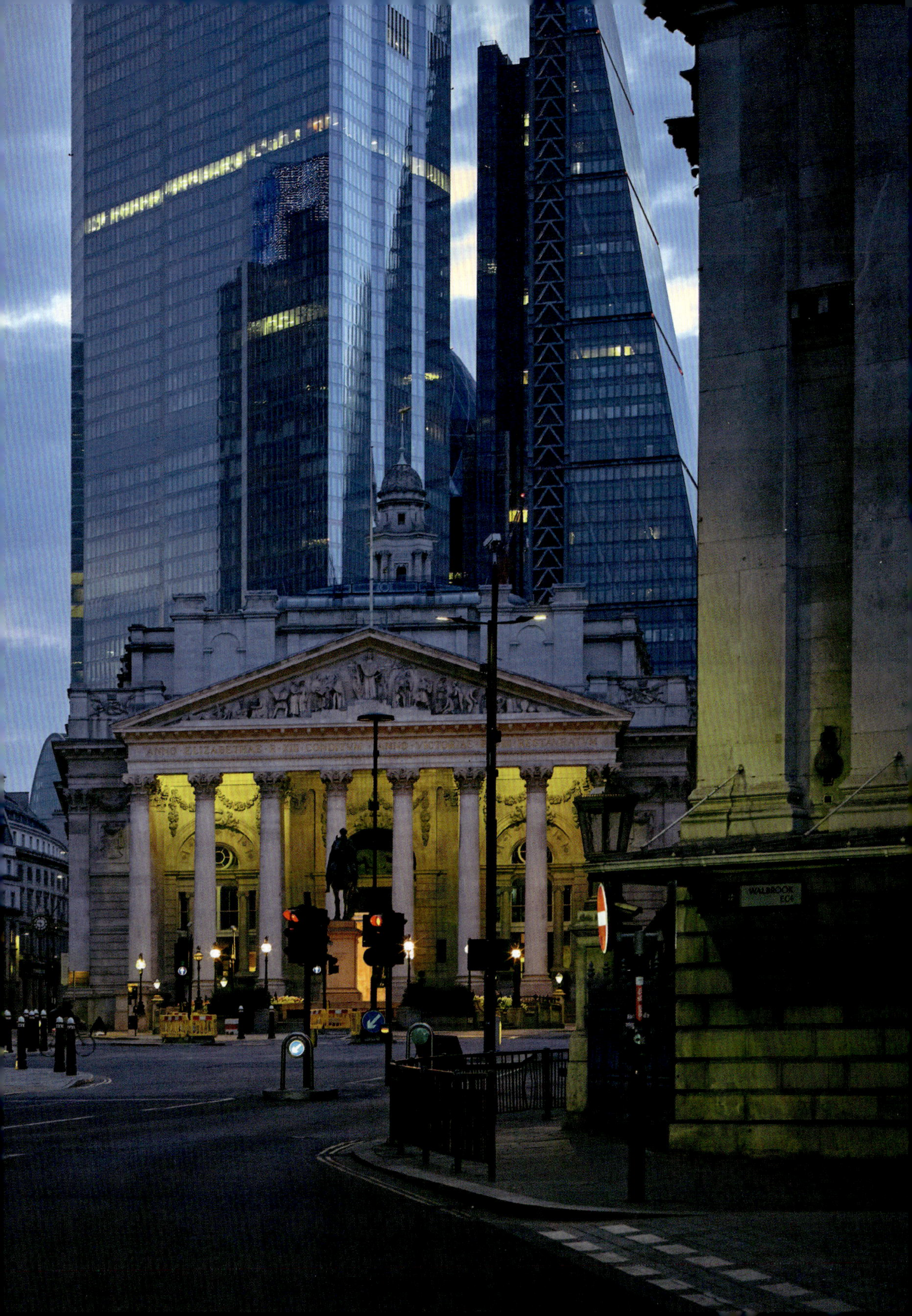

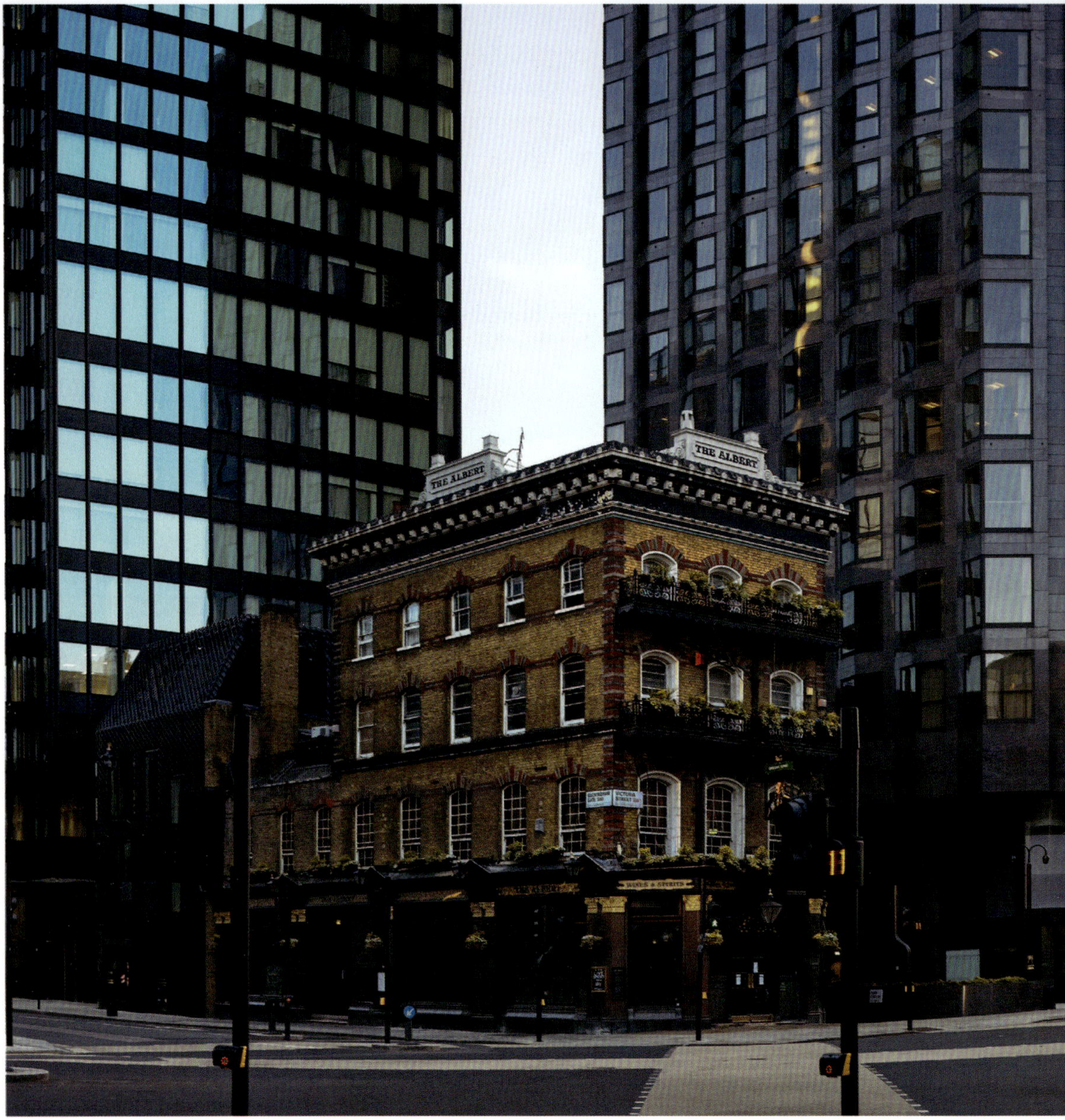
THE ALBERT
THE ALBERT
WINES & SPIRITS

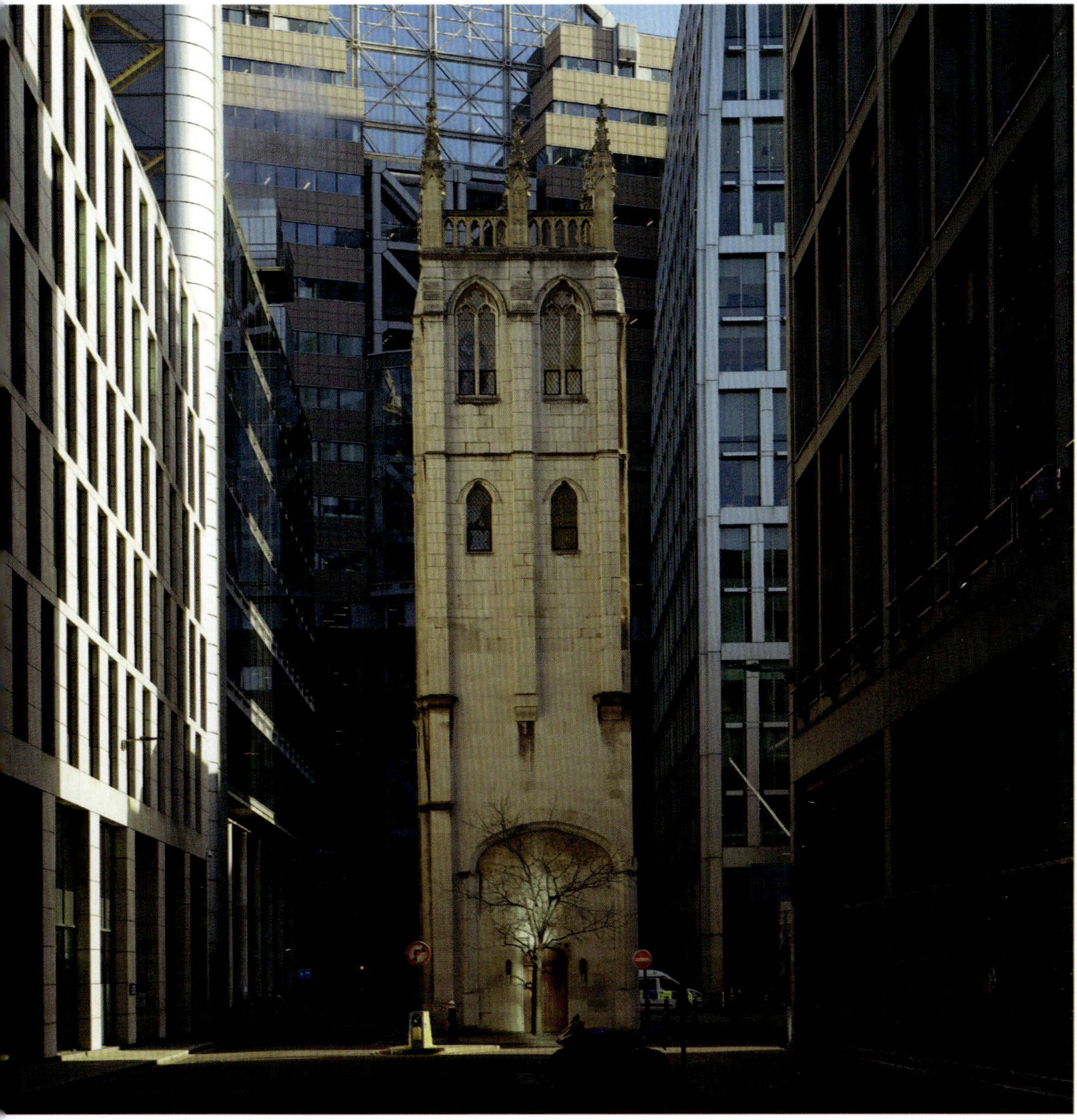

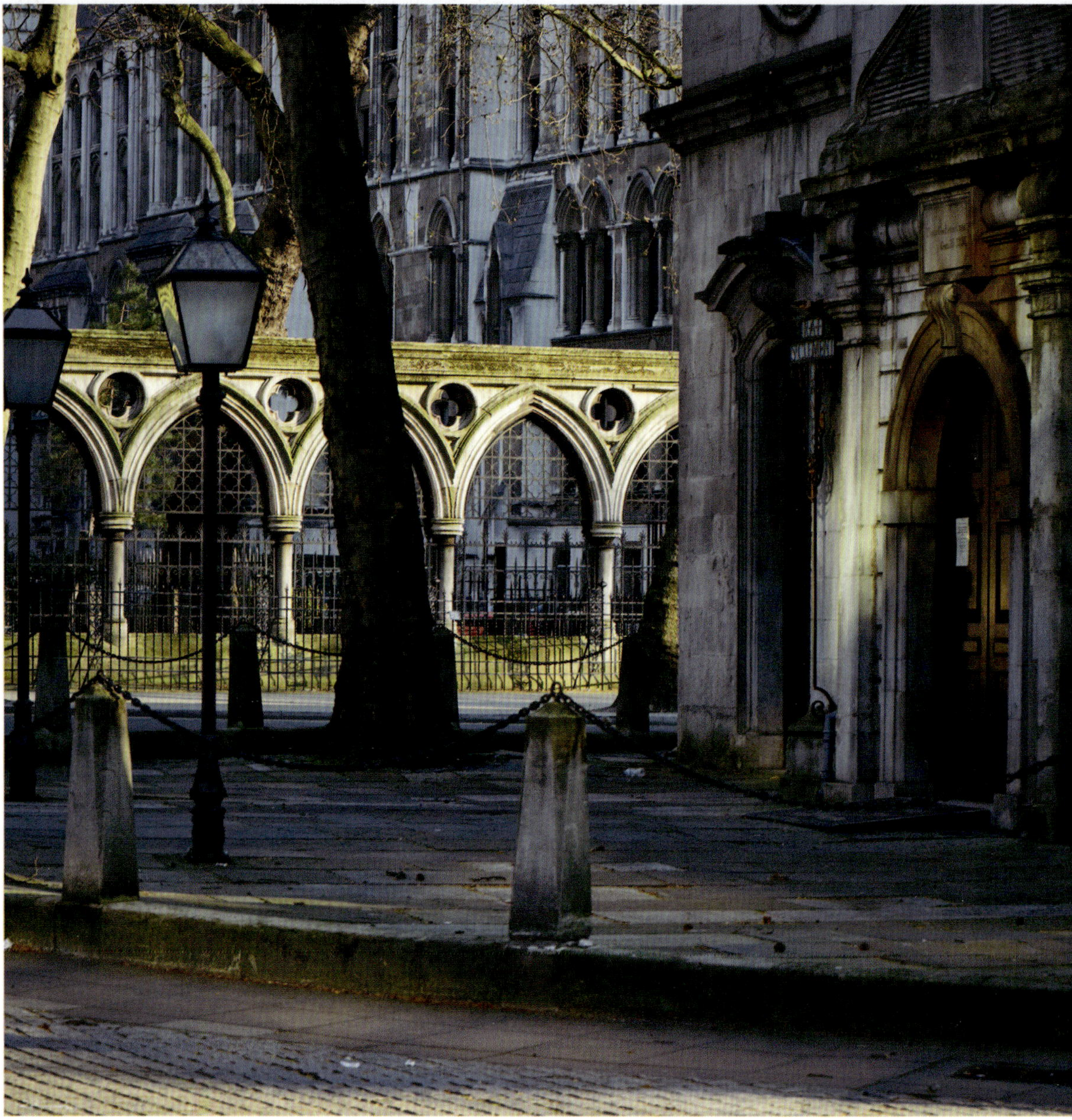

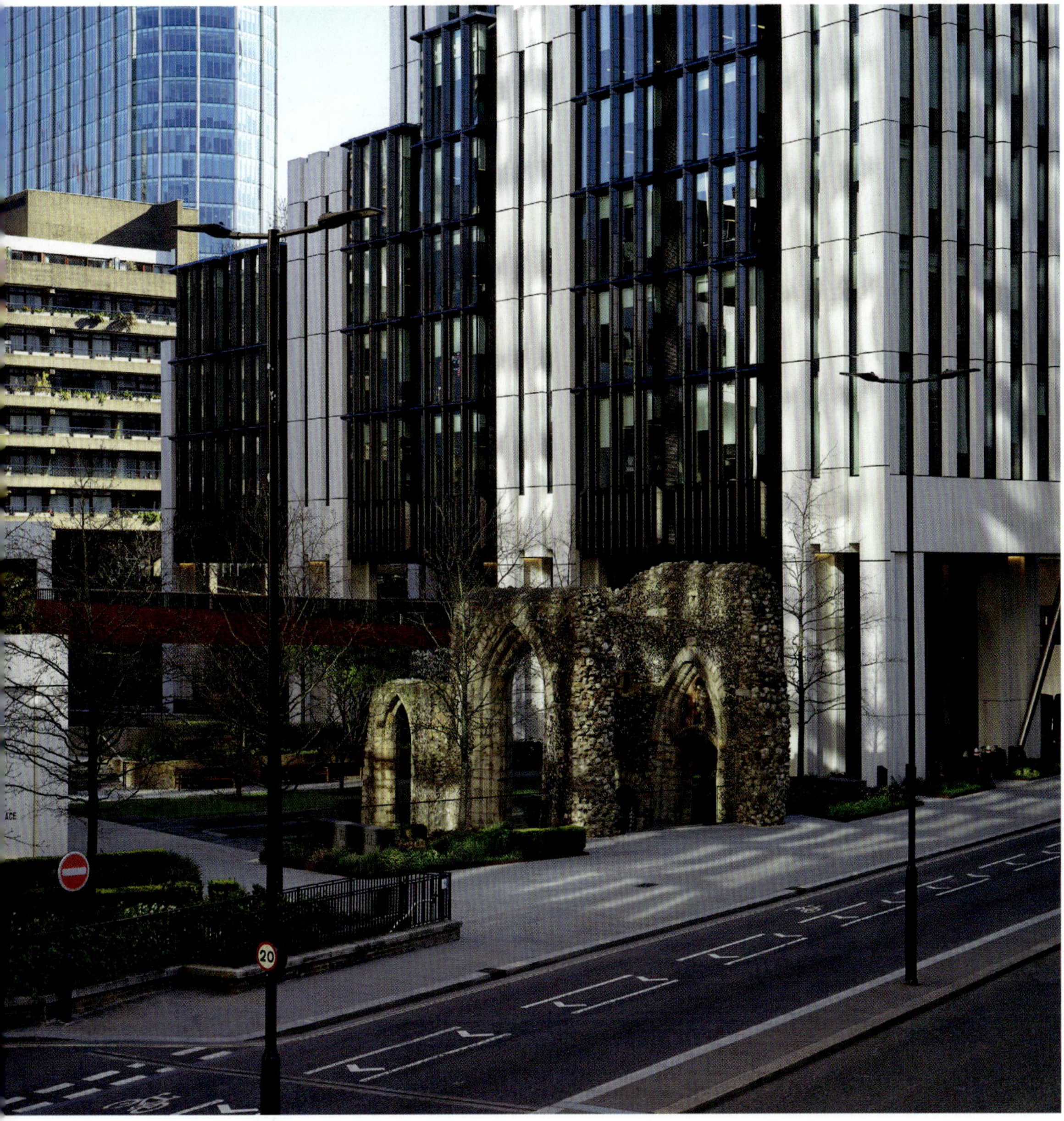
20

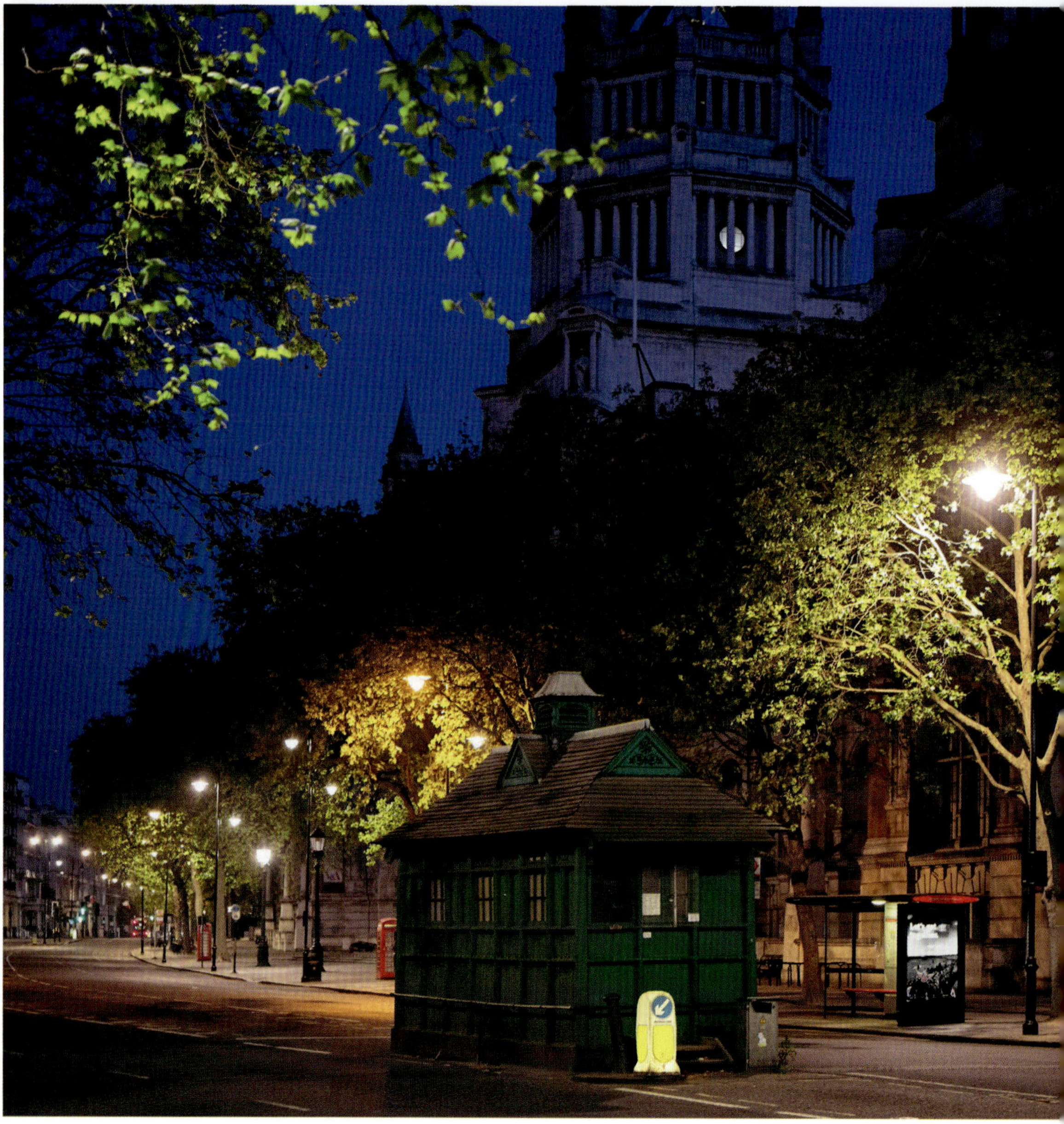

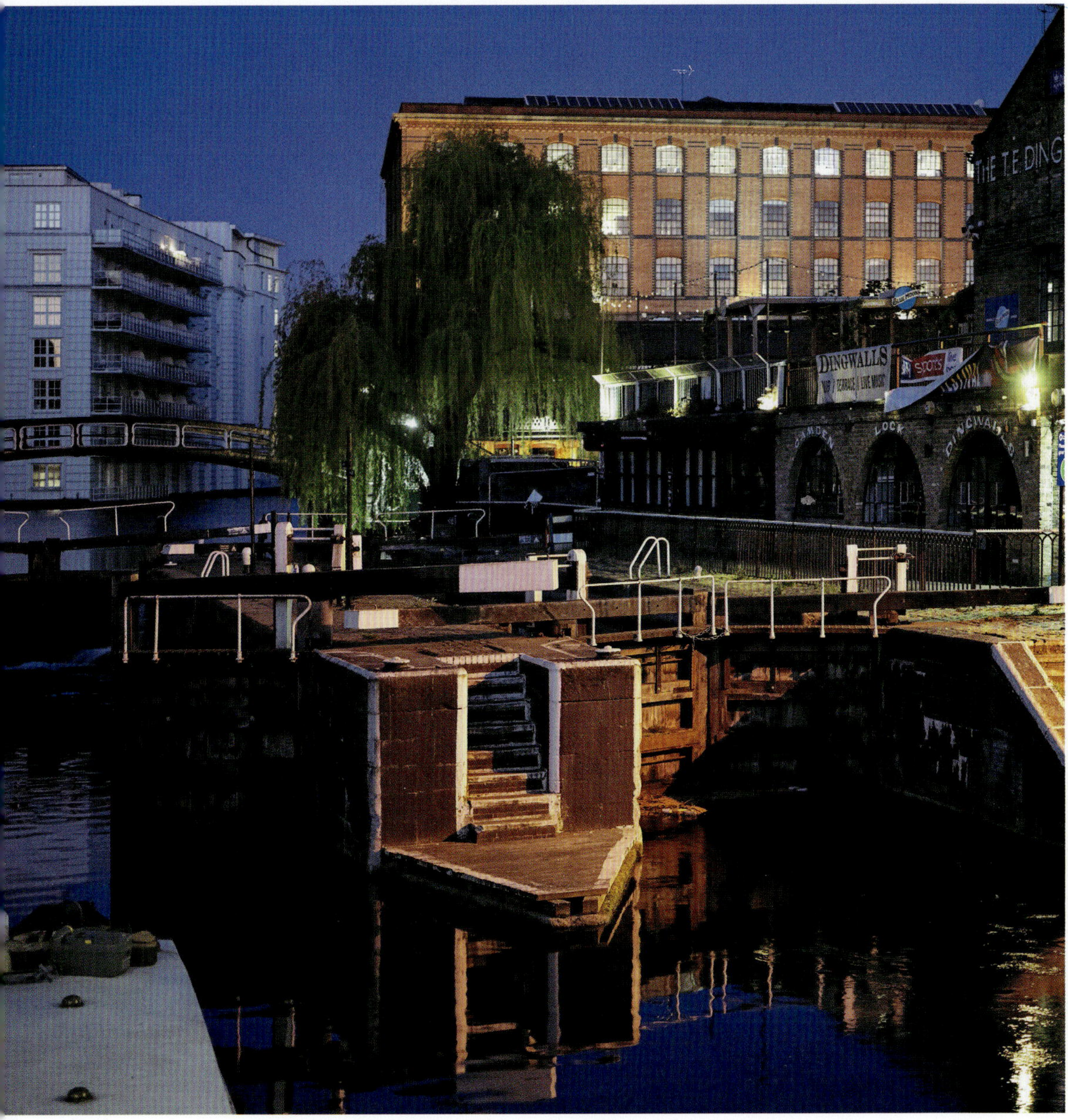
DINGWALLS
CAMDEN
LOCK
DINGWALLS

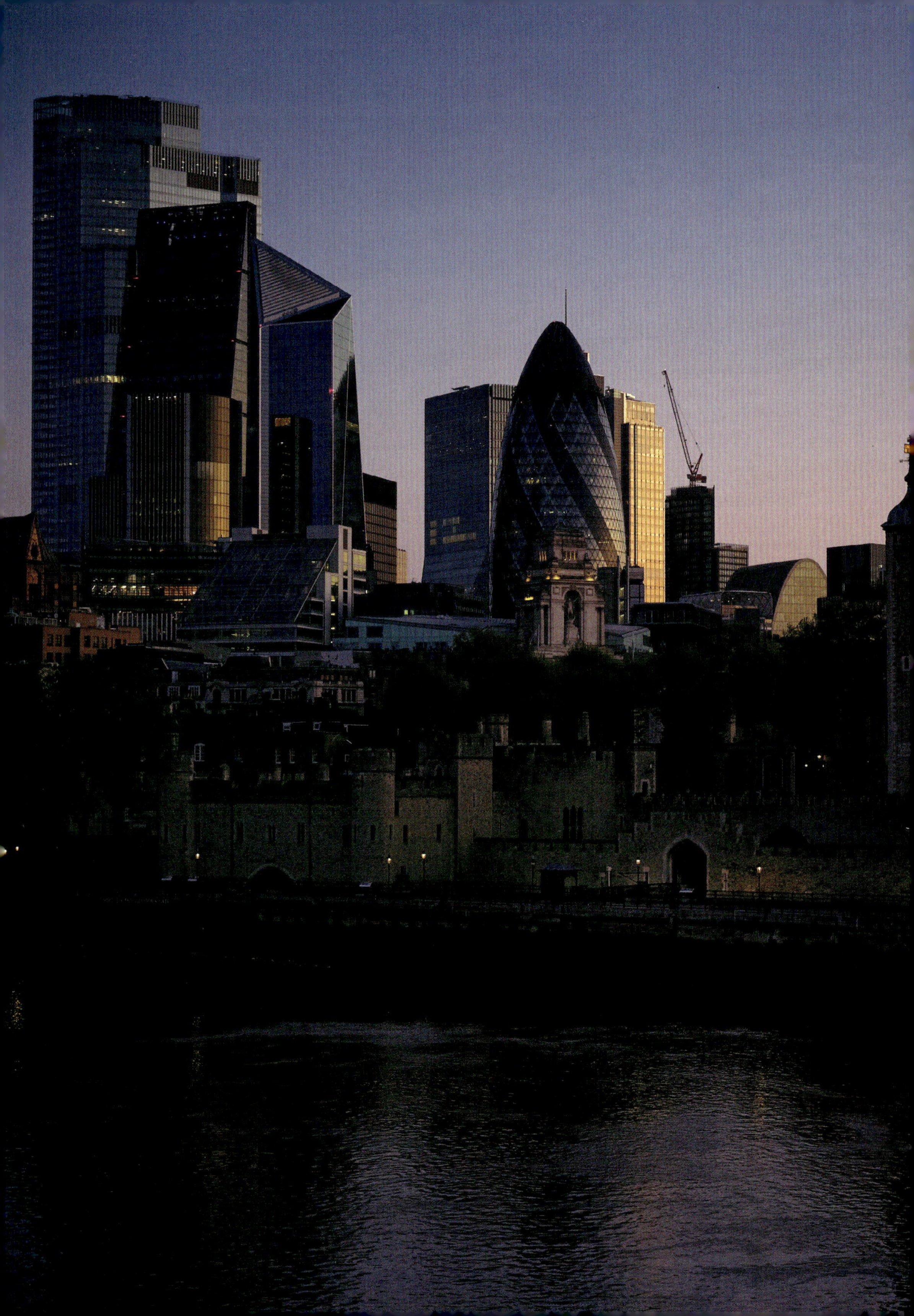

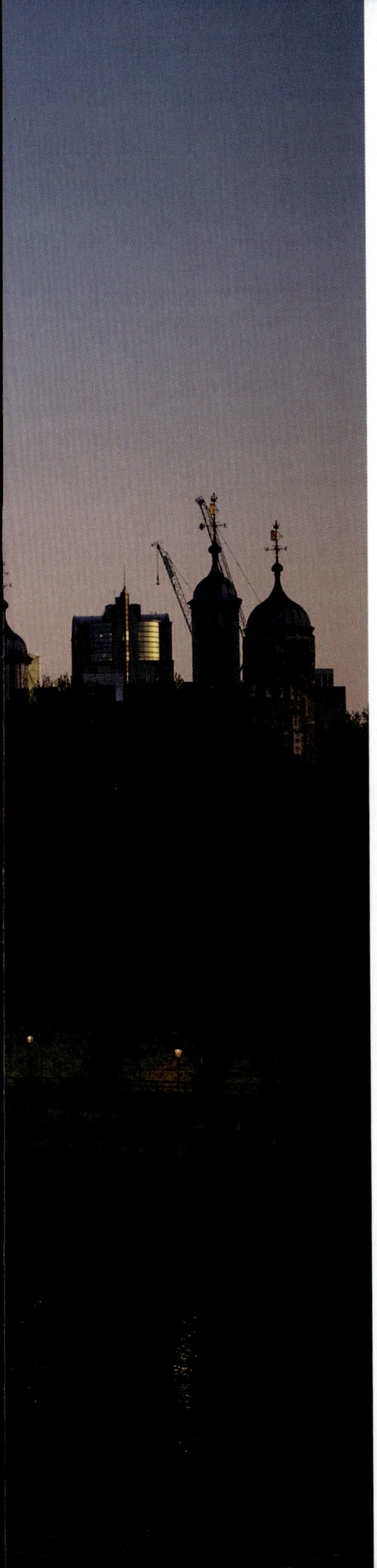

Edoardo Delille, Italy
Silence

Massimo Razzi

Santa Maria del Fiore seems straight out of an Art History book, where, to keep the eye on the architecture, people were removed. Photographing Florence at the time of COVID-19, Edoardo Delille found himself, more or less, in the same situation. It wasn't Photoshop that made people disappear, the virus of this modern plague did it instead.
"I was surprised by this experience, – he explains – photographing the squares and symbolic landmarks of Florence, emptied of the millions of tourists who usually fill the streets of the centre was a surprising experience. I found myself in a city almost ghostly in its renewed beauty, on the set of a movie that I would not have imagined watching. The silence of the streets, usually crowded with people, accompanied me in visiting, in solitude, what for centuries have been the symbols of the Renaissance beauty of the city."
And, one by one, those symbols re-emerge in a ghostly and disturbing purity. The spaces, in Delille's pictures, expand to almost abnormal dimensions such as the Belvedere in Piazzale Michelangelo or Piazza Santa Maria Novella. You can see their magnificence and also their flaws in some worn-out cobble pavement, in some rubble, in a few too many blades of grass growing among the stones. As if people actually "built" the landscape to which we are accustomed and as if this landscape today was really something else, motionless, empty and, at the same time, overwhelmingly self-sufficient.
"I shot the scene from above – says Delille – looking through the eyes of those who are now forced to see life through a window facing the street. This angle reinforced the idea of immobility, of stasis, which characterises this period of modern history. I chose to shoot at times of the day when the streets of the centre were usually crowded with people. The hours when it is usually difficult to take a good picture of the monuments' architecture. The very harsh light of these days reveals the absence of humans even more."
That's right, to the extent that seeing here and there a passerby, a runner, a delivery boy, becomes almost a relief for the eyes and heart. We human beings miss each other, even in that wonderful Florence of stones and marbles, where the "stern" of Santa Maria del Fiore emerges like a black and white ship cast in the middle of the square and doesn't seem real to us.
But Delille tells us that "the few passersby at the edges of the frame are there by chance. There are boys delivering groceries, some people jogging and others taking their dogs out. The Florentines who still live in the centre return home with shopping bags, all of them wearing masks and keeping social distance in a totally empty city". He didn't put them there on purpose, he didn't look for them, but one can believe that, by framing some of them in that eternal immobility, his heart felt almost relieved.

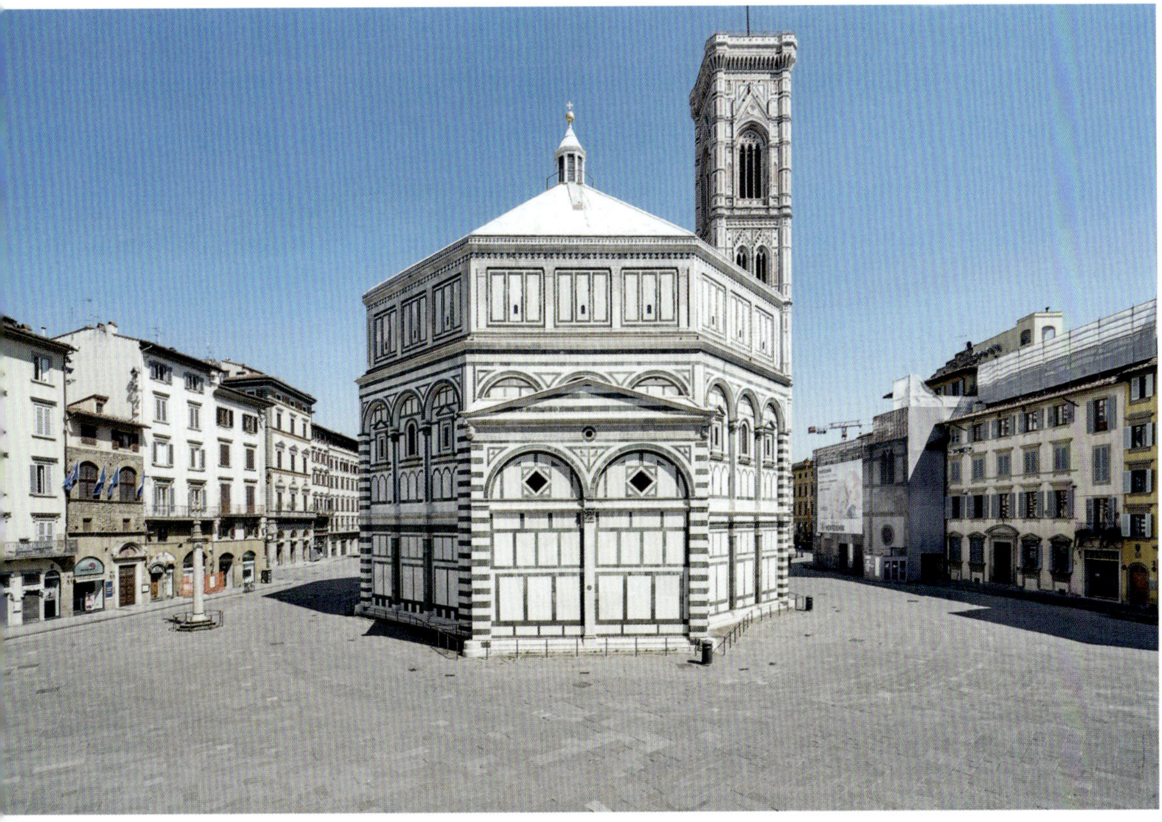

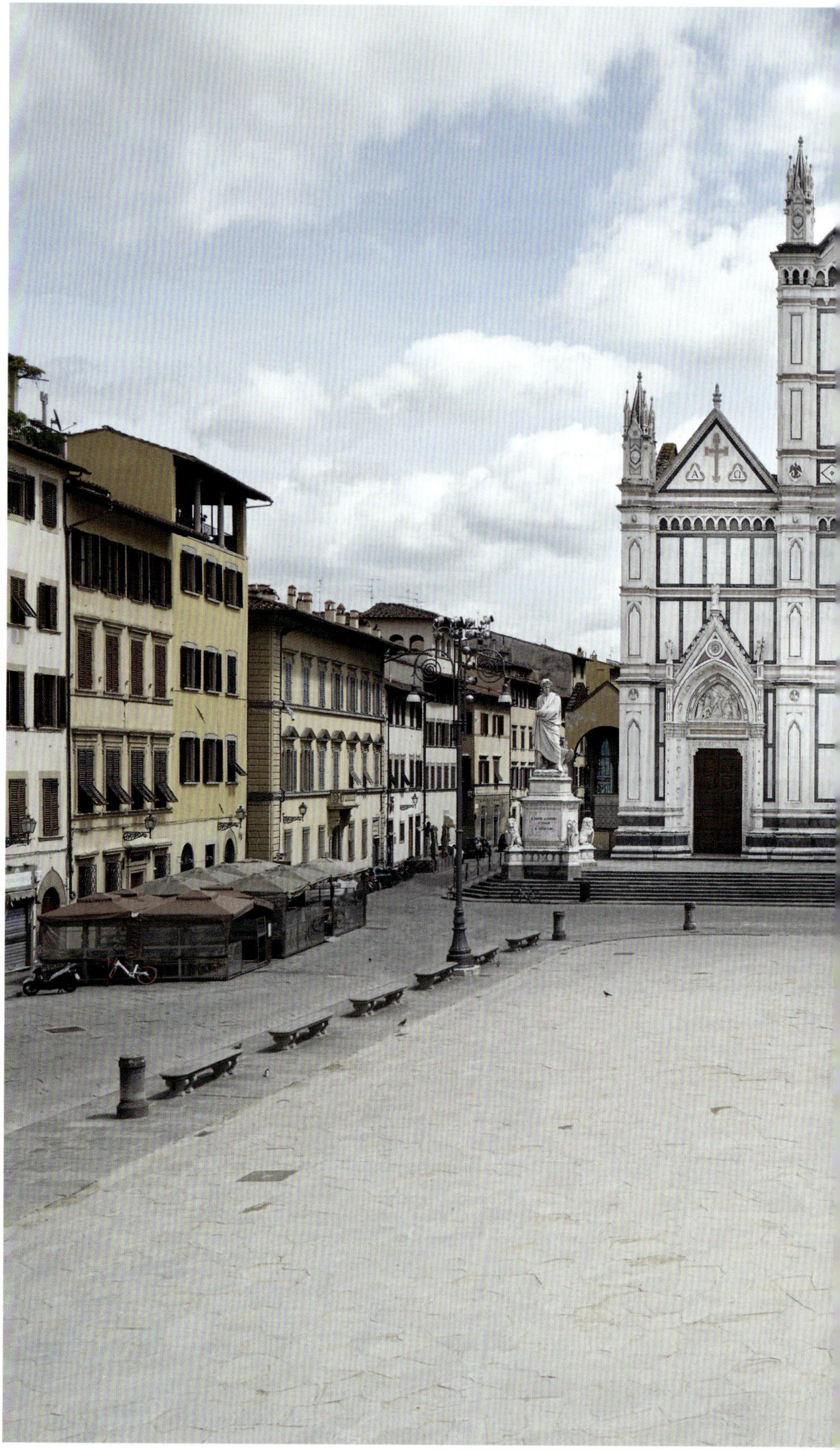

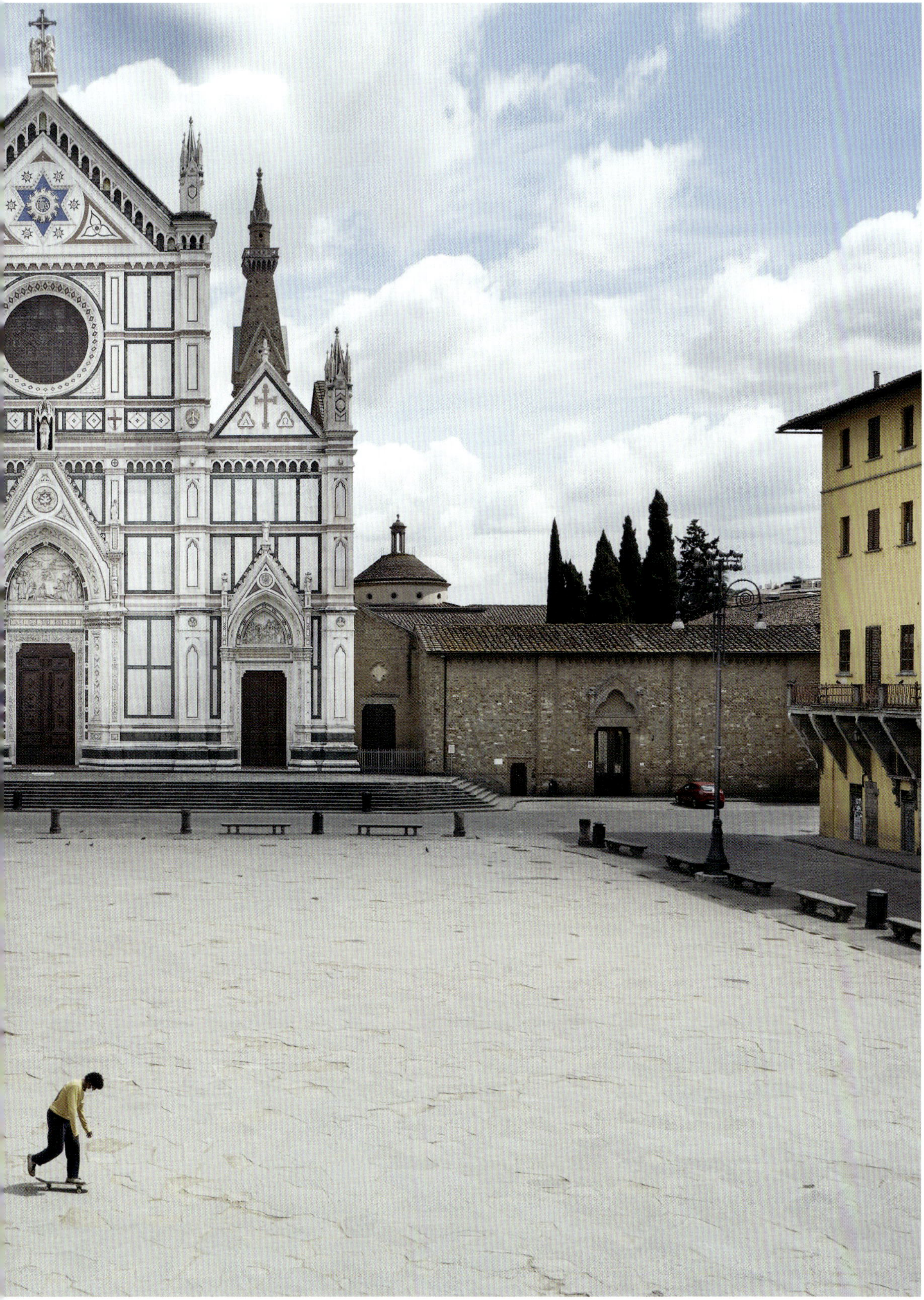

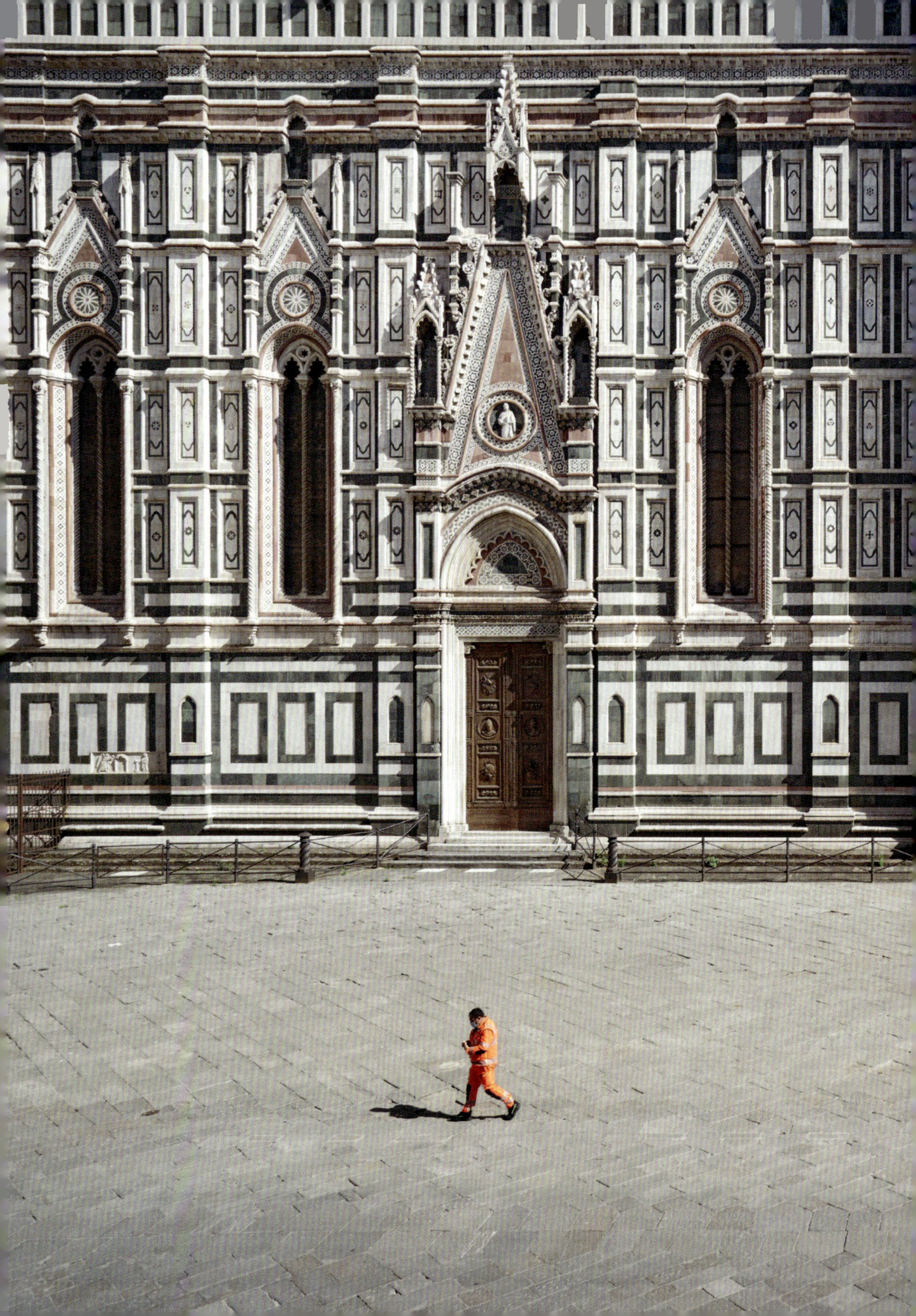

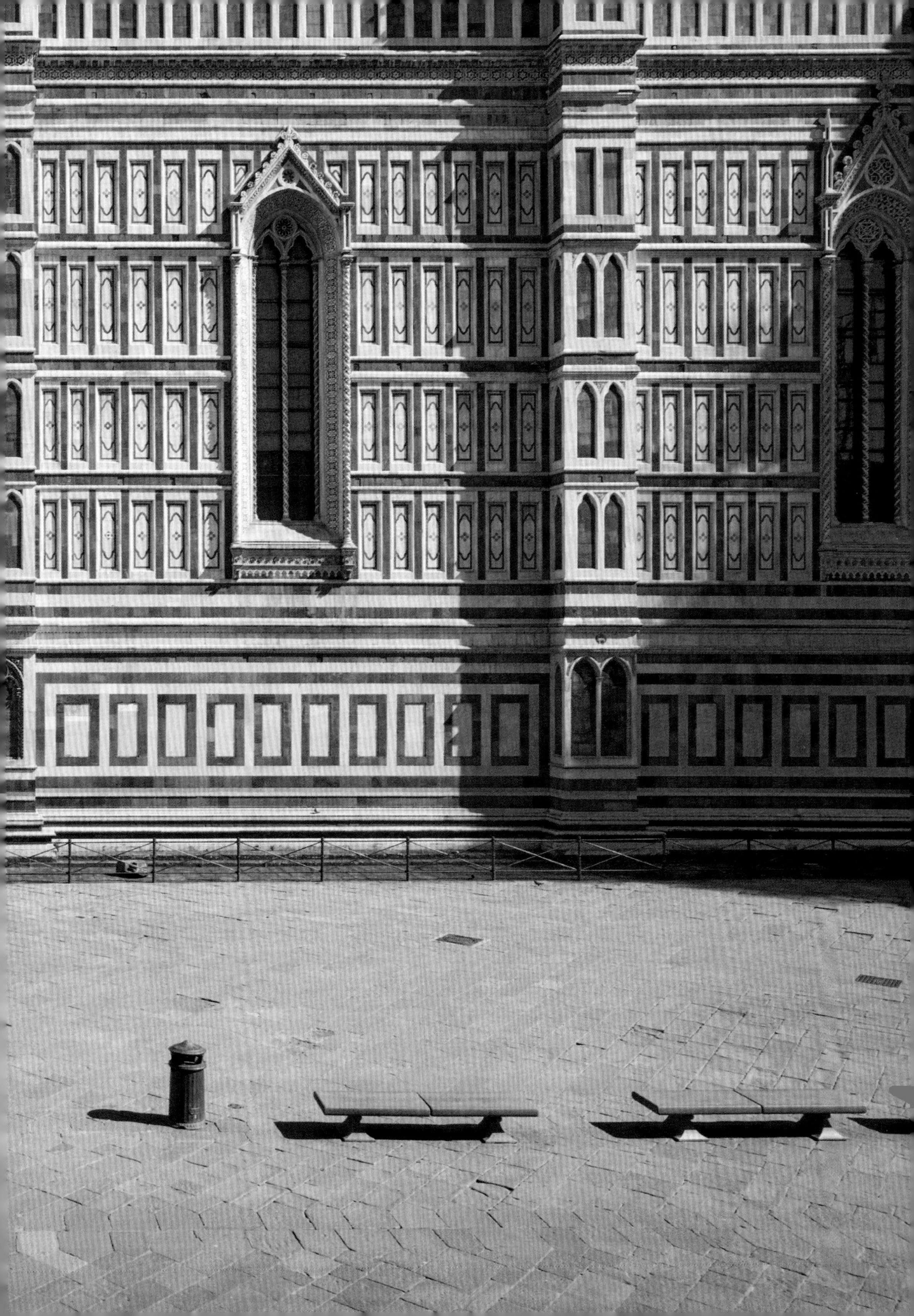

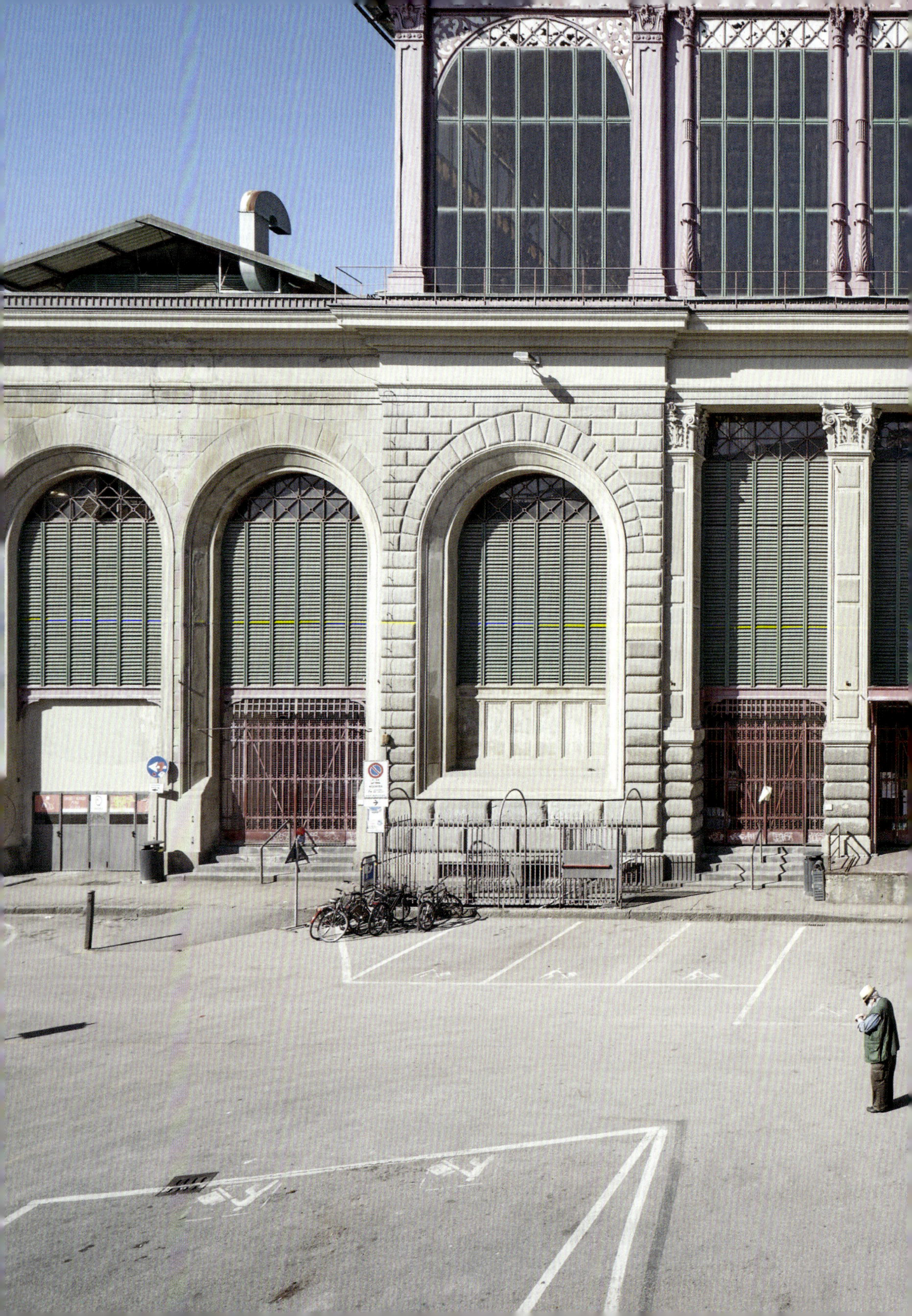

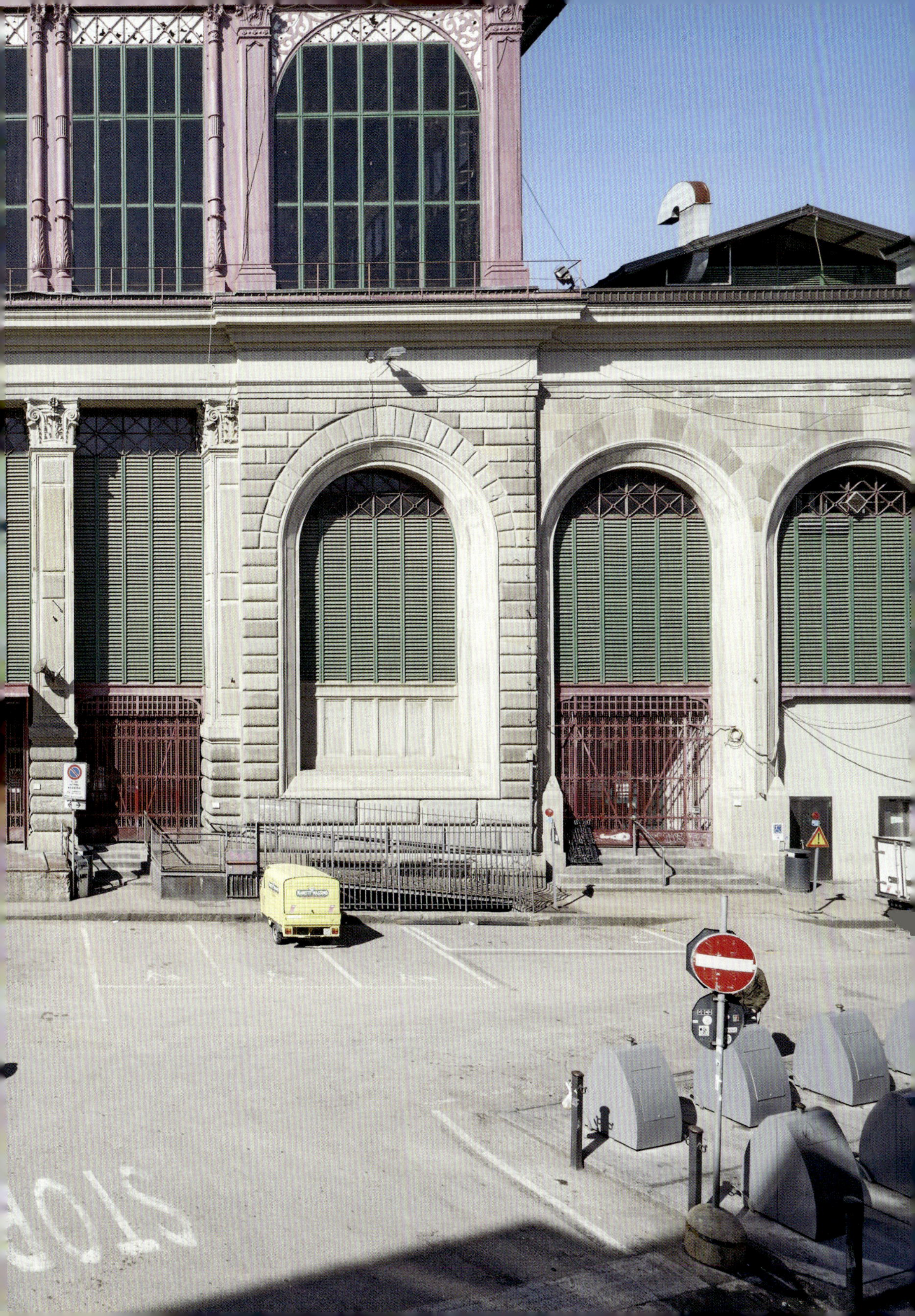

STOP

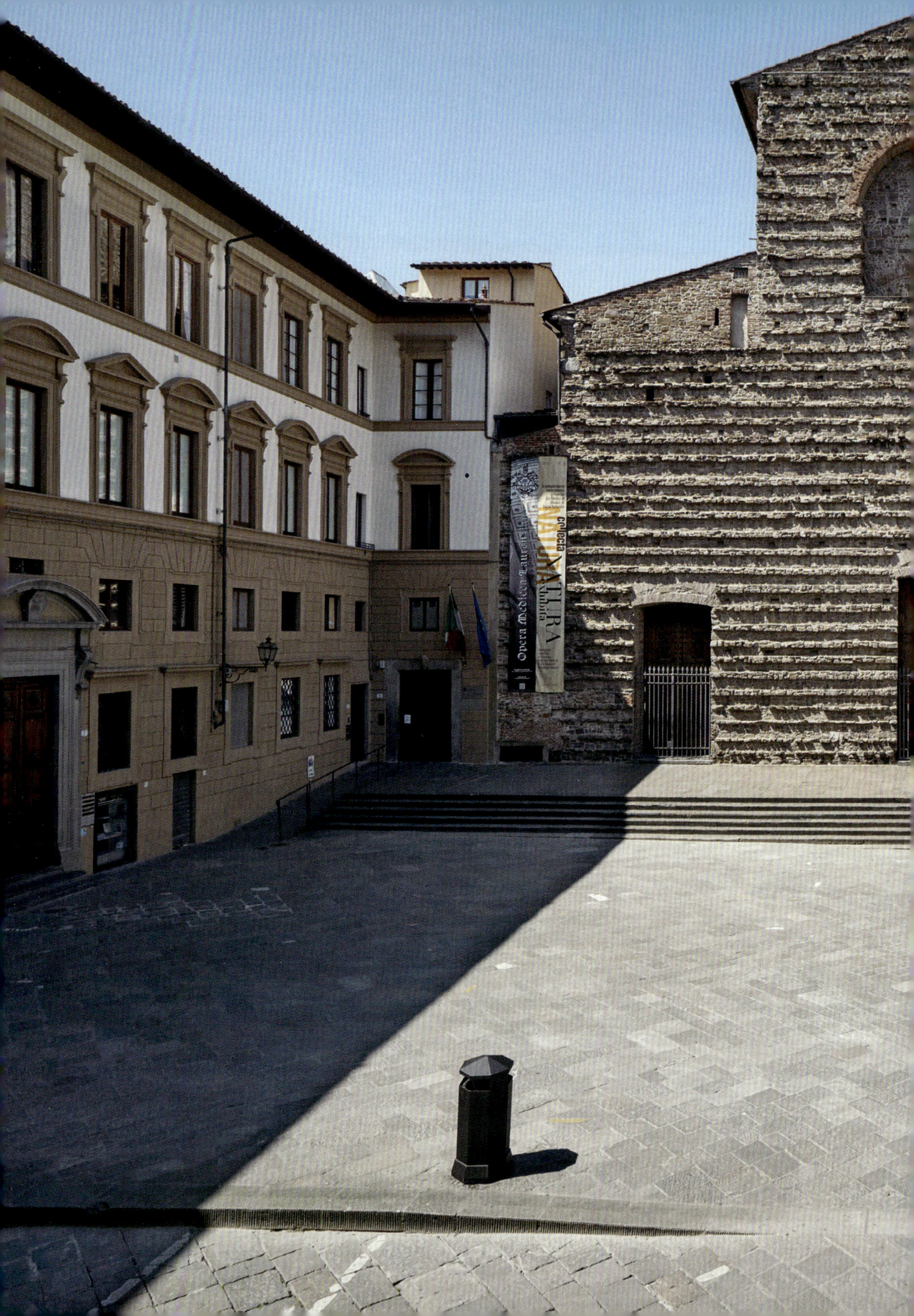
collecta
Opera Medicea

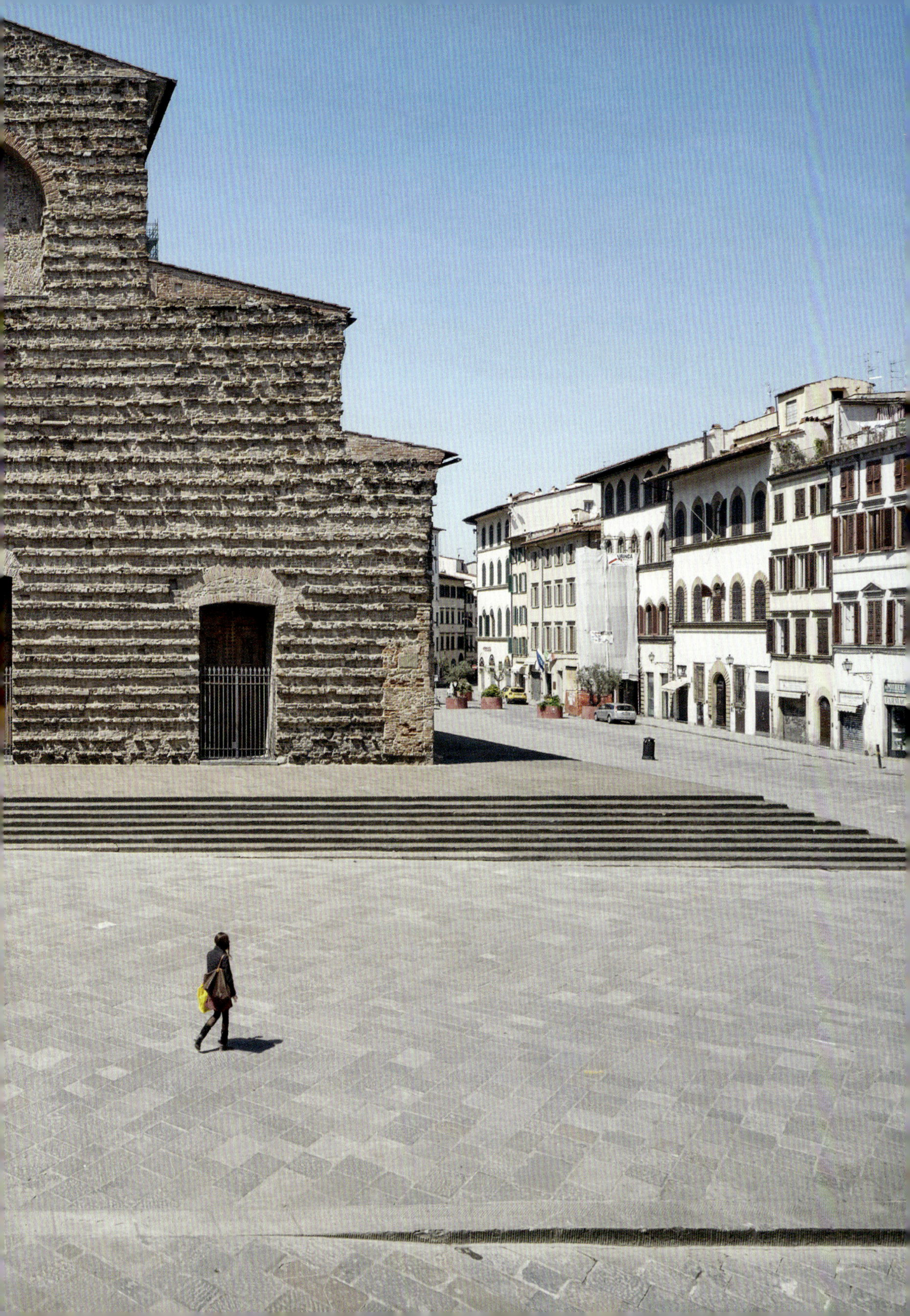

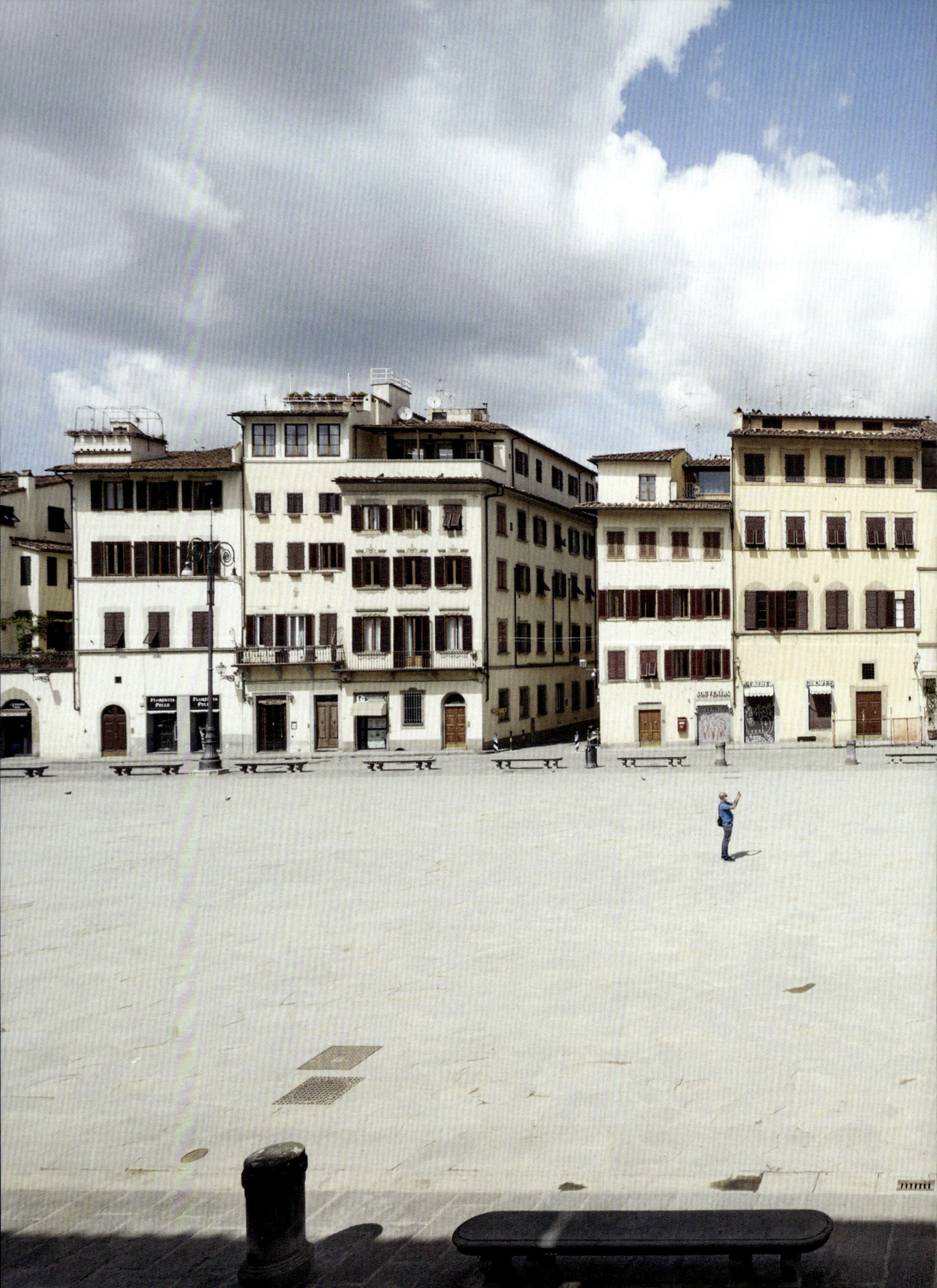
FLORENTIA PELLE
SOUVENIRS
GLOVES

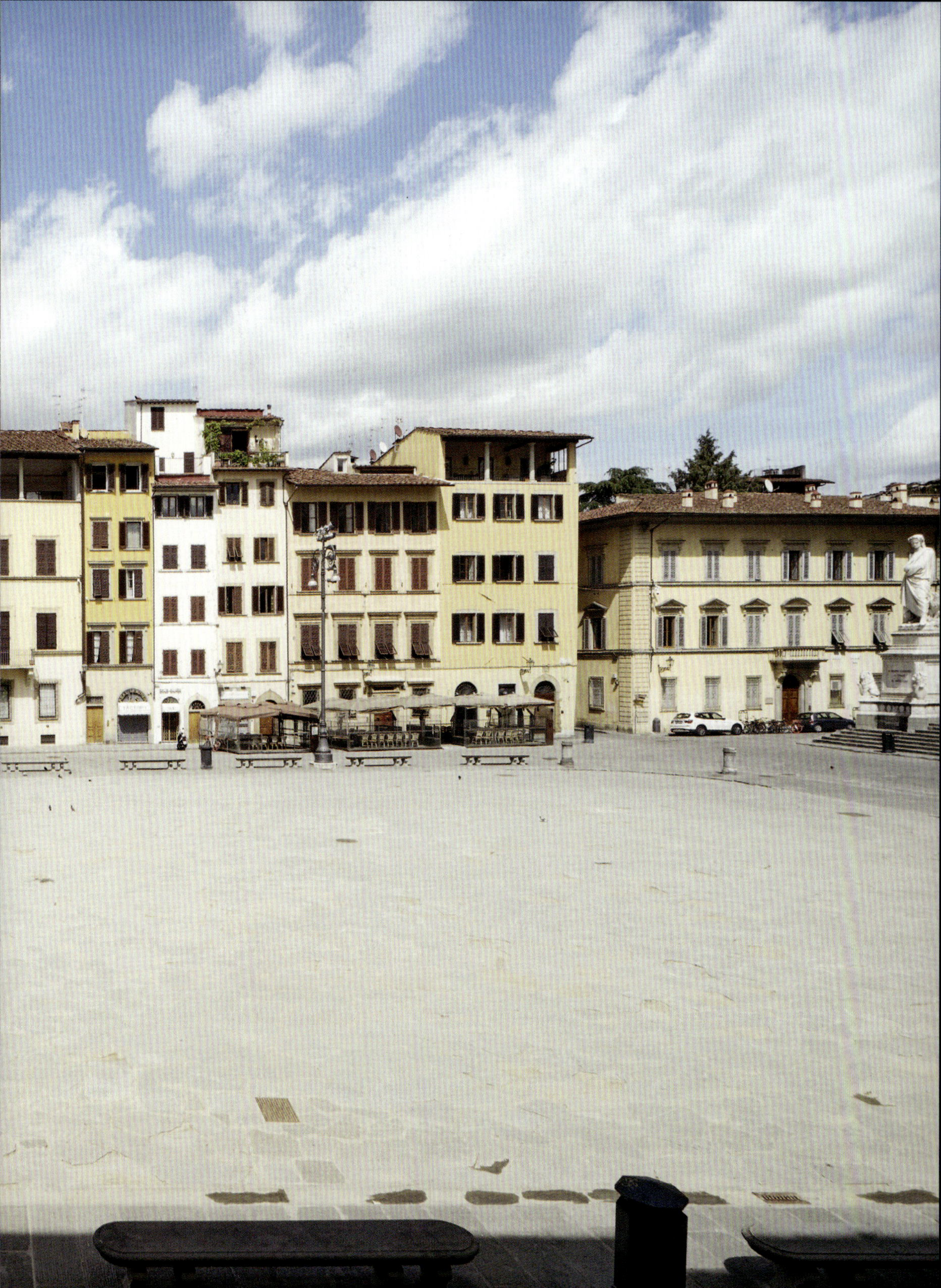

Paolo Woods & Gabriele Galimberti, Italy
Locked in Beauty

Italy's museums are closed and deserted. What do these museums look like emptied of visitors? How do the artworks fare without those that appreciate them? We had the unique opportunity to be the only visitors allowed in some of the most iconic museums in Italy. We have tried to pull them out from the darkness they are in now and reinvent them through light. The museums are haunted by the shadows of those that visited them. Italy has an immense artistic and monumental heritage, which, through tourism, is one of the main economic resources of the country. The lockdown has brought the tourism industry to a complete and painful halt. In the coming months the museums will slowly start to reopen and we thought this would be a good way to tell their story during the lockdown. We traveled the country from north to south and had the privileged to enter classics like The National Archaeological Museum of Naples with its collections of Egyptian, Greek and ancient Roman art. We discovered the precious artistic world of the Gallerie d'Italia in Milan, Naples and Vicenza. We spent hours in the shadow of Michelangelo's *David* at the Academia in Florence and let ourselves be illuminated by the whiteness of Canova's marble. Finding beauty in places that are now closed but will be accessible again and documenting what they look like devoid of visitors is a way to deal with the scope of this crisis and its implications. It is time to go back to contemplating art because it has an urgent message for all of us. Possibly without pushing through a crowd but still in the company of our renewed fellow humans.

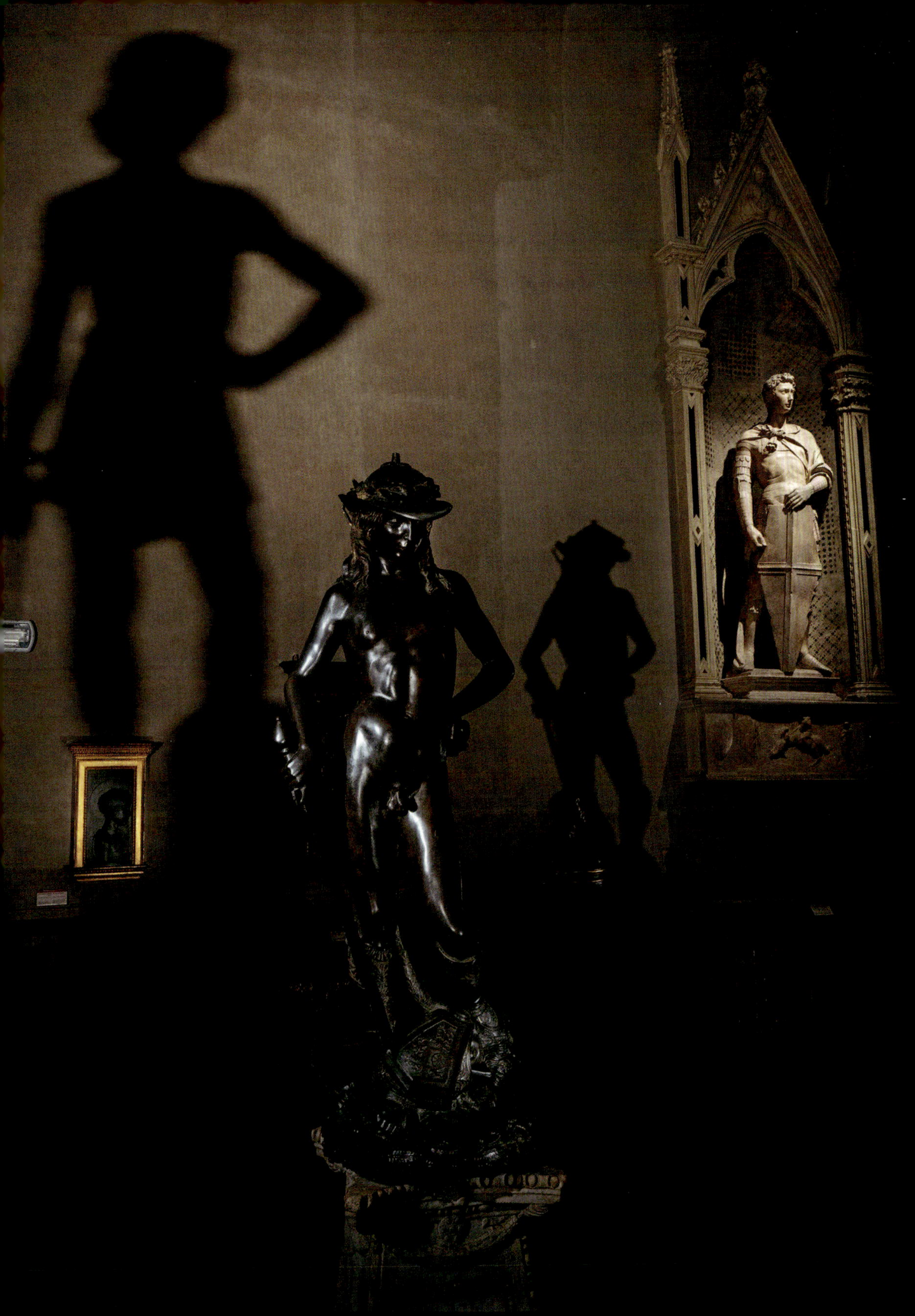

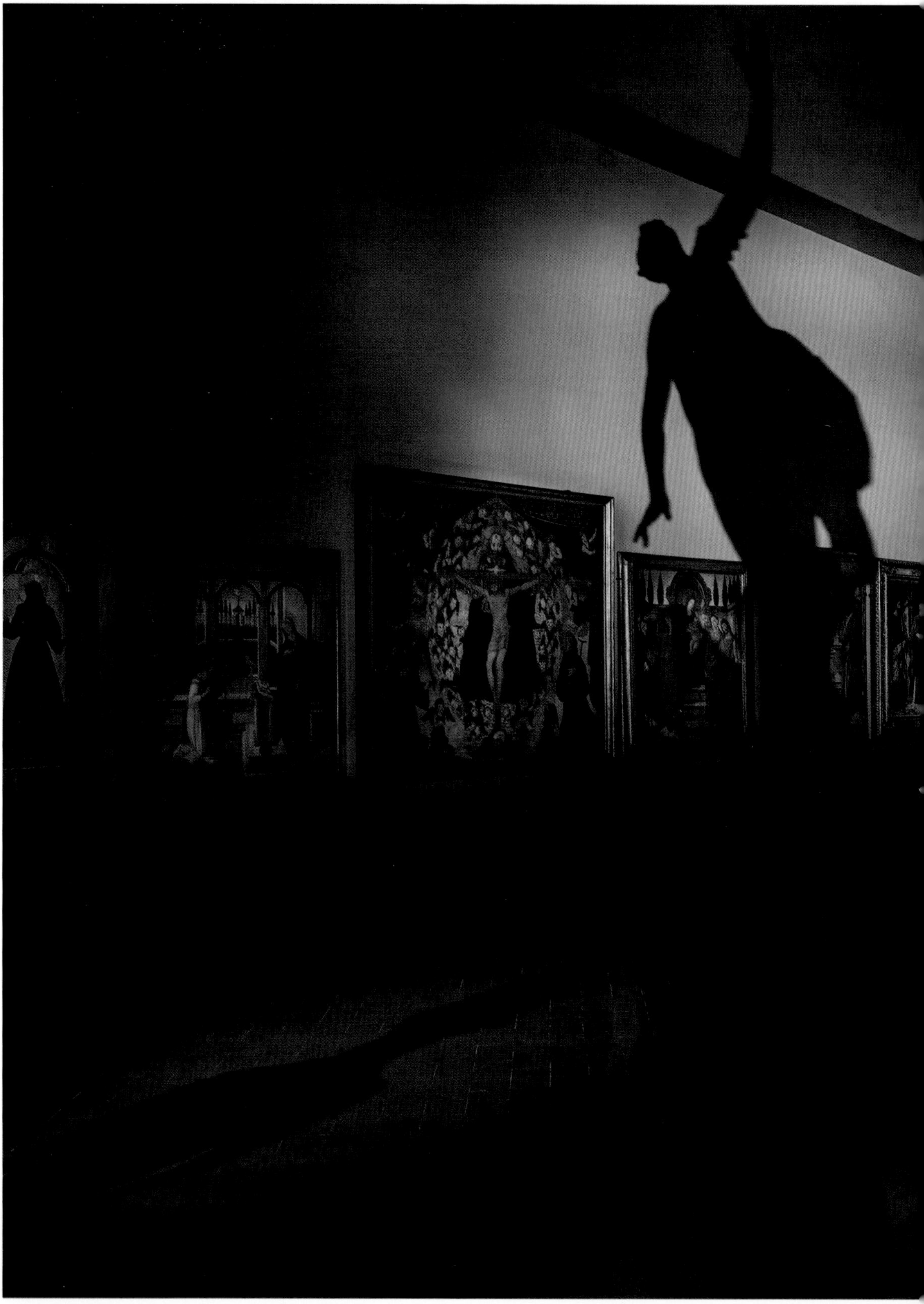

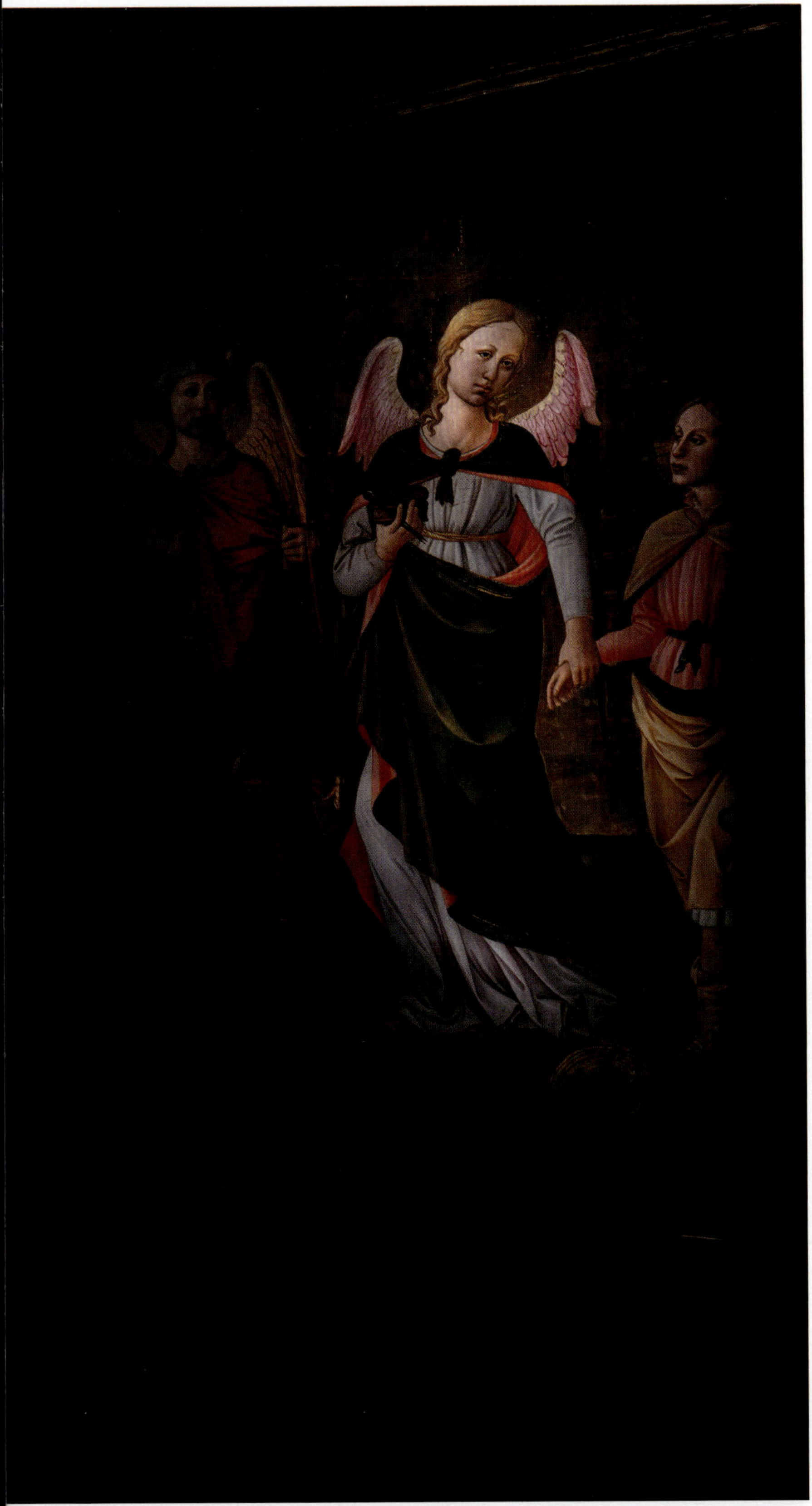

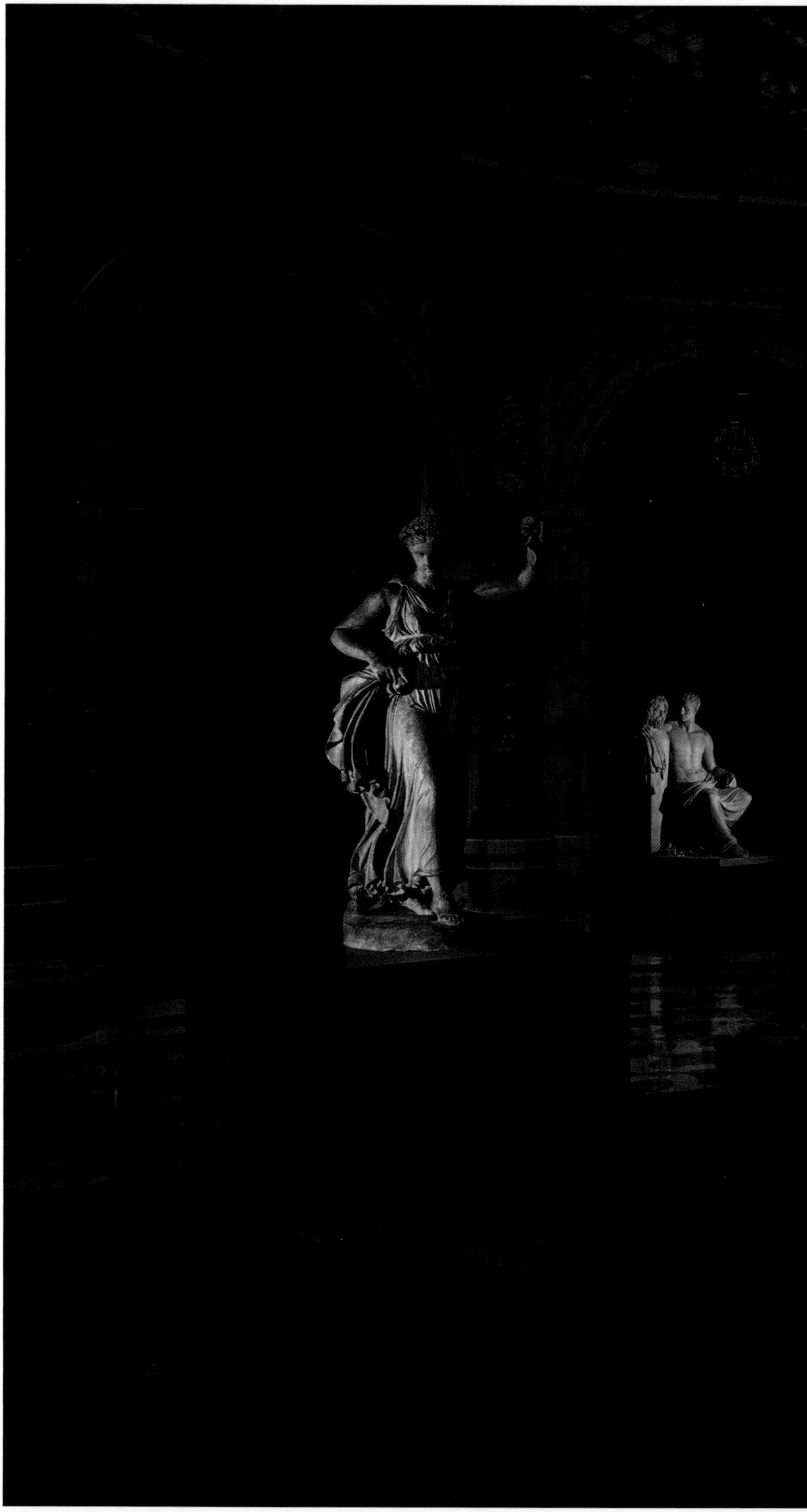

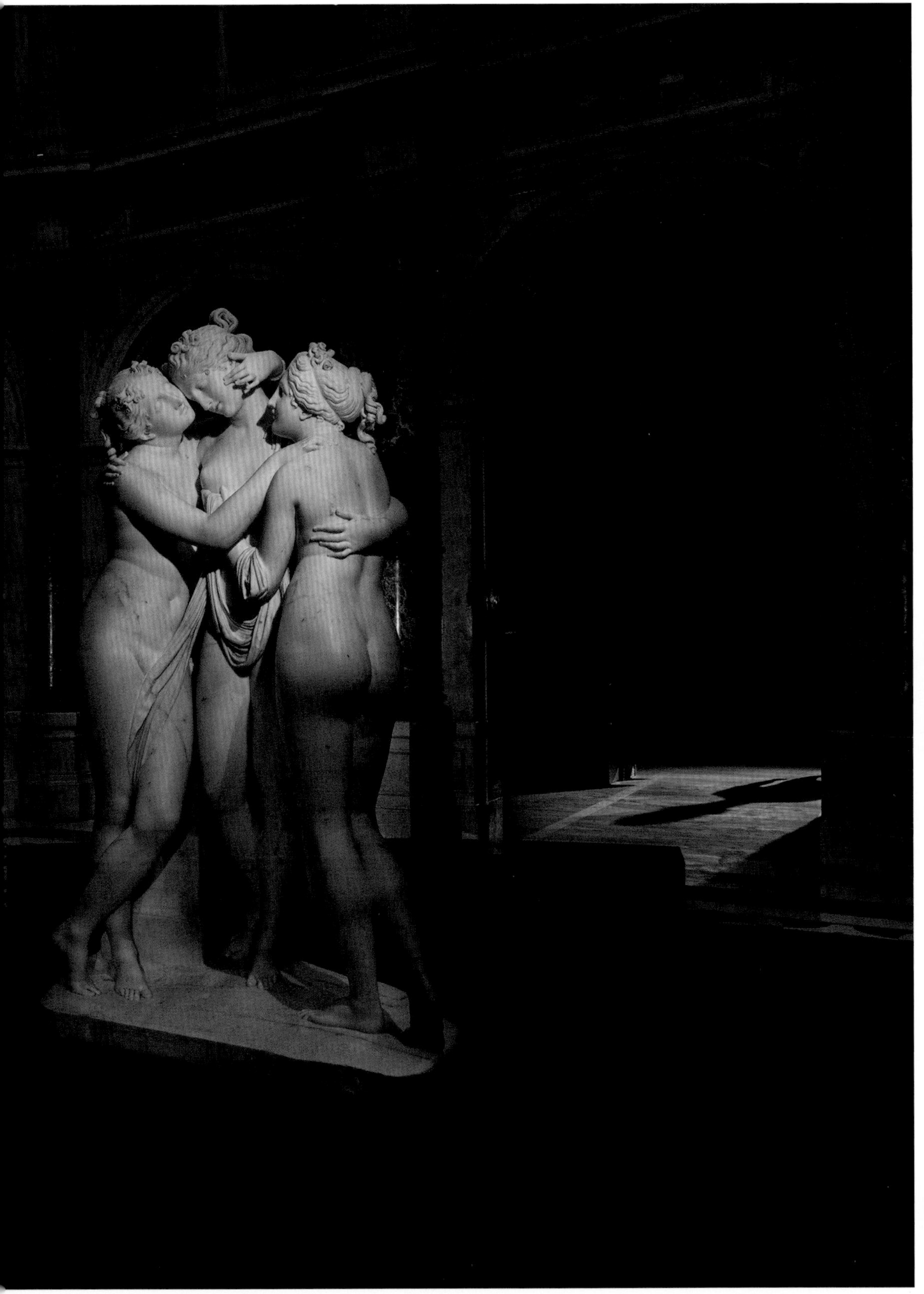

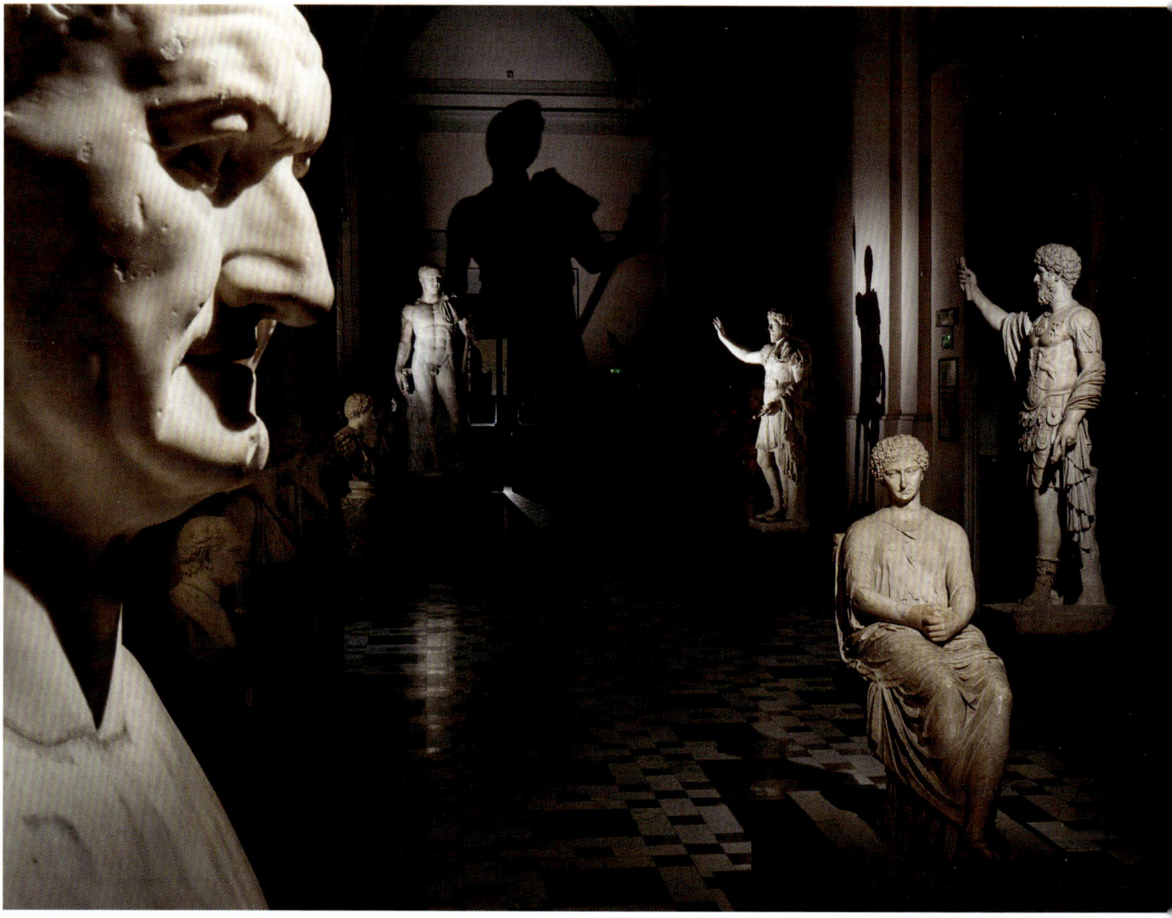

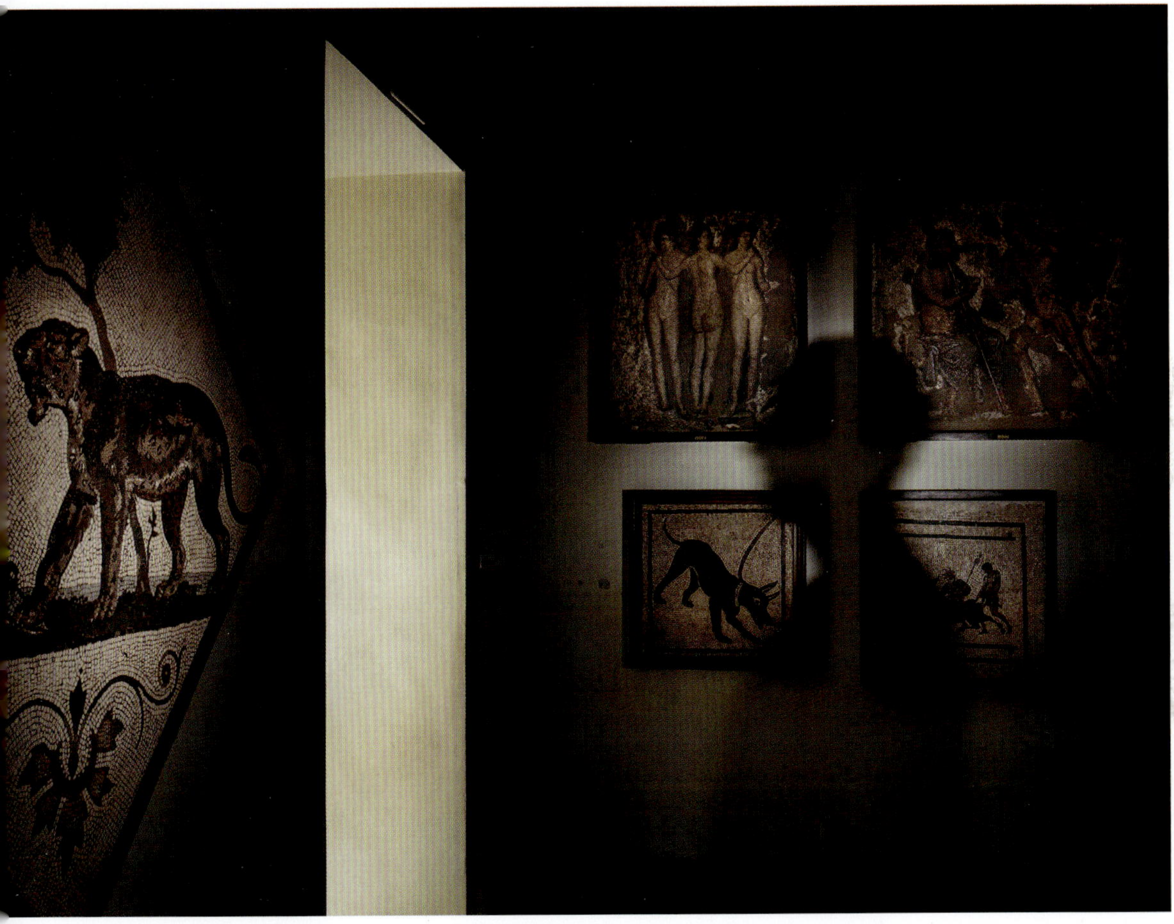

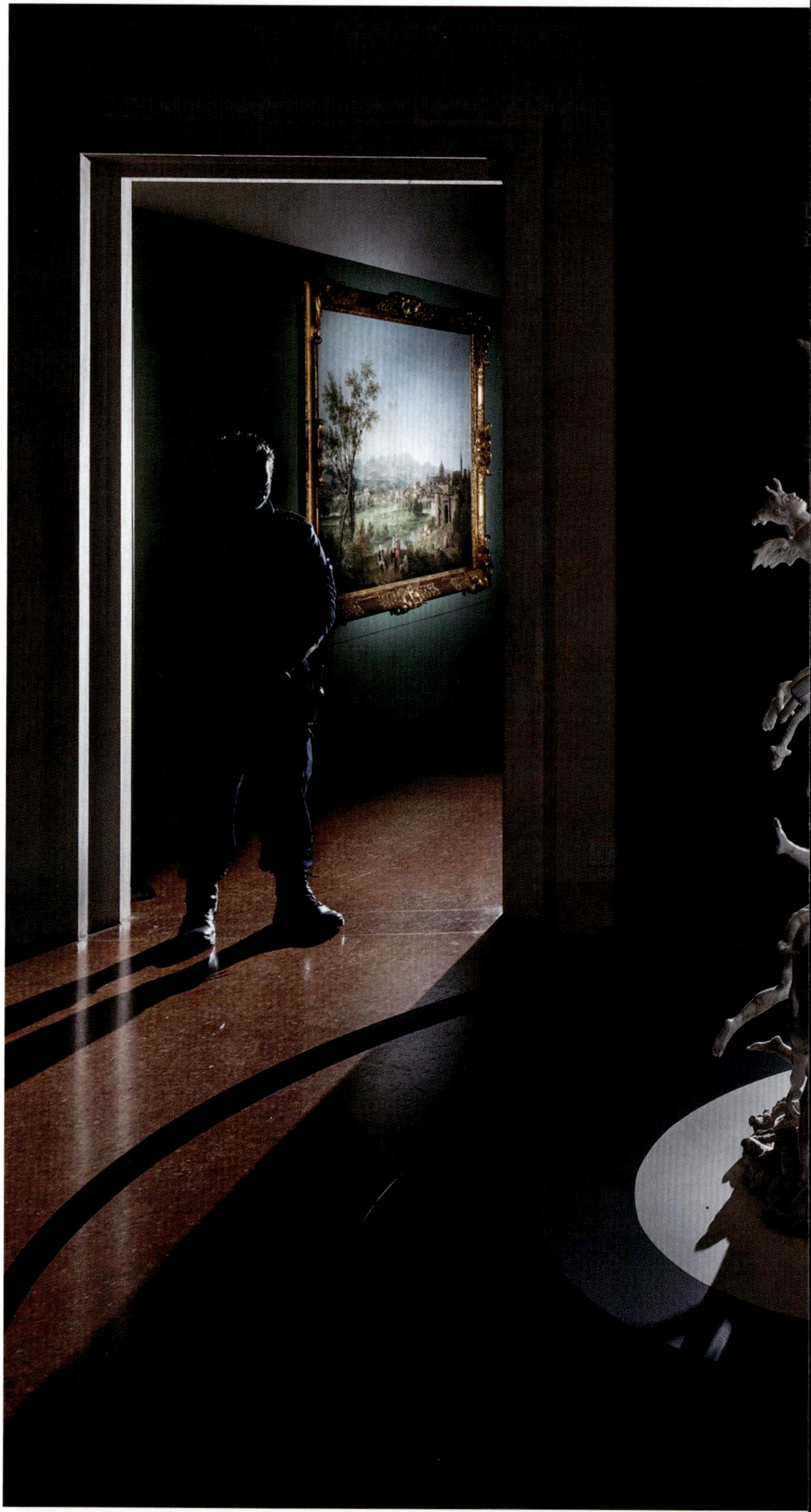

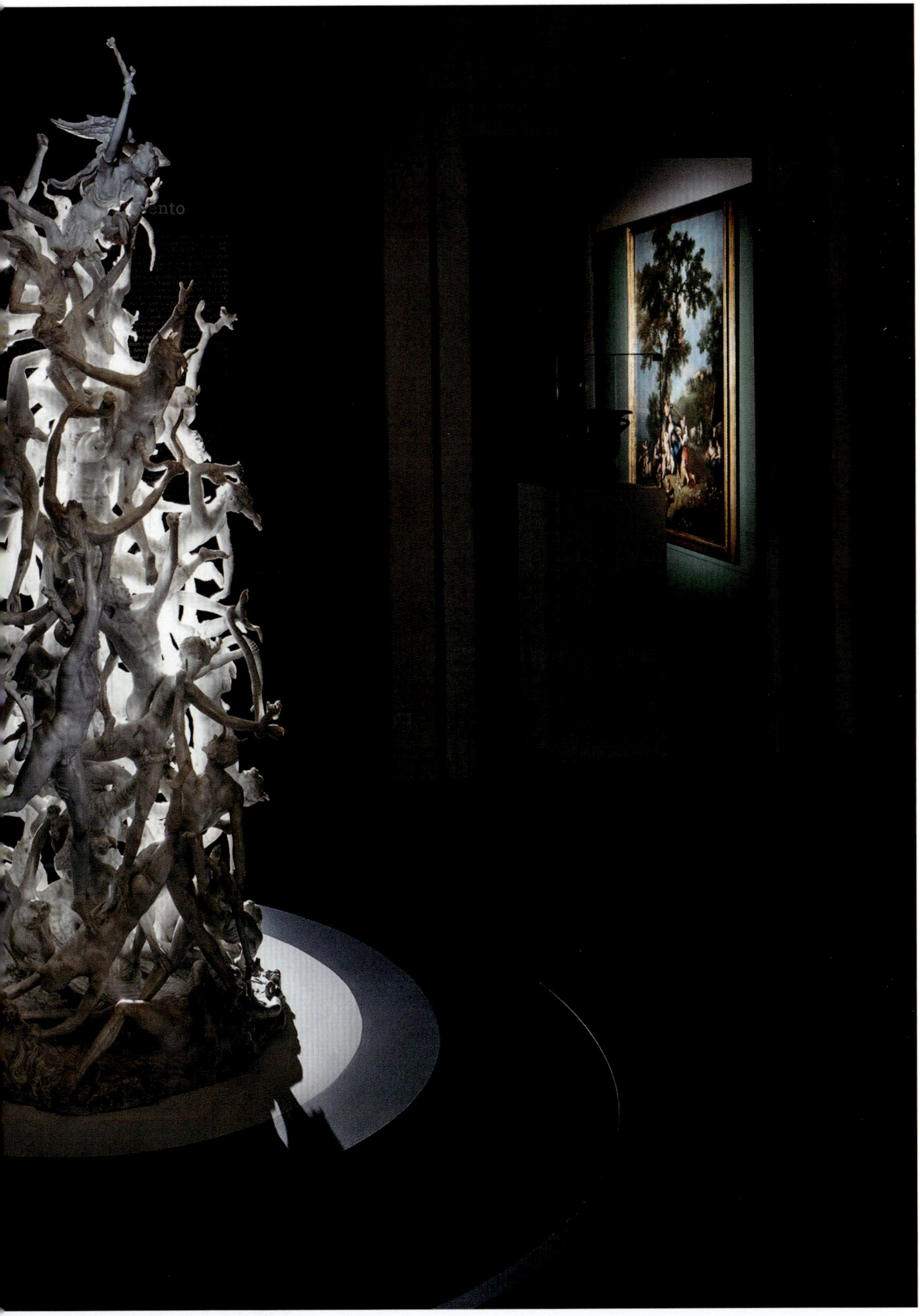

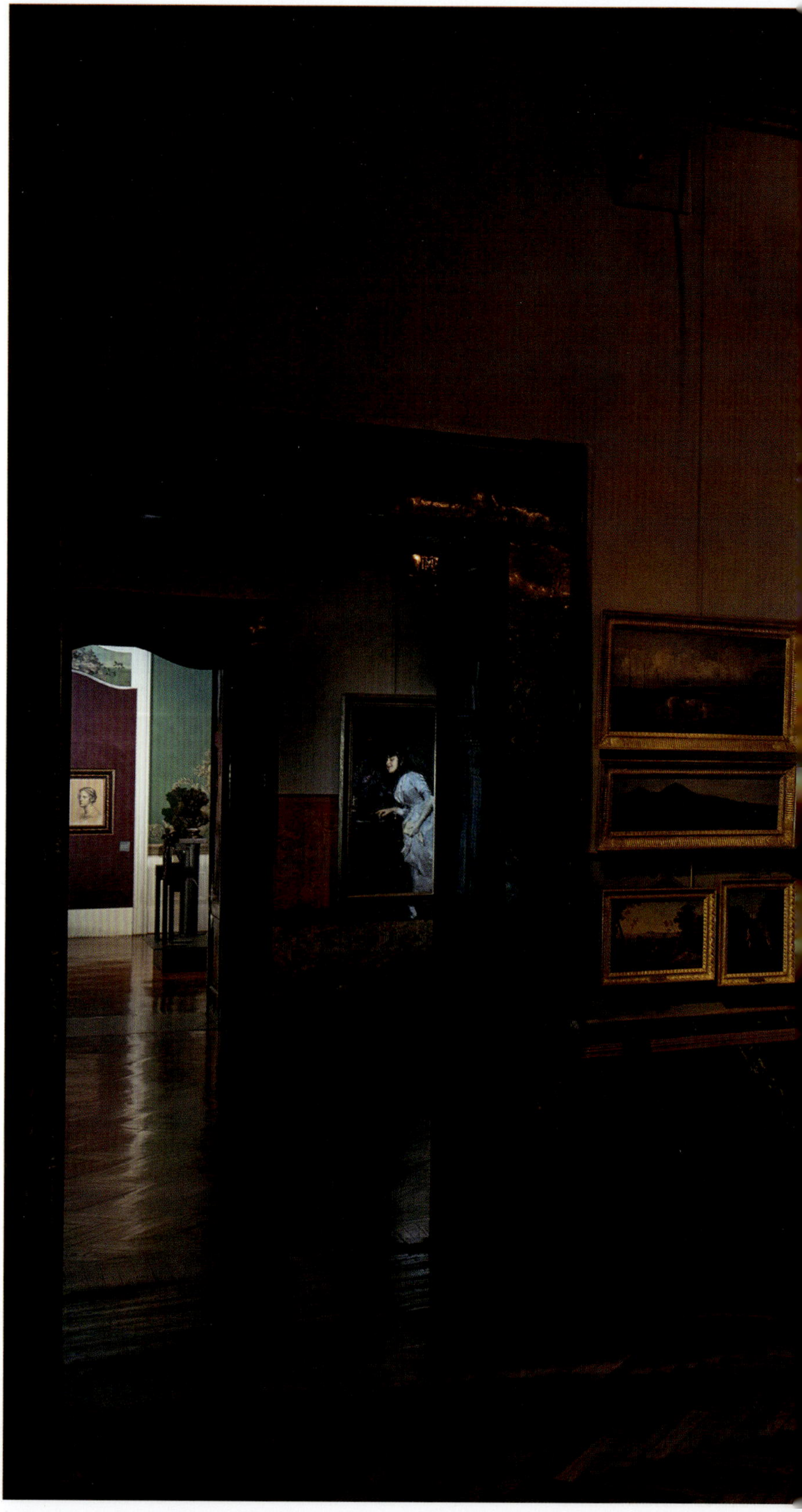

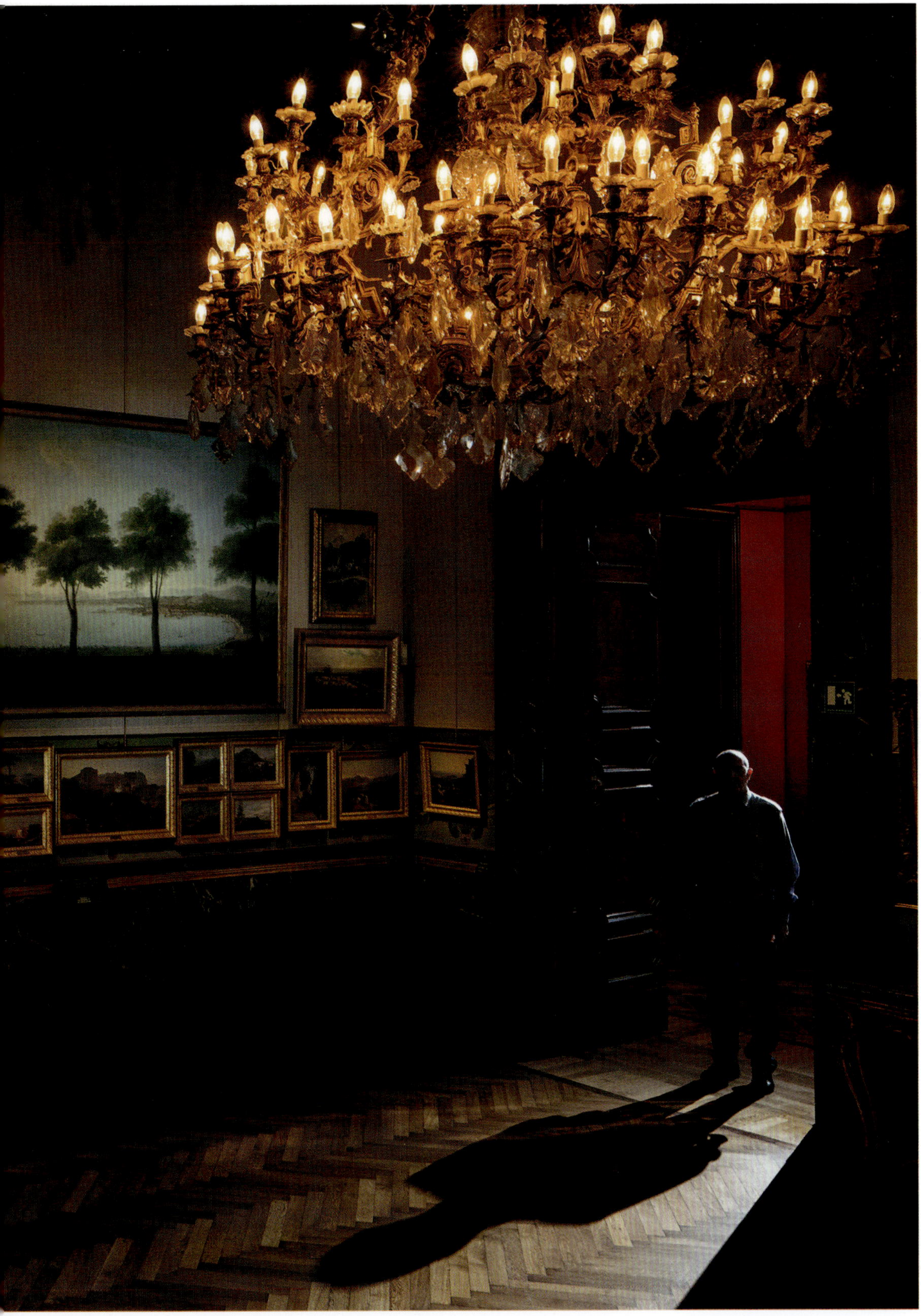

Daniele Ratti, Italy
Next Stop

Massimo Razzi

"I had to shoot a reportage on some buildings in different parts of Italy for a client, when the COVID-19 lockdown was enforced. I realised that I was one of the few who could circulate on deserted highways and that I had a unique opportunity. The motorway service stations appeared to me like cathedrals in the desert, like those ranches lost in the middle of nowhere on the great American plains that seem to be waiting for someone who hardly ever passes. And I started taking pictures of them."
This is how Daniele Ratti explains the genesis of his project on the Italian motorway service stations. For nine days he drove on the motorways that connect South to North, East to West, coming across very few cars. "Between Rome and Florence, — he says — I stopped at one point... For ten minutes no one drove by and I had time to cross the motorway on foot, walking slowly and climbing over the guardrail before a truck appeared on the horizon." He has photographed about fifty motorway service stations, these "non-places" that we are used to seeing full of people and that, at the time of the coronavirus, seem to have lost their purpose.
"Yet, many of them are also beautiful. These service stations seem to regress to before they were built, like the rendition of an architect, who imagined and drew them using a soft, almost watercoloured palette."
There they are, large, useless in their often imposing shapes, mounted astride roadways where hardly anyone passes. Parking lots wait for cars that won't stop, picnic tables wait for families that won't sit down, small playgrounds would like to welcome children who aren't there. Billboards shout out pointless "Welcome".
It almost makes you think that, as for many things, after the coronavirus, they (the service stations) and we (the travellers) will look at each other differently. As if in these days we had met, as Daniele Ratti did, in an embarrassing situation of strange nudity.
"...And anyway, in those nine days of travel, I was always driving slowly. No more than 90-110 km per hour. It came naturally to me because, without the other cars, for the first time I realised what a precious observation point the highways were. And I filled my eyes with what was flowing around me at what was once human speed."
The motorway service stations must have stayed with Daniele. So much so that he tells us: "There is one on the Milano-Laghi motorway they told me about, which seems to be very interesting also from an architectural point of view. As soon as I can I want to go and shoot it". But there will be cars and it will all be too normal again.

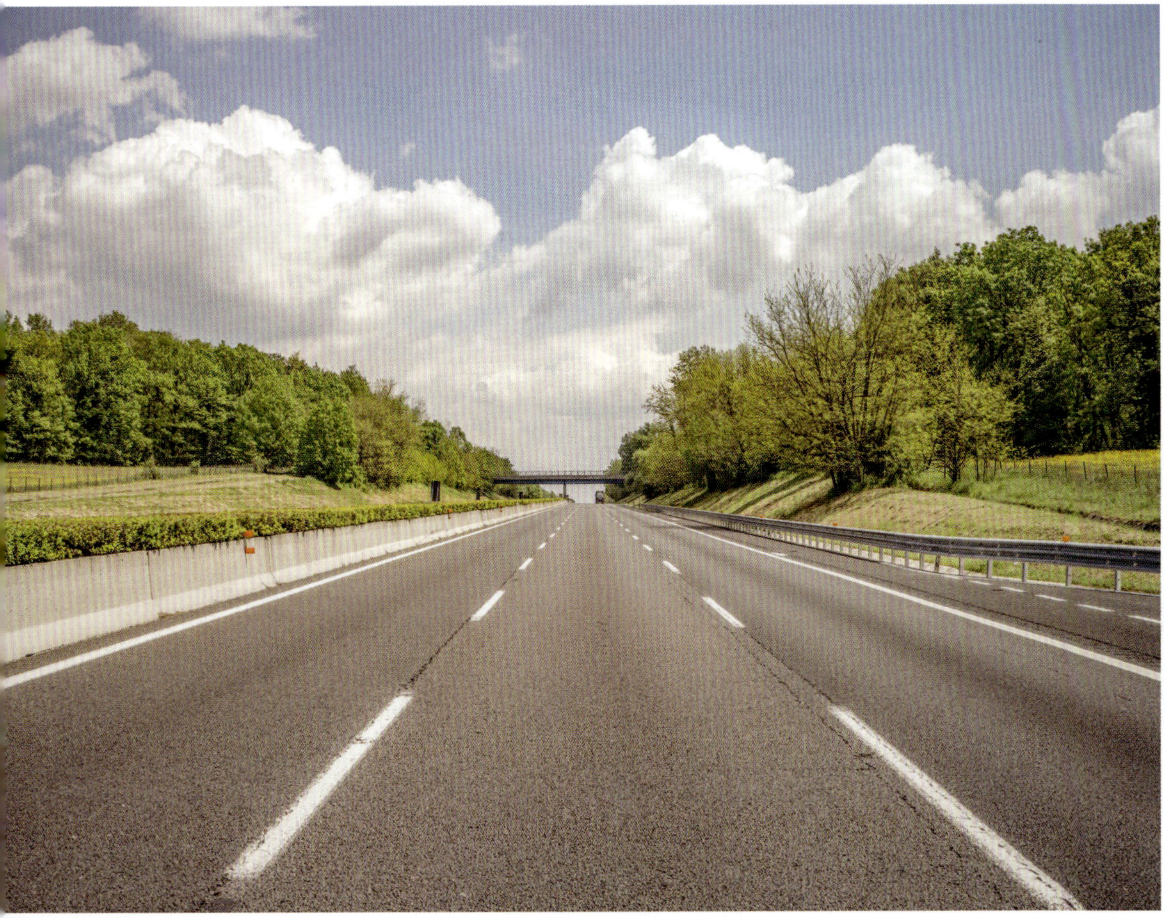

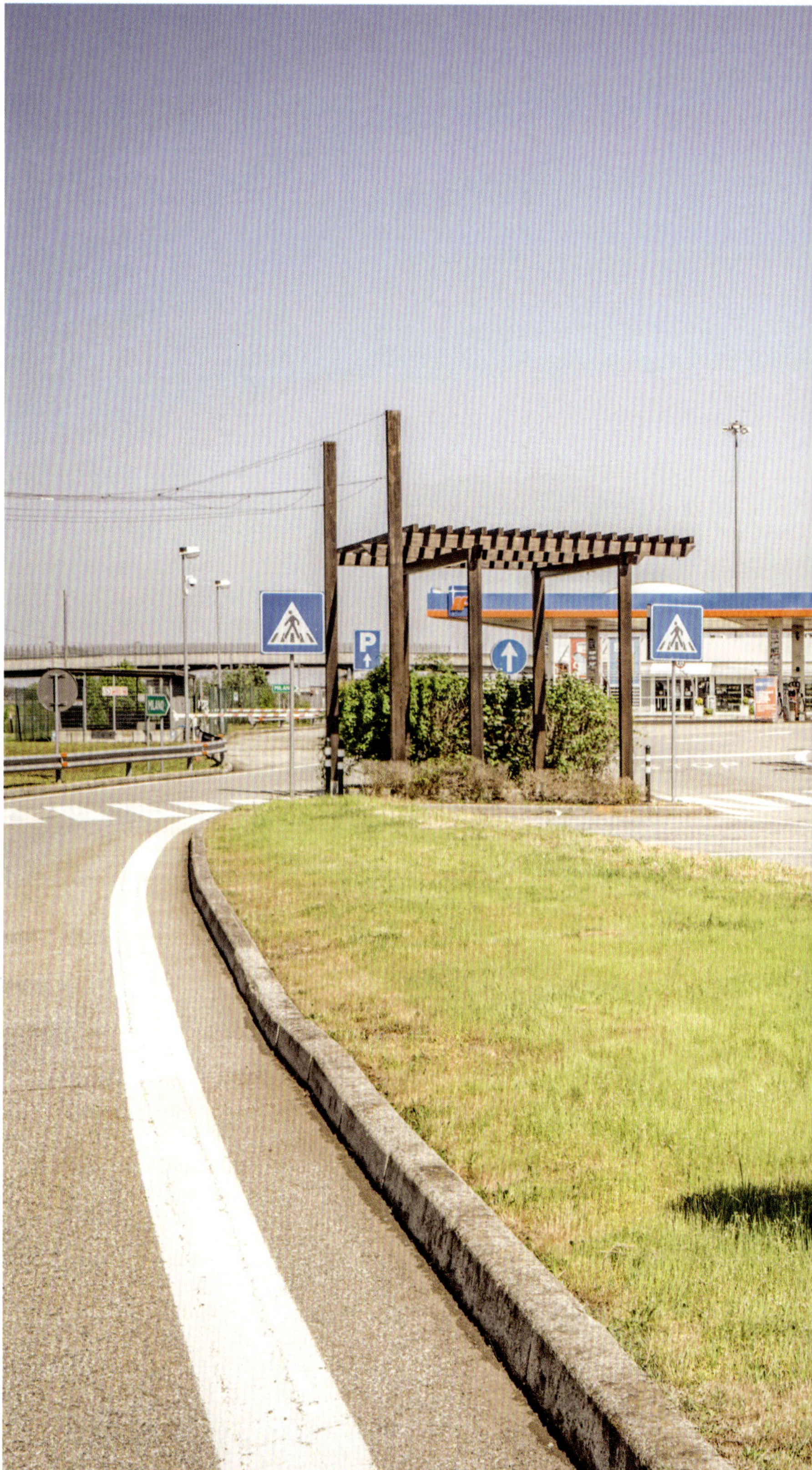

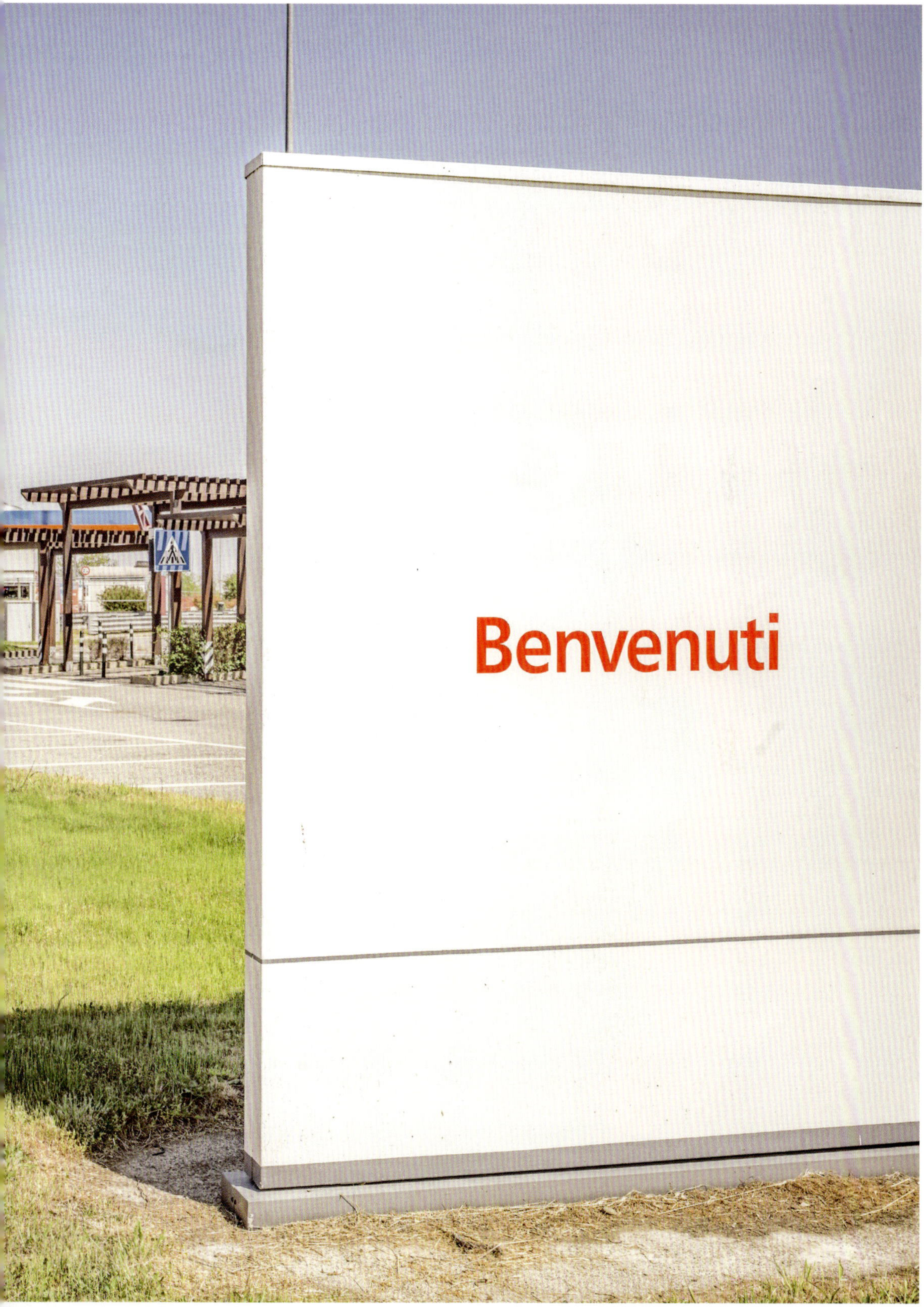
Benvenuti

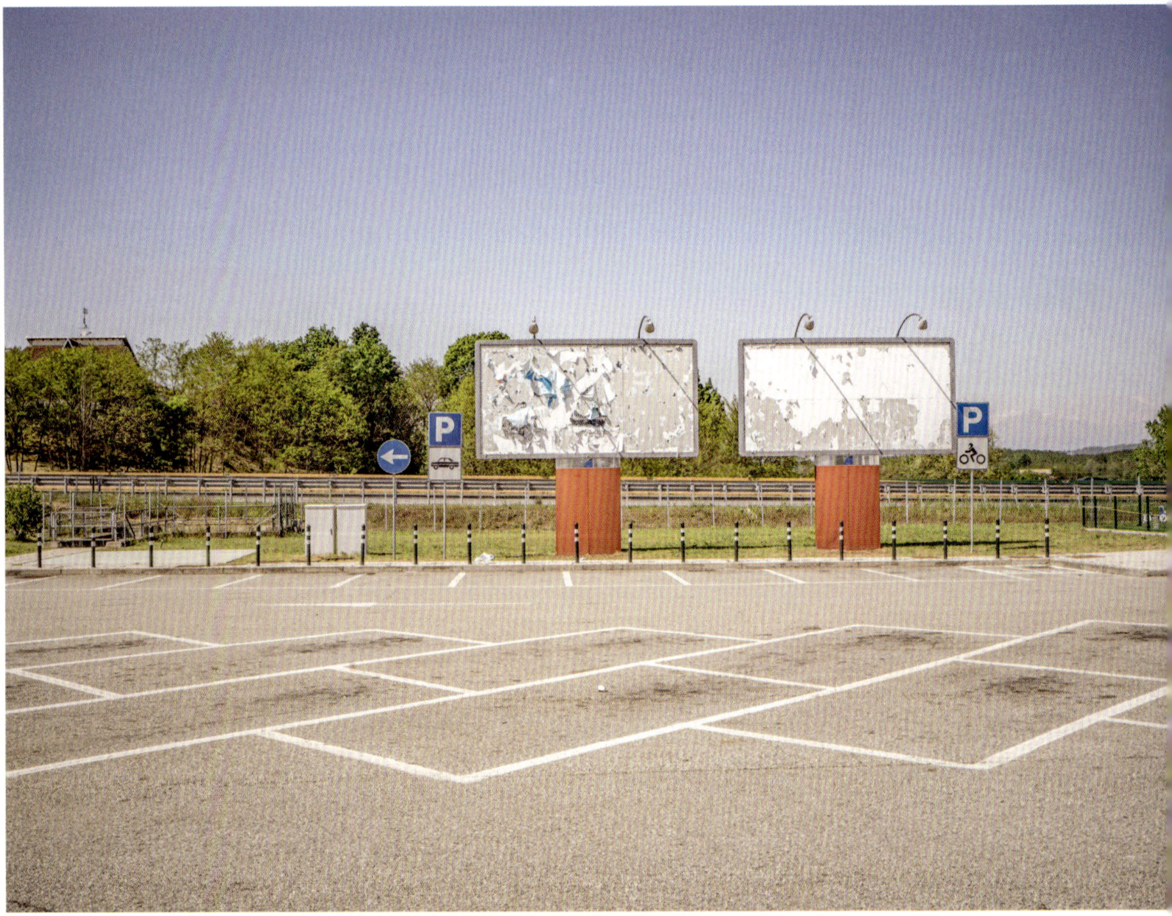
P
P

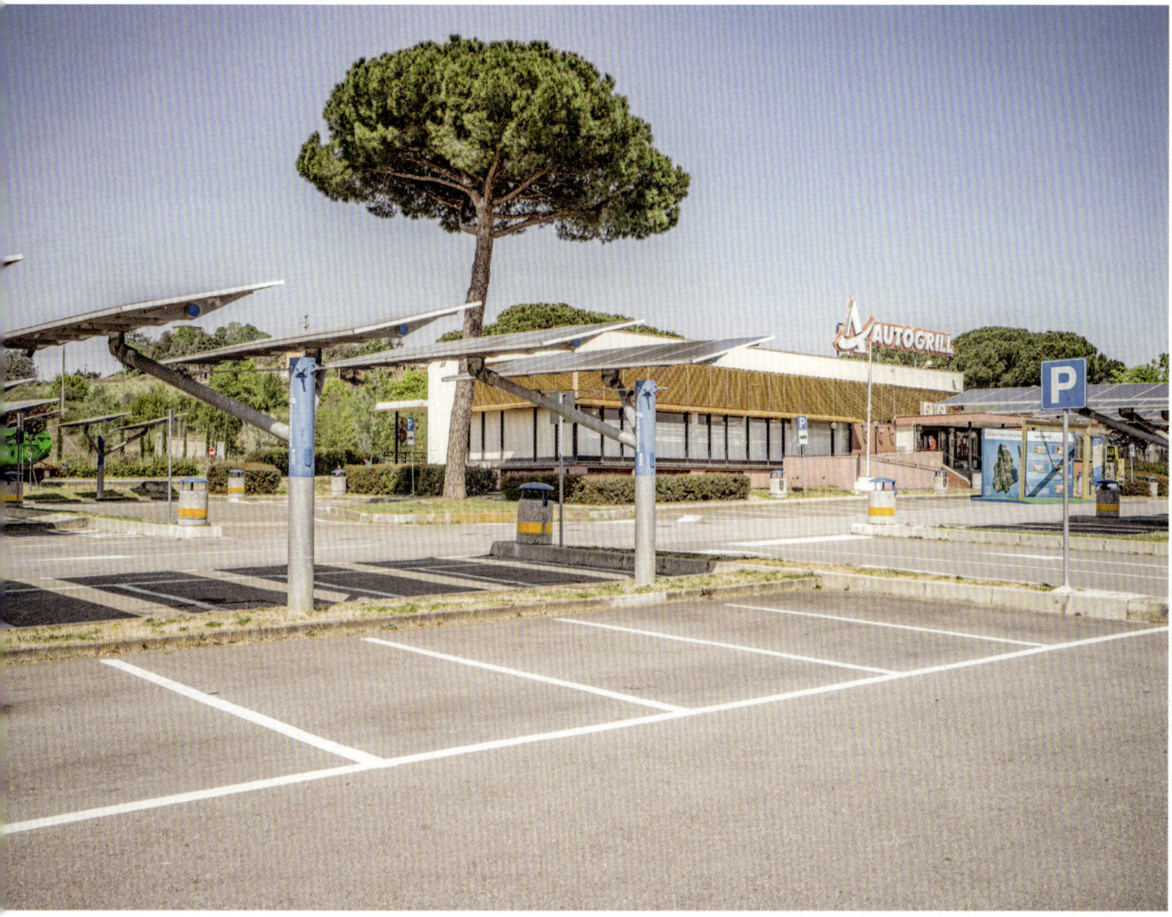
AUTOGRILL
P

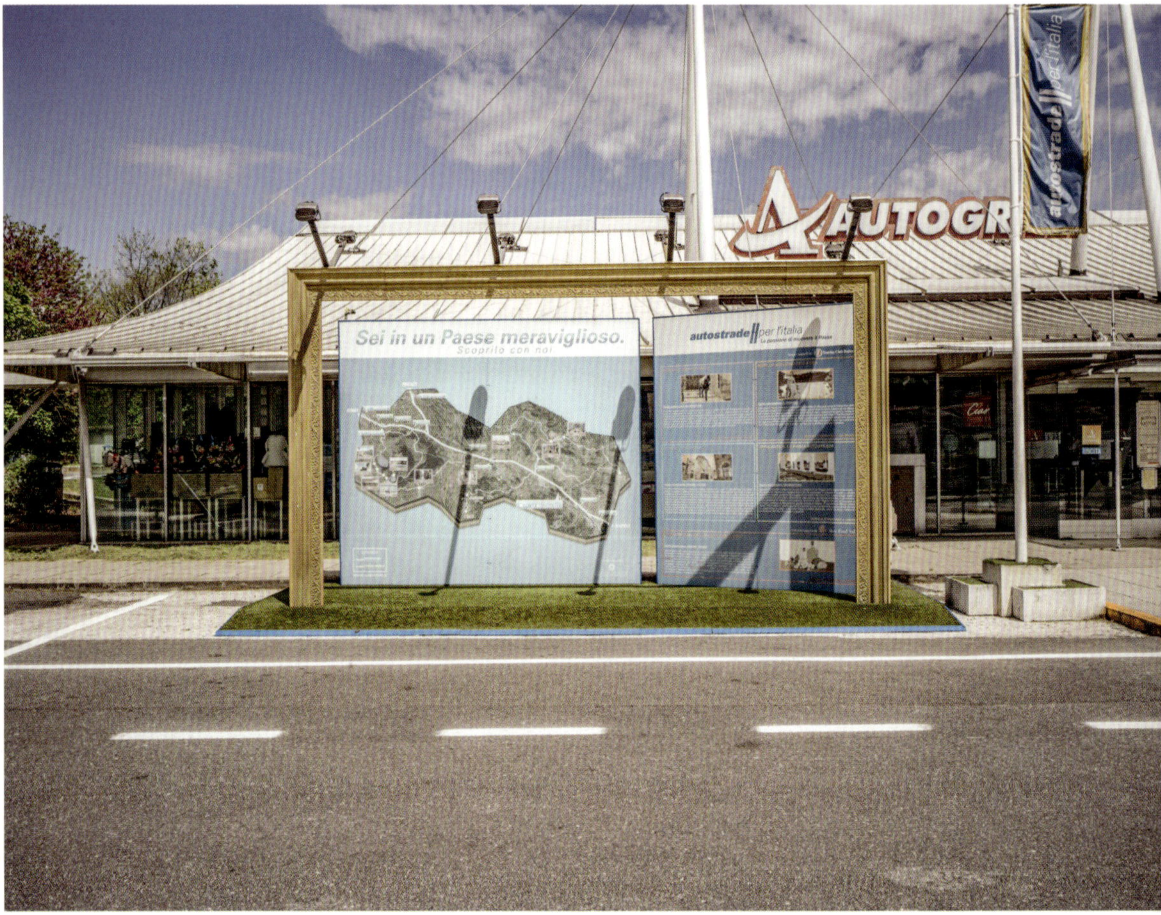
Sei in un Paese meraviglioso.
Scoprilo con noi
autostrade per l'italia

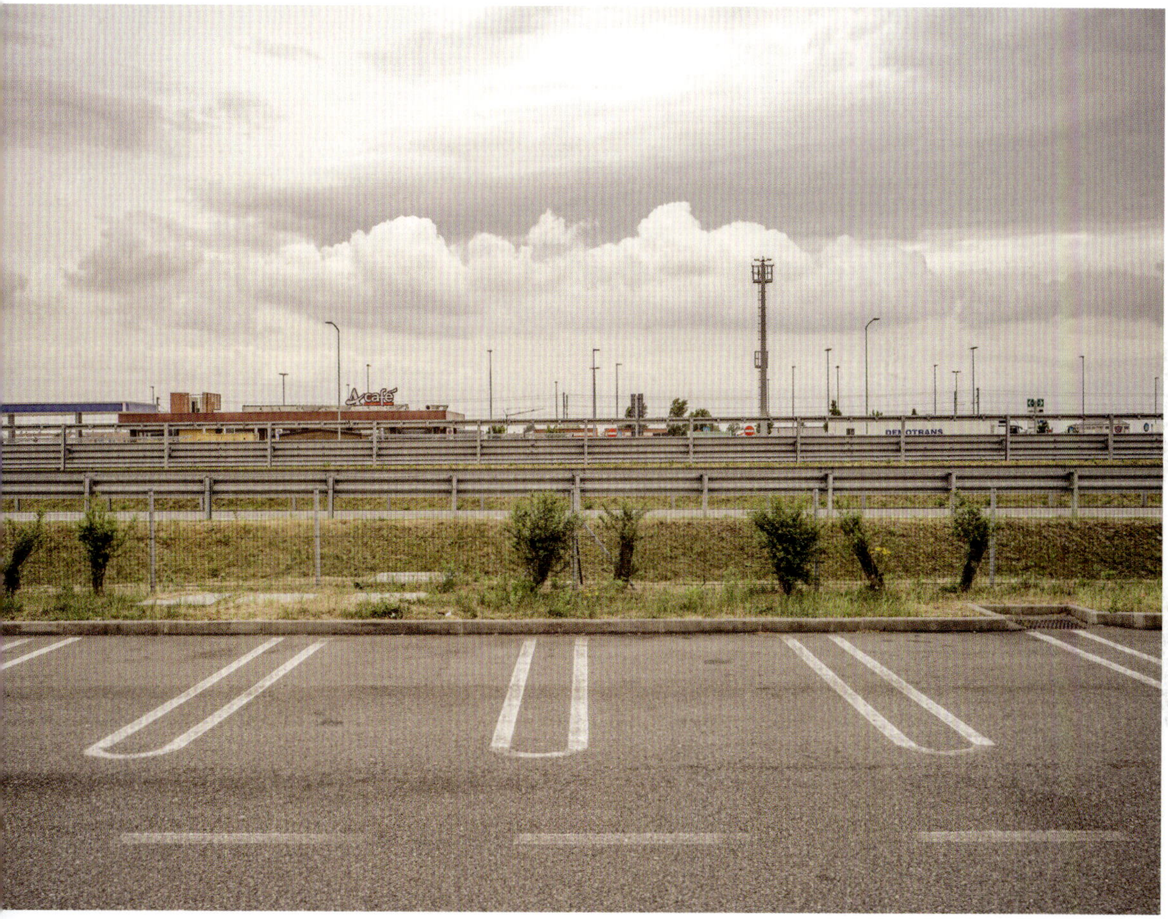
café
DEMOTRANS

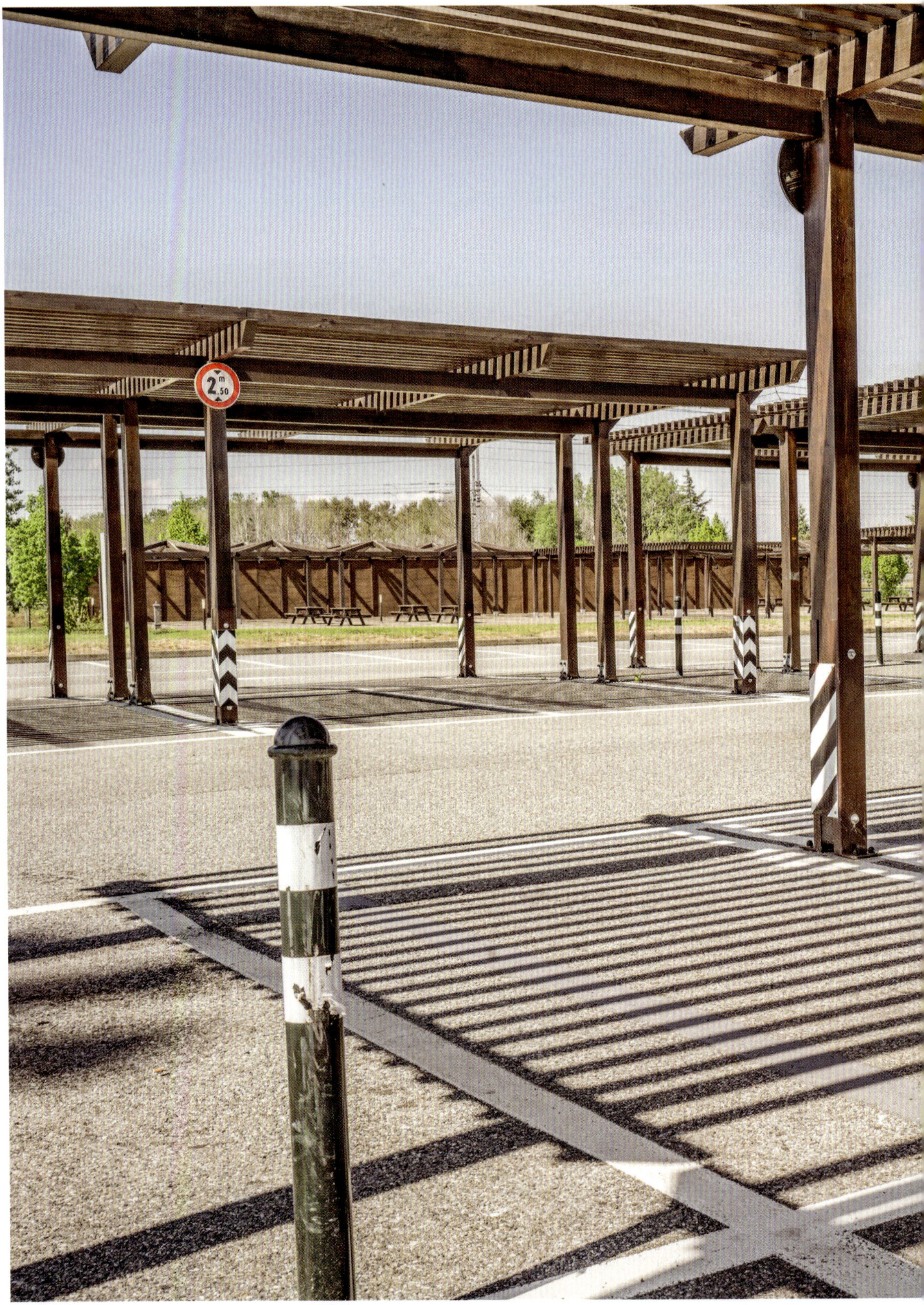
2 m 50

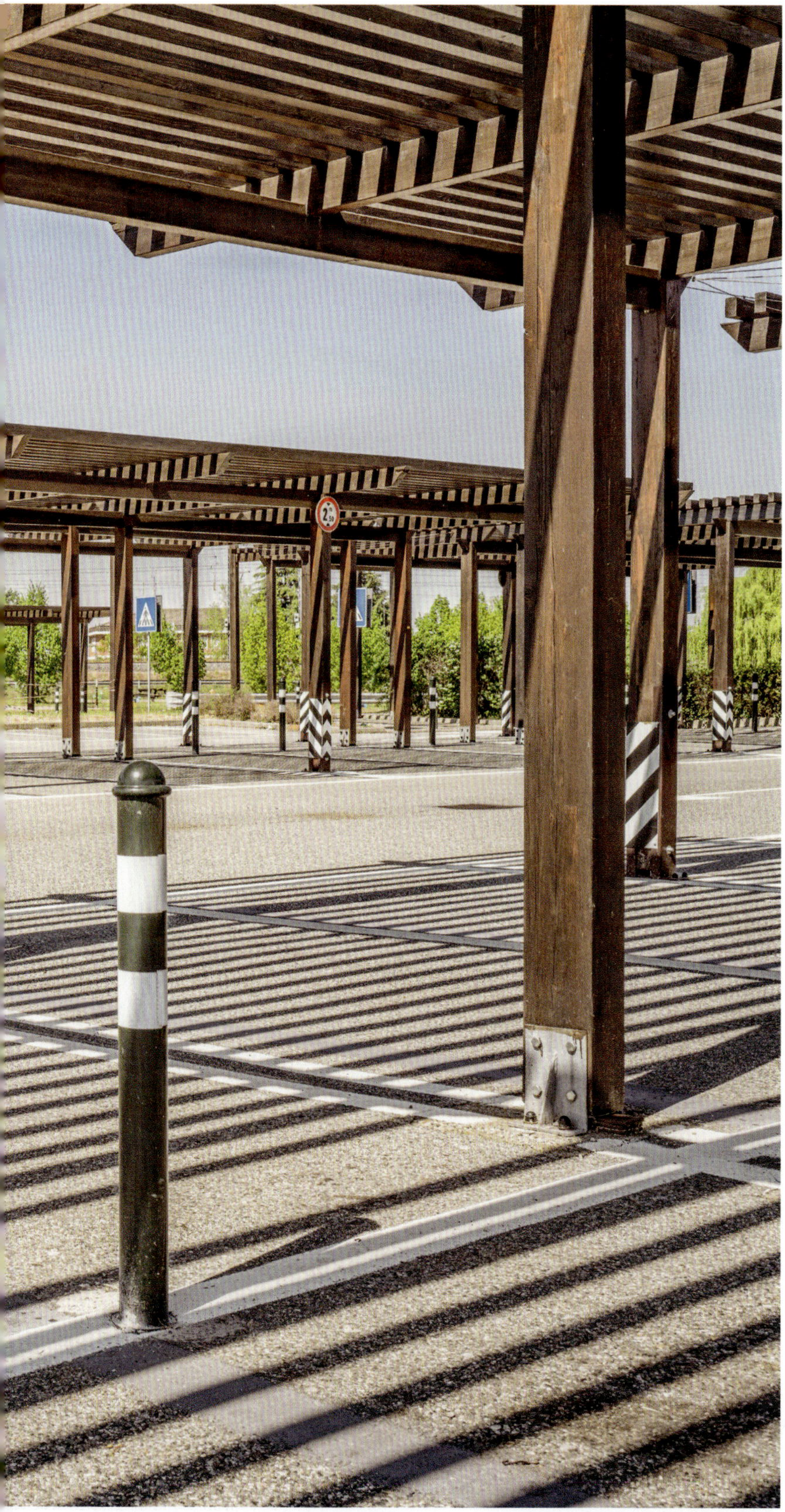

02. The Urban Void
Captions

Simon Norfolk, United Kingdom

The photographs were taken in London, in April 2020.

The Royal Exchange is the heart of the financial district of London called simply The City. Founded in 1571, it was the main marketplace for traders in every commodity although for a century or so the new "stockbrokers" were excluded for their juvenile and uncouth behaviour. During the Great Plague of 1665, where the disease was thought to transmit through "miasmas", huge bonfires were lit at The Exchange's doors to draw out the diseased air and dump it, presumably, onto the street and its pedestrians.
(Pages 148–149)

The Albert, a magnificent example of a Victorian public house, was built in 1862 as part of the redevelopment of this part of Westminster. Although one end of Victoria Street is a cathedral, a private school and a palace, much of the district was a notorious slum marked black on Charles Booth's Poverty Map of 1889: "lowest class, vicious ... occasional labourers, street sellers, loafers, criminals and semi-criminals". The few open areas, Christchurch Gardens and Vincent Square are only so because they are both on mass graves from the Plague of 1665.
(Page 150)

The Leaning Tower of London's Love Lane Leans A Little To The Left: St Alban's church in Wood Street on the corner of Love Lane, formerly a street of brothels. Who would have thought that a district of prostitutes was also a home to actors and their friends? Had it not been for local residents John Heminge and Henry Condell gathering together William Shakepeare's papers after his death in 1616, a good half of the Bard's work would have been lost to us. Three of Shakespeare's darkest tragedies, *Macbeth*, *King Lear*, and *Antony and Cleopatra* were written under lockdown during the plague outbreak of 1605–1606.
(Page 151)

St Clement Danes church (right), and the Royal Courts of Justice (beyond).
England can be rightly proud of its laws and the Royal Courts are the most imperious in the land. Here are some of our legal highlights: The Licensing Act of 1872 makes it illegal to be drunk in charge of a cow and an Act of 1603 makes it illegal to trespass on someone's land unless you are directing a boat to a shoal of fish. A statute from 1313 stops a Member of Parliament from entering either house whilst wearing a suit of armour and under an 1847 Act you can keep pigs in your back garden but it's a £1,000 fine if they're in the front. Things are improving though. Queen Elizabeth I did make it illegal to be in her presence wearing shirts with "outrageous double ruffs", or hose of "monstrous and outrageous greatness", but these laws were repealed by later kings; and the 1541 law demanding every Englishman between 17 and 60 each week do two hours longbow practice was repealed, but not until 1960.
(Page 152)

St Alphage London Wall was a church in the City built directly upon the Roman wall that enclosed Londinium so although the church has history to 1340 its foundations could be late 2nd or early 3rd century.
Over the years the church has suffered many calamities and rebuildings and today looks like a rotten molar in the midst of shiny, fake orthodontistry. The final indignities dropped on it by the Luftwaffe were topped off by urban planners from the 1950s. Other pieces of the old Roman Wall have been incorporated into nearby bank buildings as a kind of heritage lobby art.
(Page 153)

The Victoria & Albert Museum has amongst its huge collections the first photograph of London, a daguerreotype view from Trafalgar Square taken by a Monsieur de Ste Croix in 1839. Although made with a minutes-long exposure it has still caught a patient, top-hatted cab driver on his hackney carriage. De Ste Croix inadvertently also made the first ever photograph of a Londoner. In the foreground of my image is a distinctive "cabmen's shelter", one of only 13 remaining in the capital. Only licensed taxi drivers who have passed The Knowledge test (memorising every street, landmark and route in London) are allowed in for light refreshments. The idea for the shelters came in the 1870s when George Armstrong, future editor of the *Globe* newspaper, was frustrated by being unable to hail a horse-drawn cab in a

blizzard because all the drivers were huddled- up in a nearby pub. The Cabmen's Shelter Fund was conceived to steer drivers away from the beer and onto the straight and narrow.
(Page 154)

London's Victorian middle classes craved respectability and nothing said "arriviste" more than a drawing room with an aspidistra and a piano. Demand was such that the whole district of Camden was given over to piano factories; it was said each street contained at least one. And London was also a thirsty place and Camden was famous for its gin too, the Gilbey's Distillery was here, close to the bakery of the deliciously named Aerated Bread Company. With a heritage in booze and tunes it's not surprising Camden's post-industrial rebirth was as a nightlife district. Dingwall's horse-cart factory is now the famous venue played by Pink Floyd, Blondie and the Rolling Stones and in 1976 it was the scene of a famous street brawl between the Stranglers and the Clash. Camden was the haunt of Amy Winehouse, London's most celebrated overdosed addict since the last one.
(Page 155)

The River Thames, from London Bridge downriver is called the Pool of London and until about 1800 was a teeming forest of ship's masts discharging cargo right adjacent to the city's streets. The Pool was almost silent during the plague epidemic of 1665, shipping attempting to enter was quarantined far down the estuary at Canvey Island. The term "quarantena" comes from the 15th century Venetian for "forty days", being the period ships were held offshore for fear they were carrying the Black Death. Punishment could be harsh. In 1721 two vessels carrying cotton goods from Cyprus, then affected by the plague, were simply ordered to be burned with their cargoes. Despite the roughness of these measures the viruses were poorly understood. The disinfection procedure for many suspected diseases was to open the hatches of ships and expose the cargo to the morning dew. Little wonder the history of London is the history of countless epidemics.
(Pages 156–157)

Edoardo Delille, Italy

The photographs were taken in Florence, in April 2020.

Piazza San Giovanni.
(Page 159)

Piazza Santa Croce.
(Pages 160–161)

Piazza del Duomo.
(Pages 162–163)

Piazza del Mercato Centrale.
(Pages 164–165)

San Lorenzo.
(Pages 166–167)

Piazza Santa Croce.
(Pages 168–169)

Paolo Woods & Gabriele Galimberti, Italy

The photographs were taken between April and May 2020.

Bargello Museum, Florence.
Donatello, *David*, 1440, bronze.
(Page 171)

Galleria dell'Accademia, Florence.
Gianbologna, shadow of the *Rape of the Sabine Women*, 1582. Also visible are *The Trinity and Saints Benedict and Giovanni* by Gualberto by Alesso Baldovinetti, 1472
(Pages 172–173)

Gallerie d'Italia - Milan.
(Exhibition *Canova, Thorvaldsen. La nascita della scultura moderna*)
Antonio Canova
The Three Graces, 1812–1817
The State Ermitage Museum, St Petersburg
(Pages 174–175)

National Archaeological Museum, Naples.
(In the foreground left) *Emperor Vespasian*, ca. AD 80
(Page 176)

National Archaeological Museum, Naples.
Mosaics from Pompei
(Page 177)

Gallerie d'Italia - Vicenza.
(Centre) Francesco Bertos (?)
formerly attributed to Agostino Fasolato
Fall of the Rebel Angels, ca. 1725–1735
Intesa Sanpaolo Collection

(Left) Francesco Zuccarelli
Ideal View of Vicenza with the Allegorical Celebration of Andrea Palladio,
ca. 1762–1765
Intesa Sanpaolo Collection

(Right) Francesco Zuccarelli
The Rape of Europa, ca. 1740–1745
Intesa Sanpaolo Collection
(Pages 178–179)

Gallerie d'Italia - Naples.
Antonio Joli's atelier
View of the Gulf of Naples, 1765–1770
Intesa Sanpaolo Collection
(Pages 180–181)

Daniele Ratti, Italy

The photographs were taken between April 22 and May 3, 2020.

A1, along the highway.
(Page 183)

A4, Villarboit, Piedmont.
(Pages 184–185)

A4, Rondissone, Piedmont.
(Page 186)

A1, Badia, Tuscany.
(Page 187)

A1, la Macchia, Lazio.
(Page 188)

A4, Brebemi, Lombardy.
(Page 189)

A4, Villarboit, Piedmont.
(Pages 190–191)

03.

Shelter in Place

Lisa Sorgini, Australia
Behind Glass

This portrait series documents more than twenty mothers and their children experiencing isolation in their homes during a period of enforced social distancing in March and April 2020, to control the transmission of COVID-19 in Australia.
I have built a practice investigating relationships between mother and child. In this series I explore my long-held fascination with photographing through windows to frame a subject — a process I have never felt is more poignant than now. At my home in Bundjalung Country in northern New South Wales, I — like so many parents — had been spending my days learning new rhythms with my two children at home. I am fascinated with the lightness and darkness of parenting at this time. Now alone, with the absence of external support and simultaneously never alone as we spend intense one-on-one time with our children. Behind the glass, mother and child appear like living and breathing masterpieces — divine comedies of domesticity. Through this work, I hope to make the invisible role of parenting in isolation visible: the deepest tenderness, tedium, quietude, love, frustration, fear and despair.

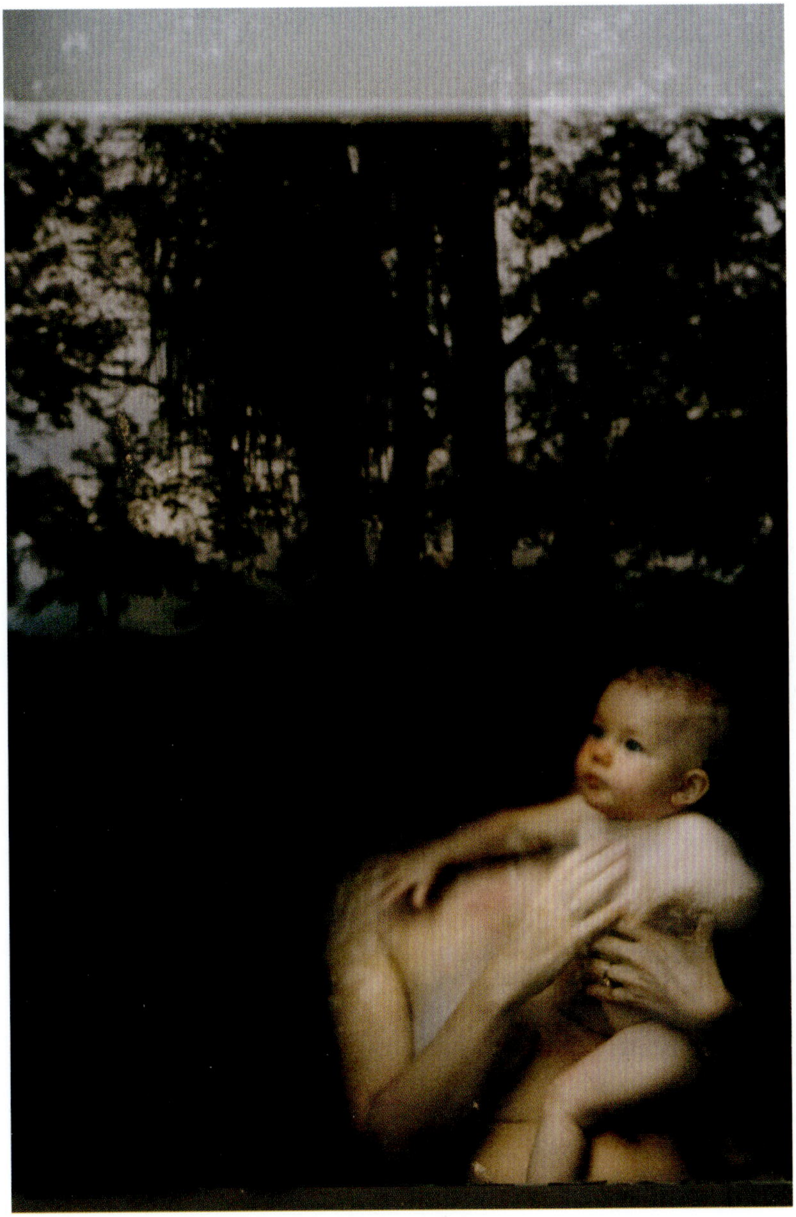

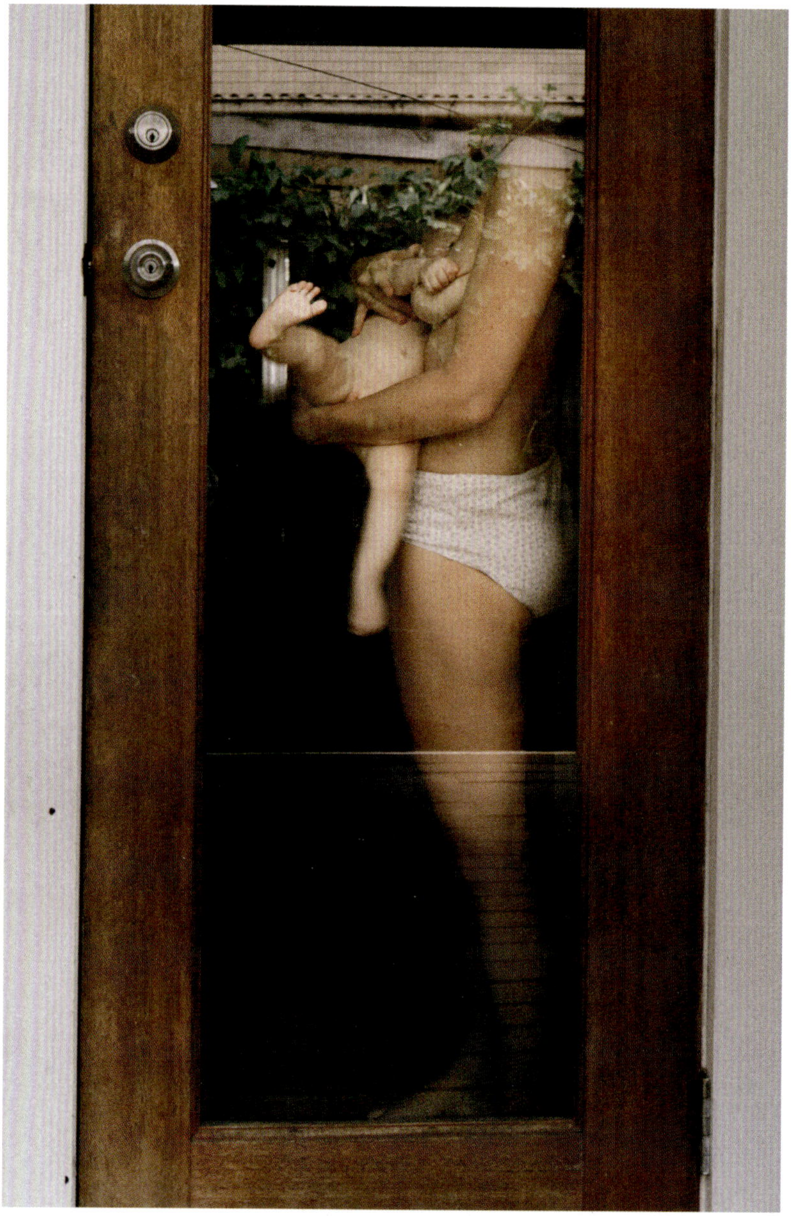

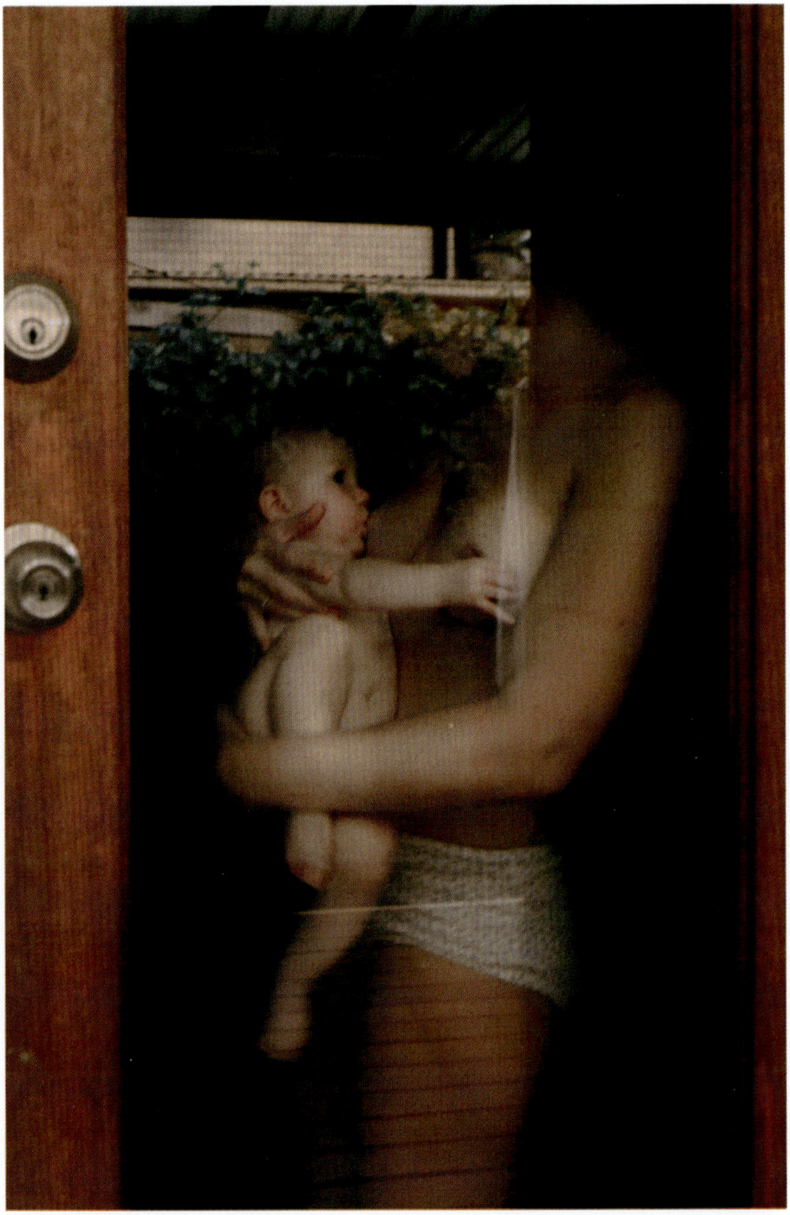

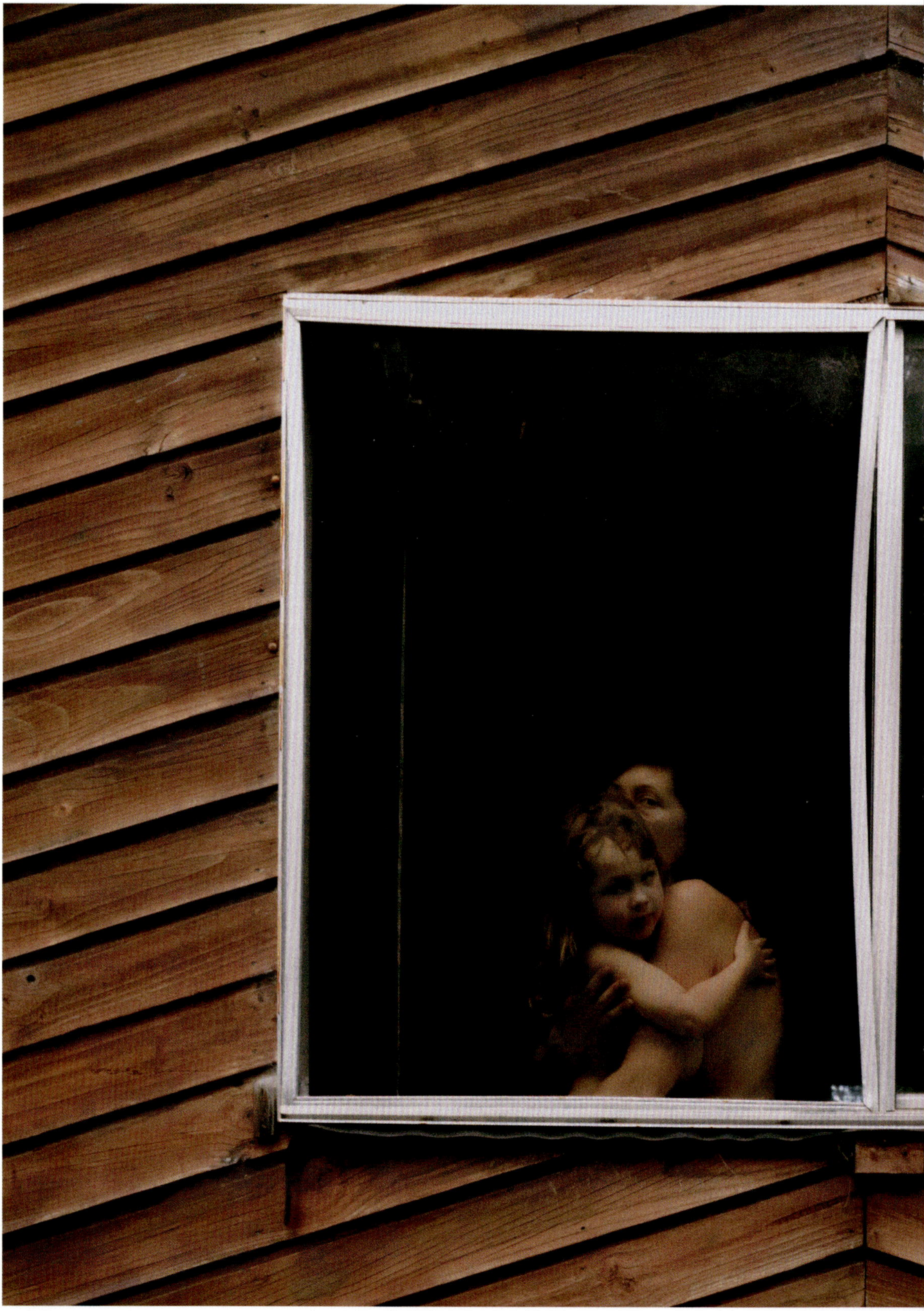

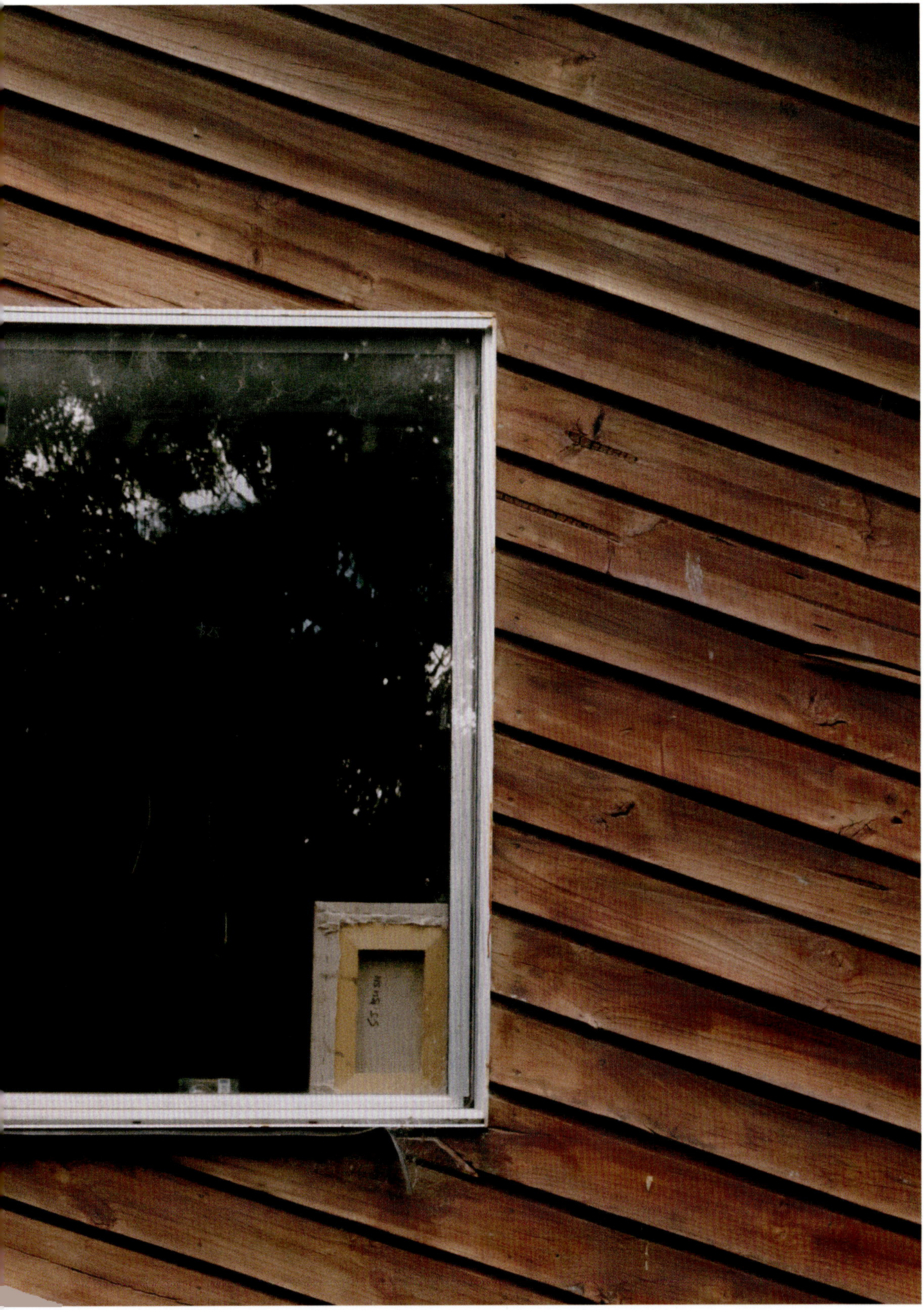

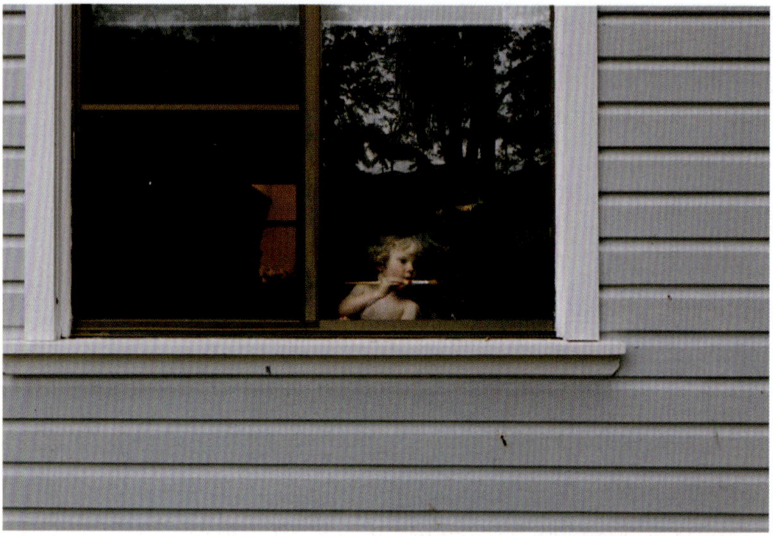
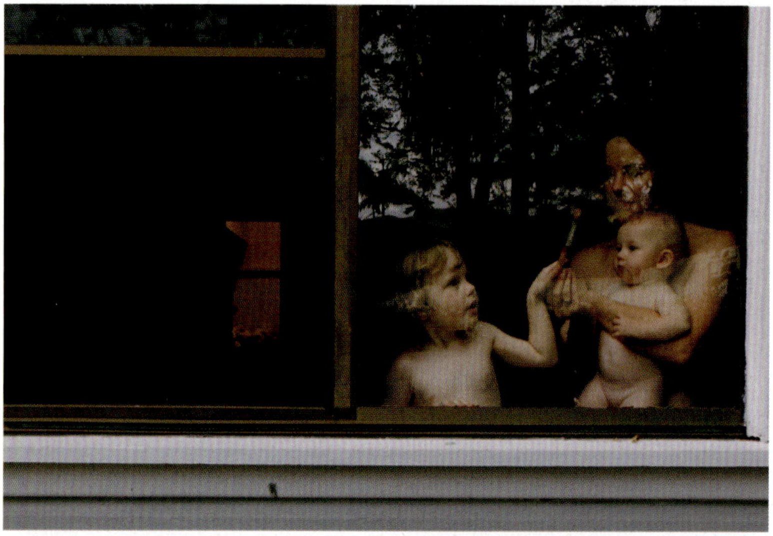
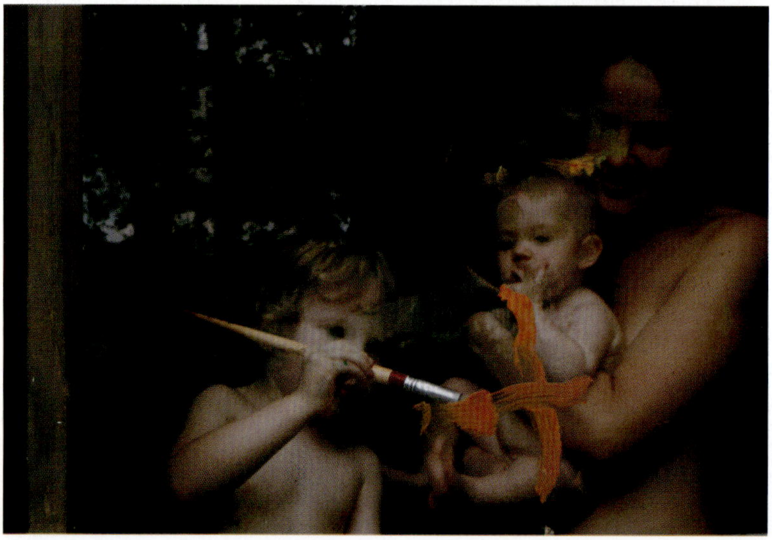

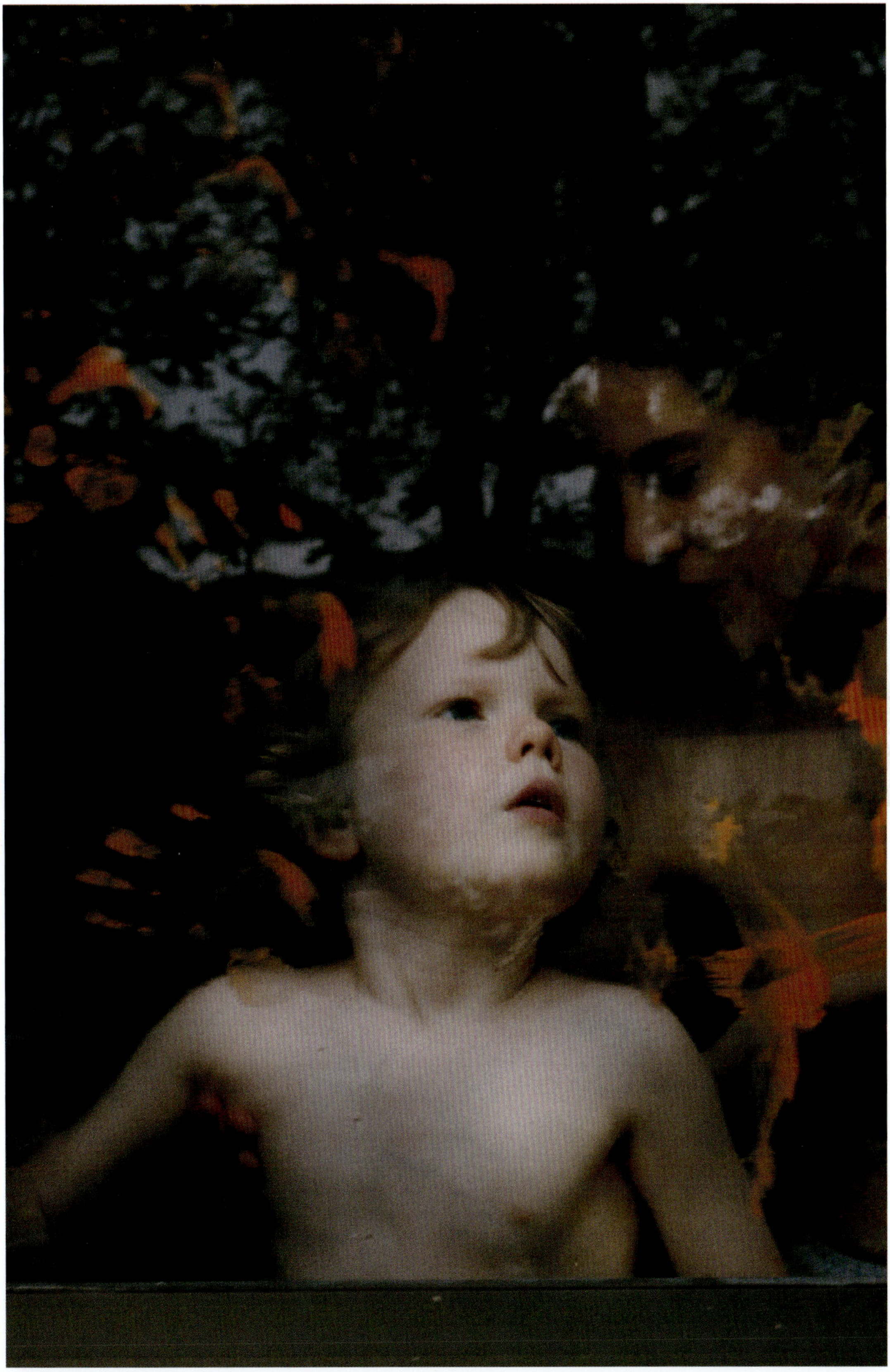

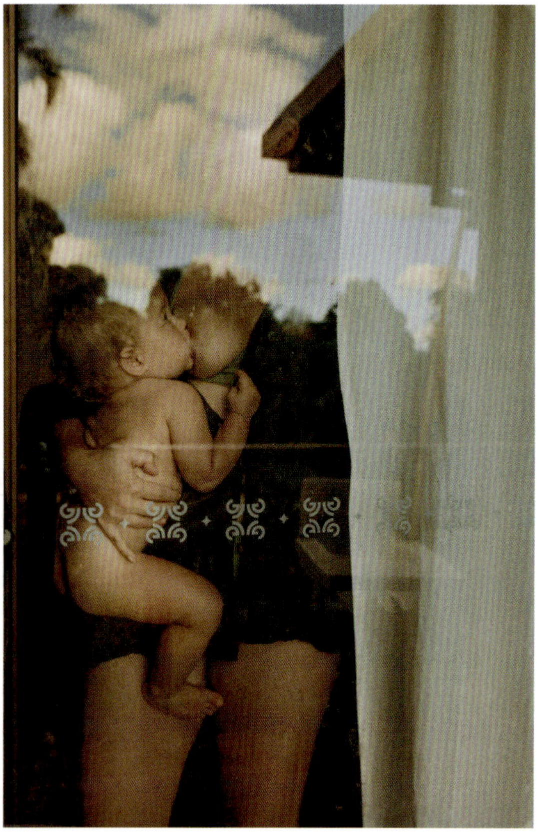

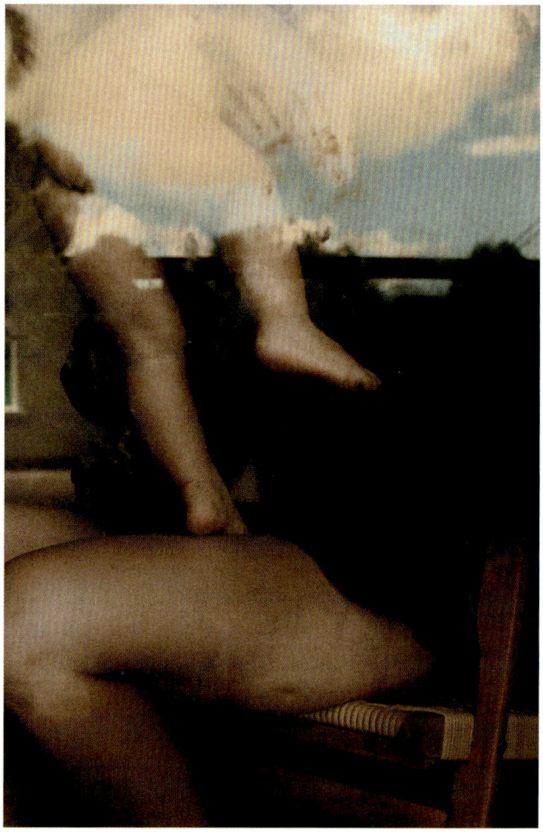

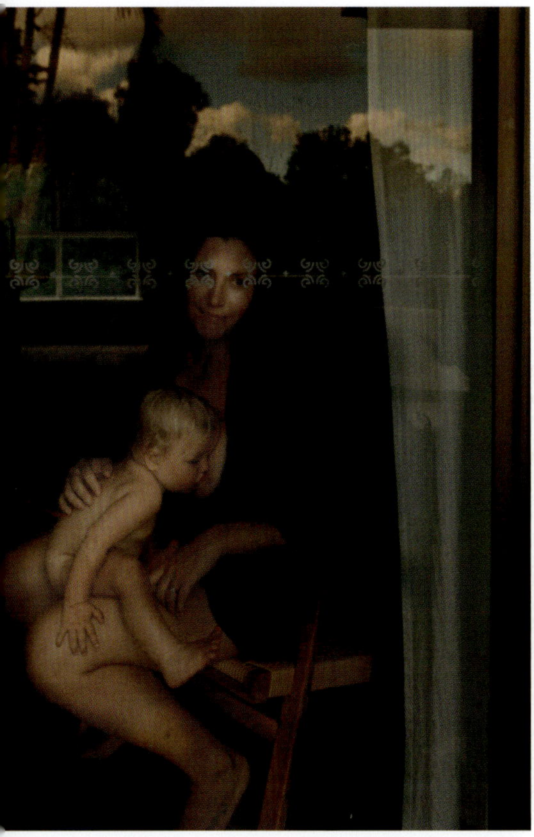

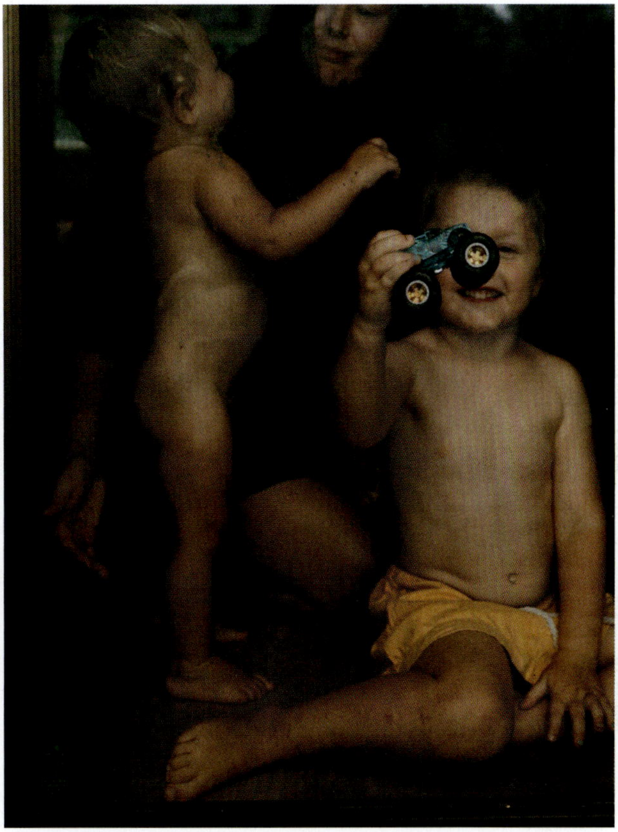

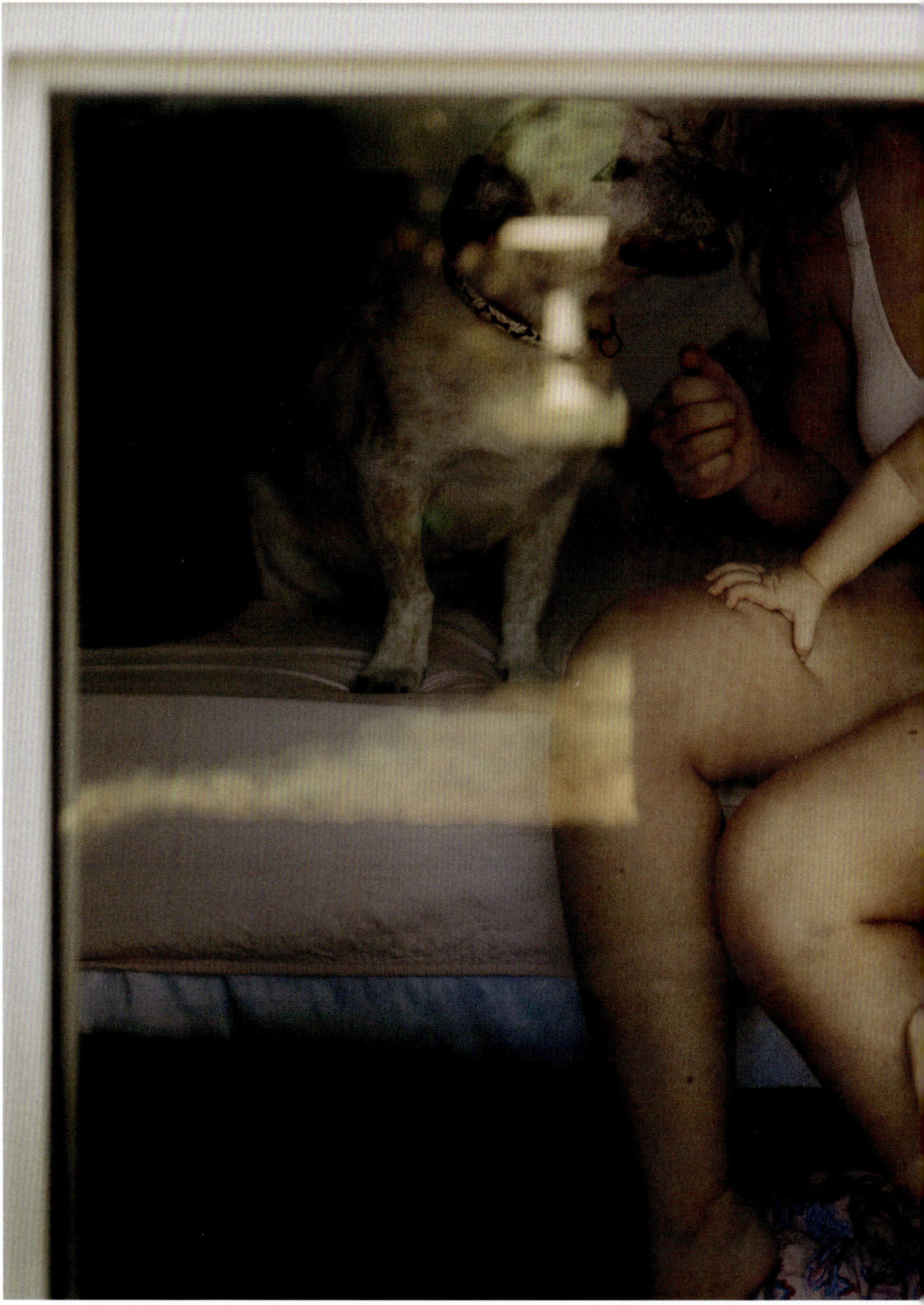

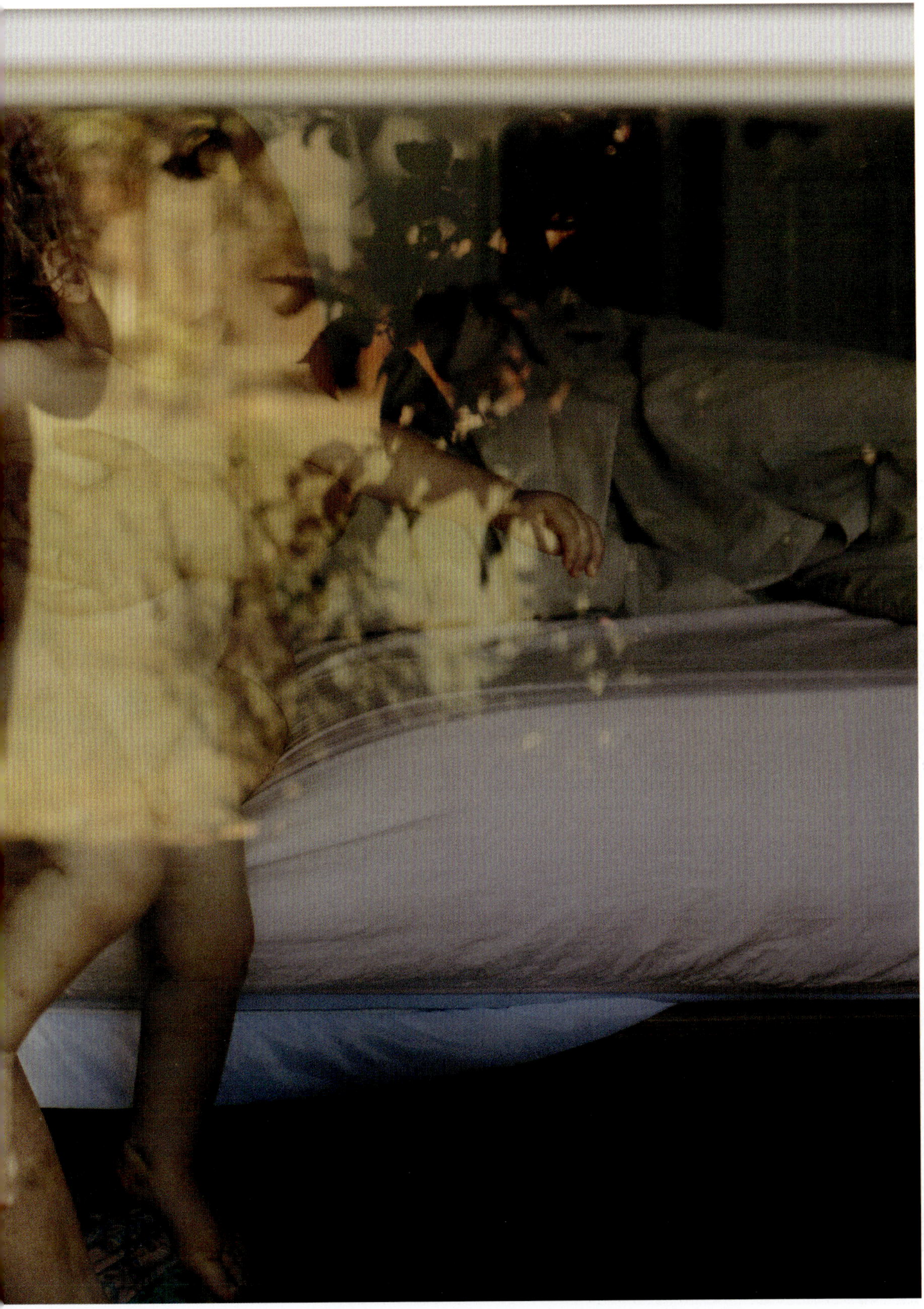

Mohammad Shahnewaz Khan, Bangladesh
Life in the Cage

In Bangladesh we held our breaths and prayed that for our impoverished overpopulated country would somehow be spared from yet another disaster, but when the government enforced a nationwide lockdown on March 26 2020, we found ourselves homebound as though we were living in a cage. This personal project about my family and me documents the interaction of our relationships during the ongoing pandemic days in our home in the coastal city of Chittagong.
I have spent my entire career as a photojournalist documenting the struggles of others for the world's major news publications and teaching and mentoring other aspiring photojournalists. Now, for the first time, I stood in front of my own camera.
I struggled to focus my lens on my own story, embracing the power of photography as a motivation to survive. This new experience felt awkward and at times uncomfortable.
My photographs show slivers of our daily life, hope, disappointments, expectations, loneliness, frustration and fears. Our joys overshadow the uncertainties we face. In these months in isolation, I also explored my relationship with my wife, Negar, and our children, Hossain and Imran. I was able to observe my family up close, and I've discovered my weaknesses deeply. While struggling to capture this moment in history, I dreamed of a downpour in the desert. I felt as though I was drowning and tried to stay alive through our story.
During the lockdown, our children became ill with fever, coughing, shortness of breath linked to allergies. We were afraid to seek treatment because of fear of being infected with the COVID-19 virus. We tried home remedies. In fact, my wife and I really had no choice. Our regular familiar family doctor has been absent from his clinic for over two months.
It was terrible because of unavailable health treatment in Bangladesh. Patients weren't getting treatment, even those who had not contracted coronavirus were dying because of panic in hospitals and lack of empty beds.
A recent survey has found that 72.6% of Bangladeshis are suffering from insomnia, COVID-19 has a significant detrimental effect on the mental health and psychological well-being of the people of Bangladesh. My two younger brothers and I lived together as a joint family, but during the coronavirus pandemic, for the first time, we became separated, each in our own cage. We can only guess what is happening inside the families of the people around us, visual observation is not possible. So I picked up my camera, where I tried to understand and disclose the crisis with honesty and bravery.

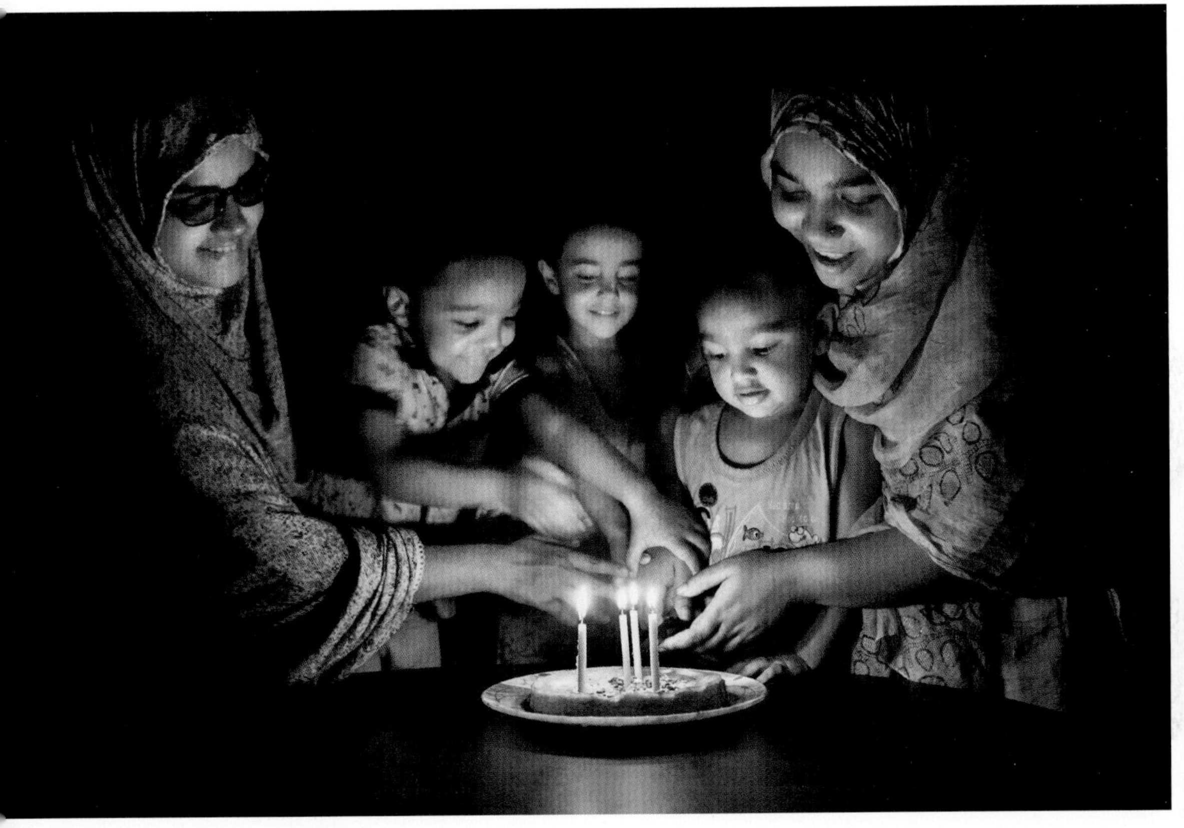

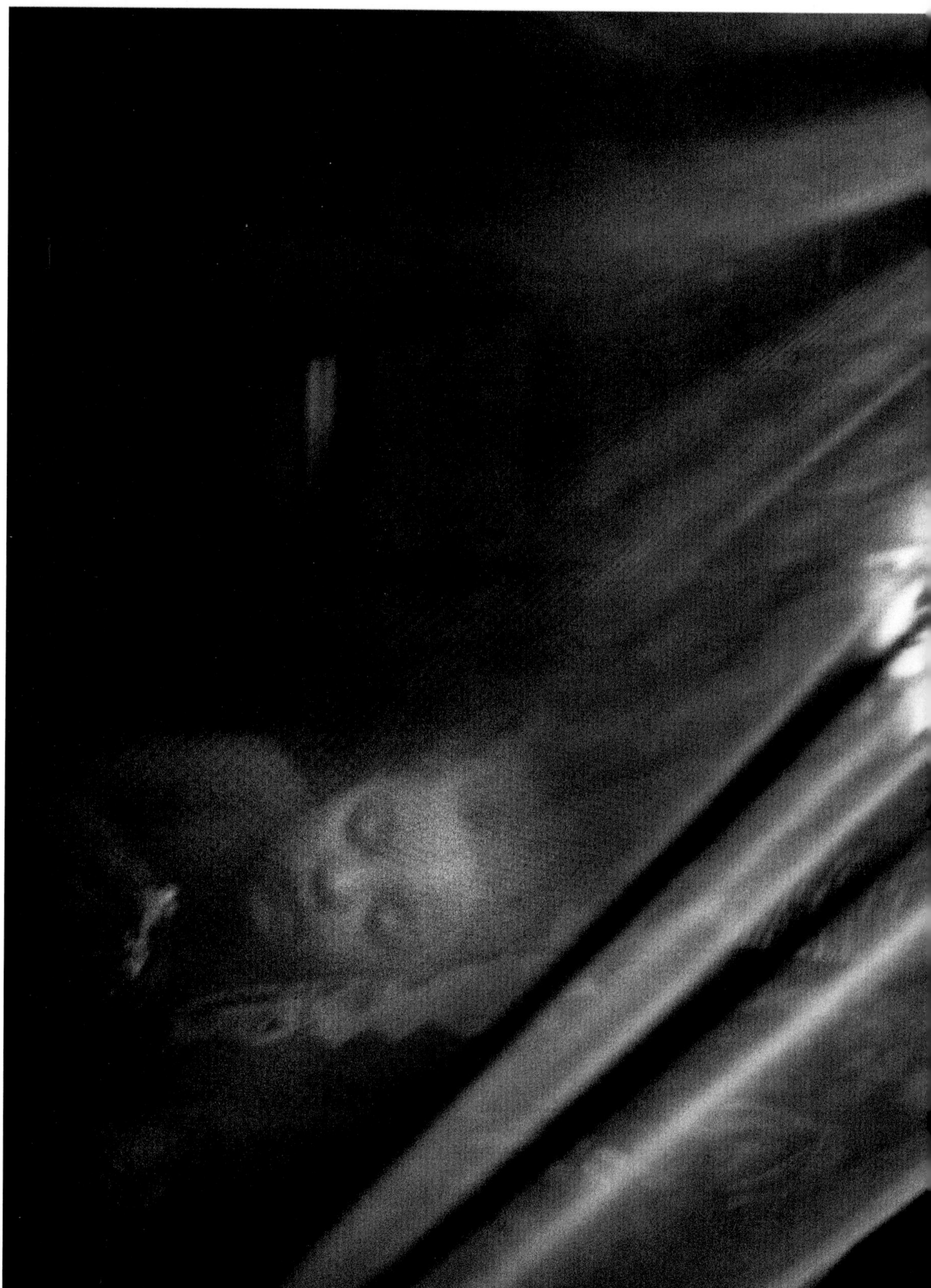

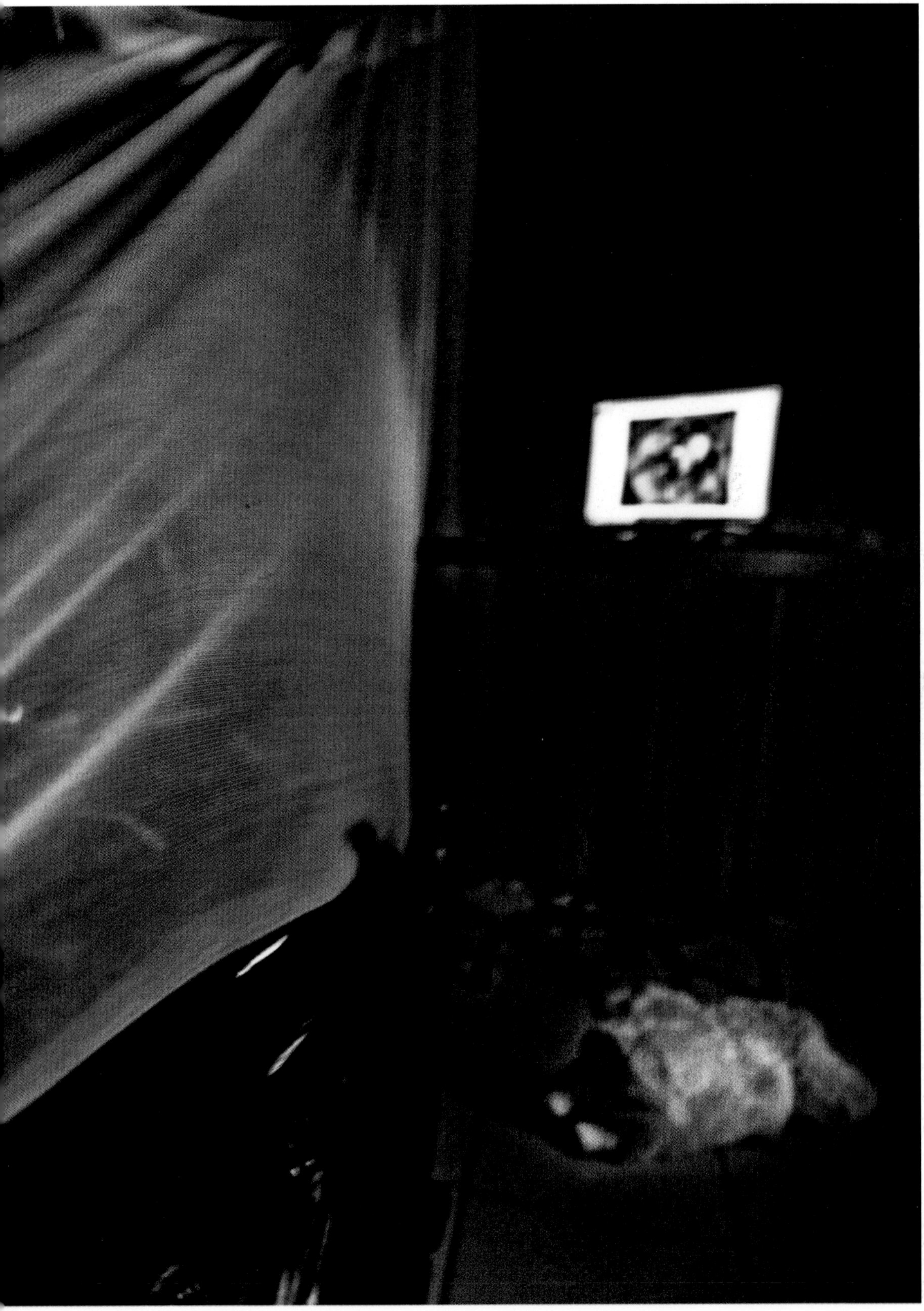

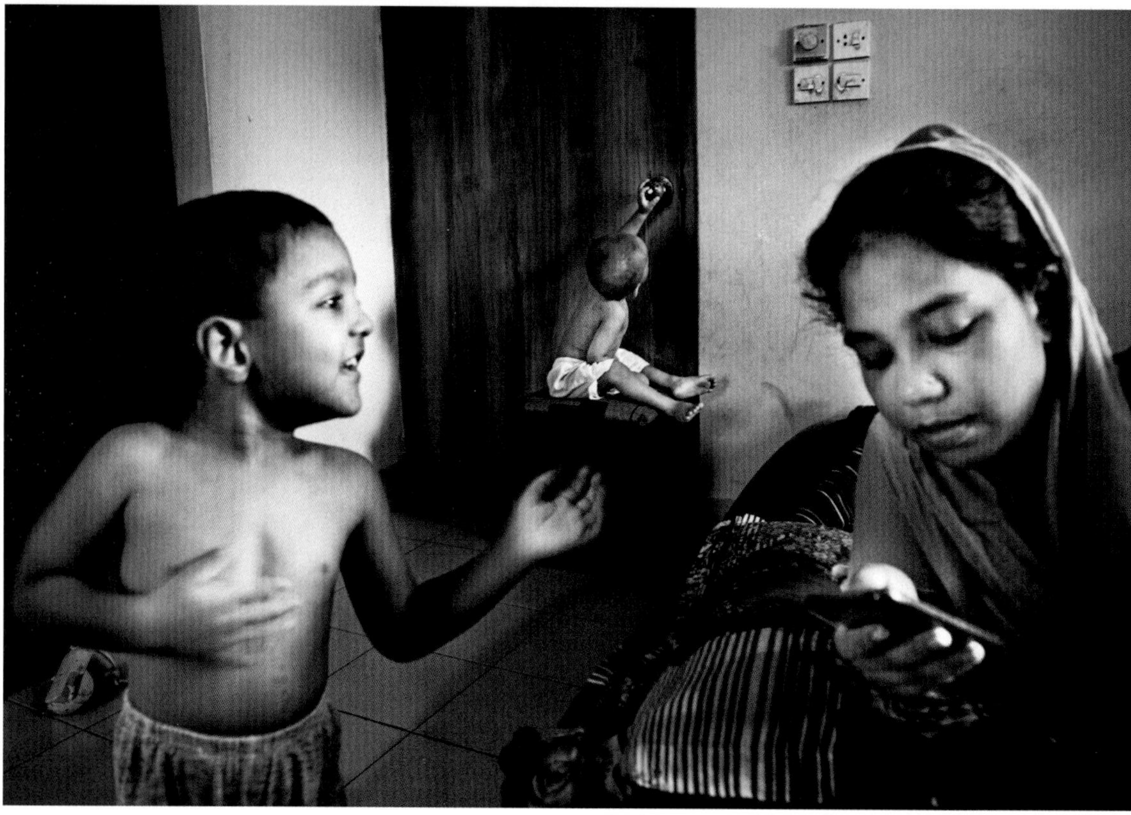

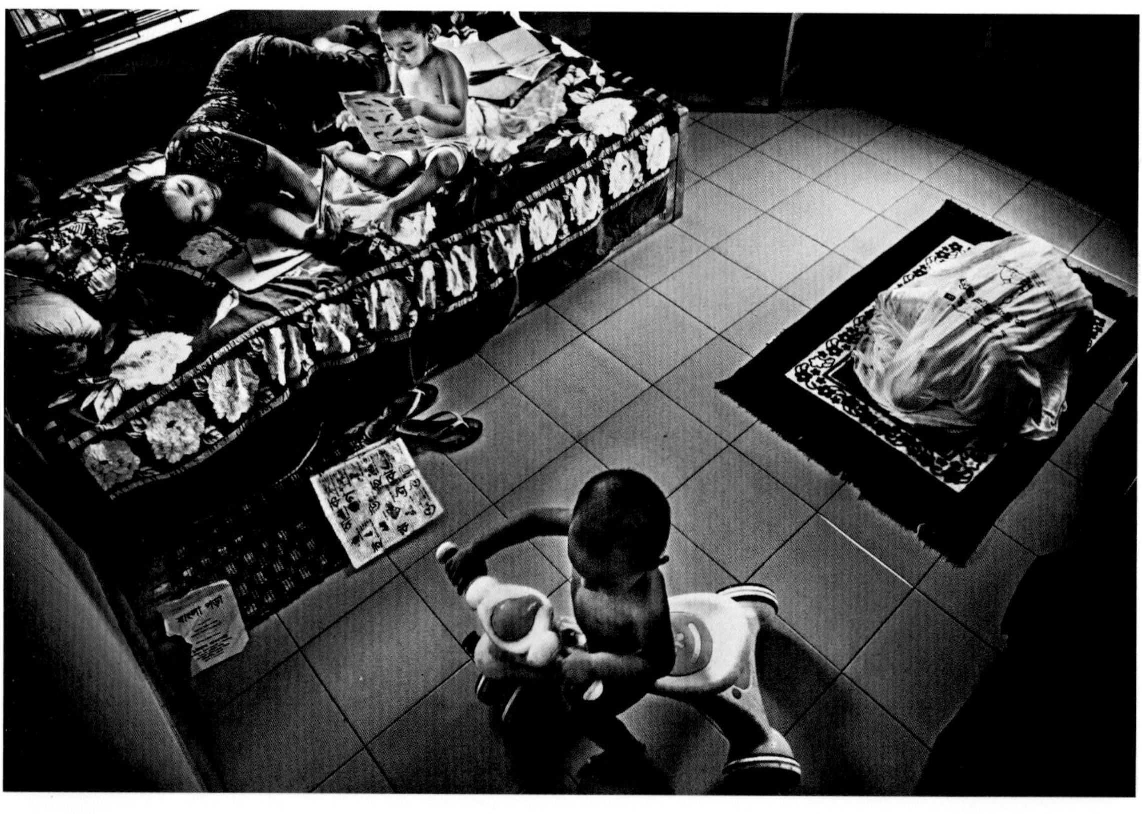

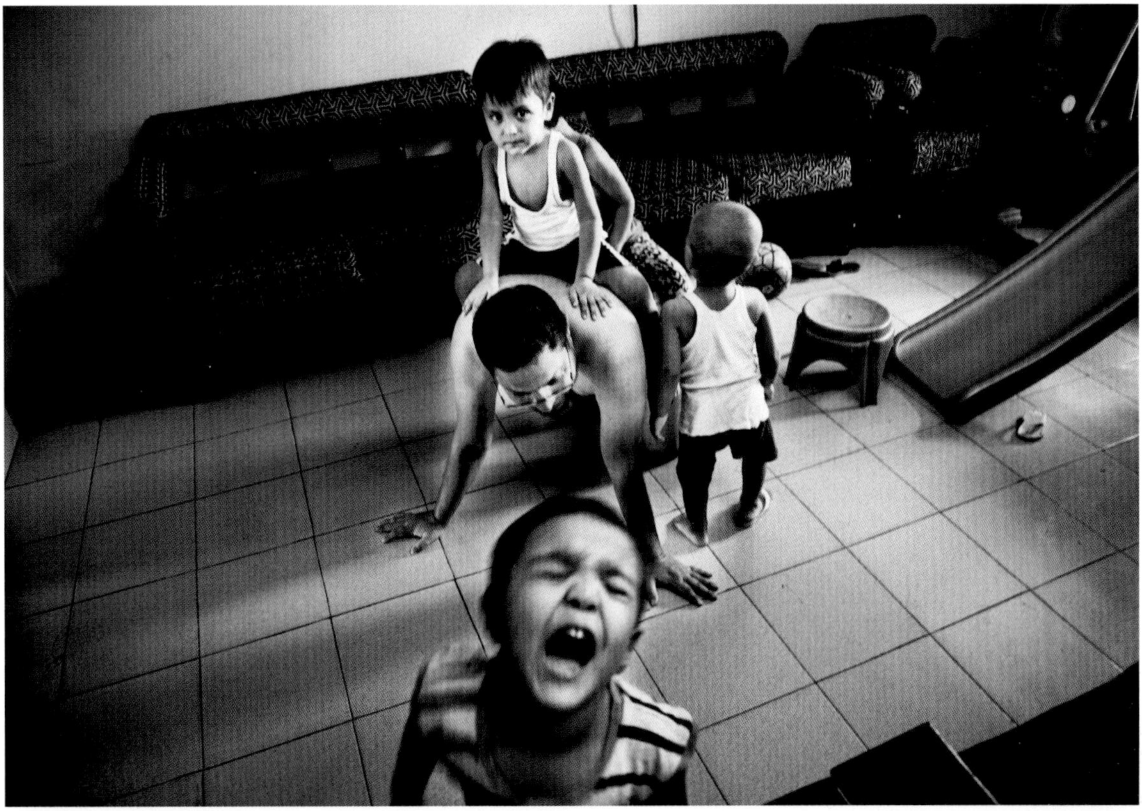

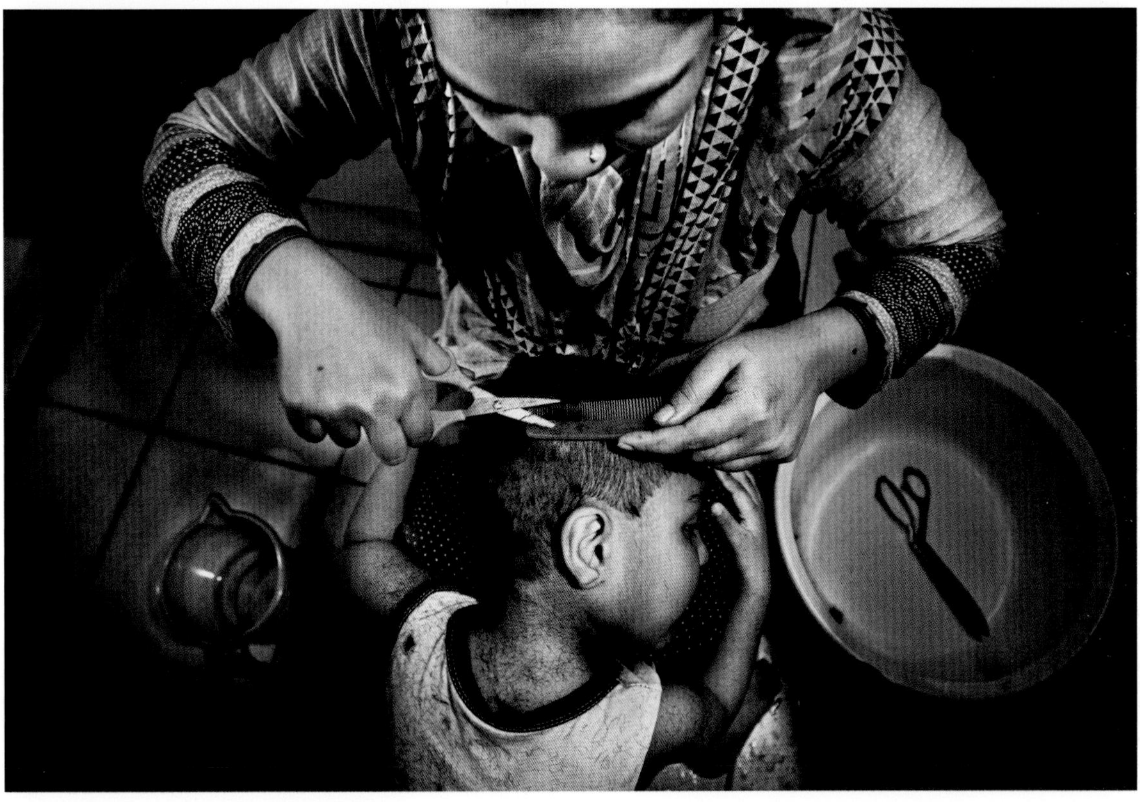

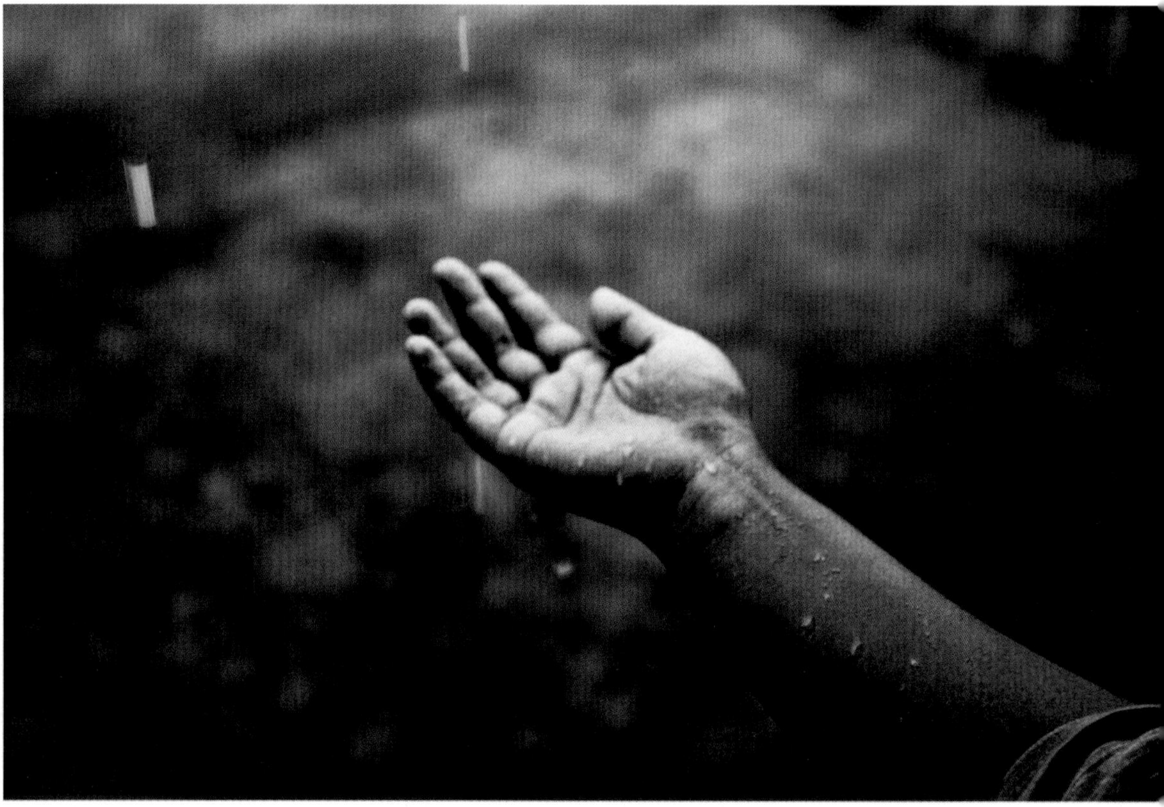

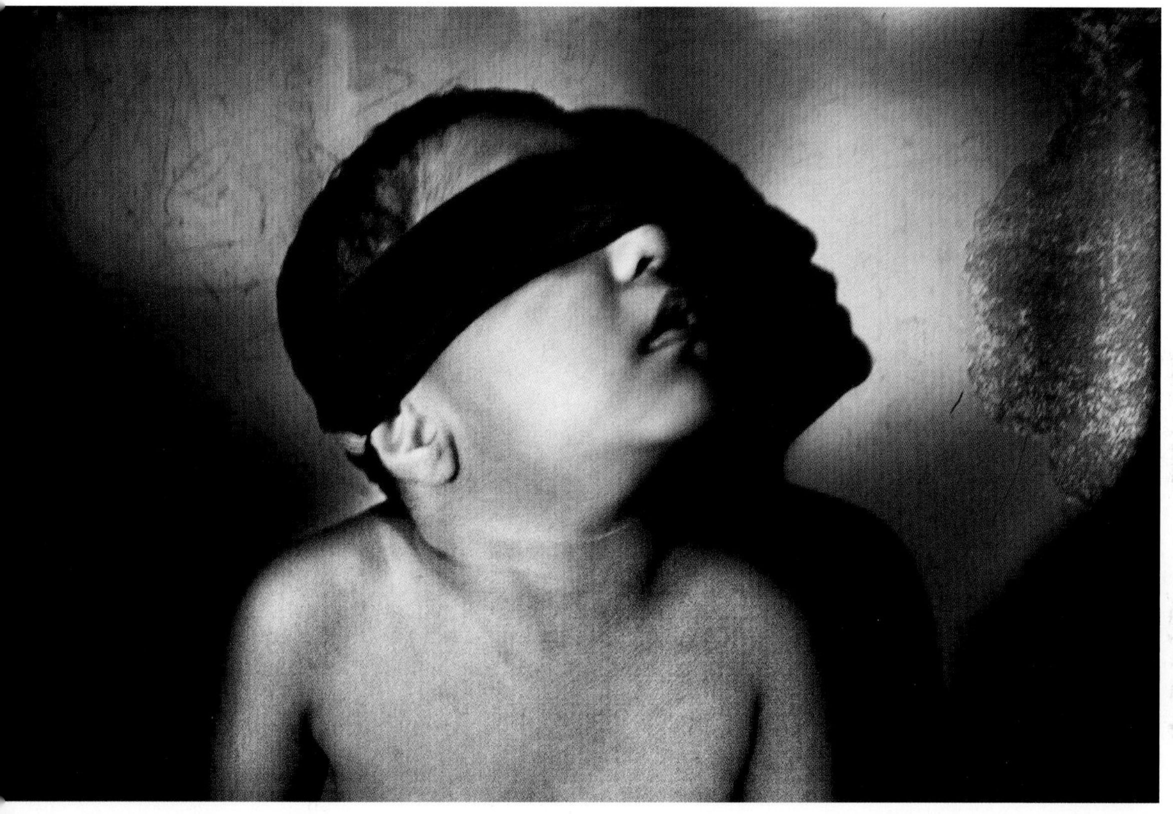

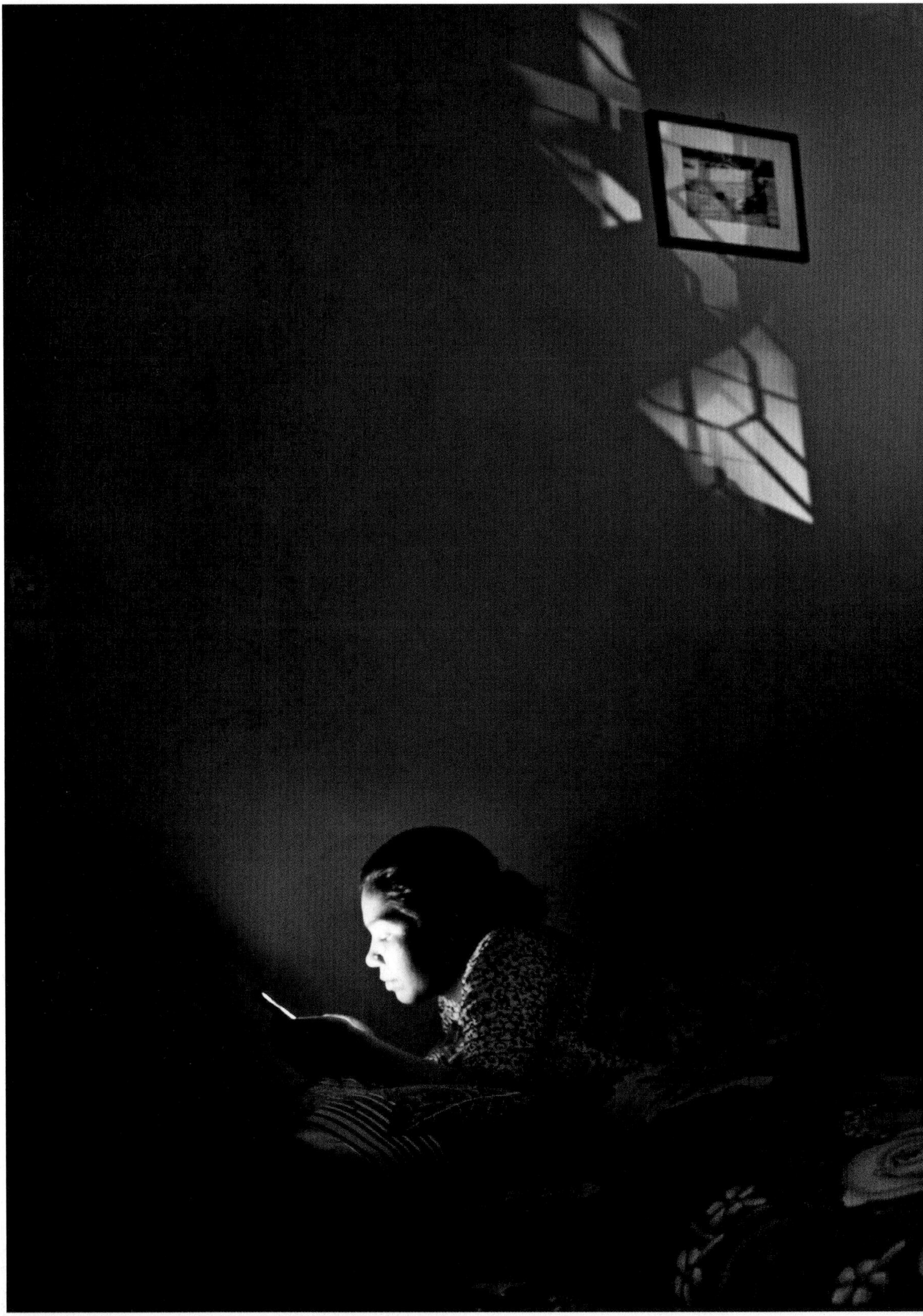

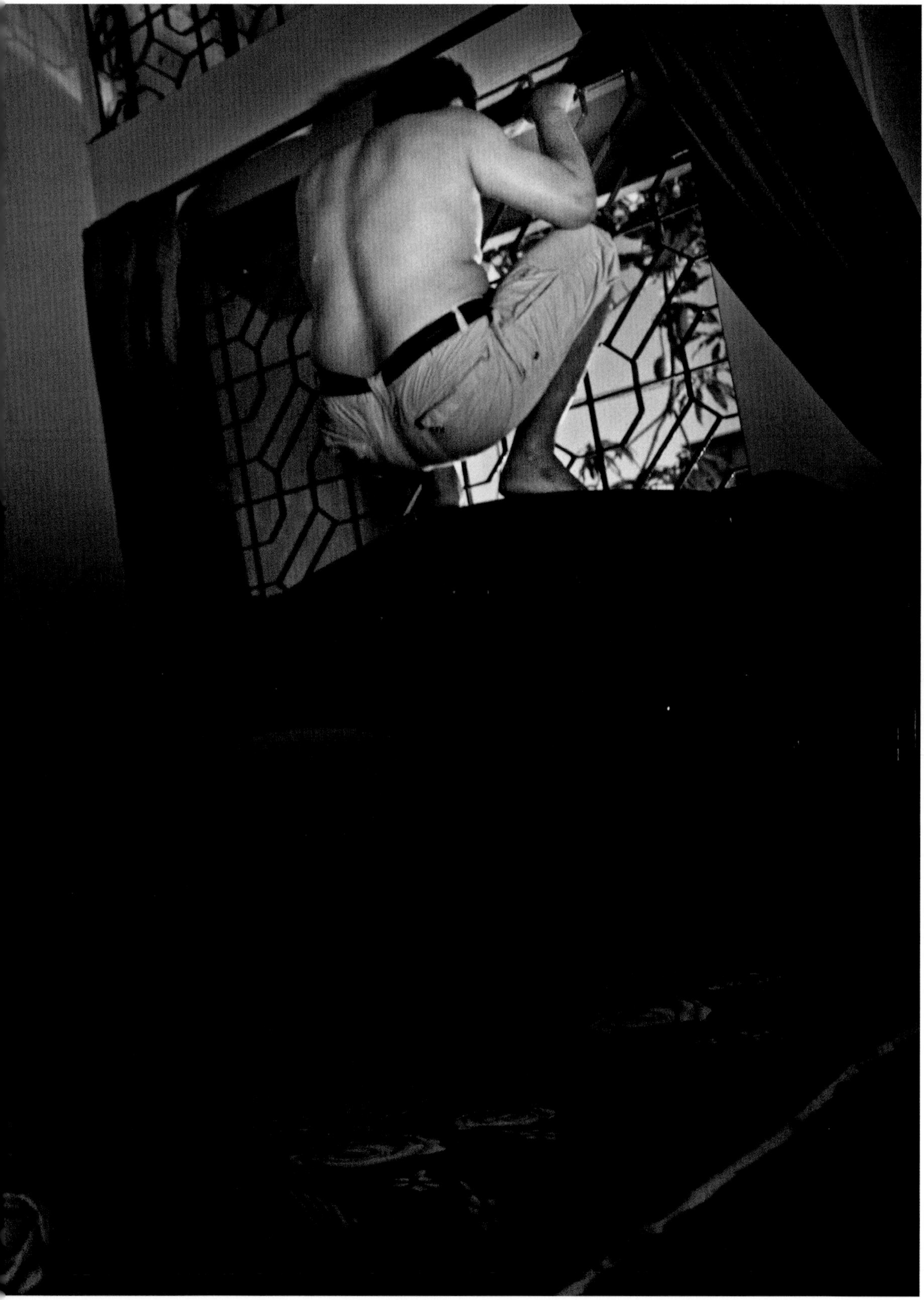

Lorenzo Pesce, Italy
Distant Tales

This project was born out of a desire to narrate our unusual everyday life during the lockdown months, filled with new discoveries but, for many of us, mostly with great absences.
As a father of three girls, I experienced first-hand what detachment meant to my daughters during that period.
My second daughter Carlotta was to complete her fifth grade (i.e. the entire primary school cycle) without seeing her classmates again. I thought she could become my assistant, she would be happy to see her friends.
Absence and a sense of lacking are the background against which the portraits are set.
The idea was to ask twenty-six boys and girls from fifth grade to tell me three things they missed during their confinement at home. As a result, I have constructed a series of portraits that attempt to represent, in a symbolic and iconic way, their state of being during those months.

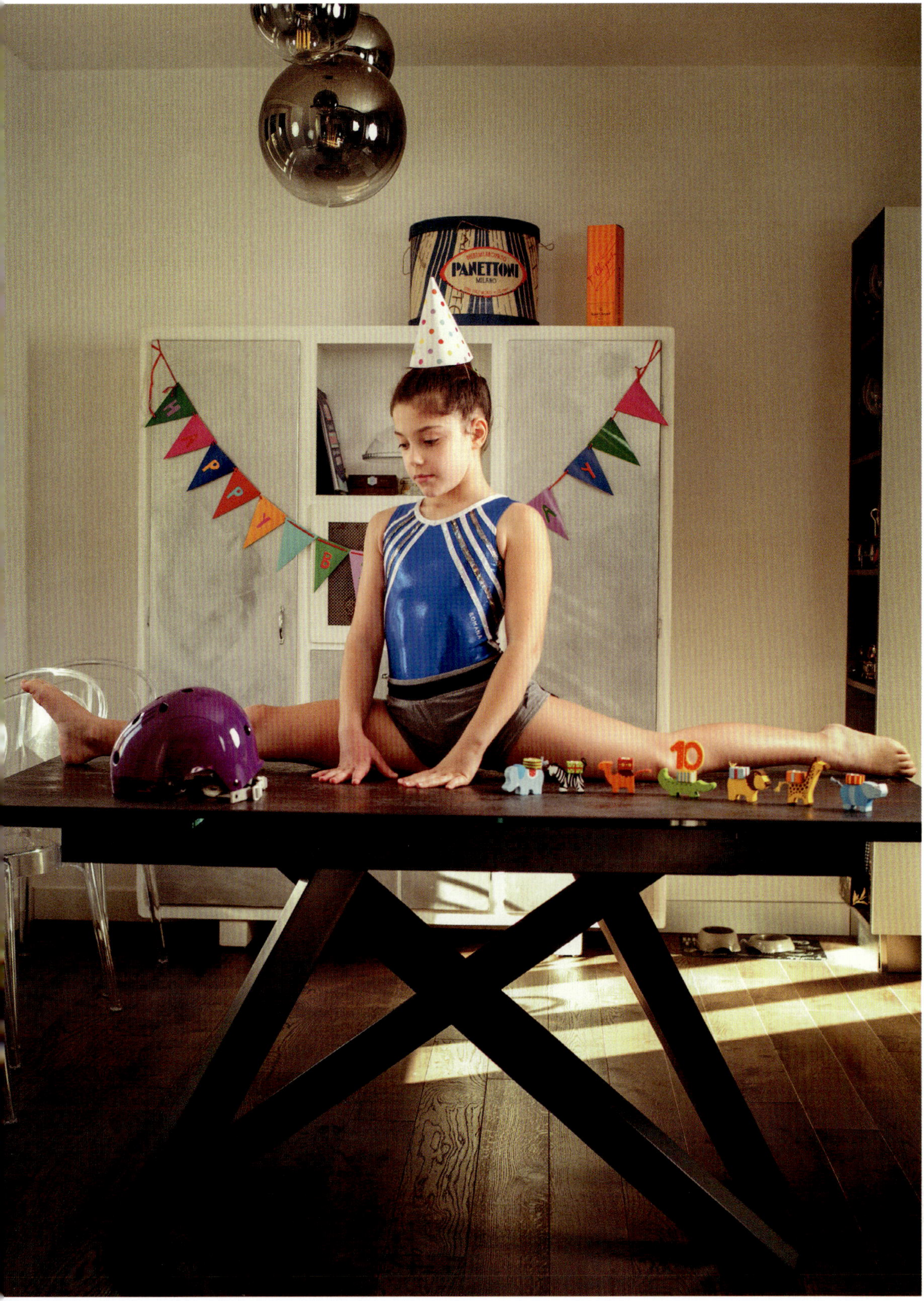
PANETTONI
MILANO

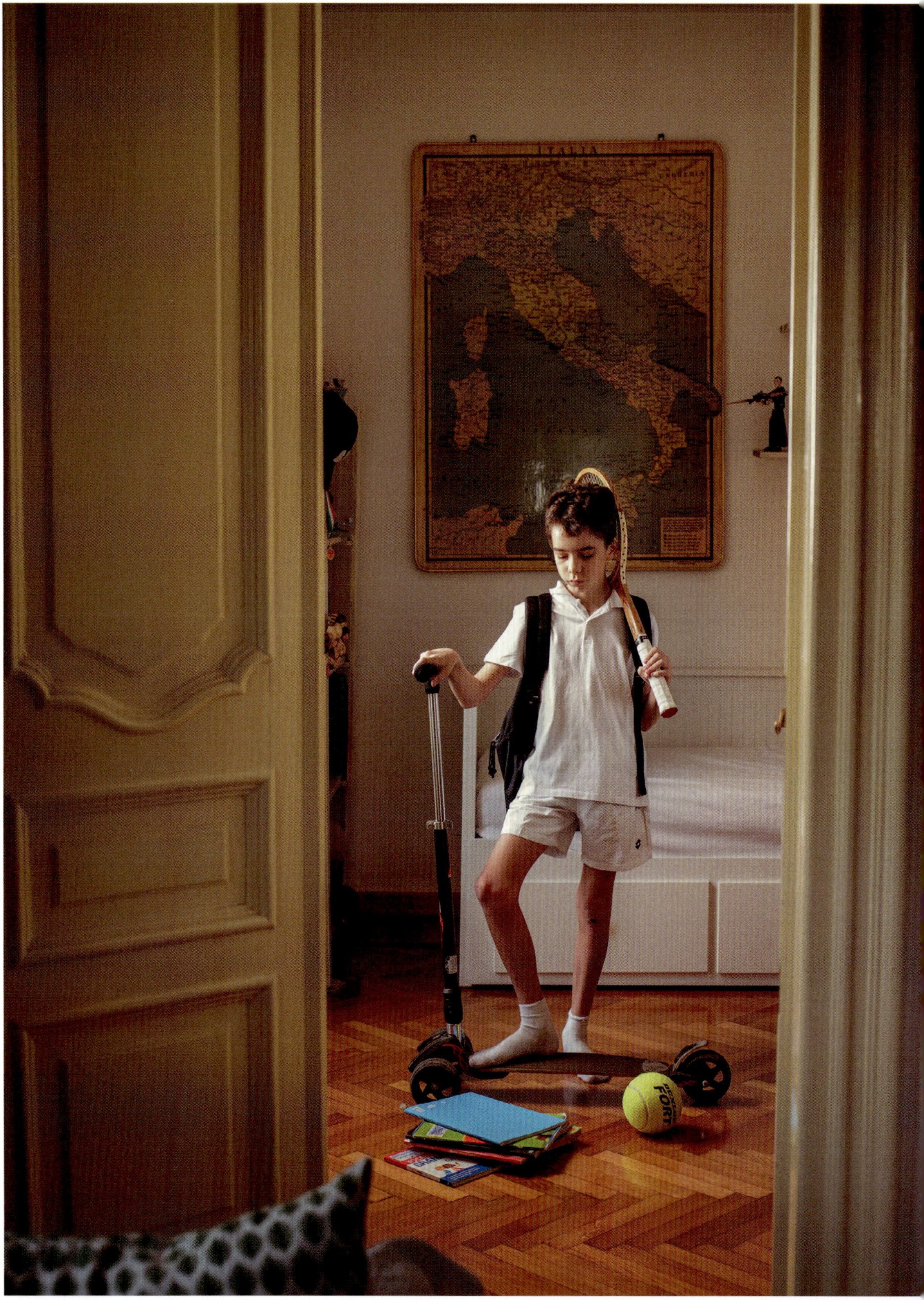
ITALIA
FORT

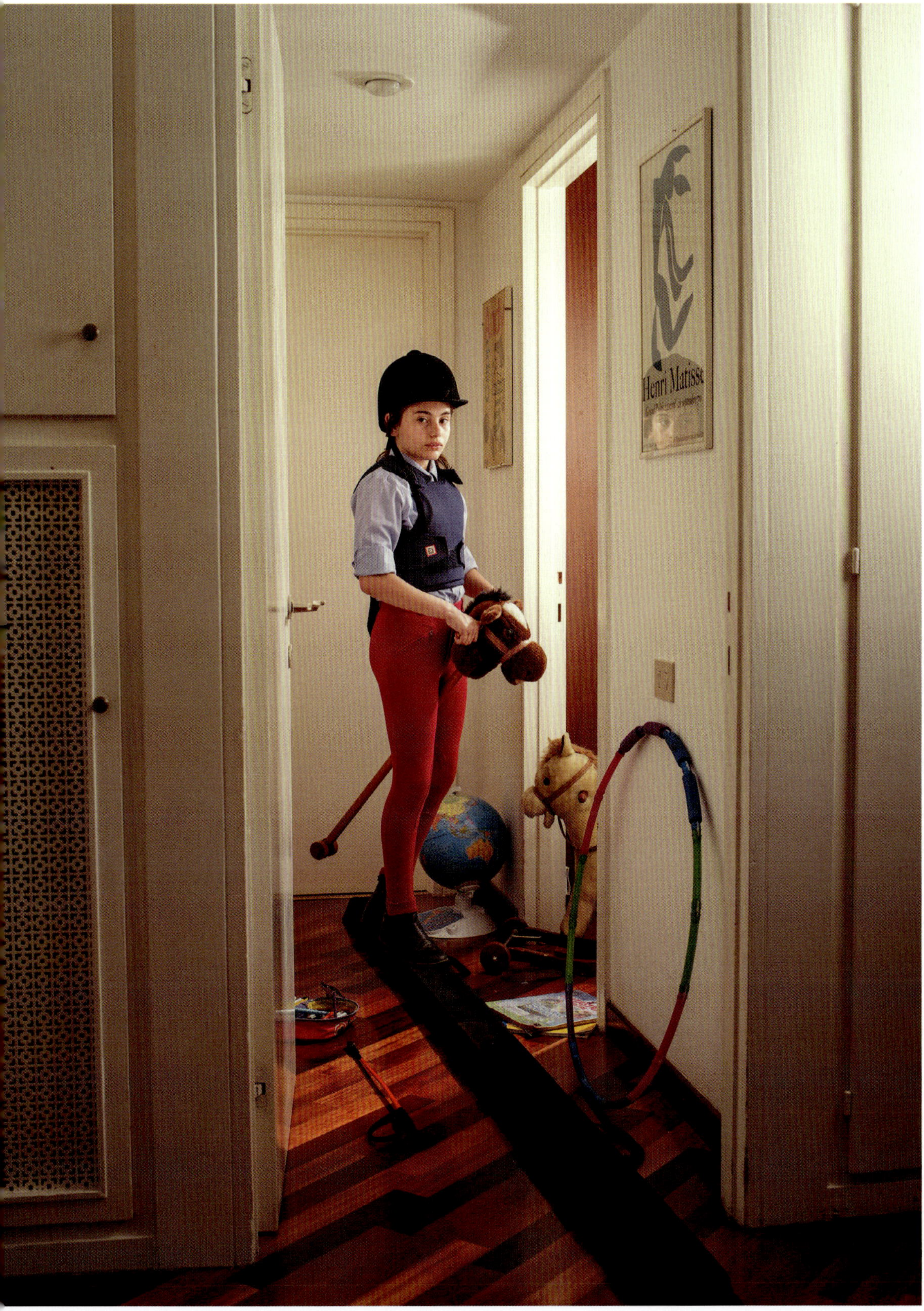
Henri Matisse

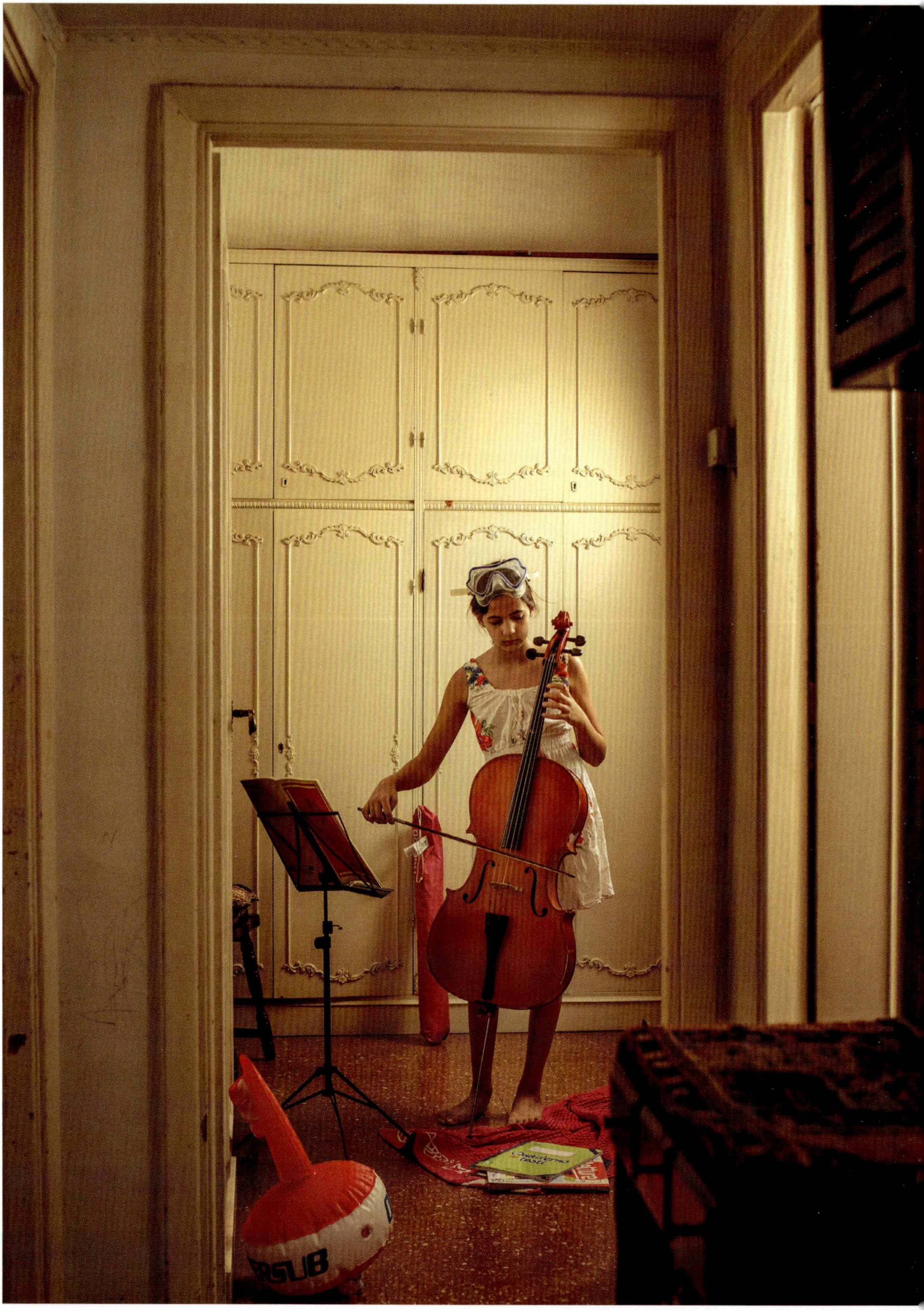

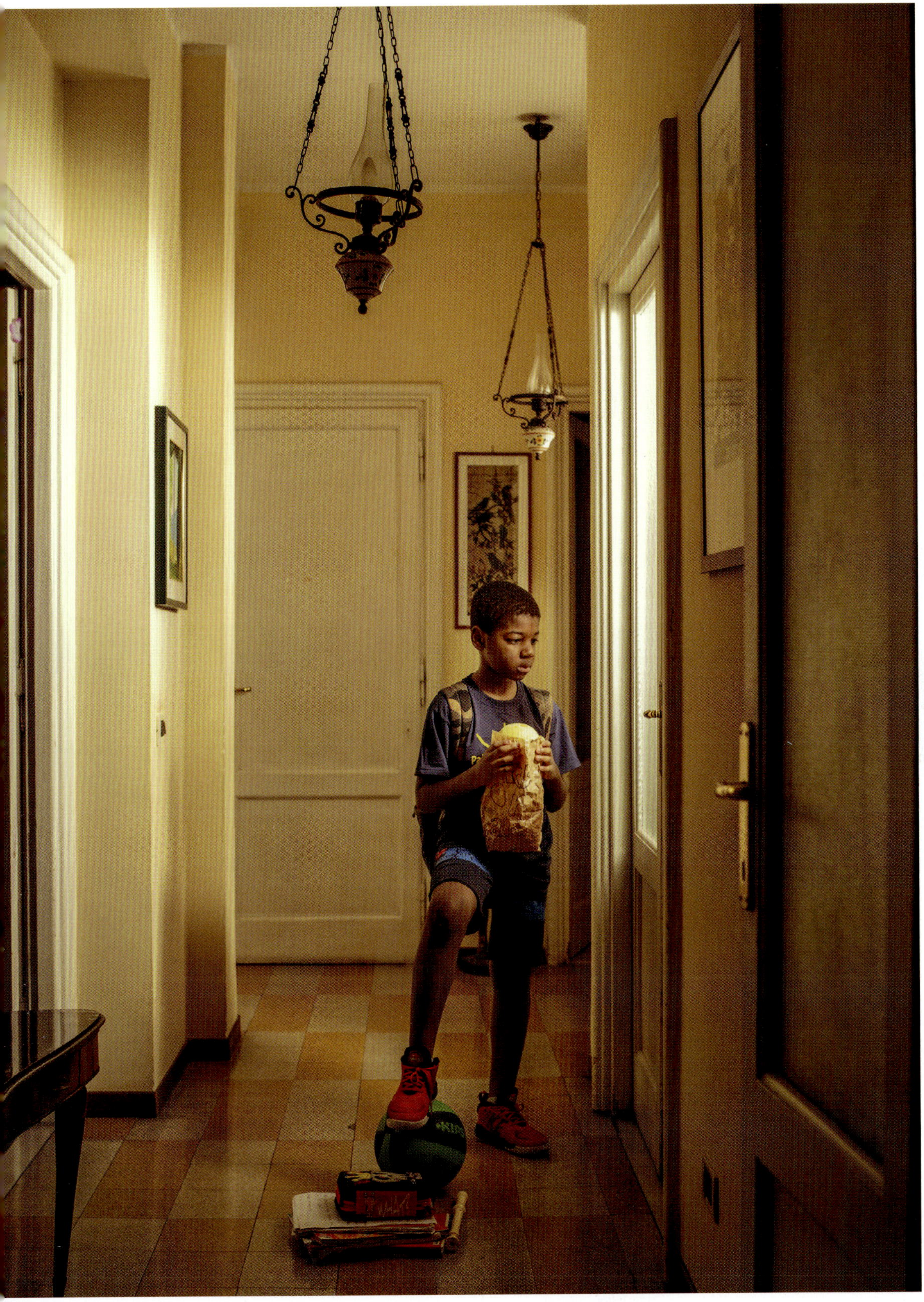

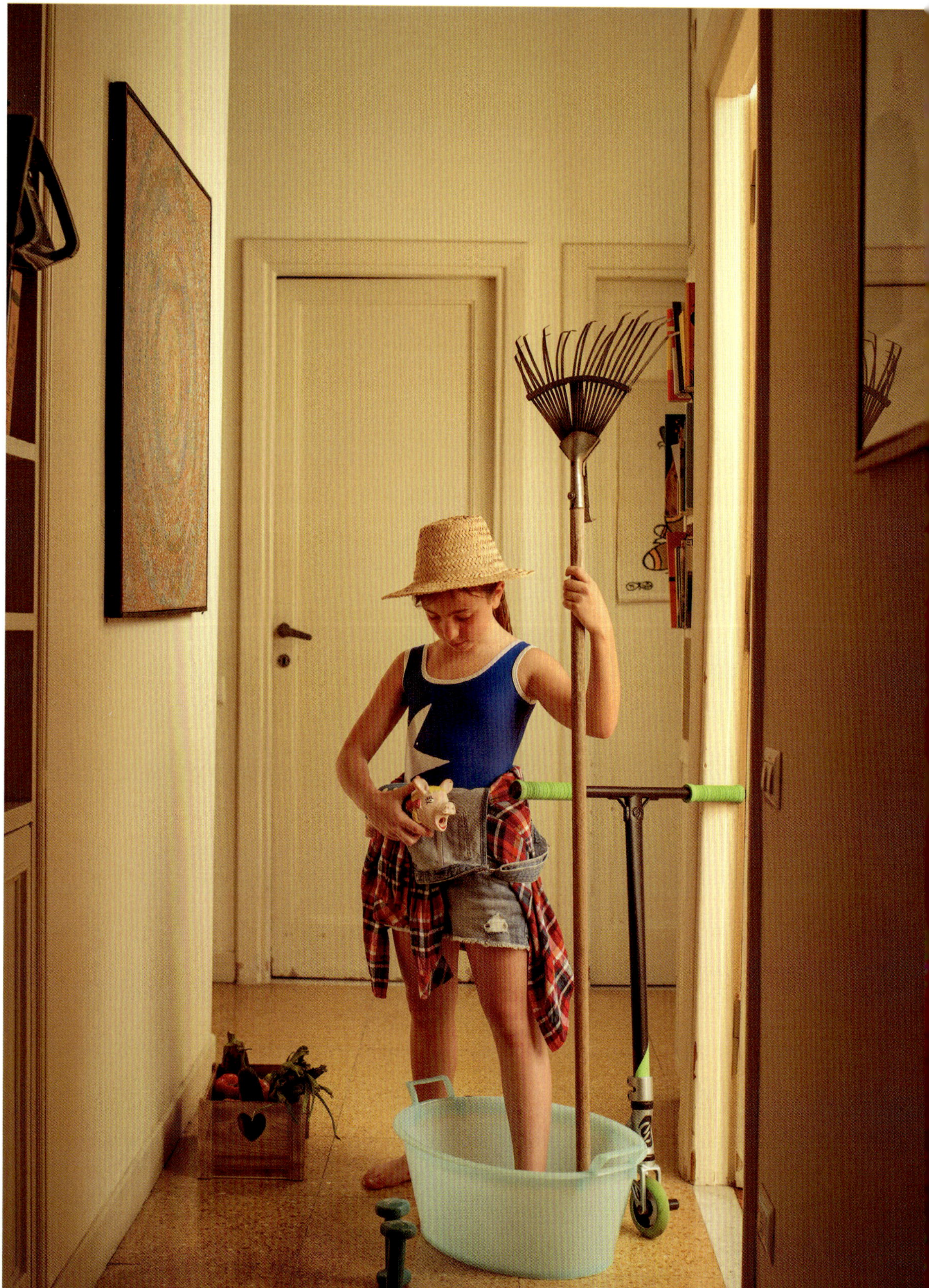

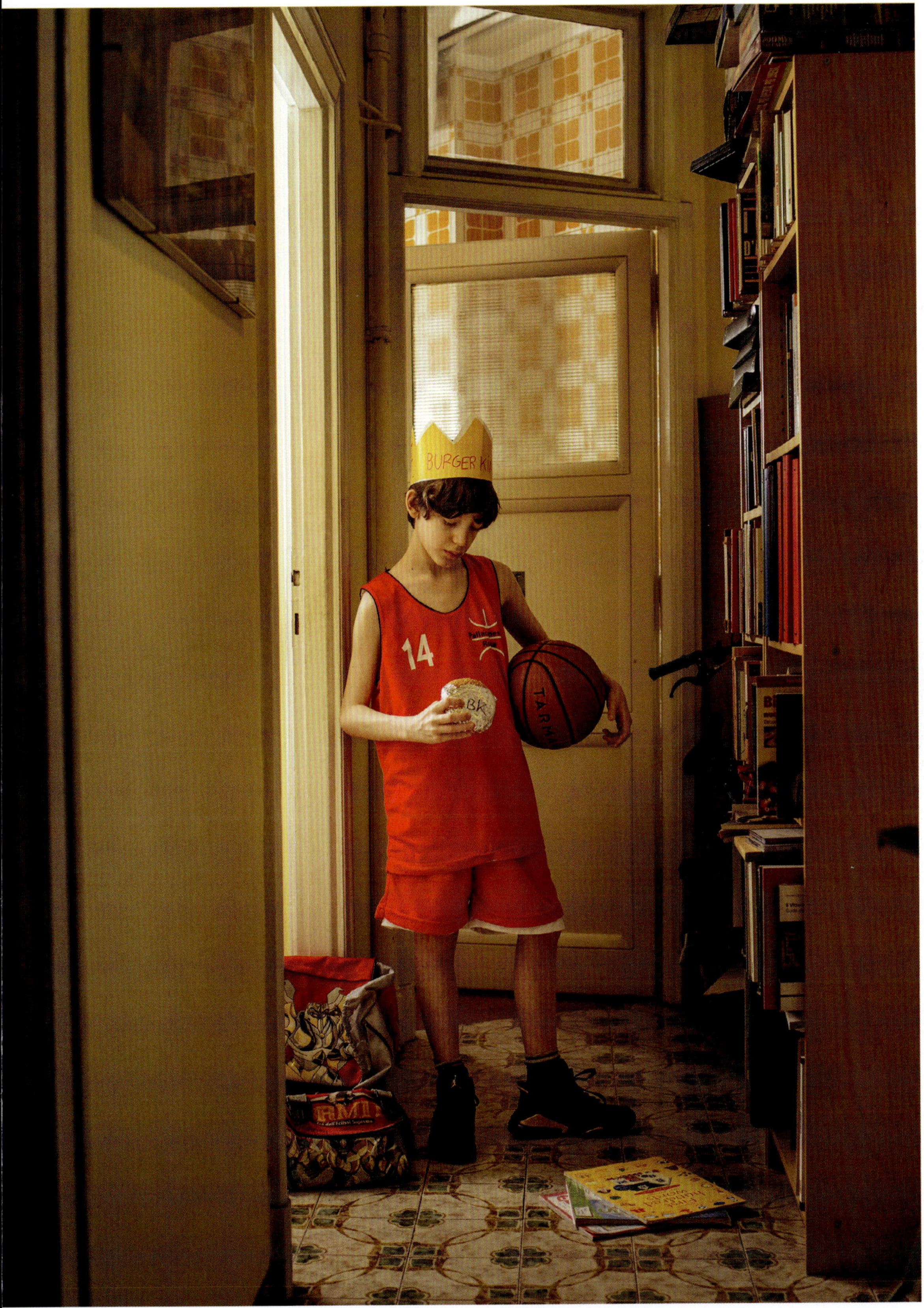
BURGER KI
14
BK

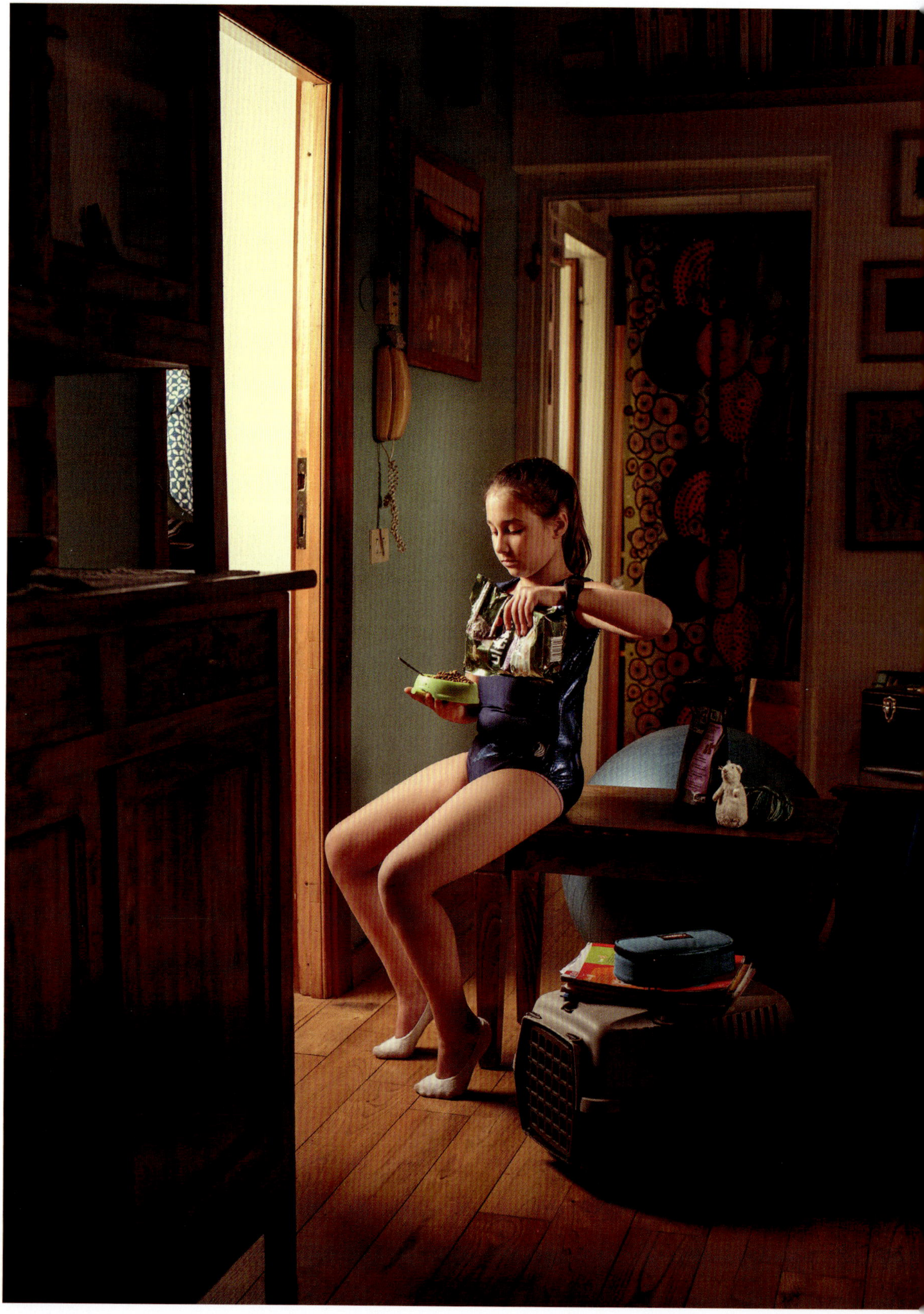

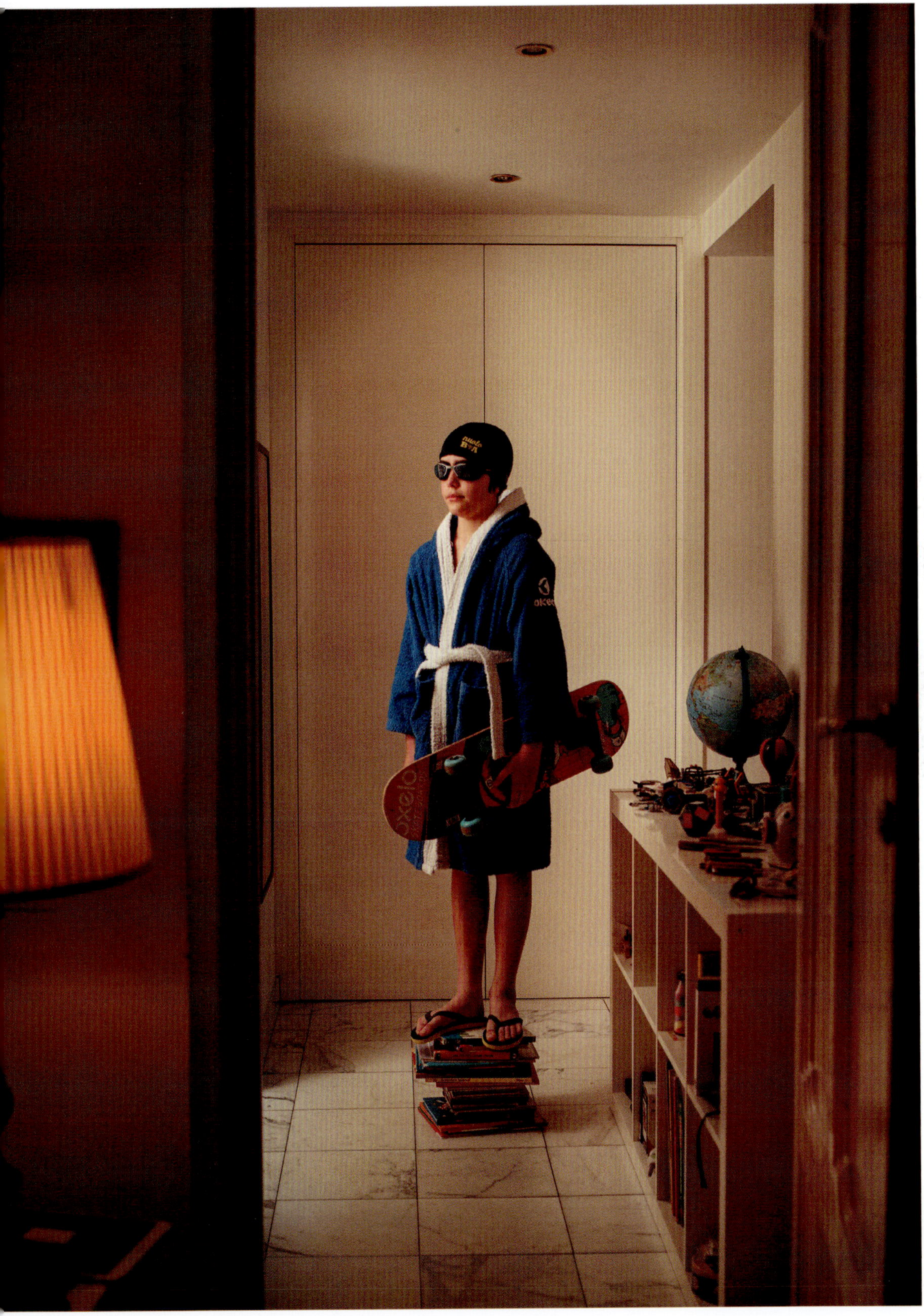
oxelo

Mattia Crocetti, Italy
COndiVIDendo 19

Following the Italian government lockdown measures imposed on March 9 2020, some families managed to reunite, possibly after a long time. Others were completely separated with some family members stranded in remote places, far away from their loved ones.
In other cases, single individuals have been forced to cohabitate with strangers, forming mixed groups, not linked by family relations. During the current health crisis, the meaning attached to the word cohabitation has changed, creating new relations from a sort of forced sharing, in particular, of spaces, habits, feelings and fears.
COndiVIDendo 19 (from the Italian "condividere" which means sharing) is a photographic and social project narrating the cohabitation of Italian citizens during the COVID-19 health crisis.
The images, like family portraits, describe groups of people living together in those environments where they are self-isolating, be that families, singles and mixed groups. Every picture has two authors: the home-based photographer and the subject as they share the whole process of creation of the final picture via a video call. The subjects share their time, their life, their intimacy and their image, first with the photographer and then with society.
From the outside the project describes the daily cohabitation of these people, in a previously unknown physical and mental state. From the inside, what stands out is the human desire to interact with society despite the isolation.

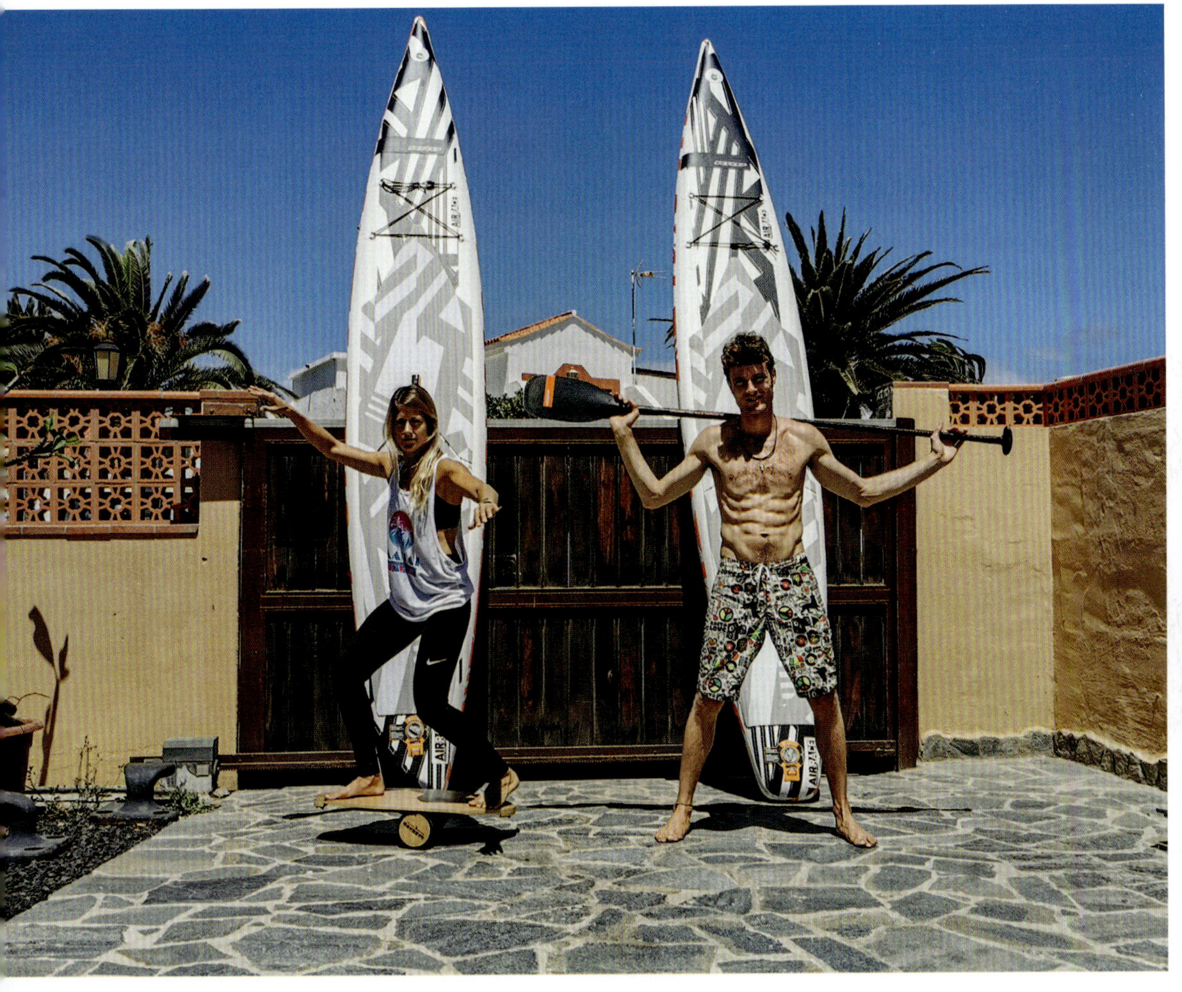

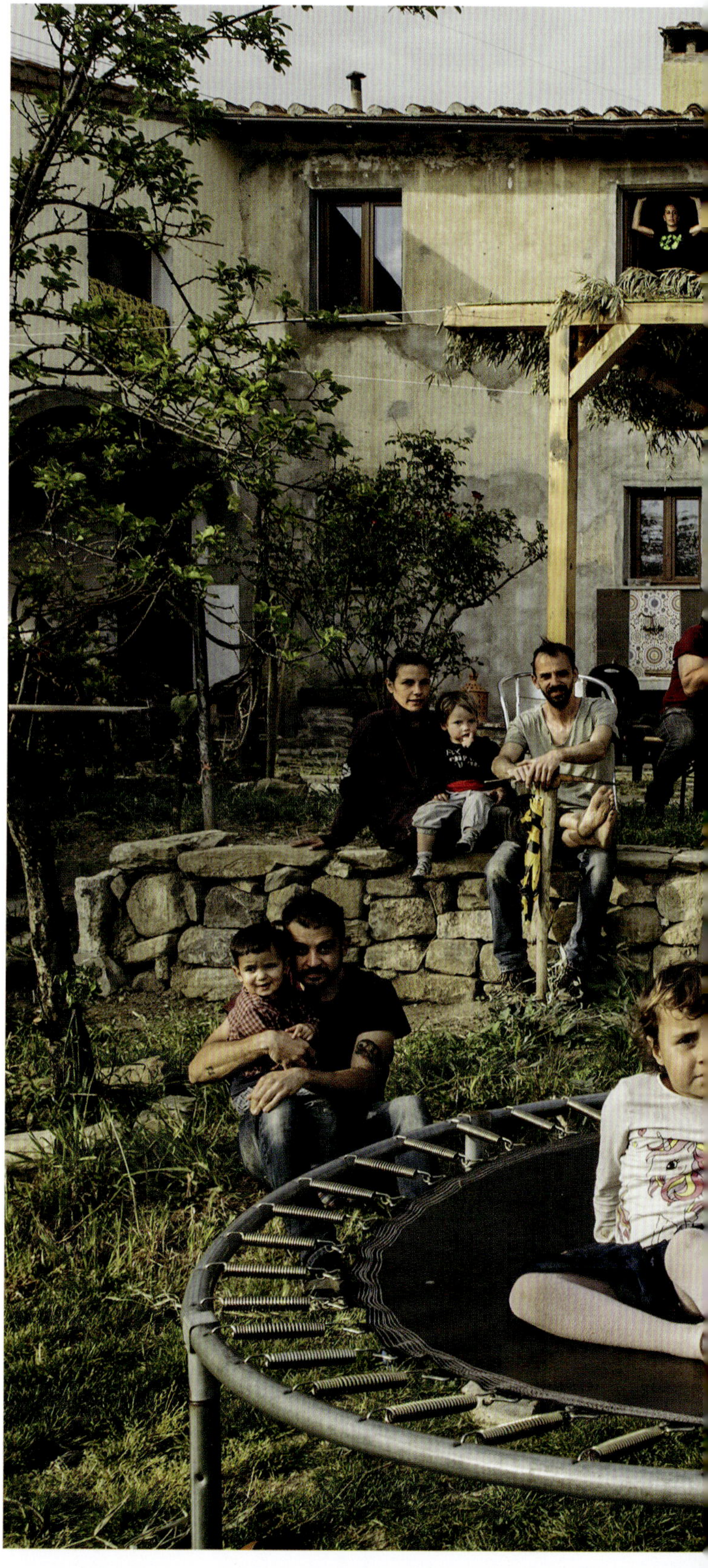

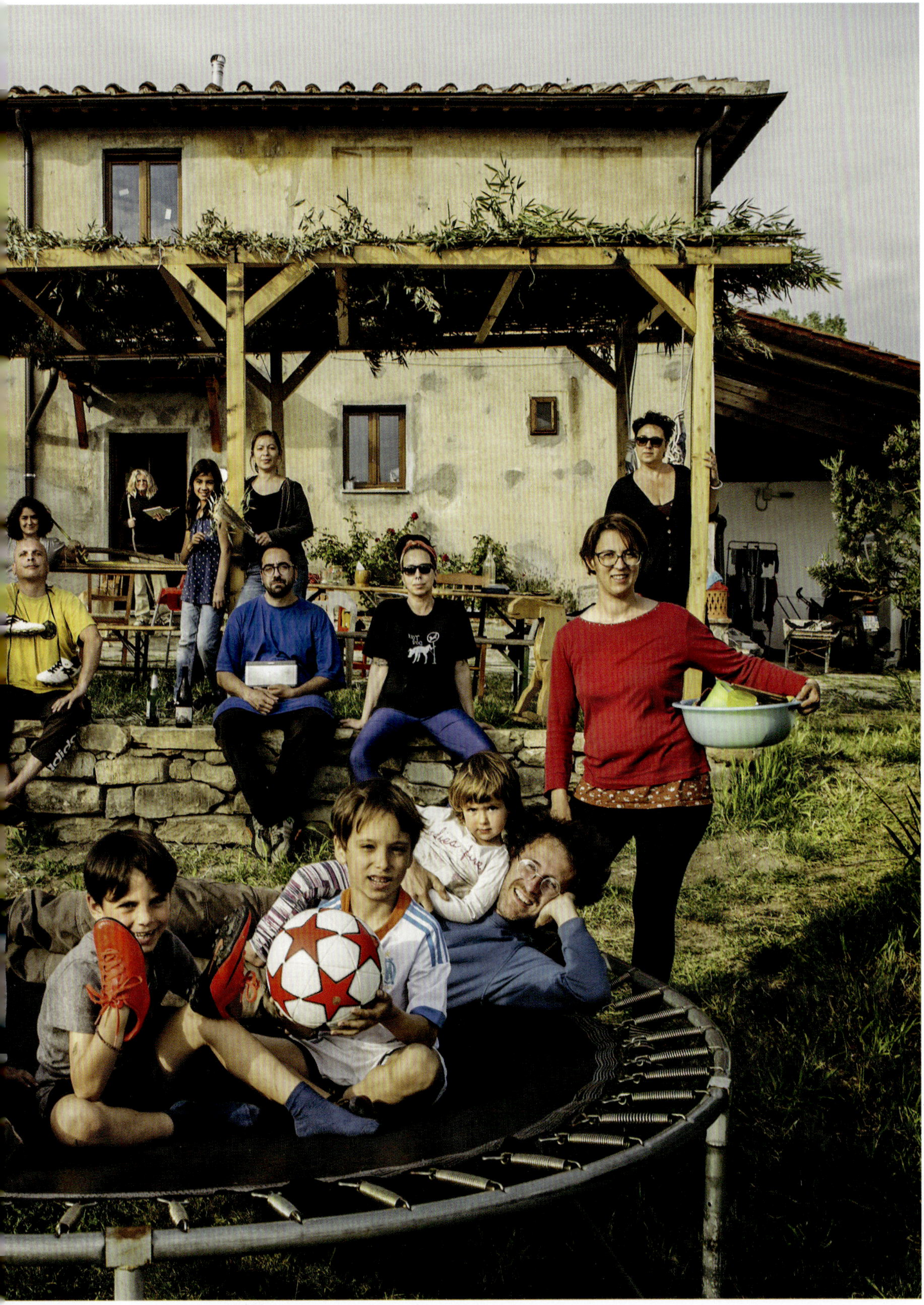

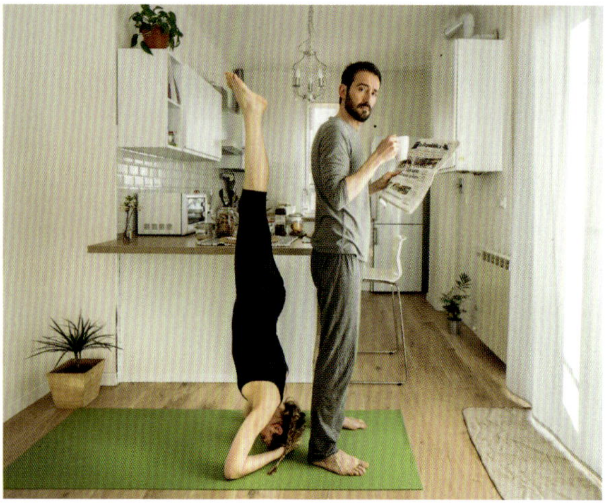
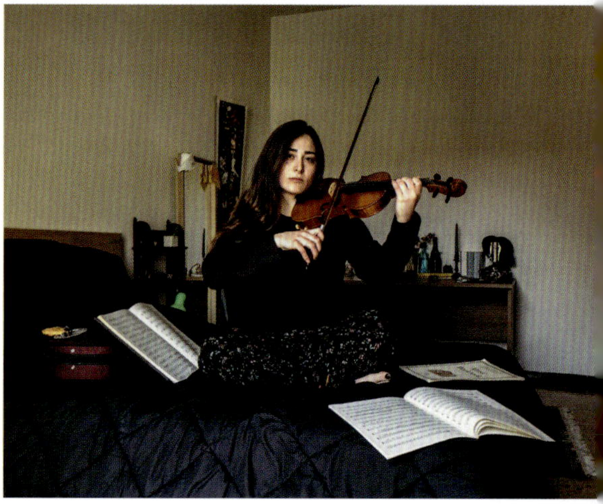
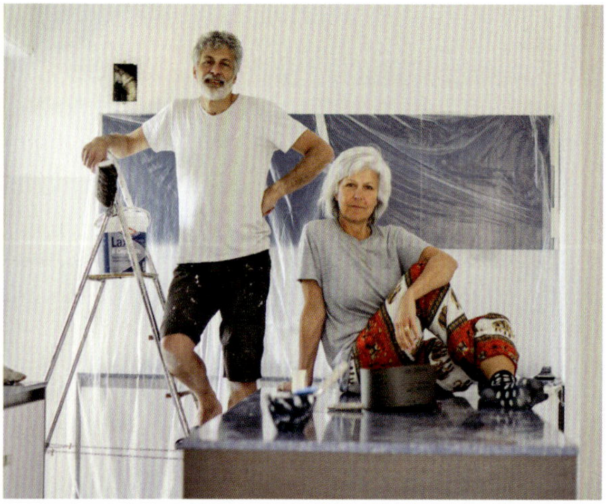
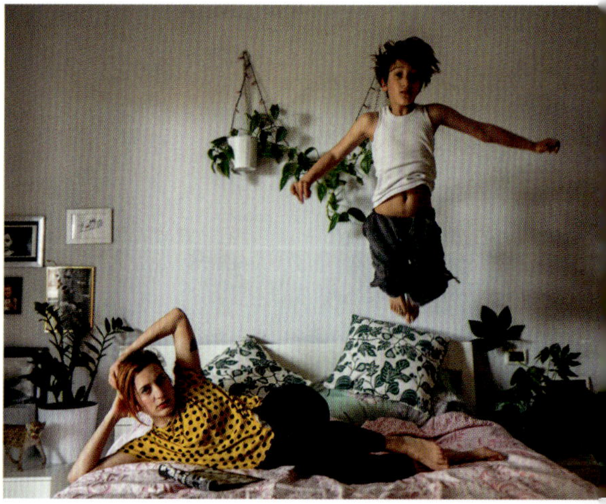
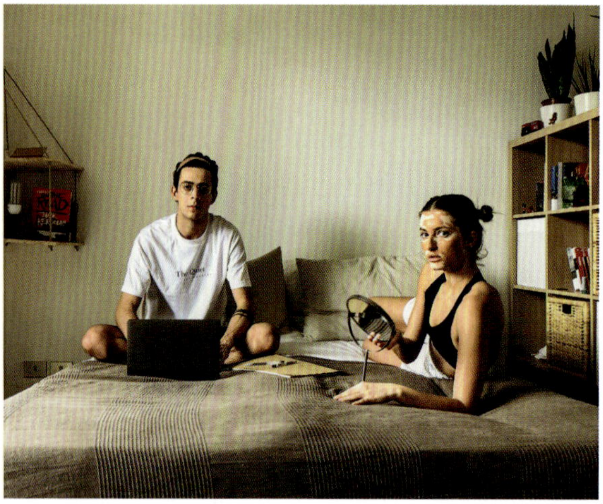
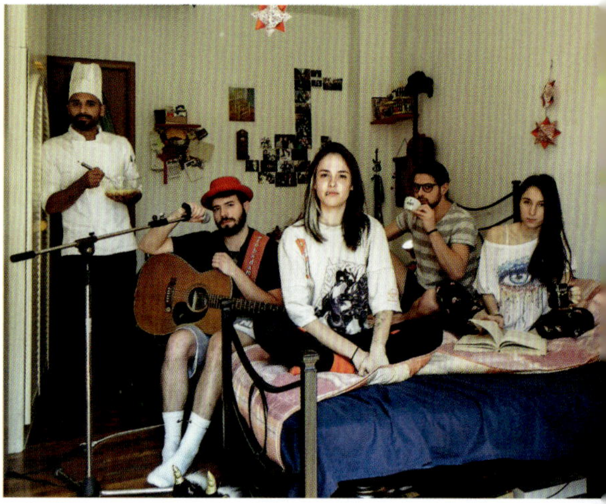

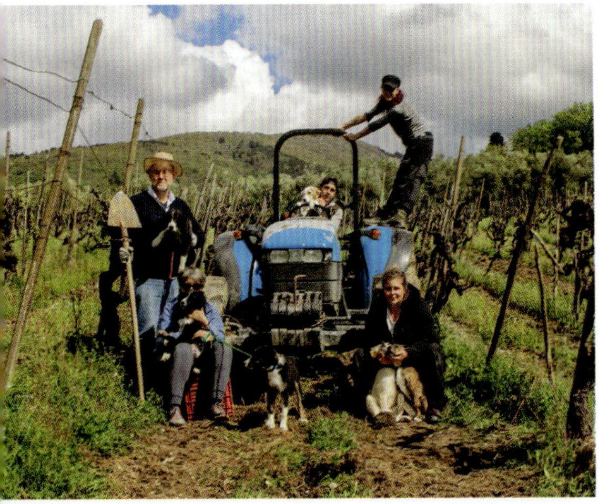
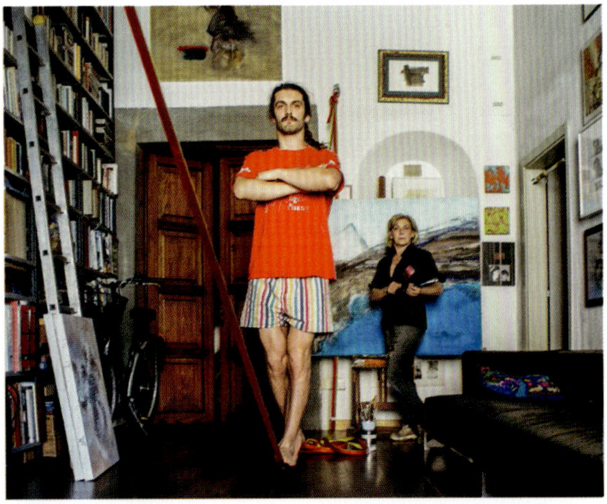
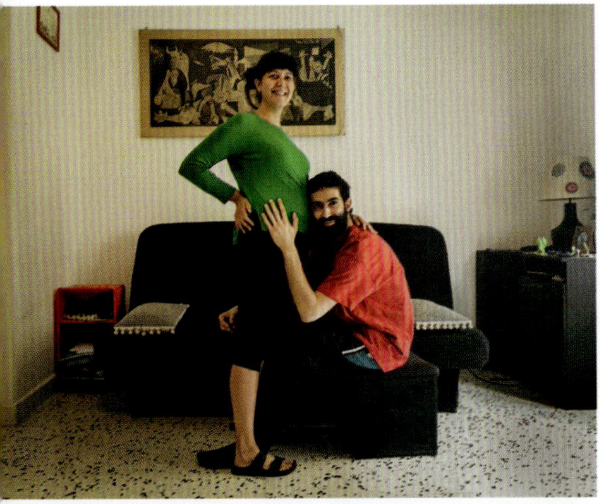
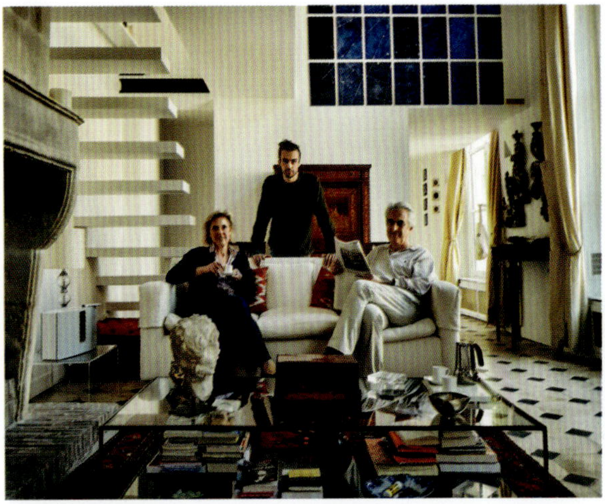
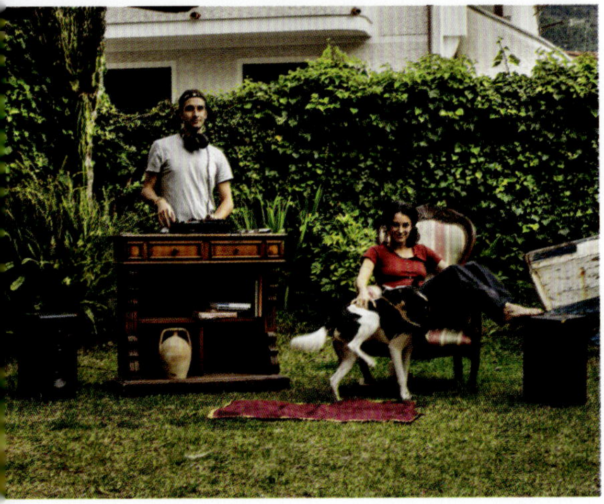
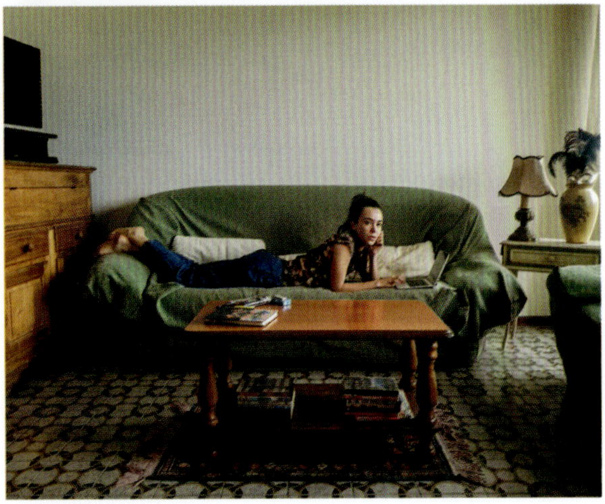

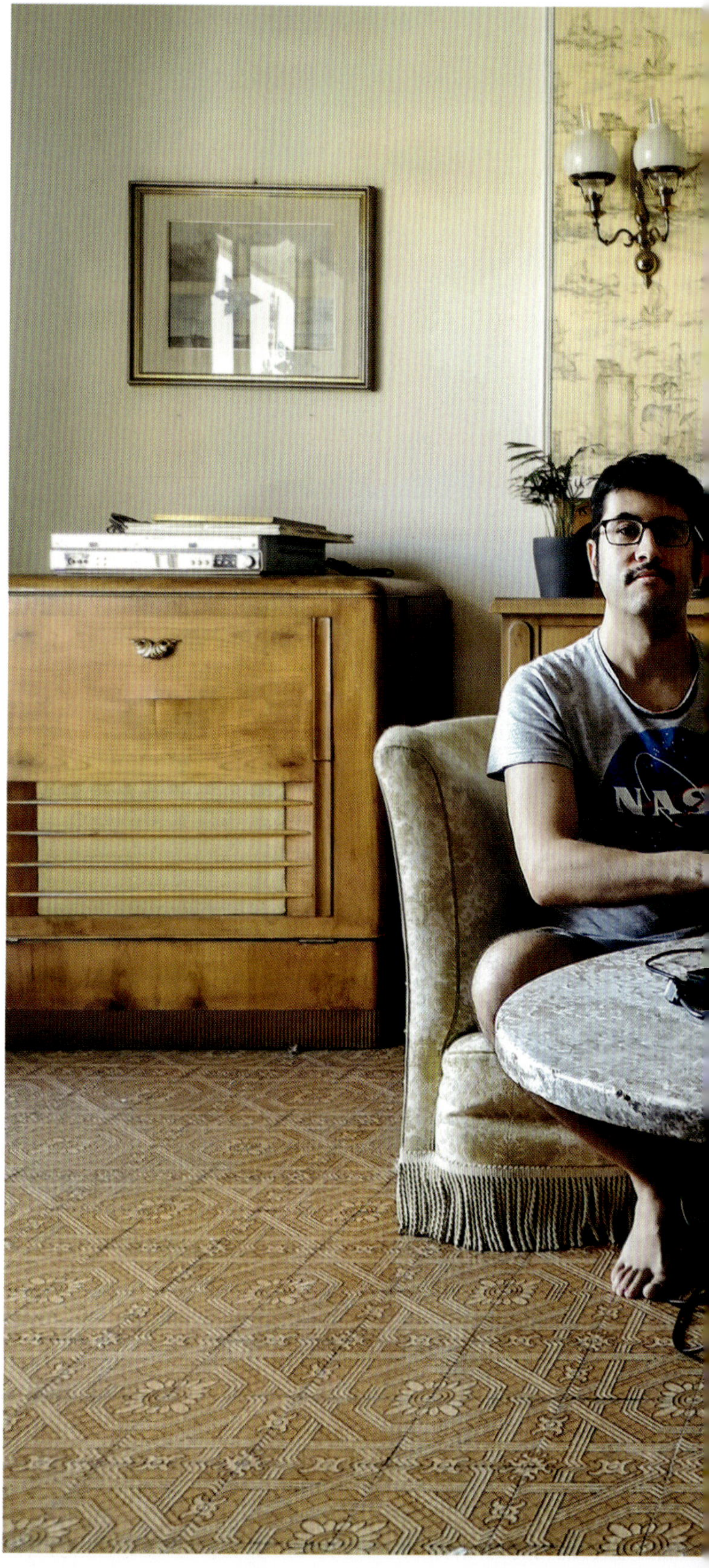
NAS

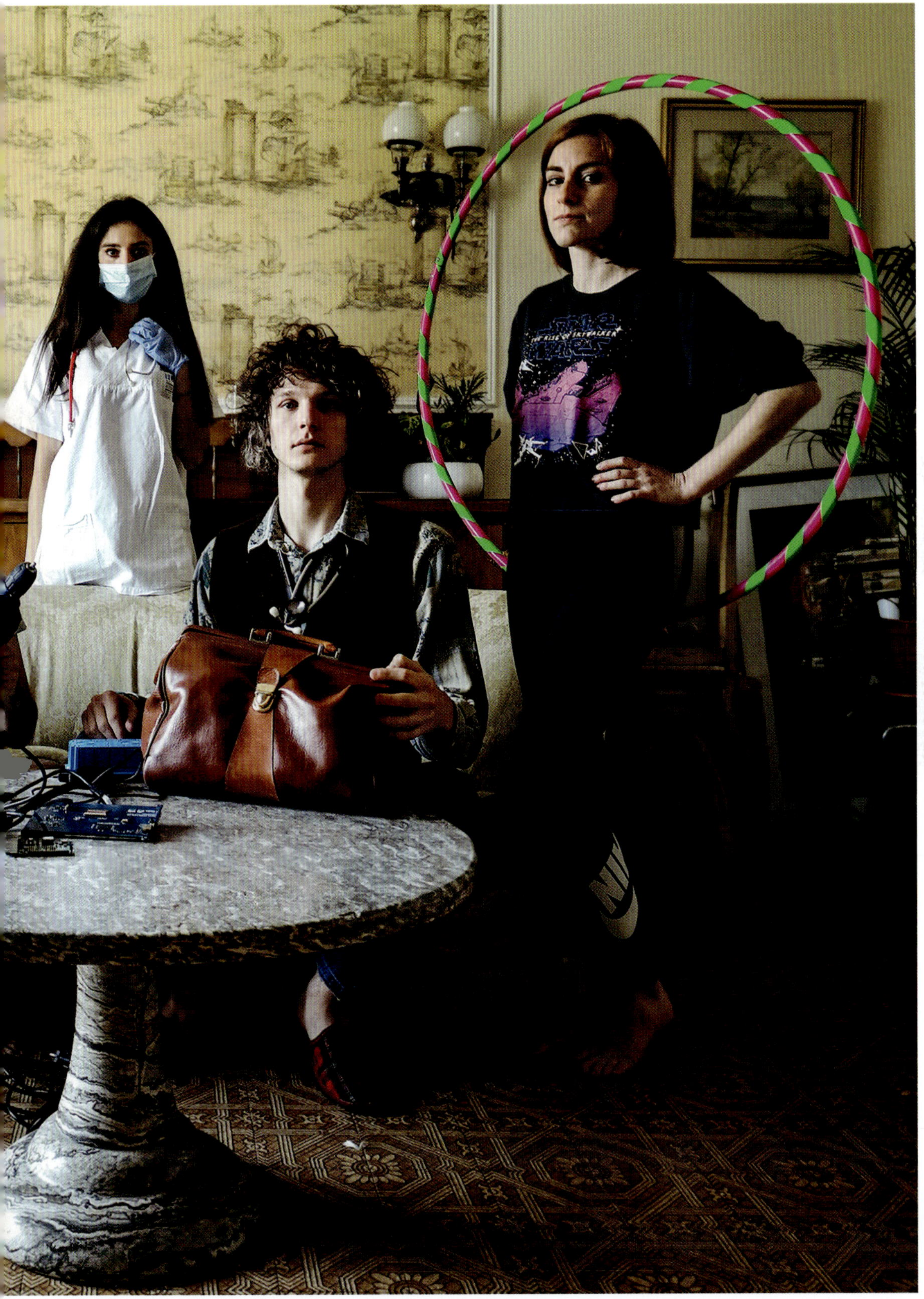

Luis Cobelo, Spain

Afuera

I was born to look.
Our outside (*afuera*) was suspended and we retired without protest. We were afraid. Suddenly the deafening noise within us became louder and we craved the external one back, to distract from it.
I look at a section of a city: Barcelona. It could have been anywhere. Without the strategic privileged position (a 180-degree view terrace) in which I find myself, I could not have done it. In fact, I never meant to, I just looked out the balcony and saw an older man walking on the roof, just like he would on the street, but without shop windows or people; only with himself. My immediate reaction was to make a video, not a photo. I was attending a unique, private, historical event. The man is doing well, he is not sitting on a couch all day. He moves, he exercises. His thoughts maybe are in the future, longing for that *afuera*.
I open my field of vision a little more and there they all were. I had a feeling that something was going to happen and I was there, with my looking machine. Life moved to rooftops and balconies. There is no precise time, although good weather lures them outside.
Contemplation and confinement became a way of survival. People with balconies look out expecting to see something that is clearly empty, some kiss or hug each other, others just talk, quite a few do some kind of exercise, look at the horizon, play ball, sunbathe, take selfies...
No one sees me. I'm hidden, they don't know that I exist. For the moment. I observe, with some nervousness: the sensation of being discovered is the excitement of a voyeur. The smartphone has become an extension of my body, it is what connects me to the world. A world in collective hysteria. So I prefer to come back to the roofs and the balconies around me. Where real people are just waiting with enormous resilience.
That older man keeps walking on the roof. This vision has become the emotional thermometer of my confinement. If I see him, I feel good. Whenever the time to go out will come, who knows, the desired routine will return and he'll go out again, watching people move, the cars, the noise of the city. Then, I will stop meddling.
It will be weird, for everyone.

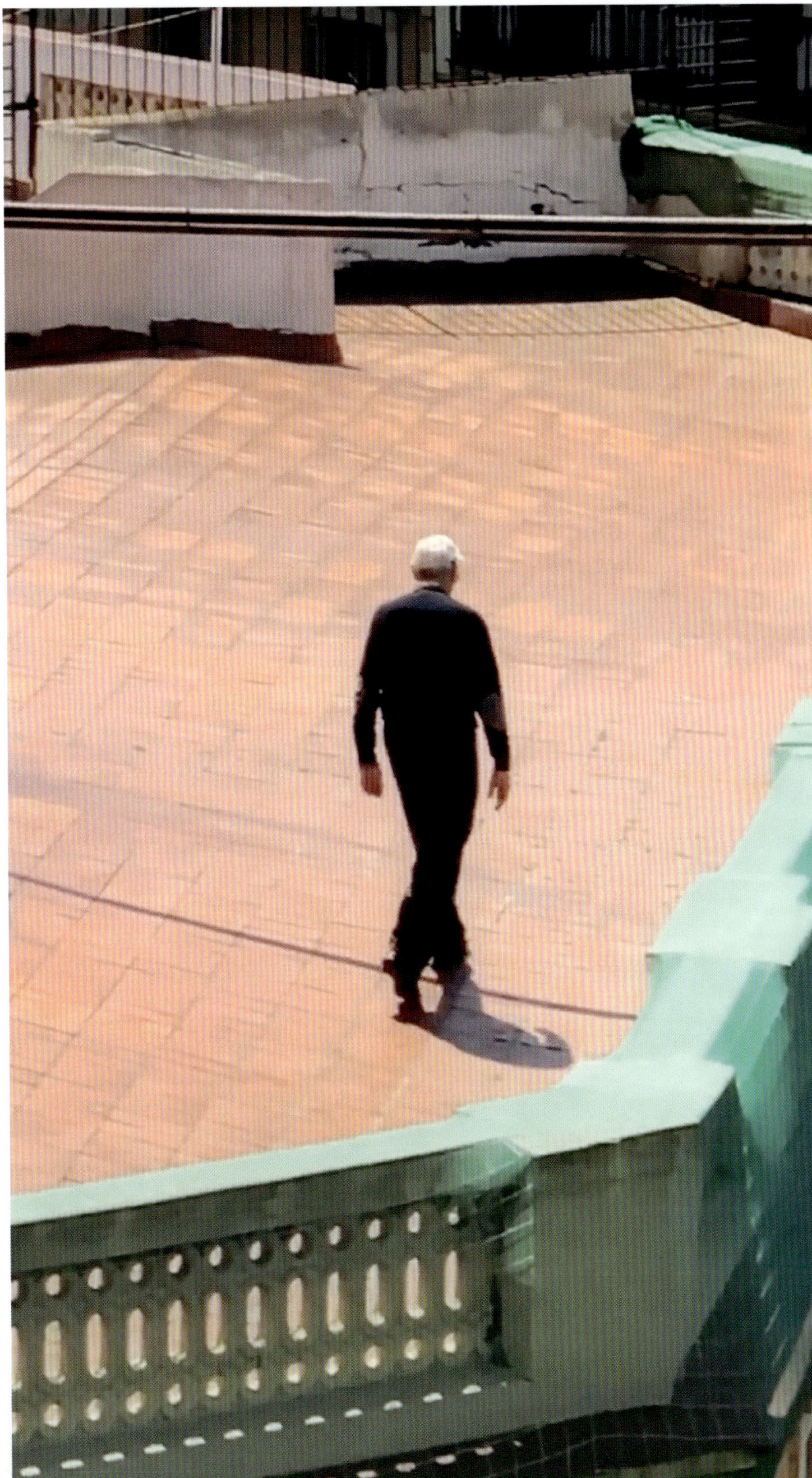

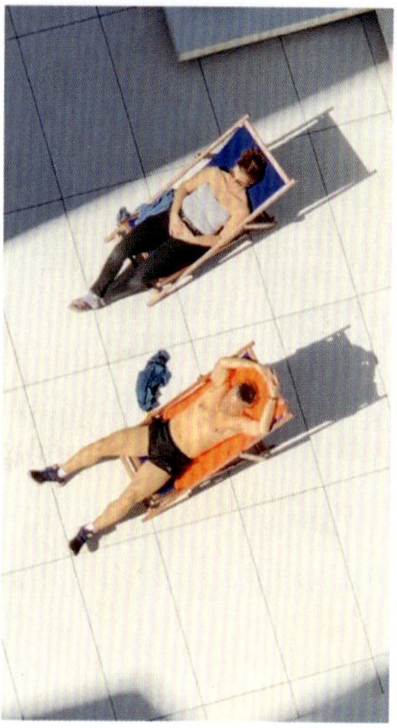
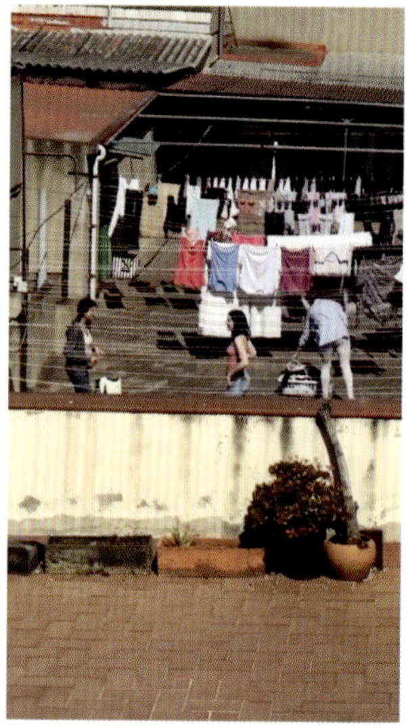
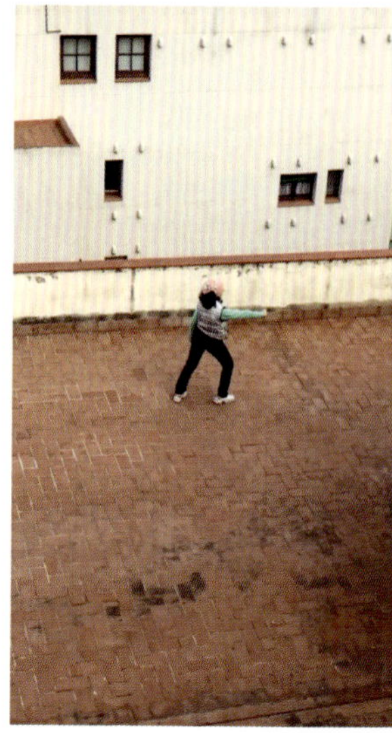
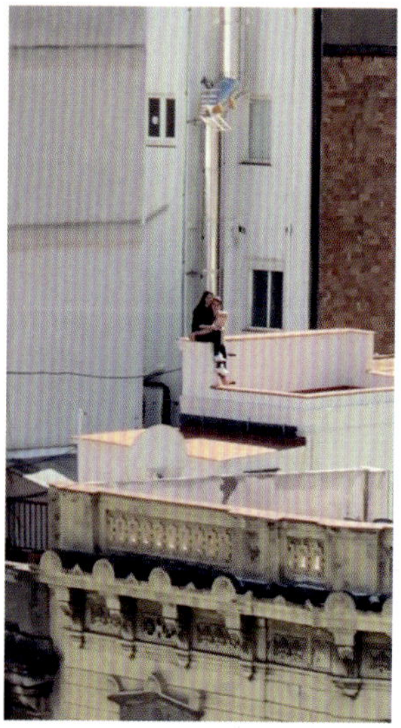
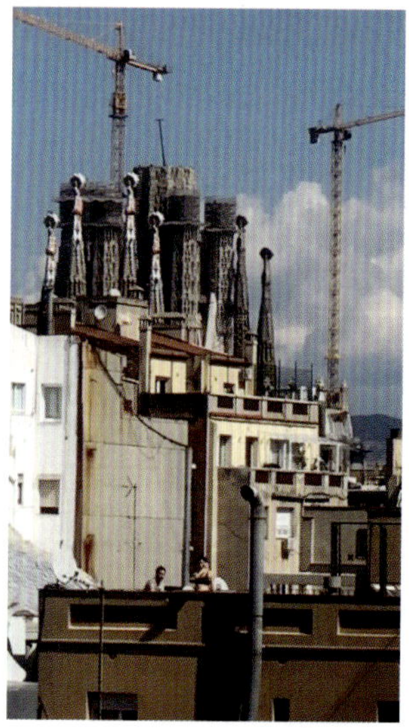
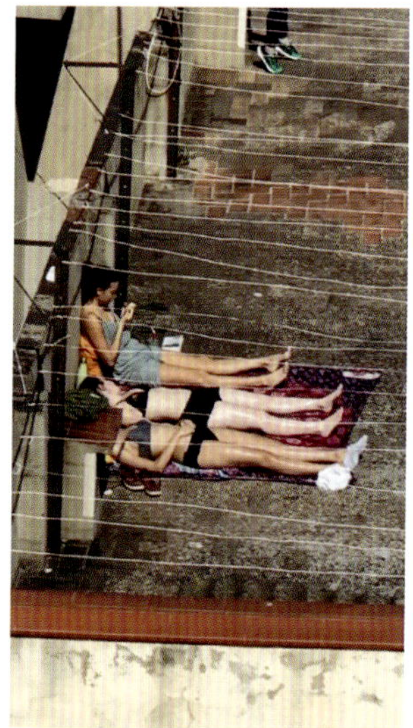
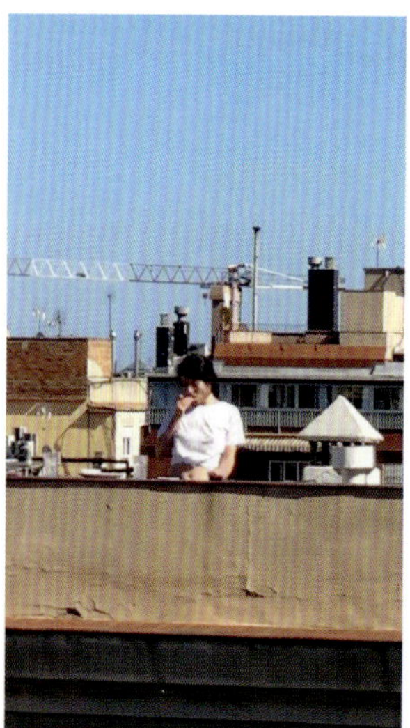
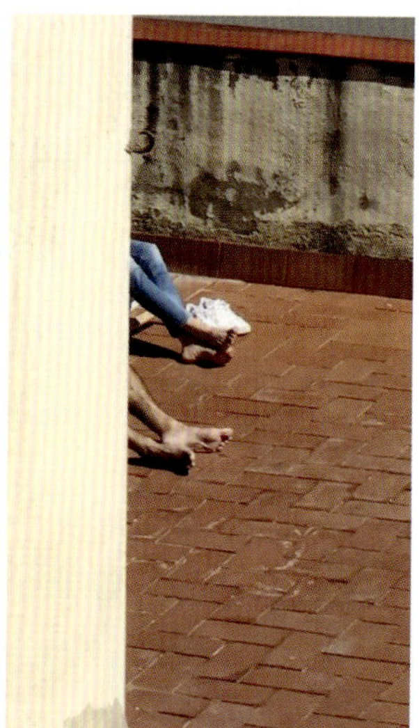
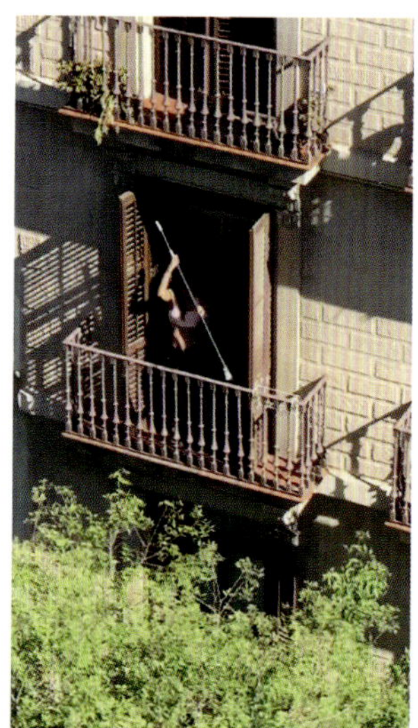

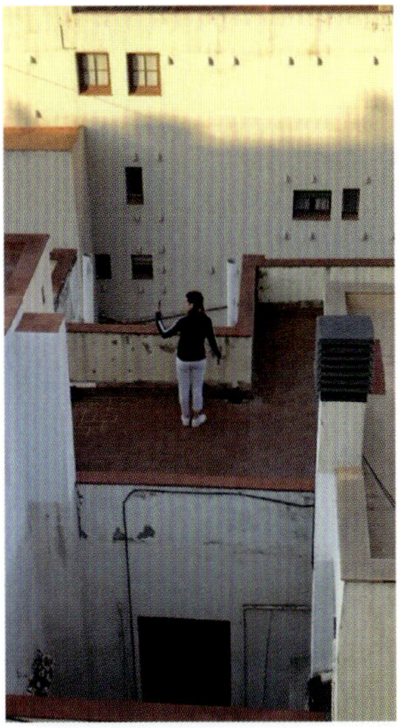
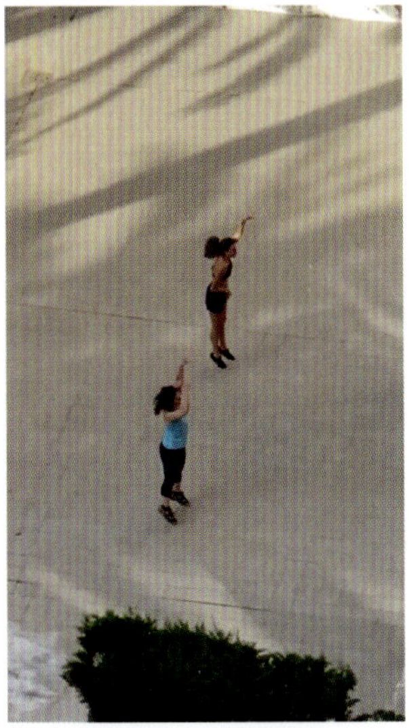
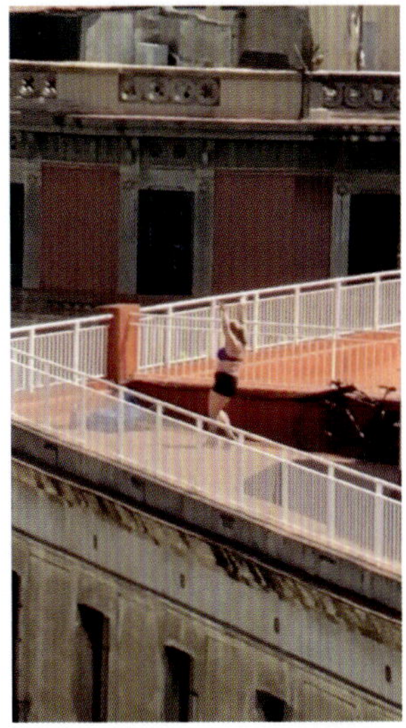
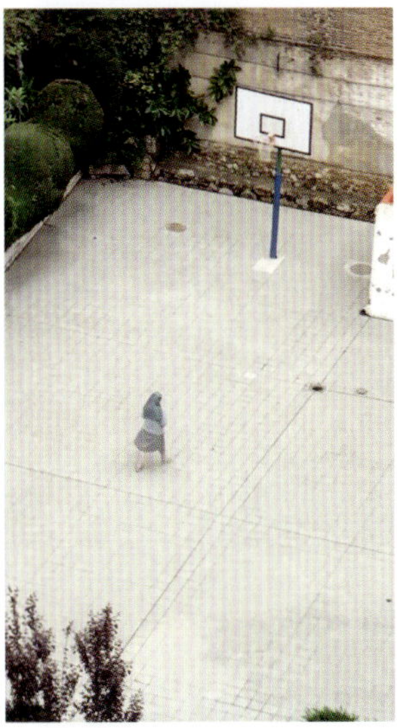
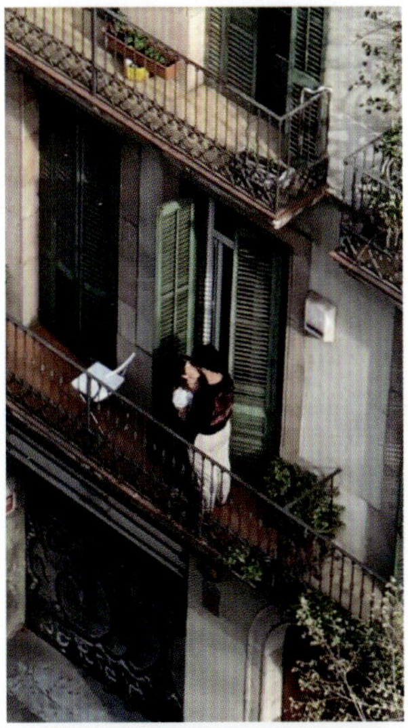
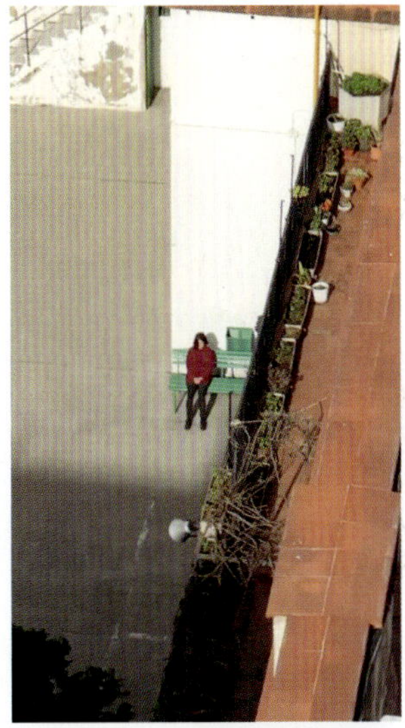
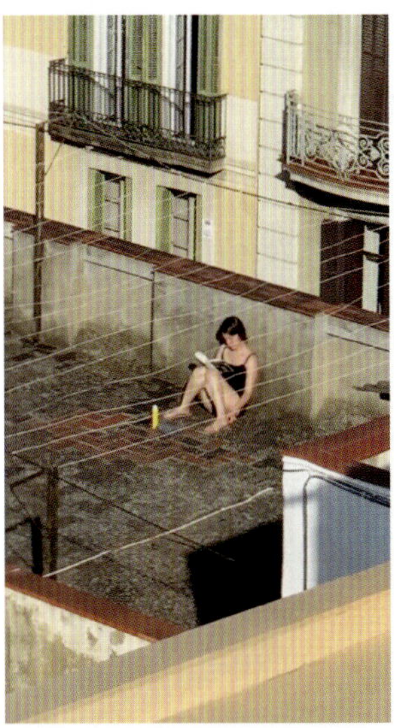
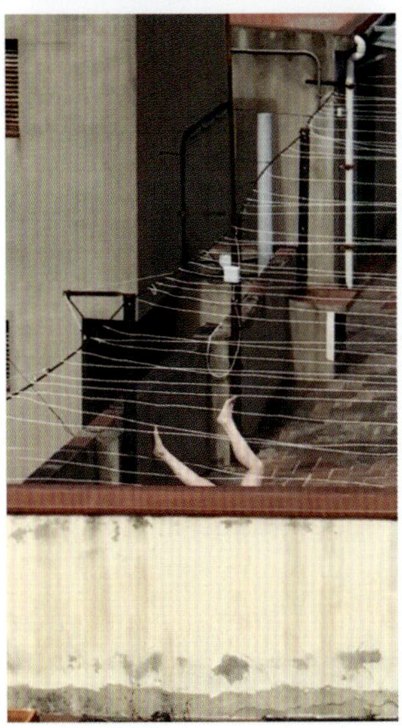
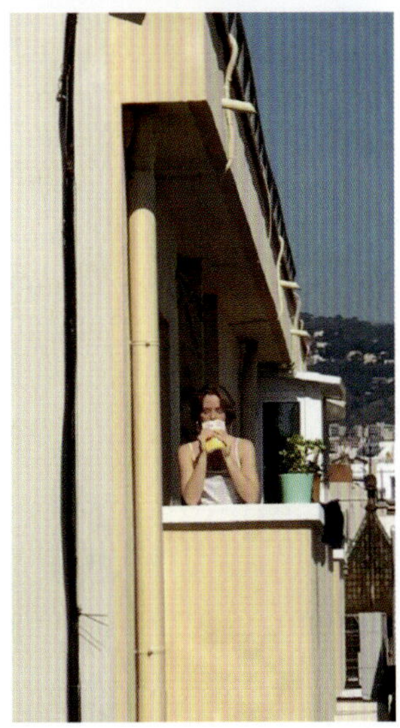

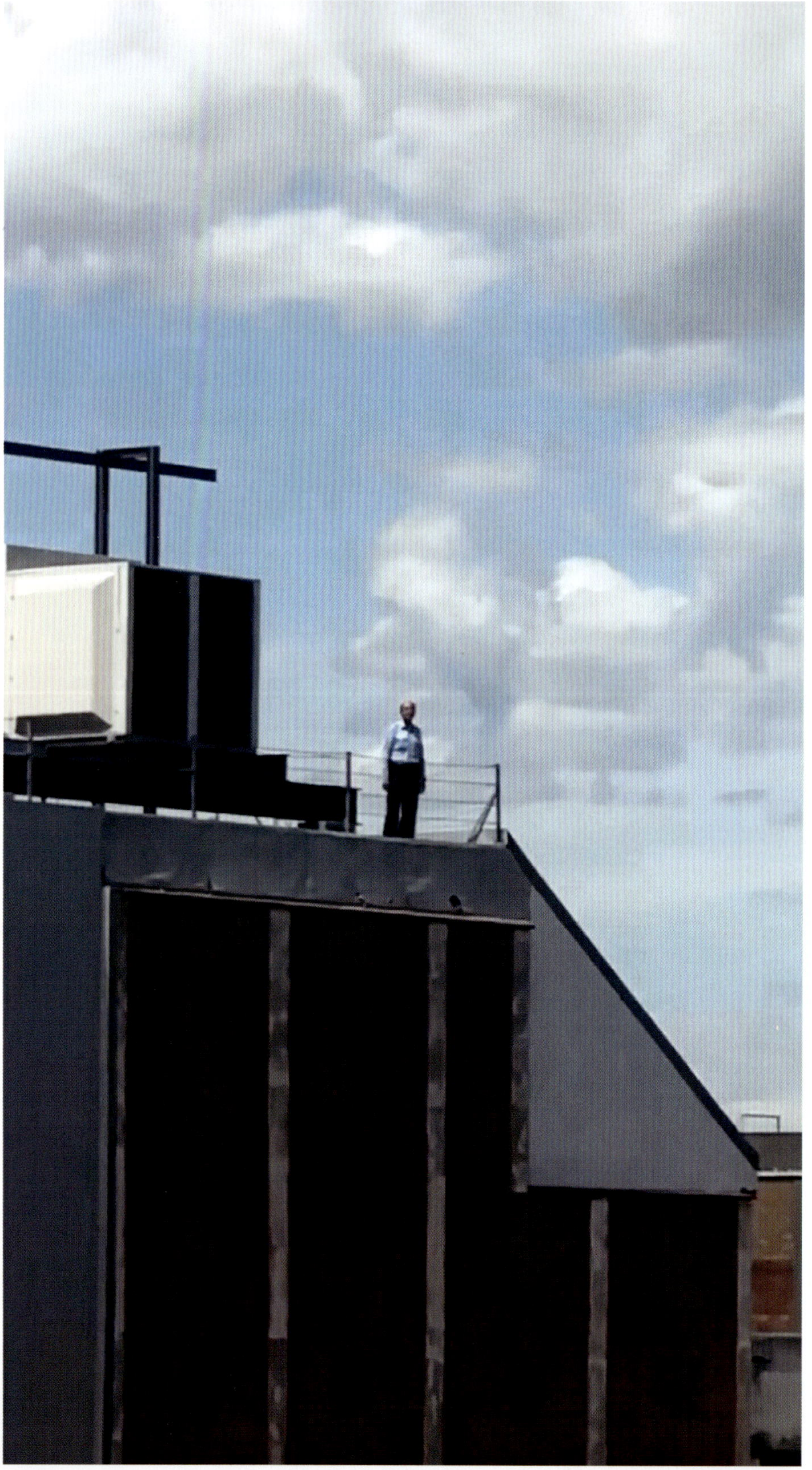

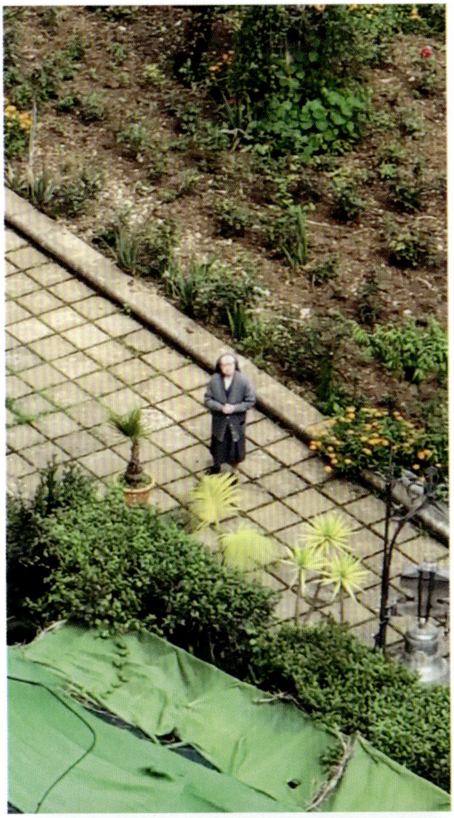
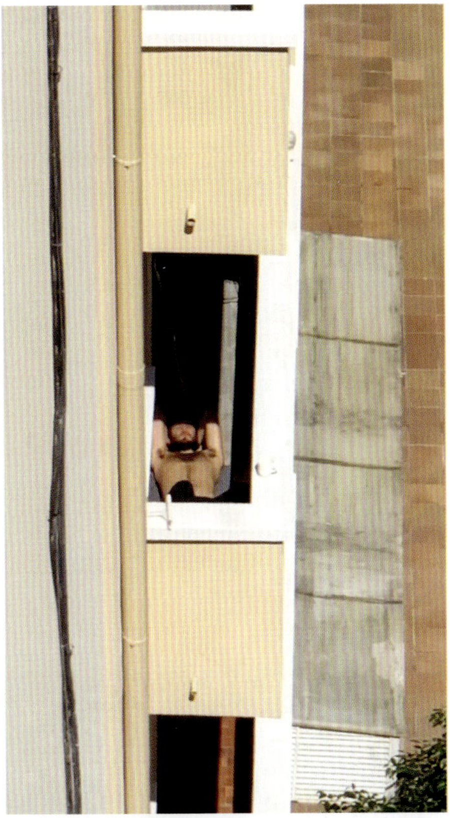
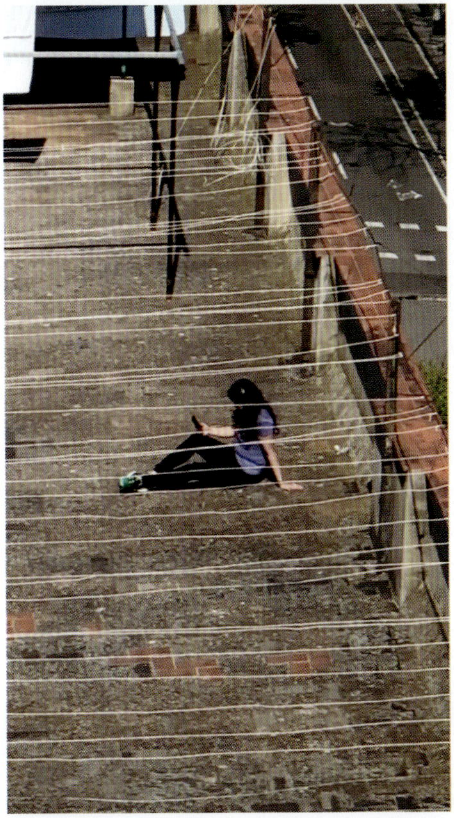
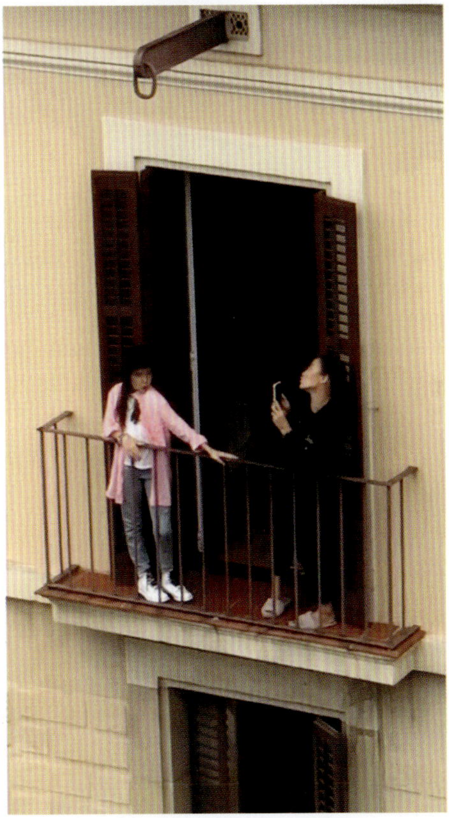

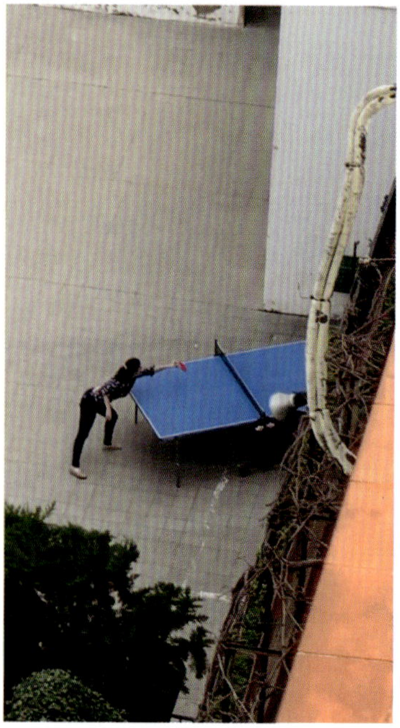
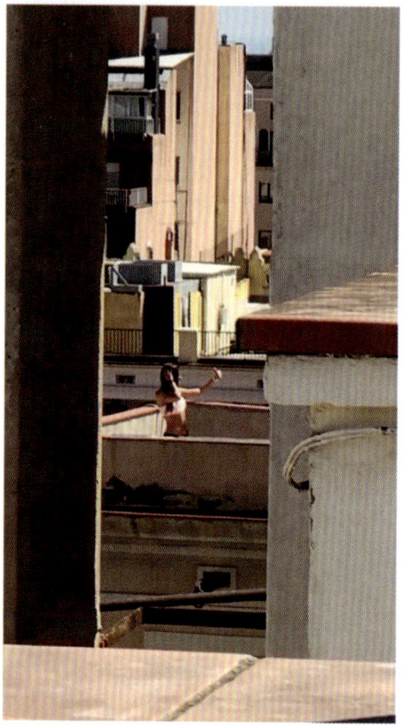
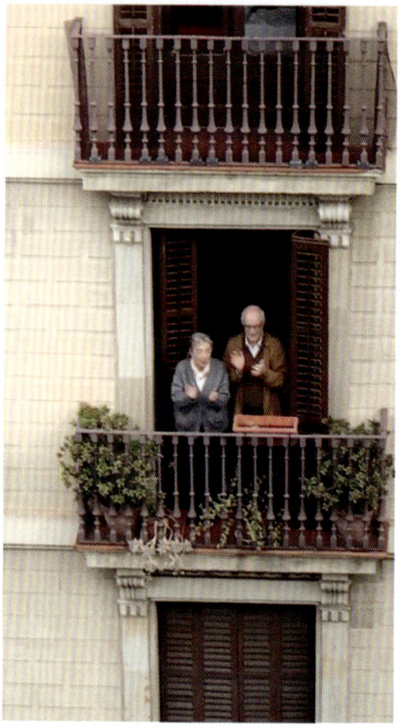
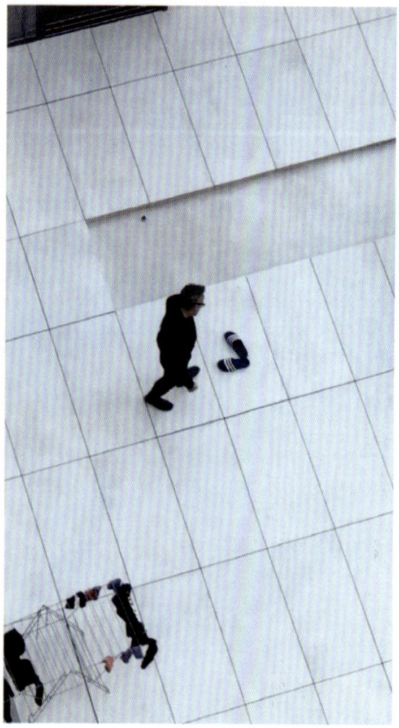
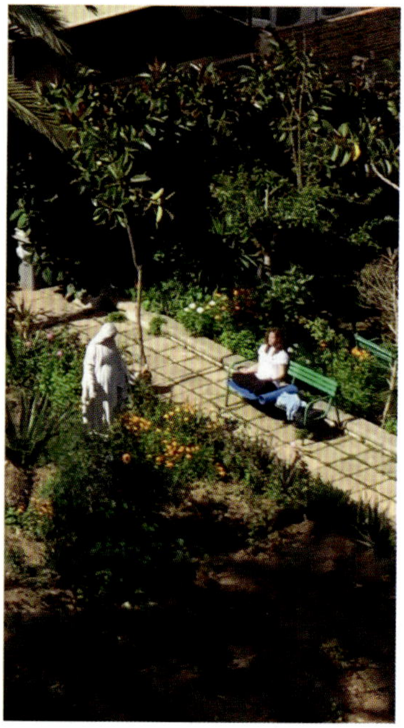
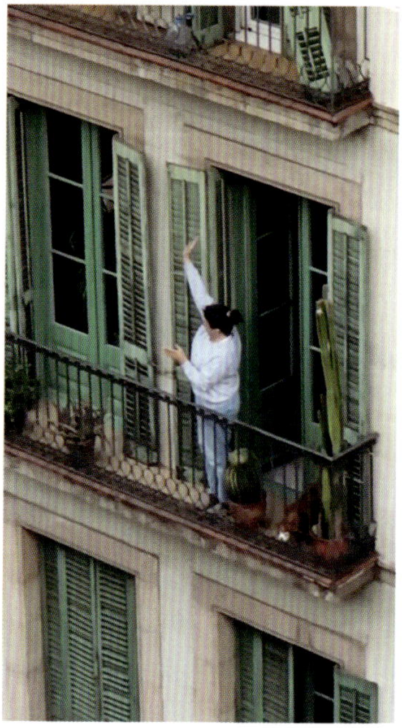

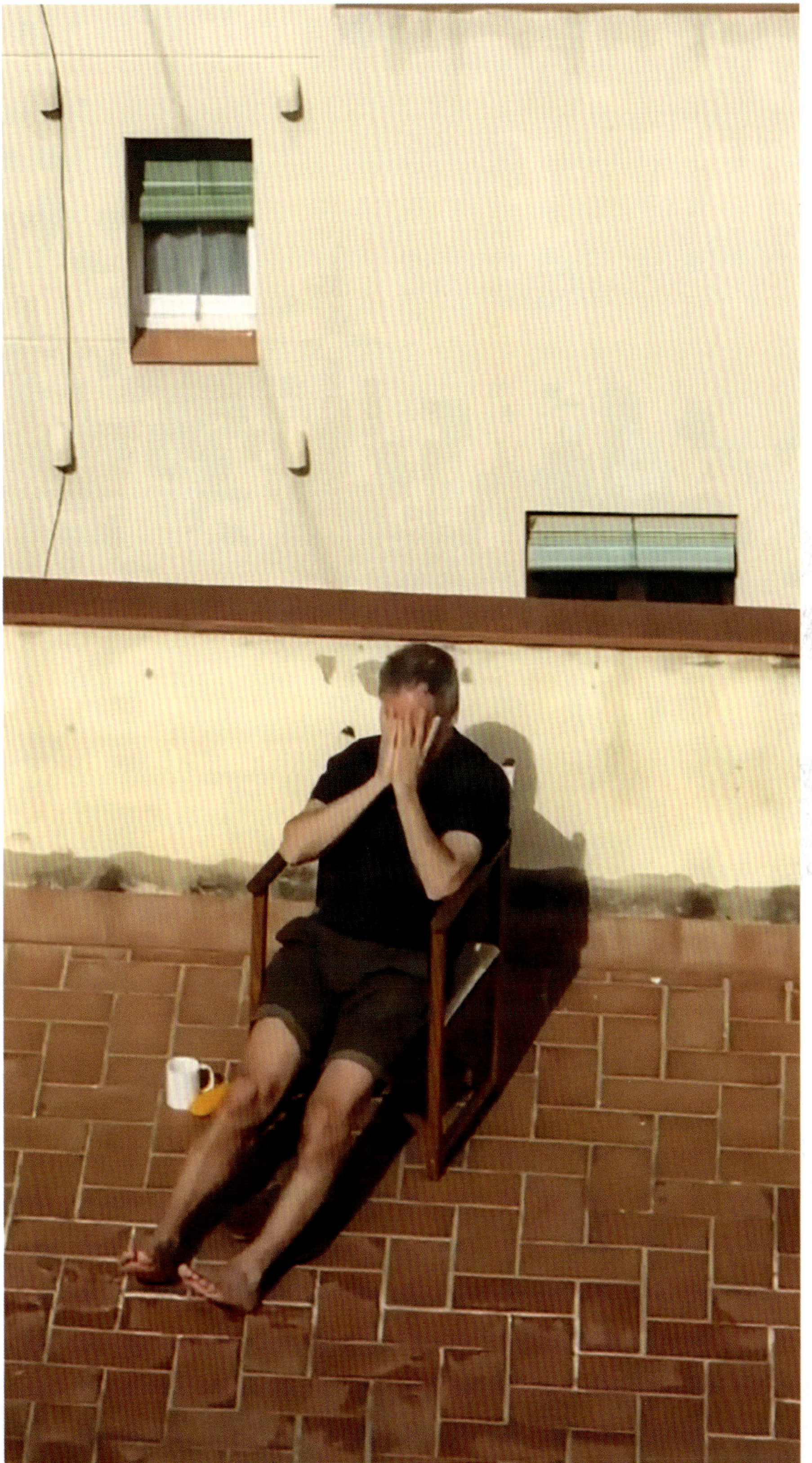

03. Shelter in Place
Captions

Mohammad Shahnewaz Khan, Bangladesh

The photographs were taken in the city of Chittagong.

Celebrating the birthday of my youngest son Imran. 19 July 2020.
(Page 211)

Daily night of Ramadan, in the month of Ramadan, we are waiting for Sehri.
12 May 2020.
(Pages 212–213)

There is no sleep in the eyes of the children. During this pandemic lockdown days, they are restless to play and go out. 11 May 2020.
(Page 214, top)

My son Hossain (three-and-half-year-old) is studying with his mother and Imran (22-month-old) is playing. My wife's aunt is praying Salah in the month of Ramadan. She is here to help us and now staying in my late mother's room. 12 May 2020.
(Page 214, bottom)

I have two kids, and two of my younger brothers also have children. During this time, the kids are restless and out of control, always trying to go out and crying all the time. I just try to make them happy. 13 April 2020.
(Page 215, top)

Daily family life during the coronavirus pandemic lockdown. 3 May 2020.
(Page 215, bottom)

Negar is trying to touch the raindrop. After intense heat; it was raining a little after many days. My wife Niger was running and went to the roof, Hussein and I followed her.
24 April 2020.
(Page 216)

Portrait of my three-and-half-year-old child Hossain, here I tried to show the reality of children during this COVID-19 pandemic, isolation and lockdown days. 15 May 2020.
(Page 217)

For a time it seemed that I could no longer be worldly. It would have been better if there was no family, I wanted to escape from family life, I felt stuck, I wanted to be free from all family ties. 20 May 2020.
(Pages 218–219)

Lorenzo Pesce, Italy

The photographs were taken in Rome between May and June 2020.

Angelica missed celebrating her birthday, artistic gymnastic and playing with her friends.
(Page 221)

Gregorio missed his friends, school and playing tennis.
(Page 222)

10-year-old Anna Corapi posing in her apartment. During lockdown she missed horseback riding, gymnastic, and her class.
(Page 223)

Anna F. missed school, the seaside and her orchestra.
(Page 224)

Michel missed his friends, basket and going to McDonald's.
(Page 225)

10-year-old Gaia Spinozzi in her apartment. During lockdown she missed the weekends at her grandma's house in the countryside, friends and gymnastics.
(Page 226)

10-year-old Mario Lombardi posing in his apartment. During lockdown he missed school, basket and going to Burger King.
(Page 227)

10-year-old Ada Pescio posing in her apartment. During lockdown she missed her cat, gymnastic and her class.
(Page 228)

10-year-old Enrico Modigliani posing in his apartment. During lockdown he missed his friends, school, and the swimming pool.
(Page 229)

Mattia Crocetti, Italy

The photographs were taken in the 56 days of lockdown in Italy, beginning on March 9 2020.

Paolo and Susak, couple, Fuerteventura, Spain.
(Page 231)

Cecco Rivolta family, Sesto Fiorentino, Italy.
(Pages 232-233)

Stefano and Laura, couple, Bologna, Italy.
(Page 234, top left)

Silvia, Ferrara, Italy.
(Page 234, top right)

Adriano and Lucia, husband and wife, Trento, Italy.
(Page 234, centre left)

Francesca and Giulio, mother and son, Pescara, Italy.
(Page 234, centre right)

Caterina and Daniele, couple, Milan, Italy.
(Page 234, bottom left)

Giuseppe, Giuseppe, Giovanna, Giuseppe, Camilla, mixed group, Milan, Italy.
(Page 234, bottom right)

Vannucci-Becattini family and Valentina, Reggello, Italy.
(Page 235, top left)

Anita and Francesco, mother and son, Pisa, Italy.
(Page 235, top right)

Beatrice and Maria Teresa, Portoferraio, Italy.
(Page 235, centre left)

Pantaleone family, aunt, uncle and nephew, Paris, France.
(Page 235, centre right)

Arianna and dj Lostdogz Krw, couple, Sapri, Italy.
(Page 235, bottom left)

Matilde Giannini, Pisa, Italy.
(Page 235, bottom right)

Silvia, Mattia, Pablo, Alice, roomates, Florence, Italy.
(Pages 236–237)

04.

The Economic Effects

Mattia Balsamini, Italy
Contingency Plans

Raffaele Panizza

When Italy hit 60,000 infections (out of which one third were in Lombardy) and 5,000 fatalities, on March 22 2020 a decree issued by Prime Minister Giuseppe Conte imposed the lockdown of a large part of the Italian productive apparatus, as well as prohibiting any form of unjustified displacement and enforcing confinement of the population to their homes.
On the one hand, the necessary and permitted activities, ranging from food to energy production. Companies were ready to multiply efforts to ensure that the country did not lack resources in the coronavirus emergency. On the other hand, those considered non-strategic, which with reactivity, resourcefulness and a spirit of solidarity have made themselves available to be reinvented and to support the common effort. Sudden industrial reconversions, emergency production, collaboration between manufacturers from different cities to print protective visors in 3D, volunteer shifts of workers who have accepted the risk of making closed factories live to develop sanitising gels and masks for the Civil Protection Department.
And then hundreds of medical oxygen cylinders forged twenty-four hours a day in ovens at a thousand degrees so that the convalescents who were fighting the virus at home wouldn't run out of air. And finally, the incredible scene of military and civil engineers united in support of a company in the Bologna area, to produce – in record time – the lung ventilators for intensive care units, which had required 5,000 additional beds in just two months.
From fashion to high-precision mechanics, from chemistry to software, to automotive (even Ferrari's prototype section in Maranello has created valves for personal protective equipment), here are the stories of a country that has never stopped behind its lowered shutters. And from a distance, it has united even more.

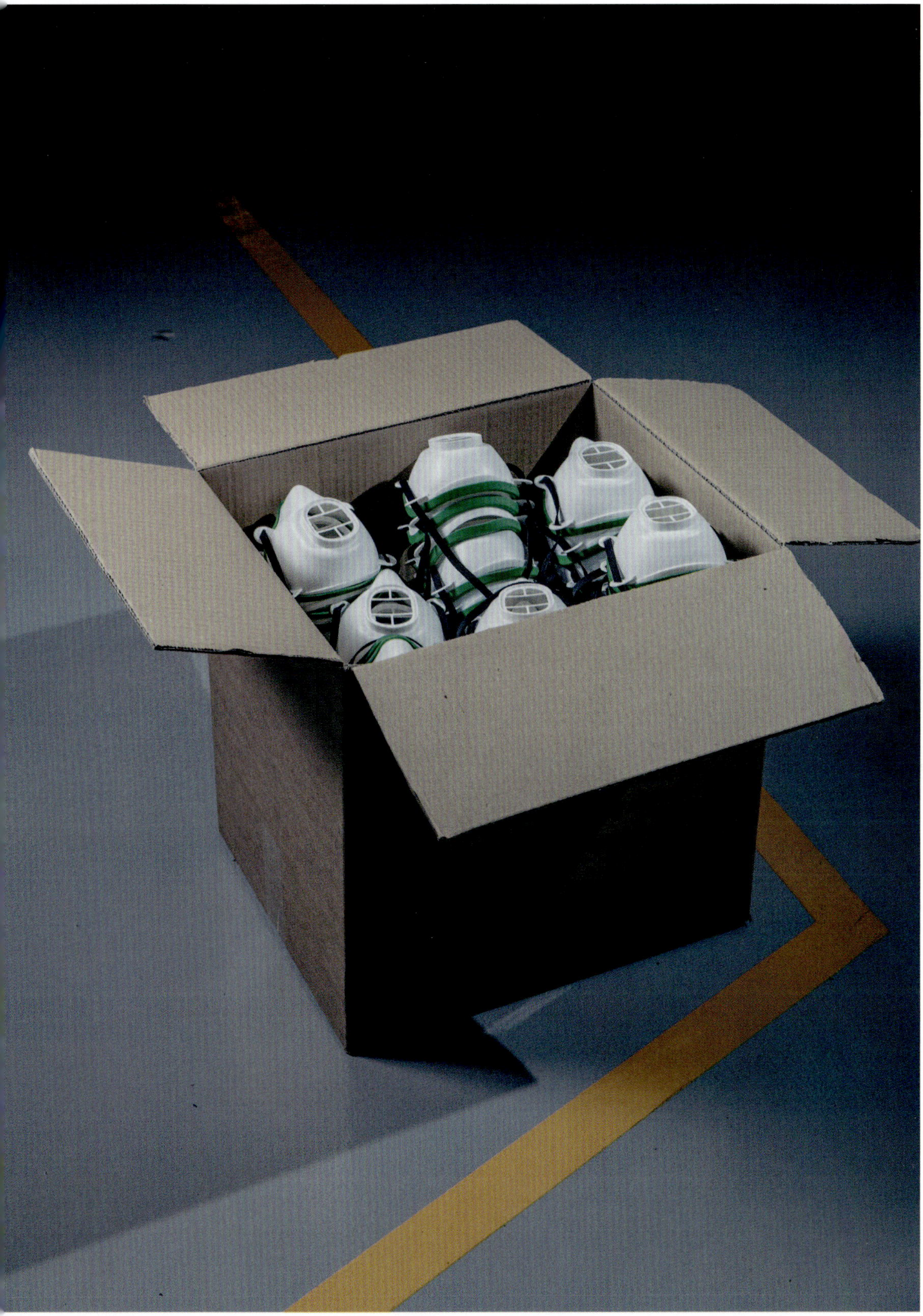

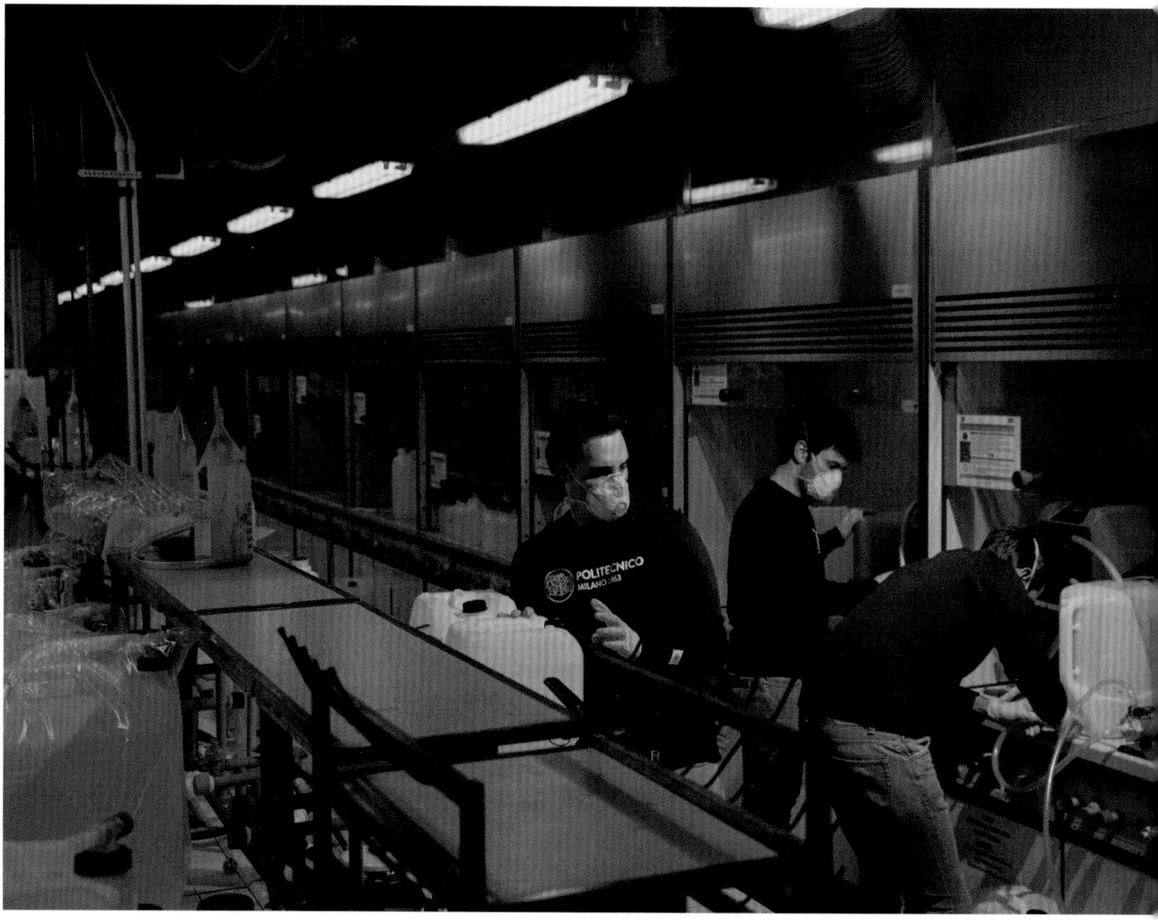
POLITECNICO
MILANO 1863

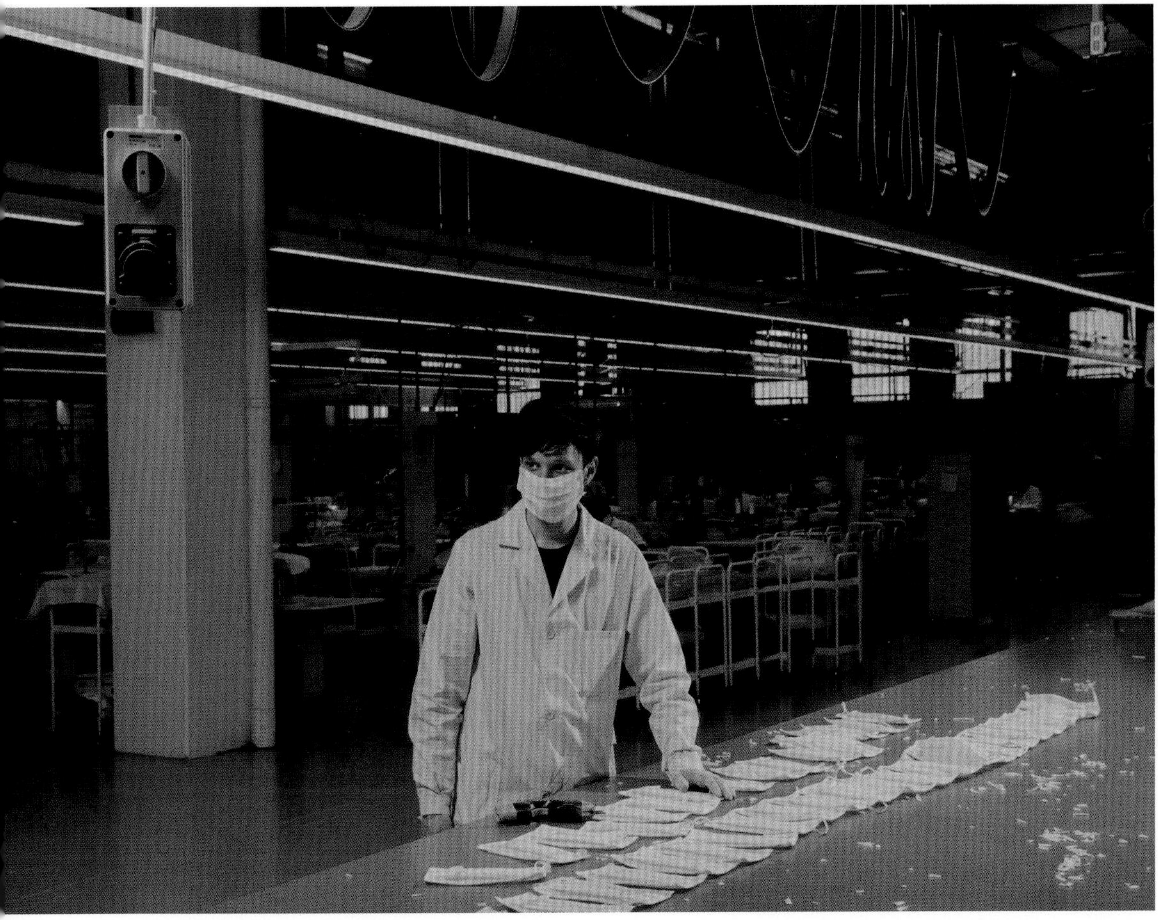

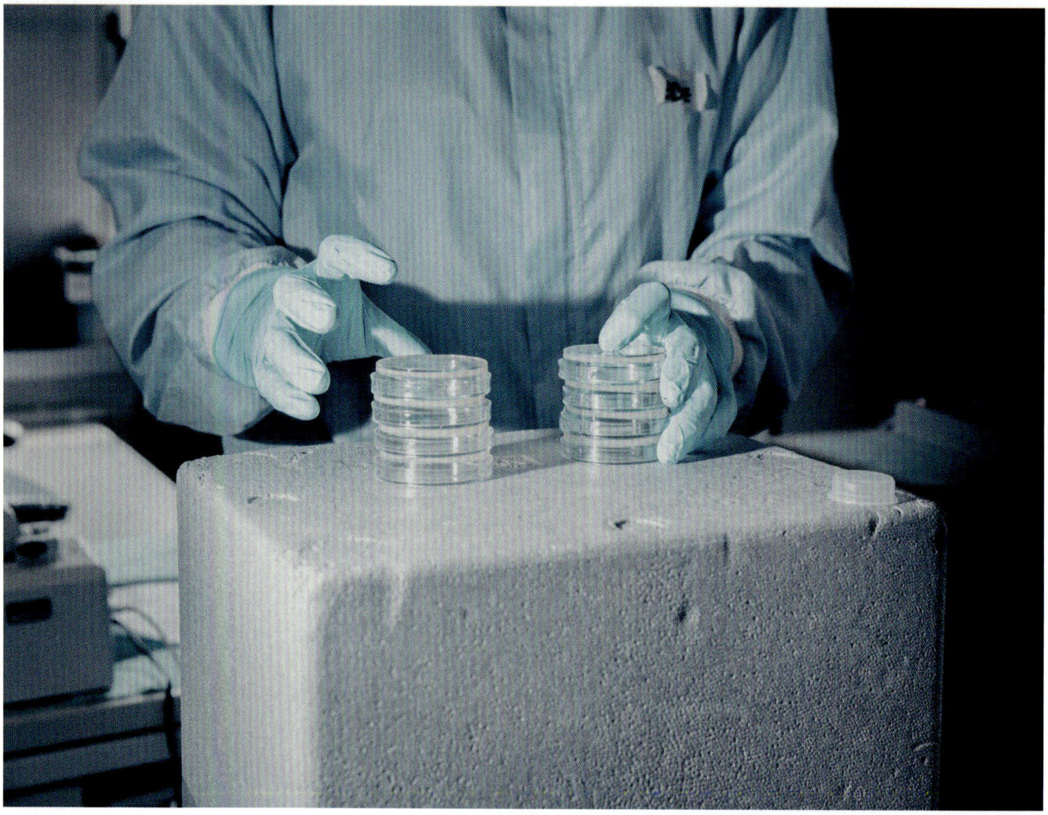

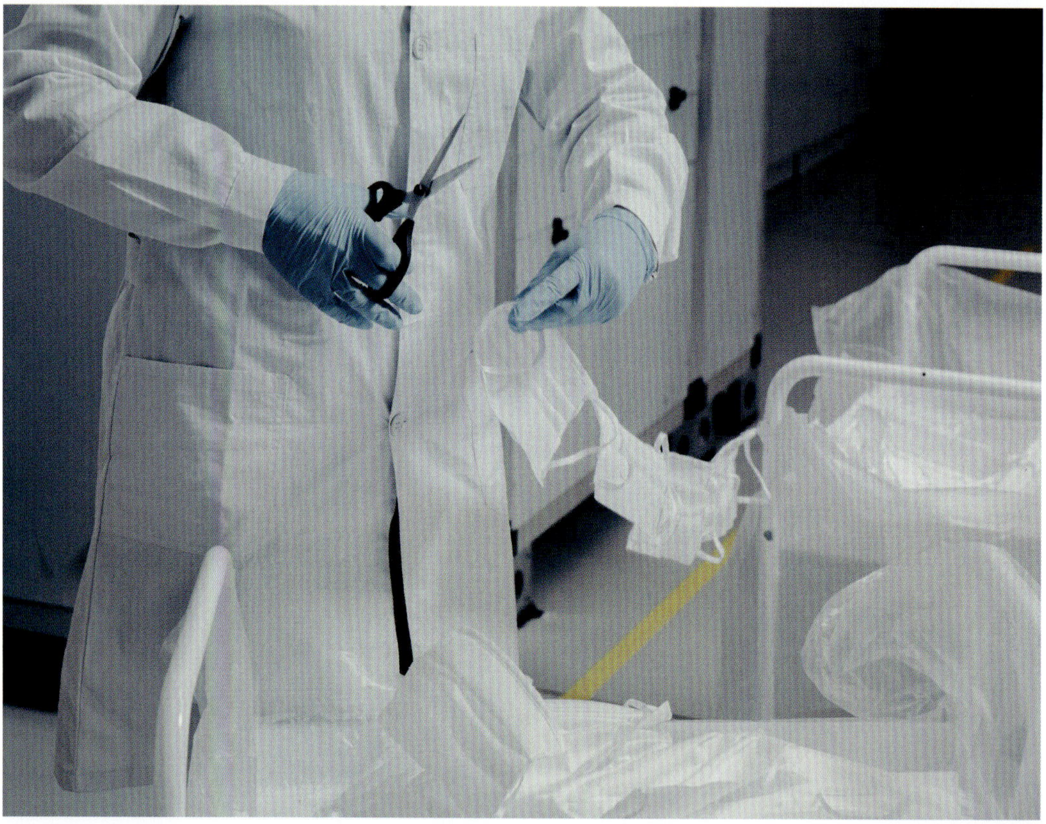

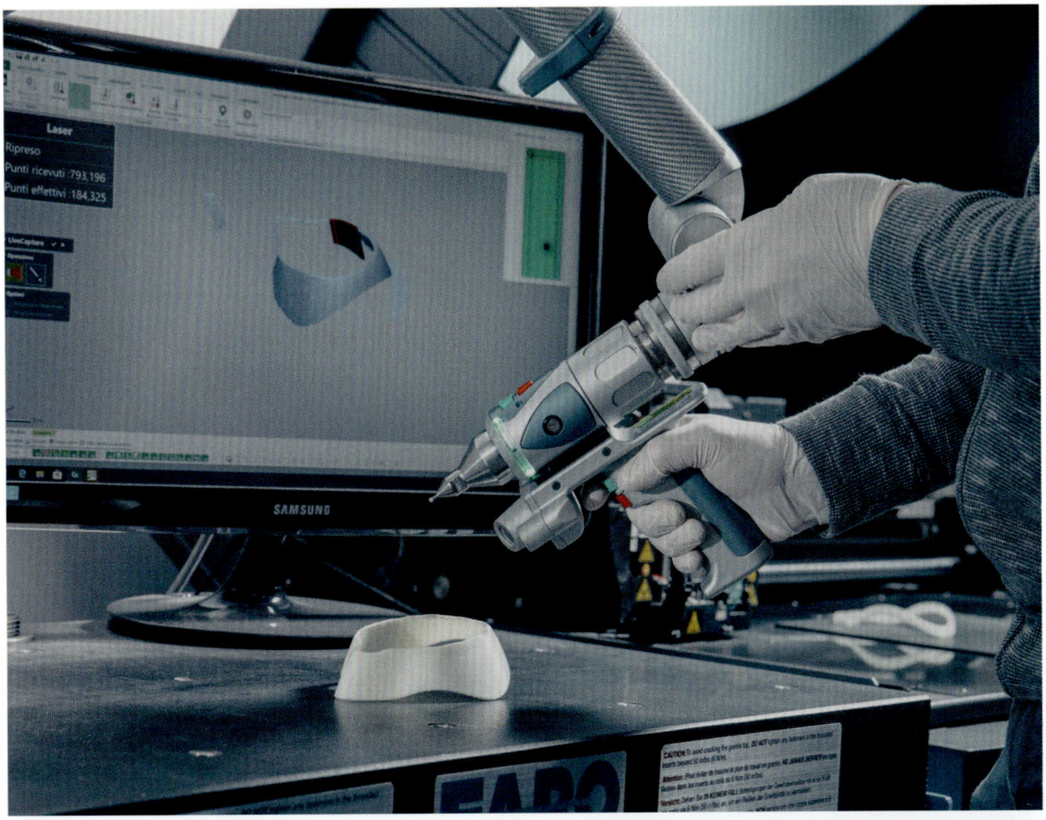
Laser
Ripreso
Punti ricevuti :793,196
Punti effettivi :184,325
SAMSUNG

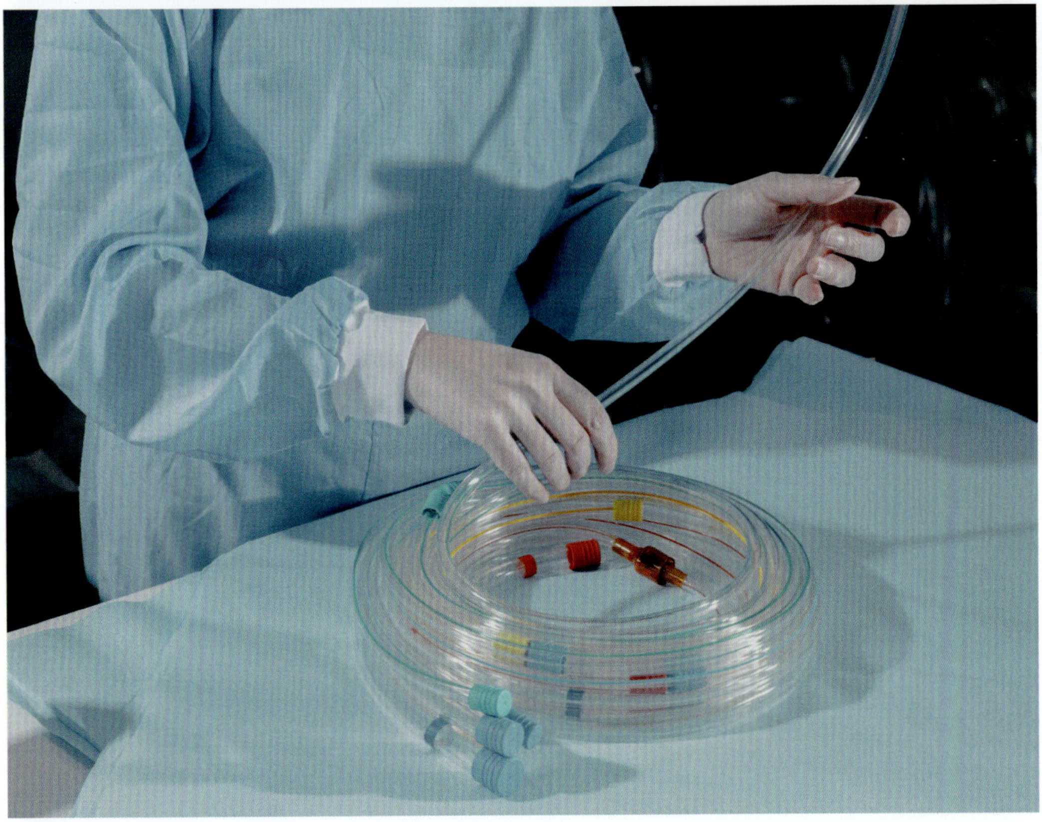

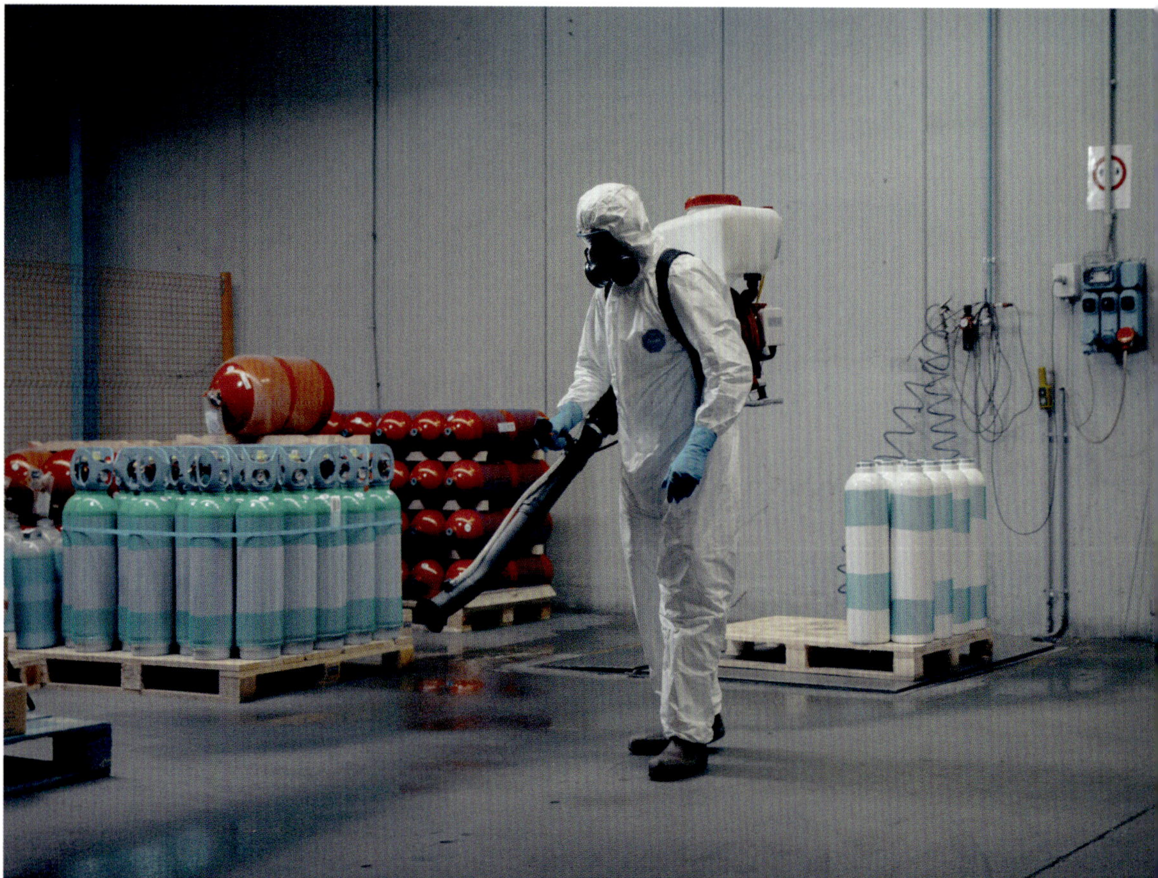

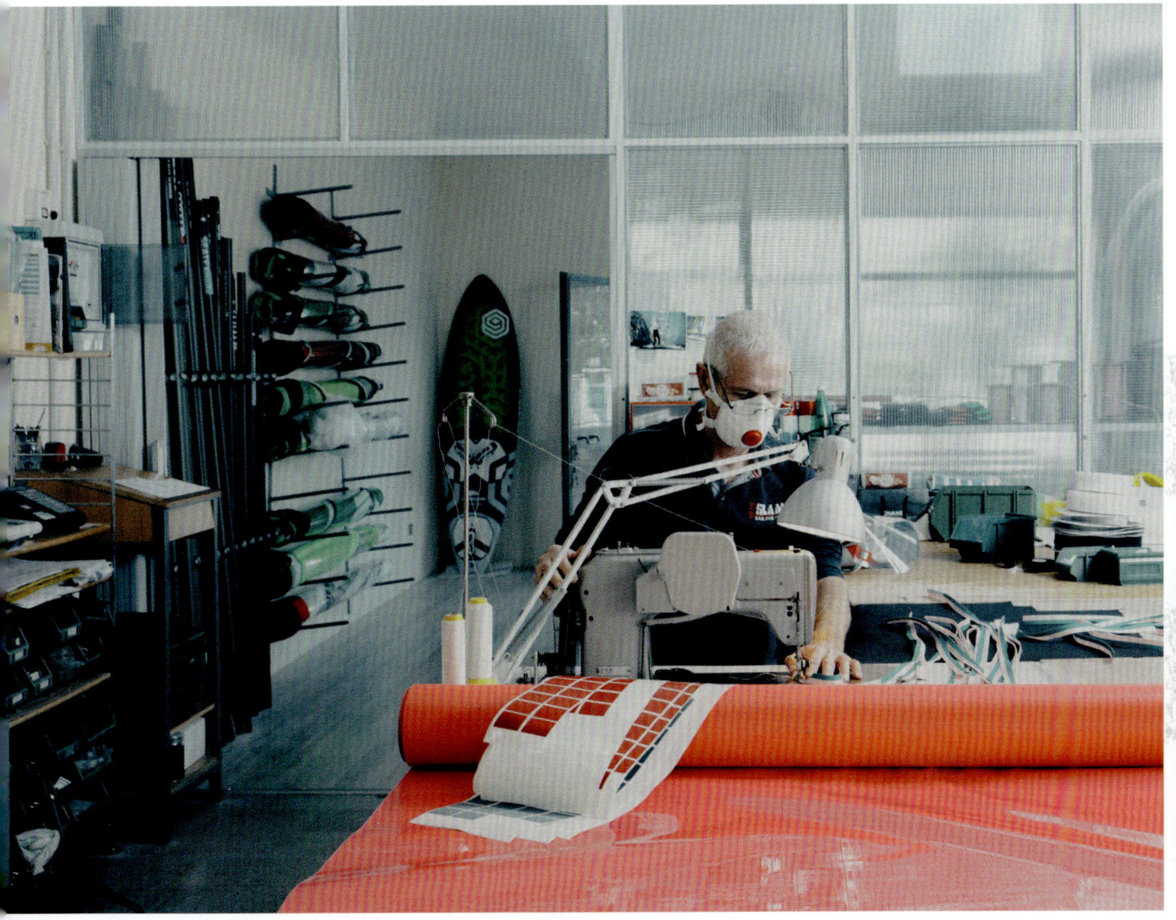

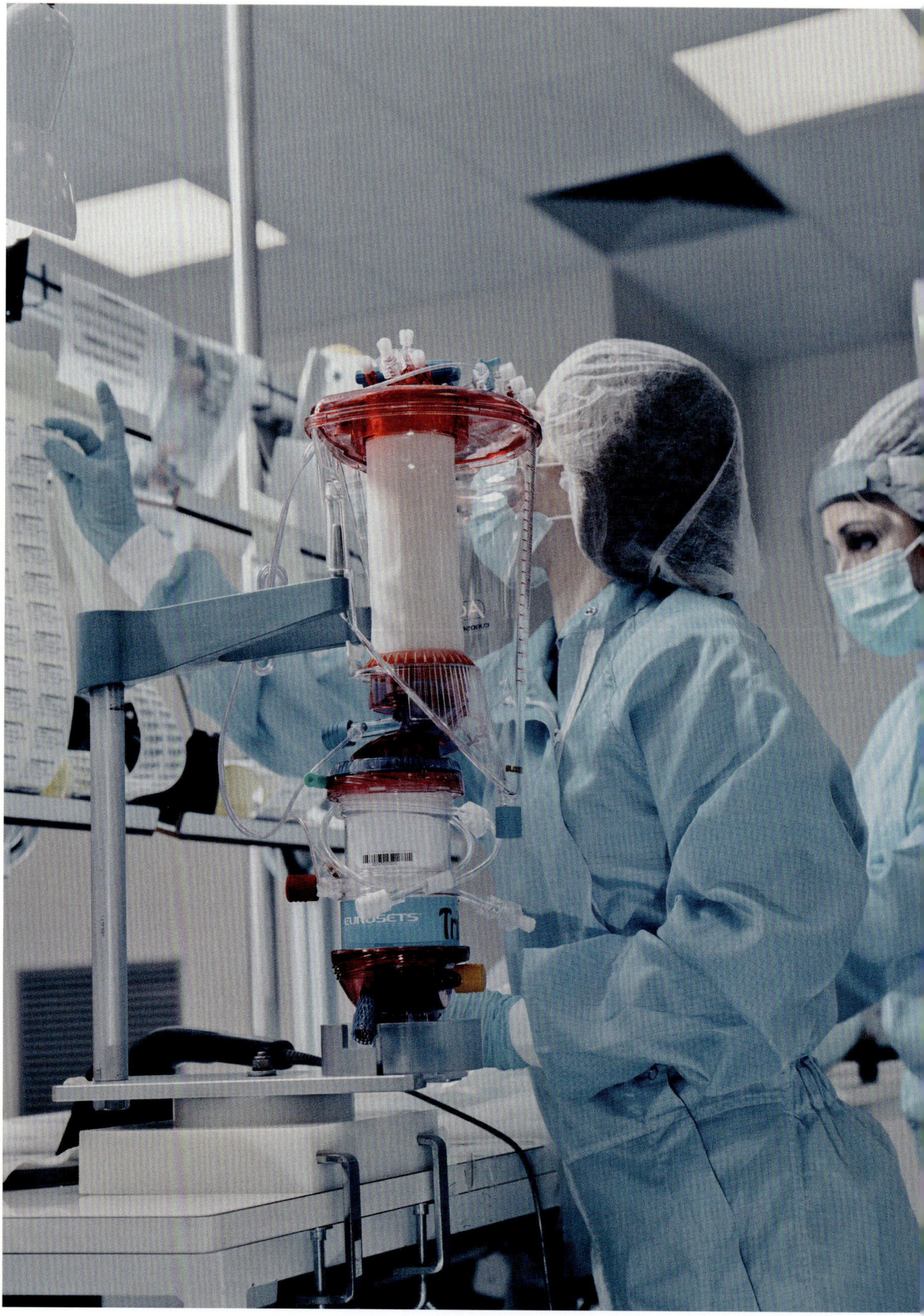
EUROSETS

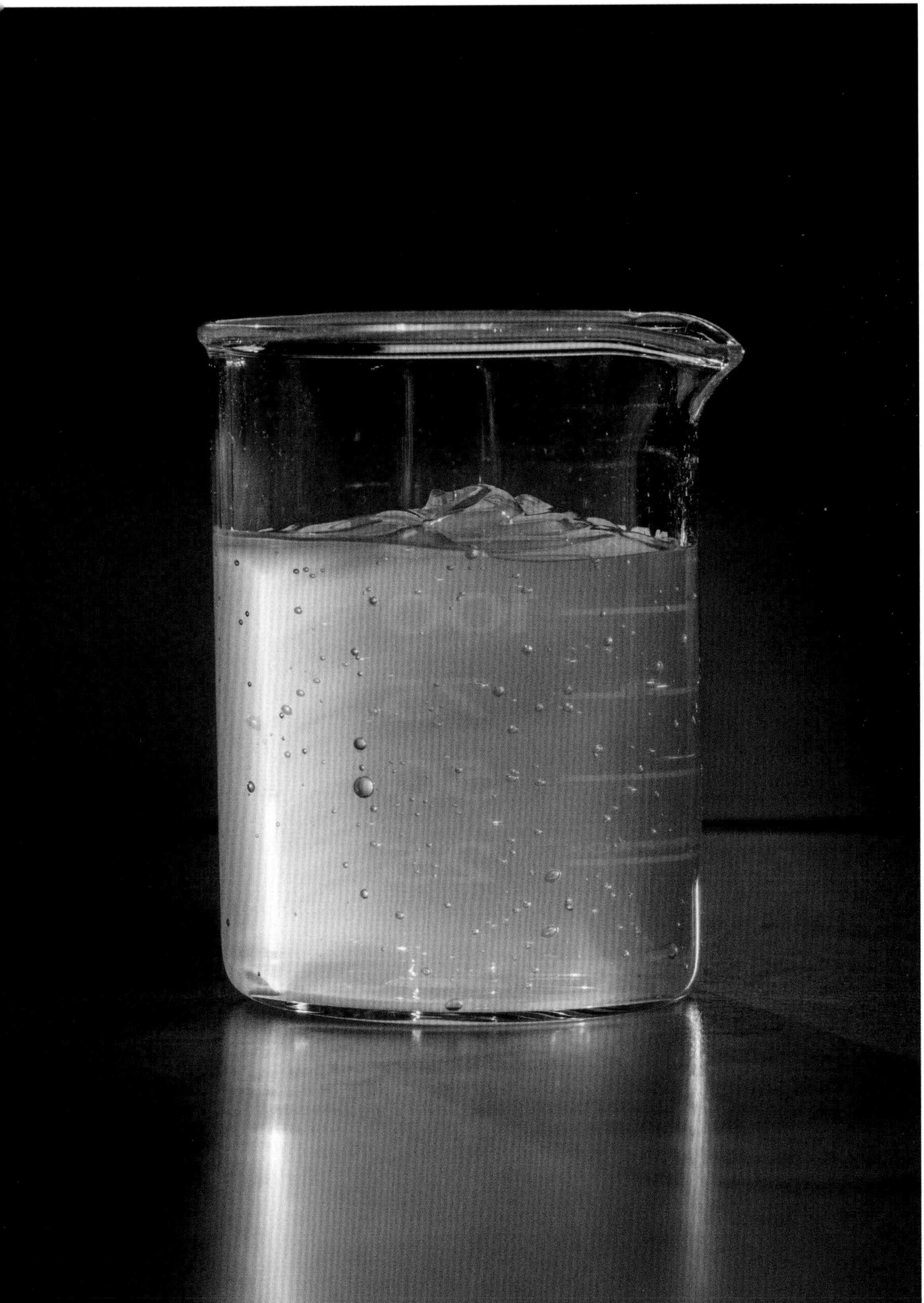

TerraProject, Italy
The State of the Art

With the lockdown imposed to curb the coronavirus pandemic, the Italian tourist sector has been heavily impacted, and the prospects for a recovery in the near future are feeble. Even as travel restrictions are slowly lifted, hesitation to travel outside national borders remains high.
According to ENIT, Italy's national tourism agency, airplane reservations to Italy dropped by 95.2% in June, 82.4% in July and 76.4% in August compared to the same period of 2019. Assoturismo, Italy's tourism federation, fears that the expected steep fall in visits could trigger the worst ever recorded drop in revenues of the sector. Recent reports calculate a 70-80% reduction, equal to about 120 billion euros. According to the Centre for Tourism Studies, Italy is now expecting 56 million fewer overnight stays.
Before the global health crisis, tourism was one of Italy's fastest growing and most profitable industrial sectors, with 63 million tourists visiting each year and an estimated revenue of 230 billions, covering about 13% of the country's GDP and employing 14% of the national workforce.
Hotels, short-term rentals, restaurants, transport, shops, tour guides and agents. These are the businesses that are mainly affected by the paralysis of the entire value chain. And larger cities, which depend more on tourists, are the most affected. ENIT expects to return to the 2019 rate only by 2023.
However, this crisis could be an opportunity to rethink the model on which the tourism sector is based. This is the opinion of Gabriel Zuchtriegel, director of the Archeological Park of Paestum. "We must focus on another type of tourism, another relationship with visitors, more intense, more 'one-to-one', and who knows, I think this could be a model for developing a model of 'slow tourism' in the future."
This project is a documentation of the effects of the coronavirus pandemic on the Italian tourism sector in Florence, Venice and Rome, cities which all heavily rely on tourism for their economy.

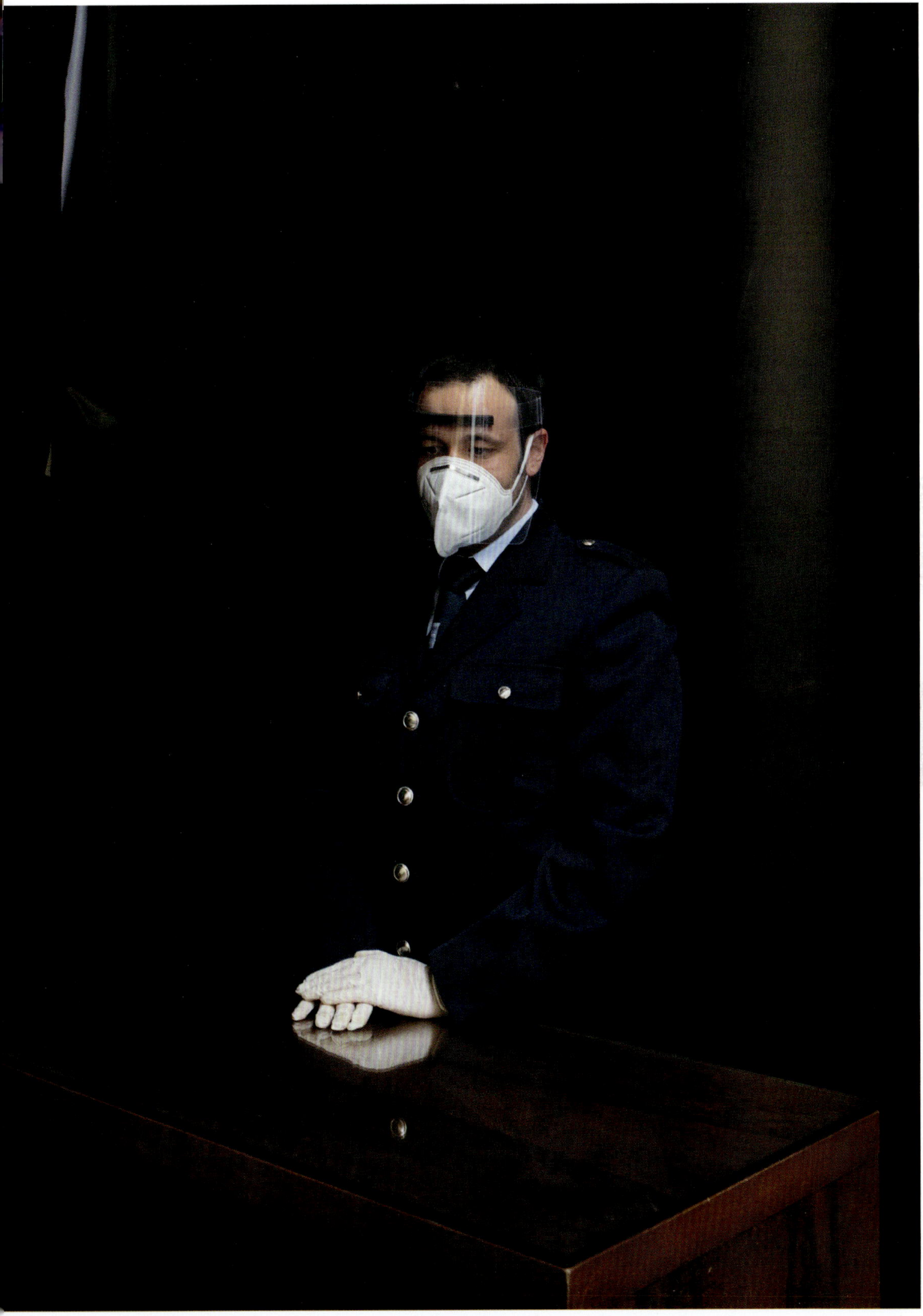

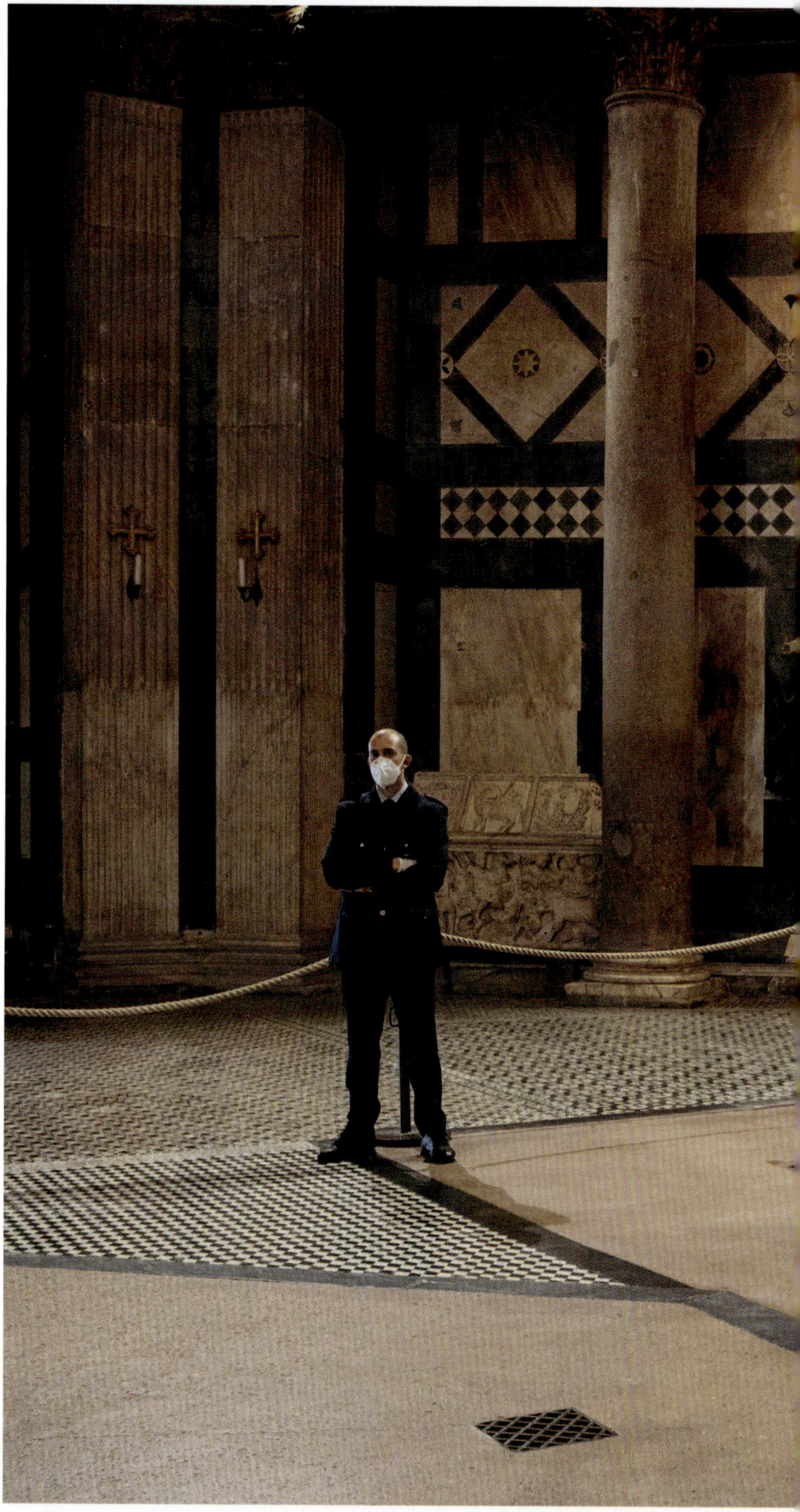

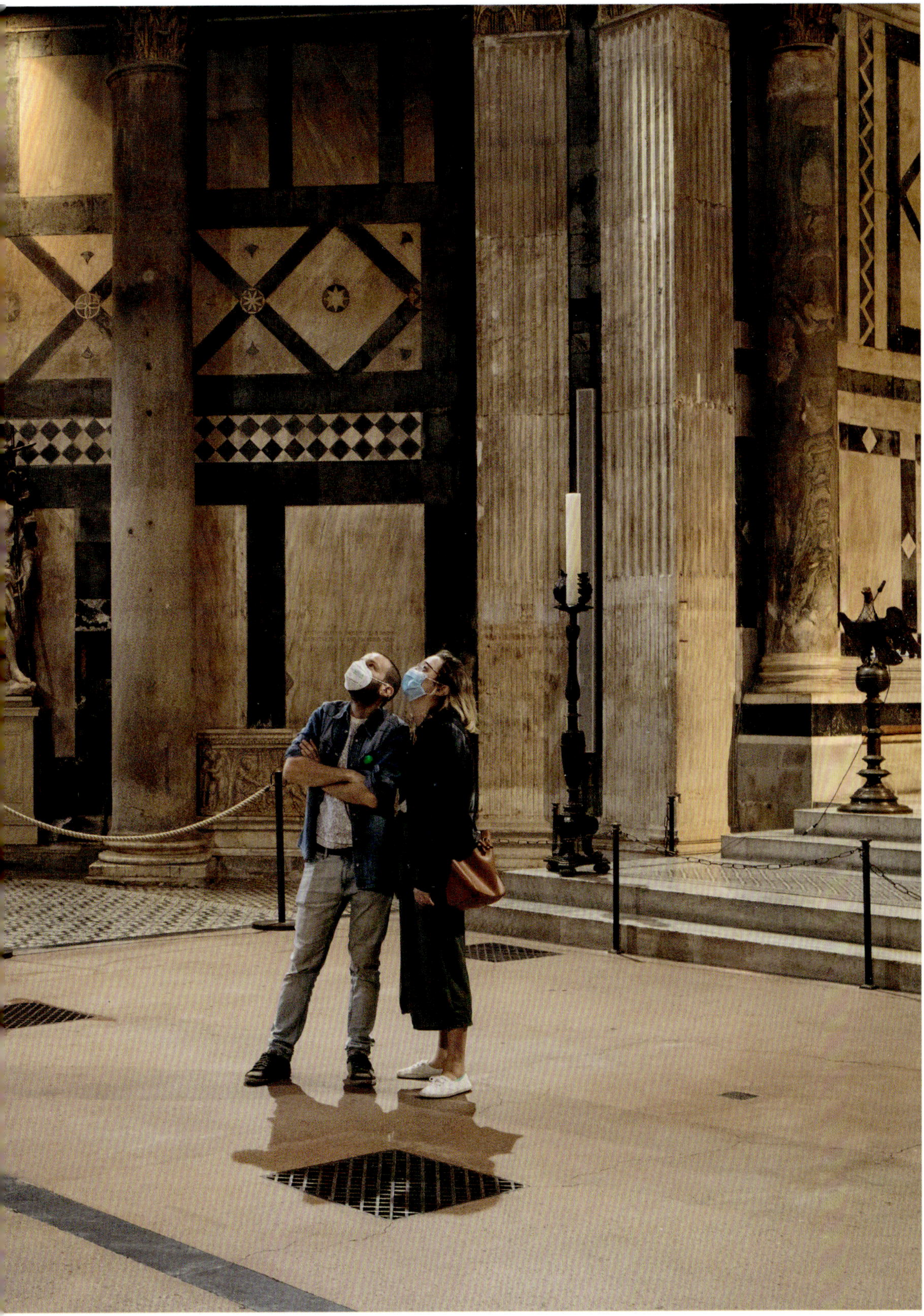

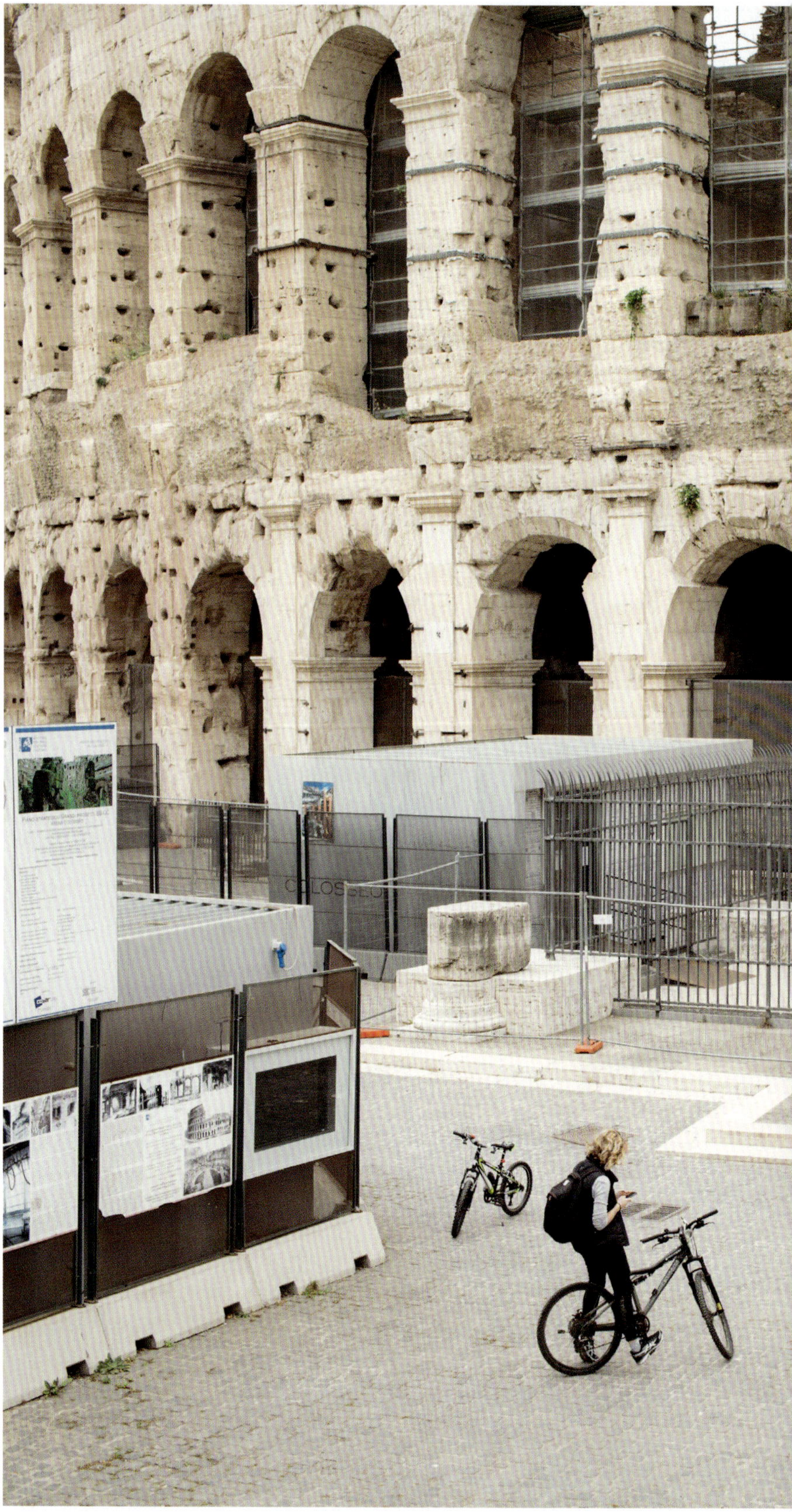

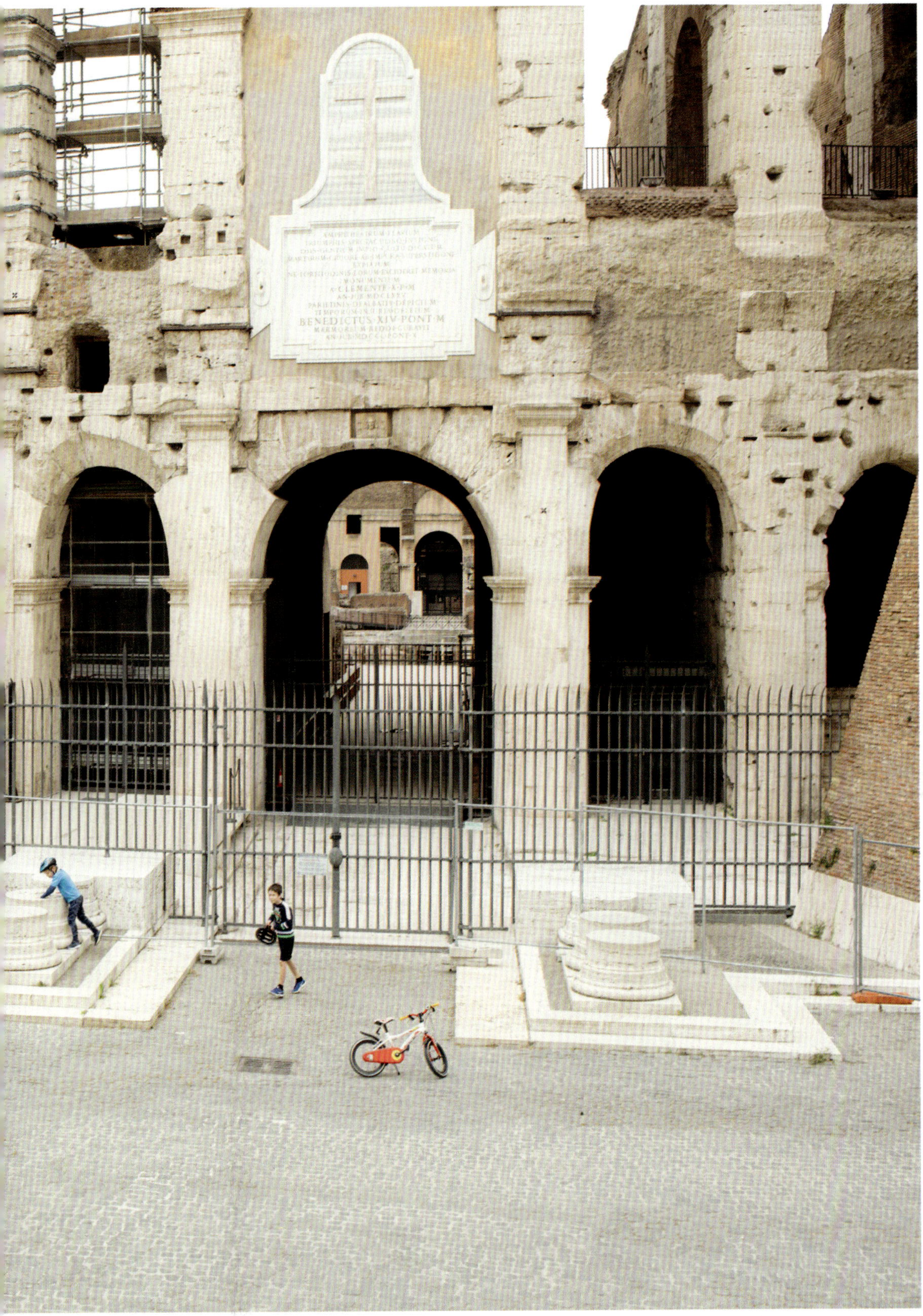
BENEDICTUS XIV PONT M

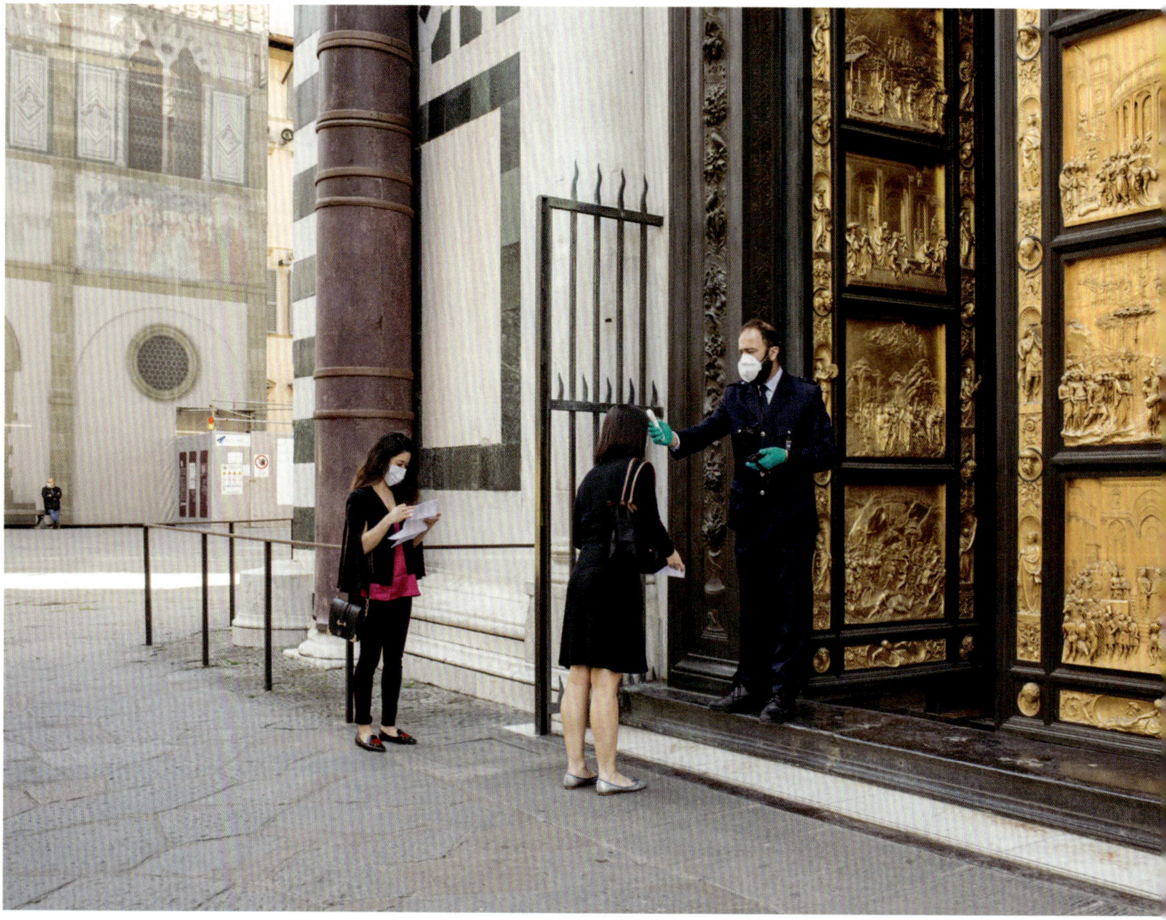

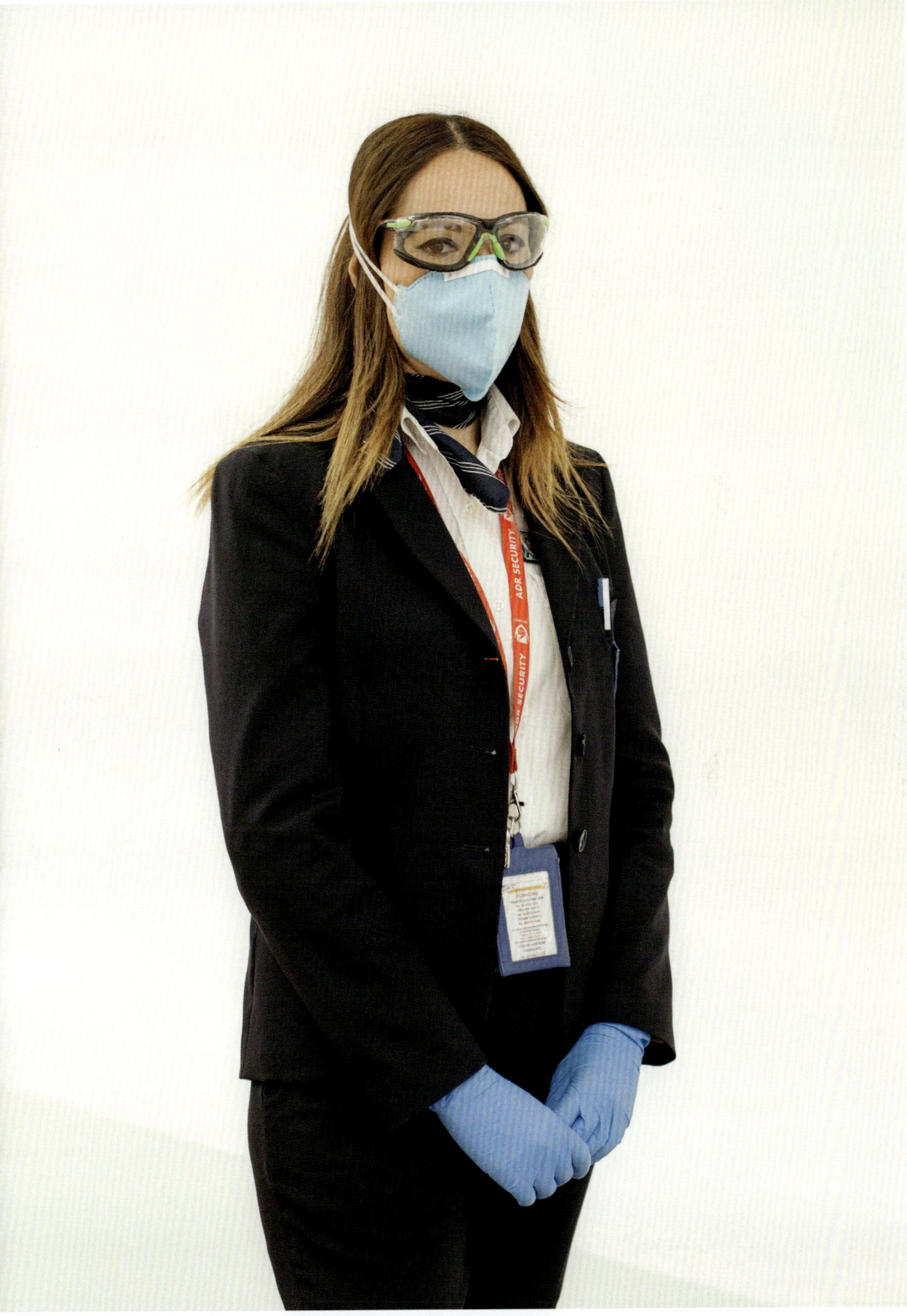
ADR SECURITY
ADR SECURITY

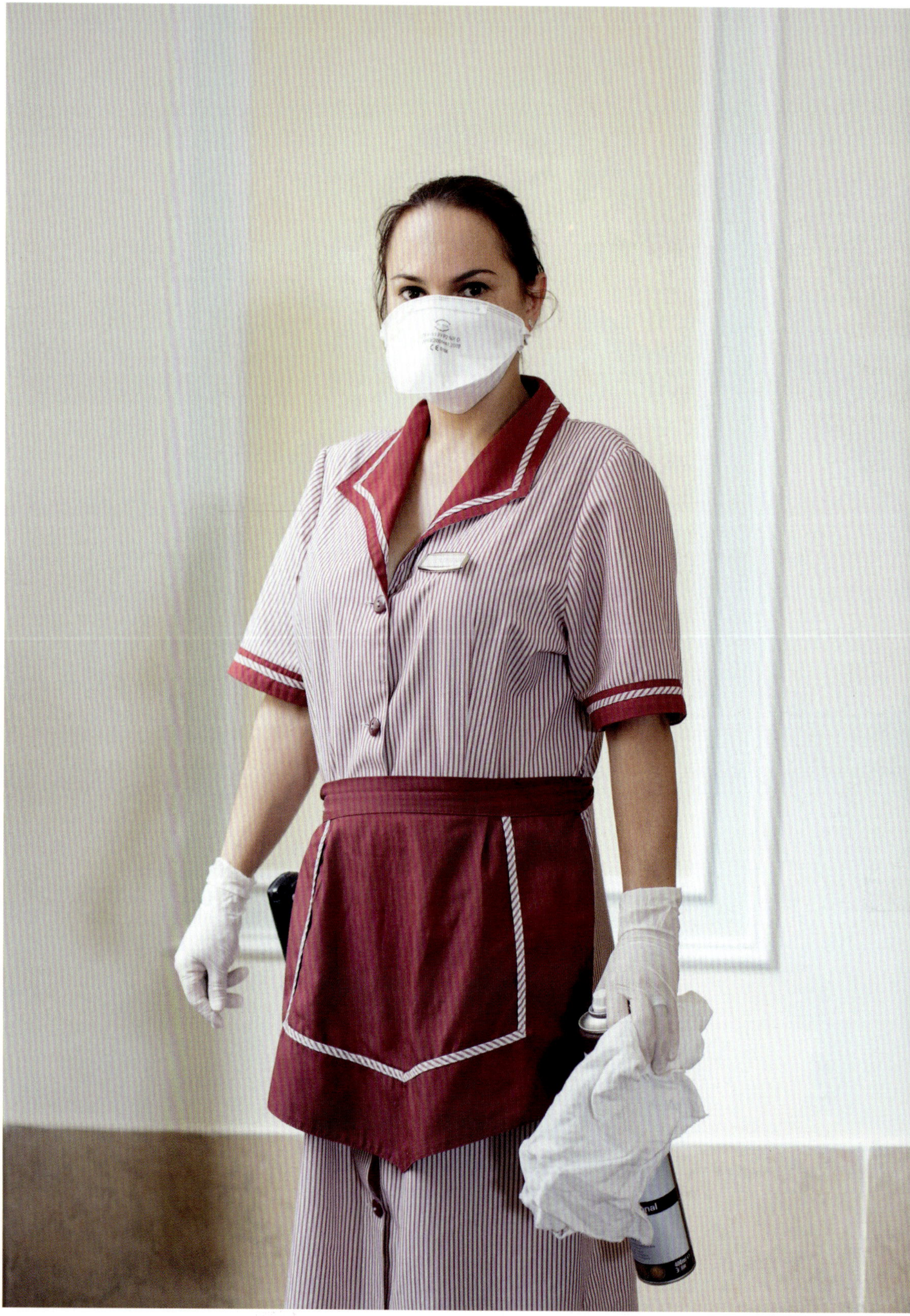

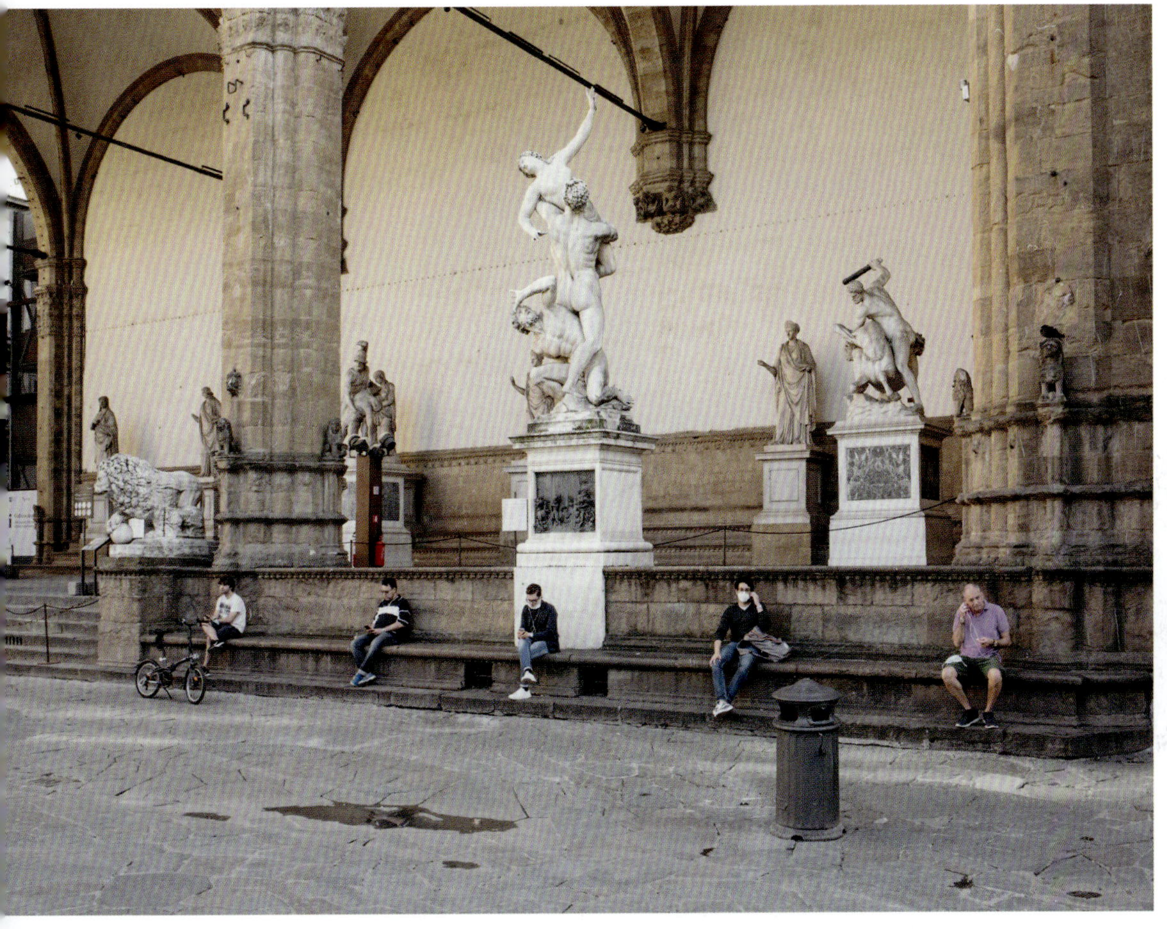

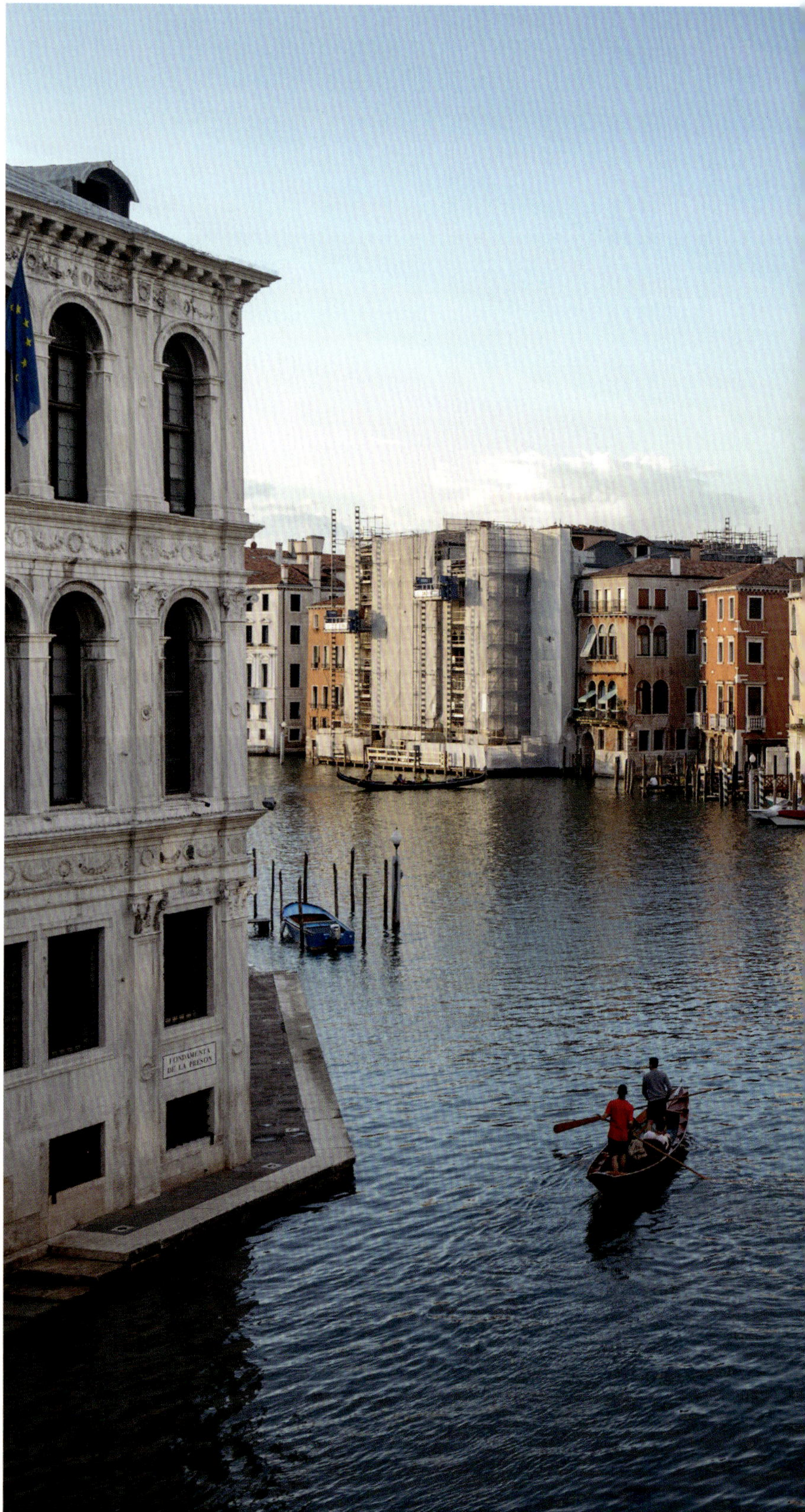
FONDAMENTA
DE LA PRESON

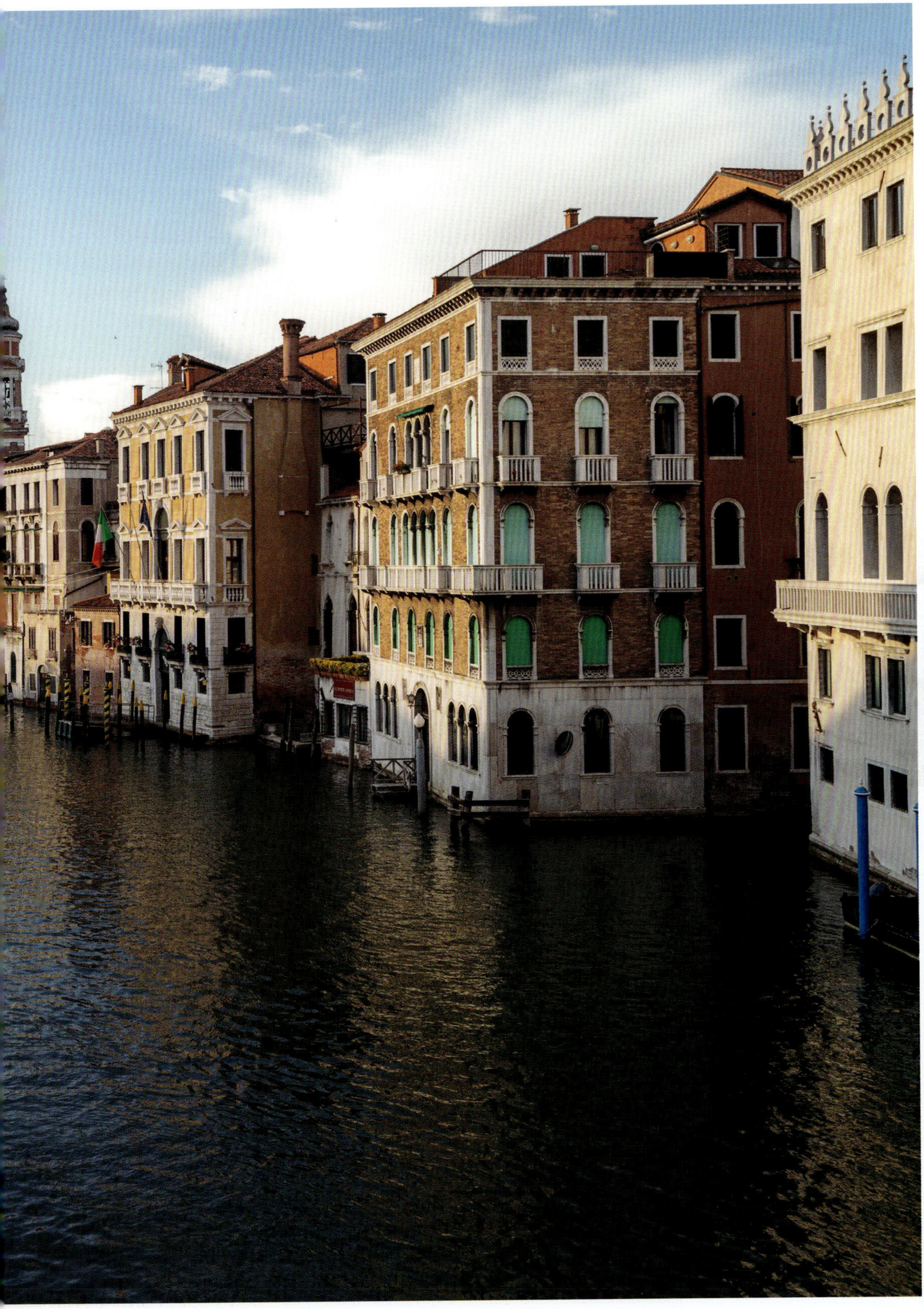

Daniel Etter, Germany
The Indispensables

Who are the people that keep a country running? COVID-19 has shown us the importance of essential workers, those who produce and deliver our food, care for our health and our children, come to our rescue. People all over the world have collectively applauded nurses, cashiers, doctors and other essential workers from their window sills. Many of them are the most exposed to the virus and often they work long hours for a low pay and lack of social standing. Most are first generation immigrants. Daniel Etter has portrayed some of these indispensable workers in Germany. The long term goal is to explore if their situation will change once the COVID-19 crisis has passed or if the appreciation was just symbolic.

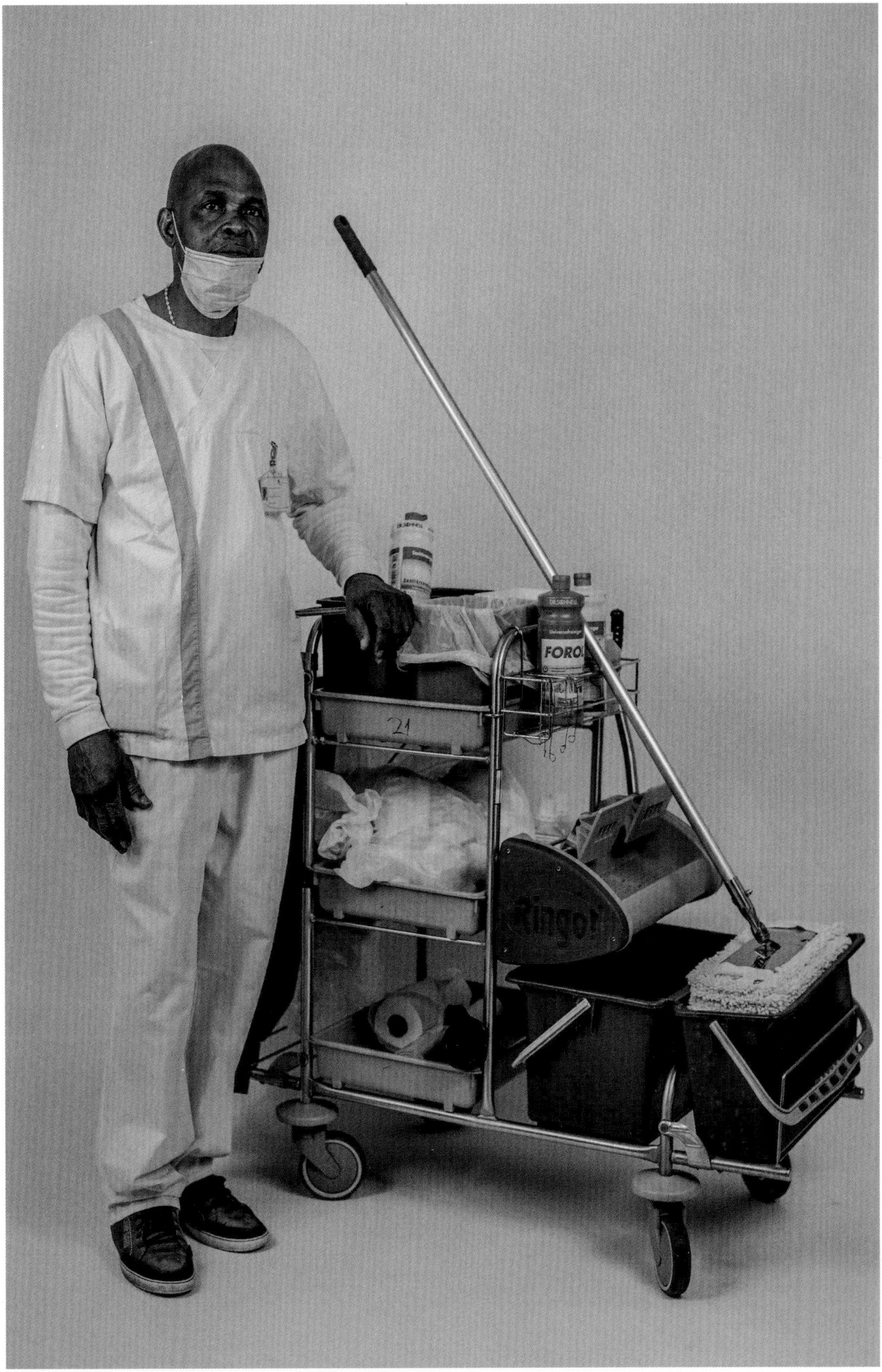
FOROL
21
Ringo

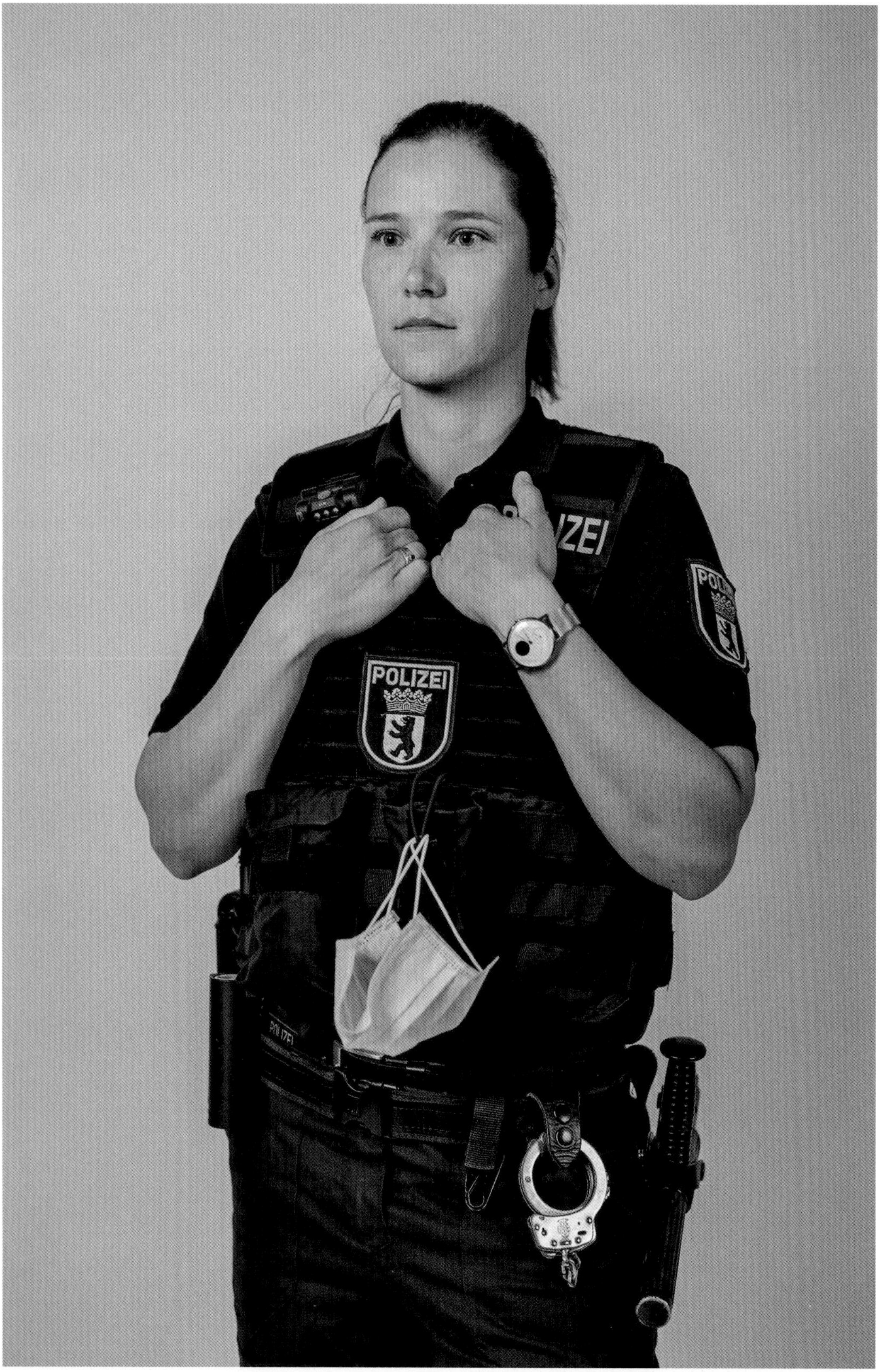
POLIZEI

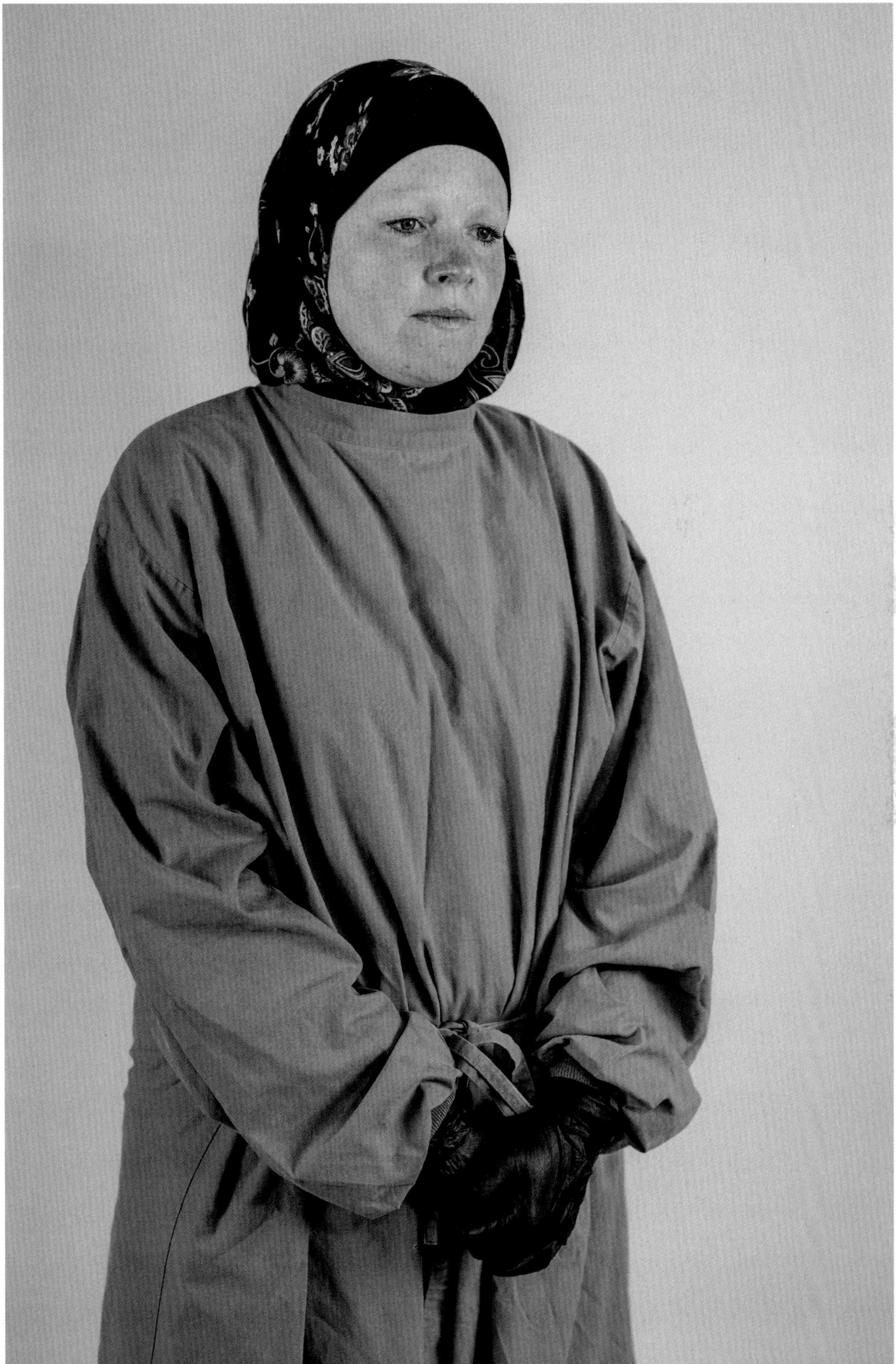

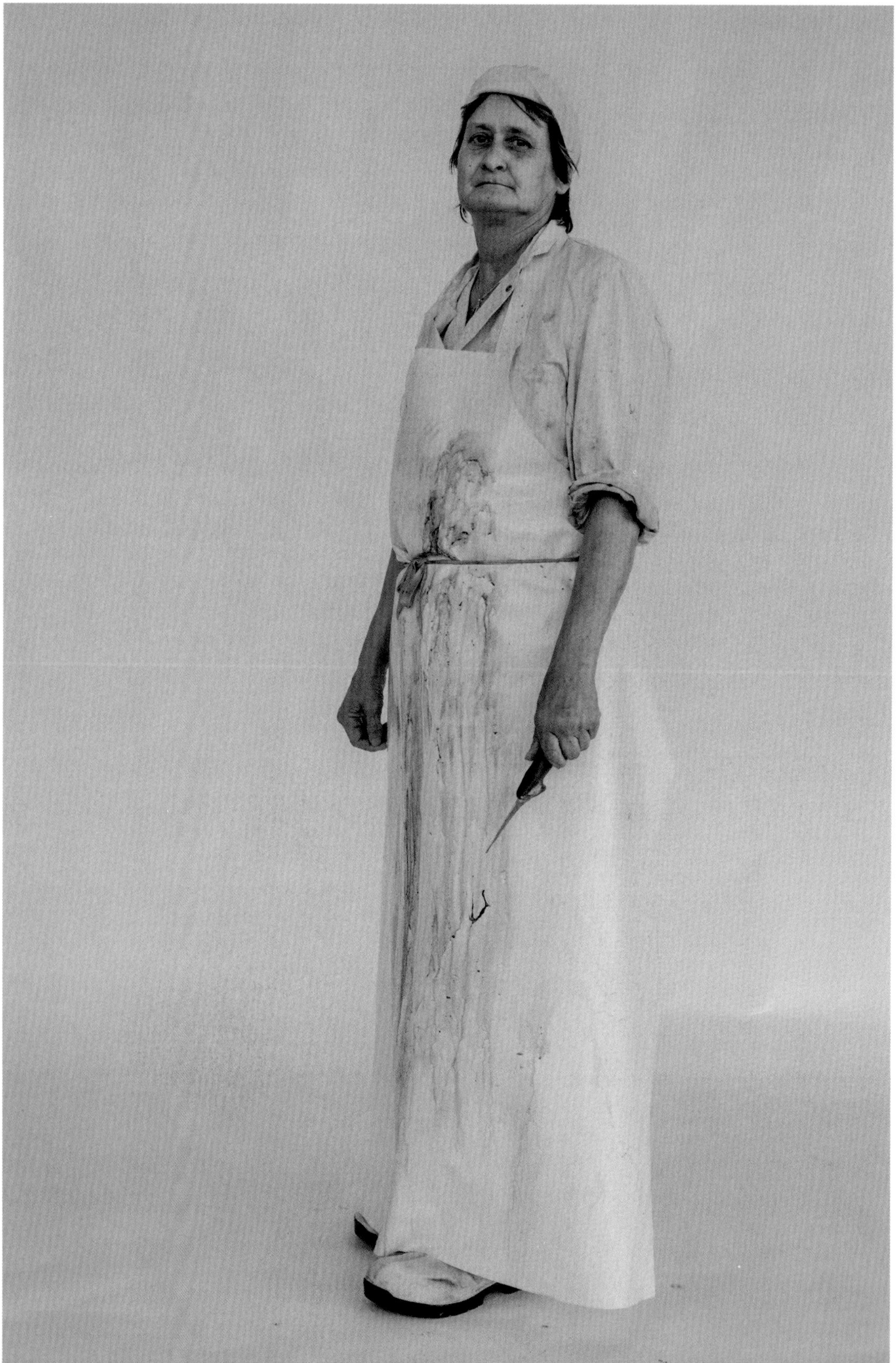

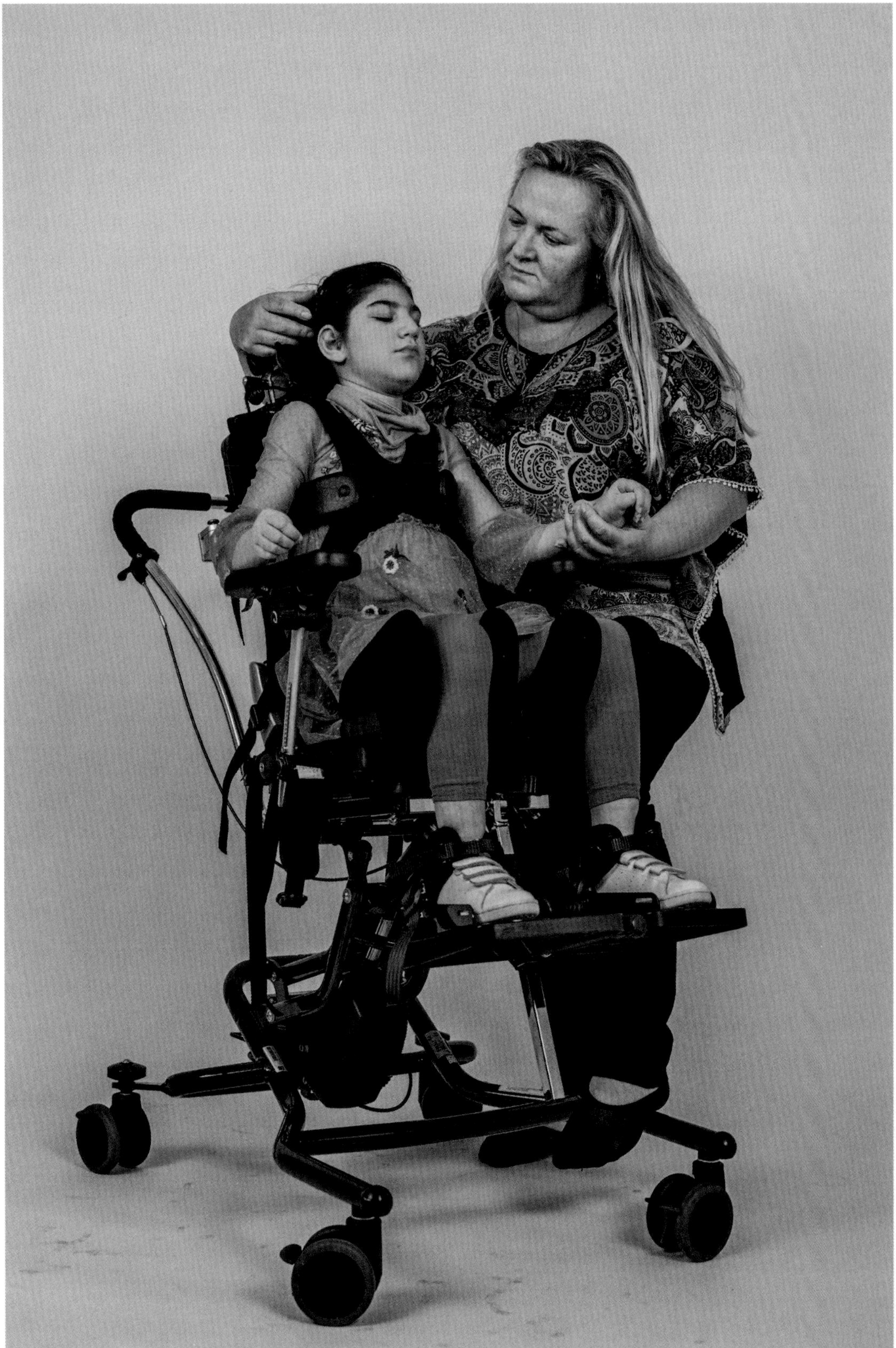

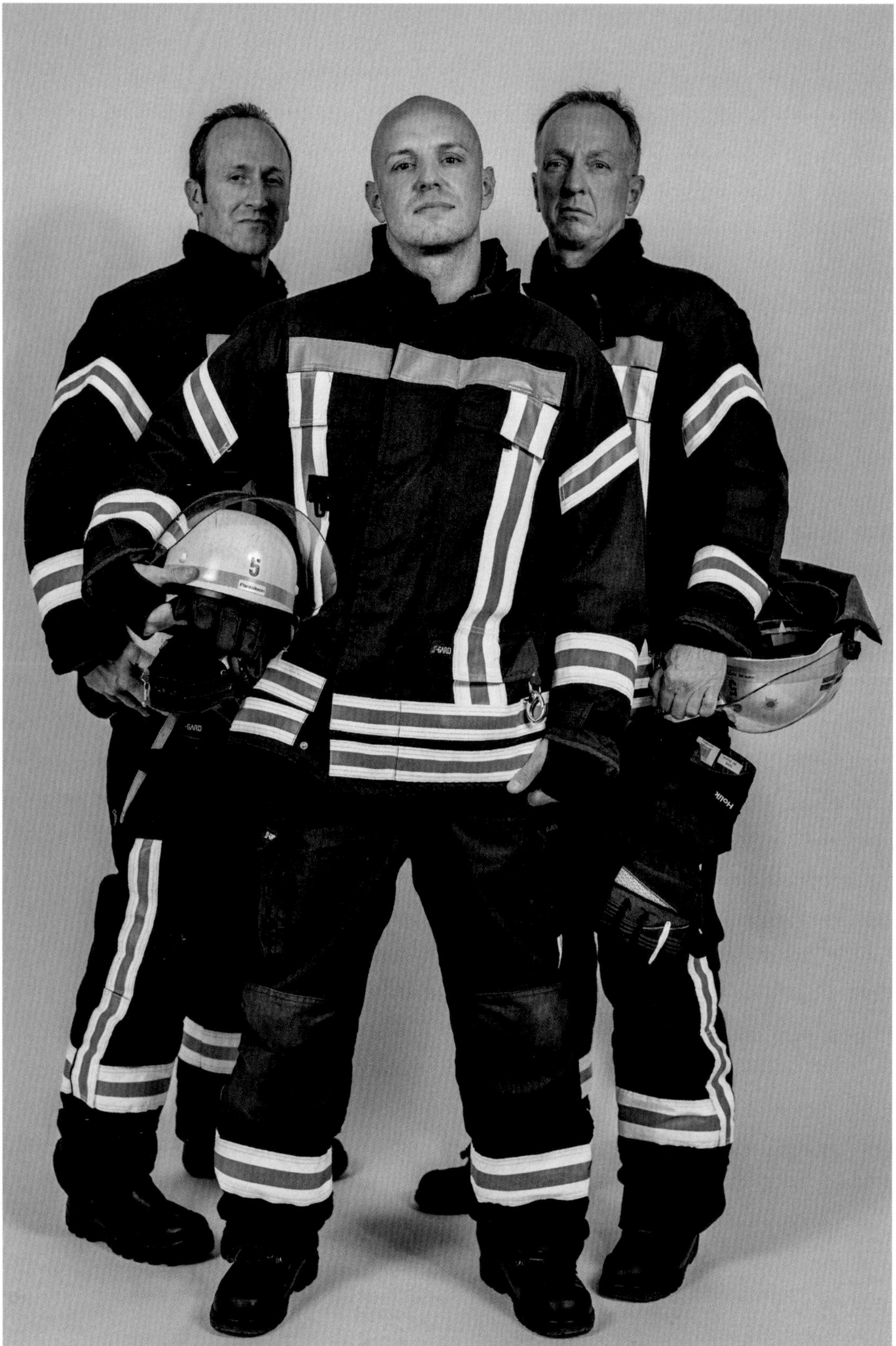
5

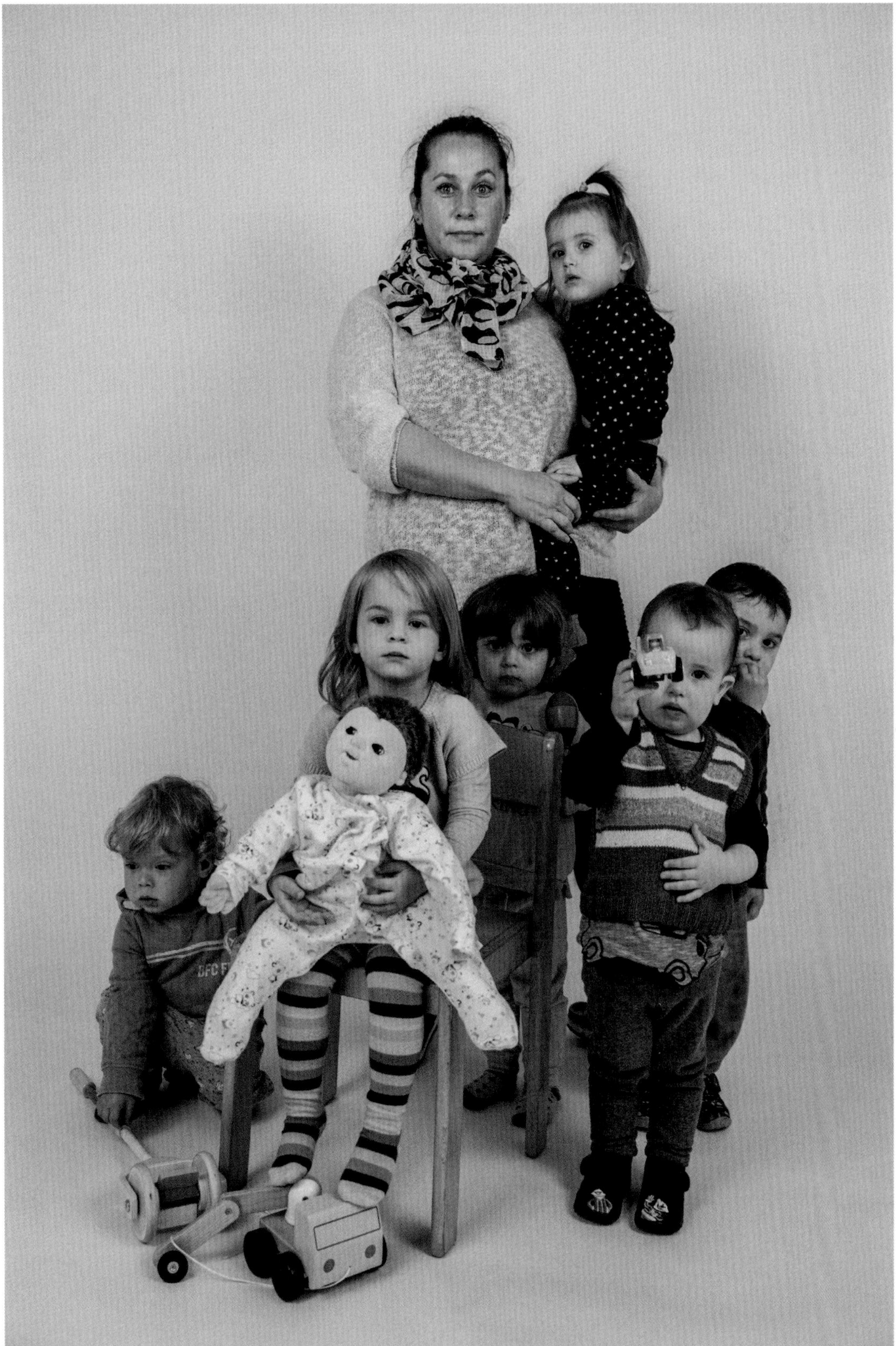

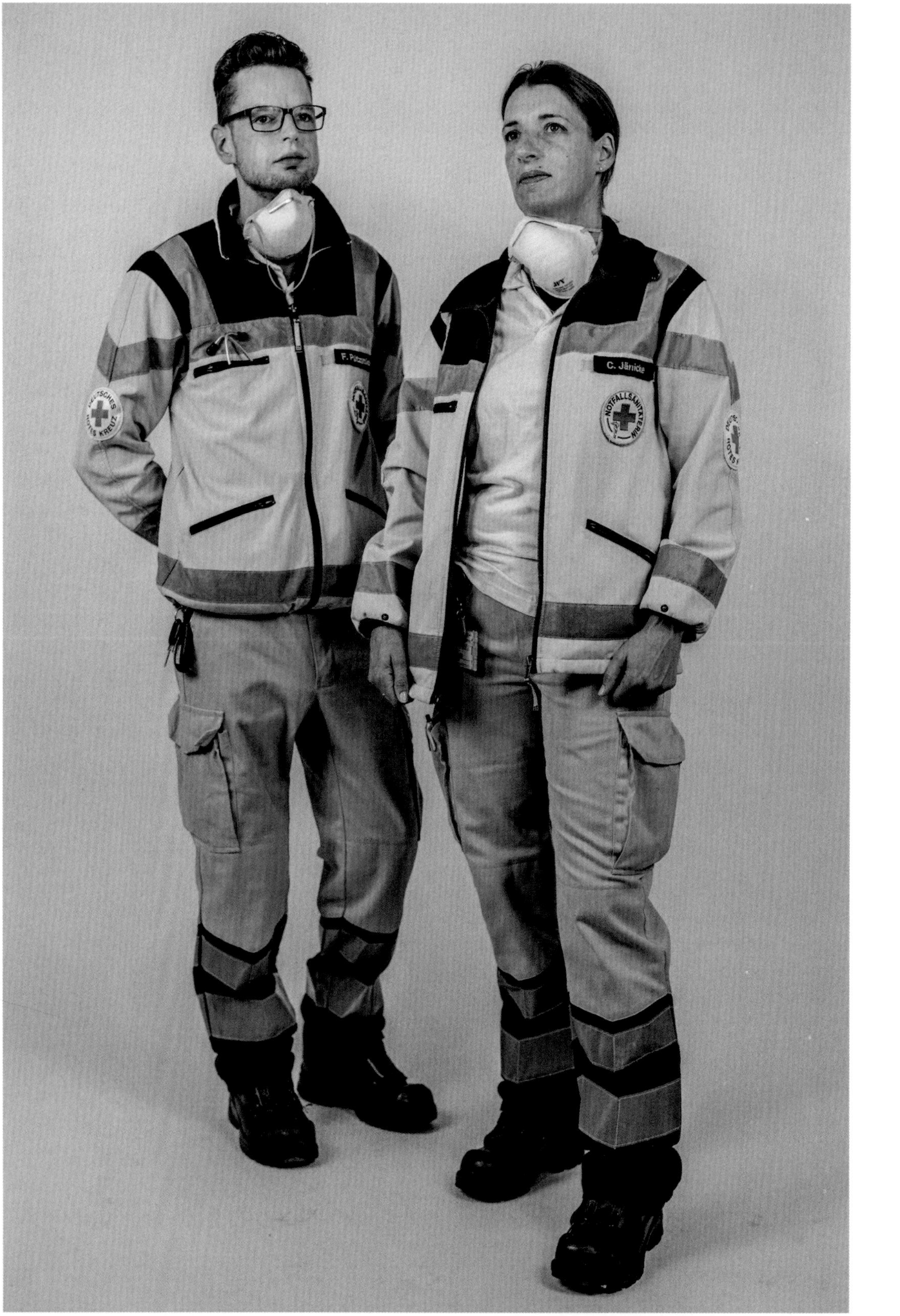
DEUTSCHES ROTES KREUZ
C. Jänicke
NOTFALLSANITÄTERIN

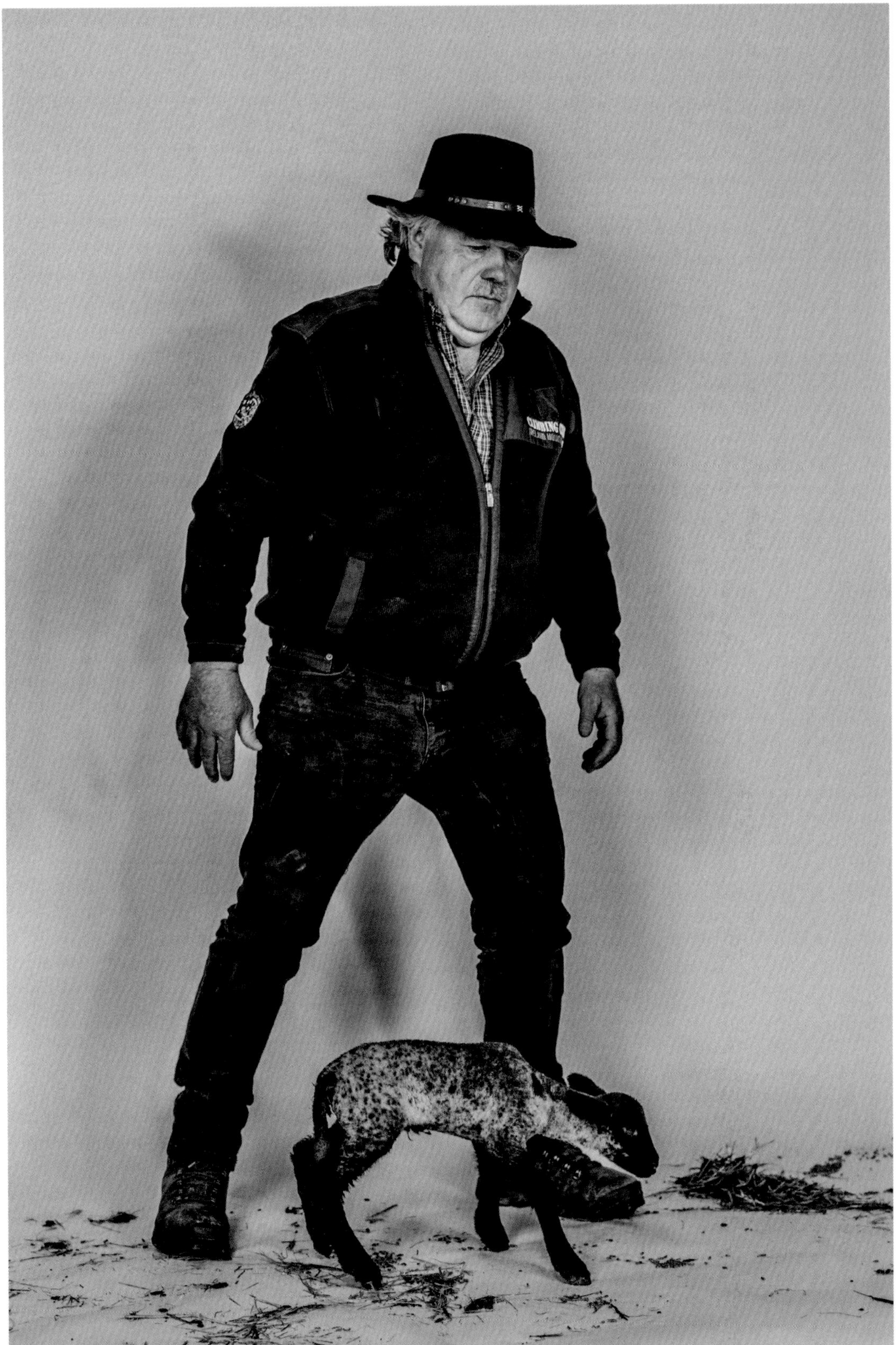

Lou Lou D'Aki, Greece
Summer Moved On

Greece was lauded for its swift and effective response to the novel coronavirus threat in early 2020. Immediately following the confirmation of the first three cases on February 27, and before a single death was recorded, Greek authorities started putting in place restrictions on large gatherings, including in educational and religious institutions. By March 23, restrictions on all non-essential movement throughout the country were enacted, officially commencing a full lockdown in Greece.

Over the following six weeks, people wanting to leave their residence were required to send a text message to a government-issued phone number with a code — a number from one to six — stating the reason for their movement. Among the acceptable reasons were: travel to or from one's workplace (during work hours), going to the pharmacy or supermarket, visiting a doctor, and personal exercise.

For the most part, everyone followed these measures without complaint. But with the approach of the summer tourist season, compliance quickly turned to worry. More than a quarter of Greece's GDP comes from tourism and the thought of losing out on the much awaited and much needed income from the millions of tourists who would arrive in Greece this year was terrifying for some.

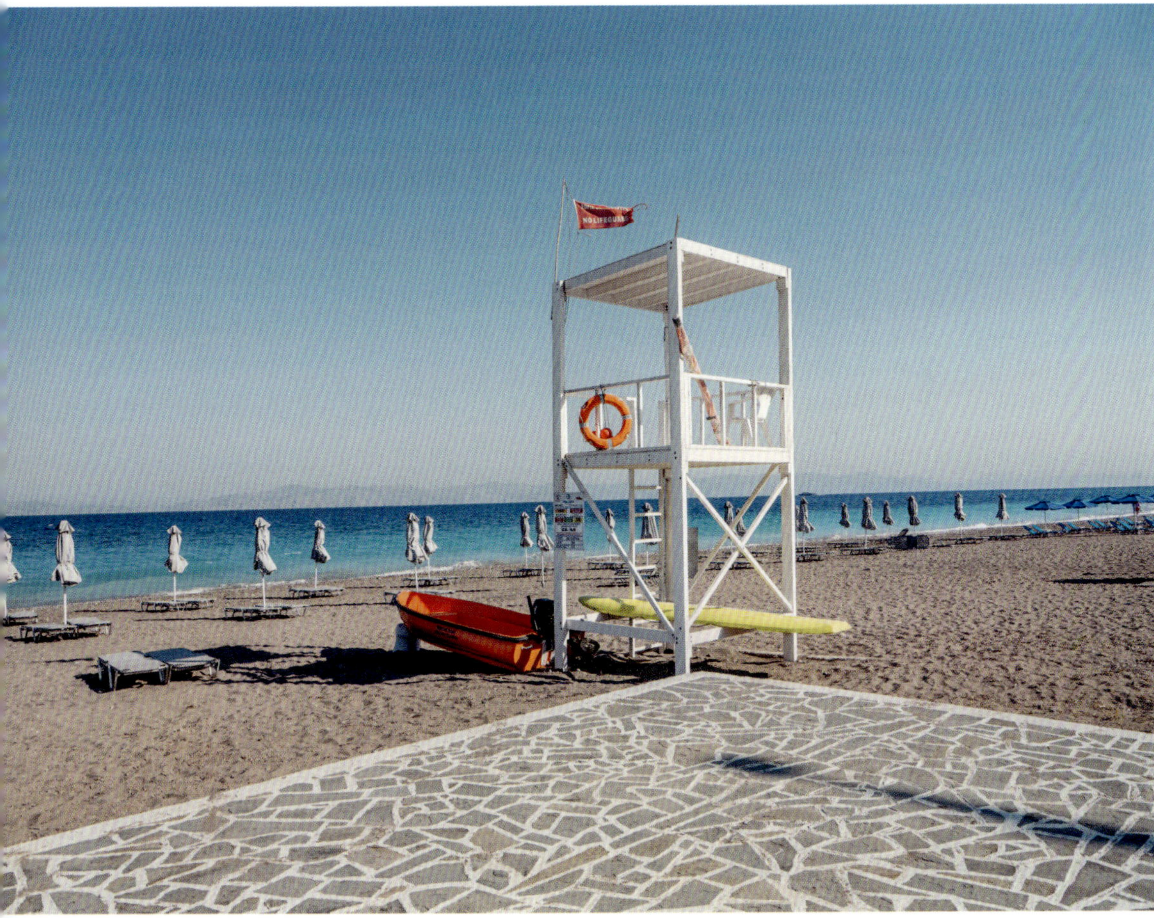

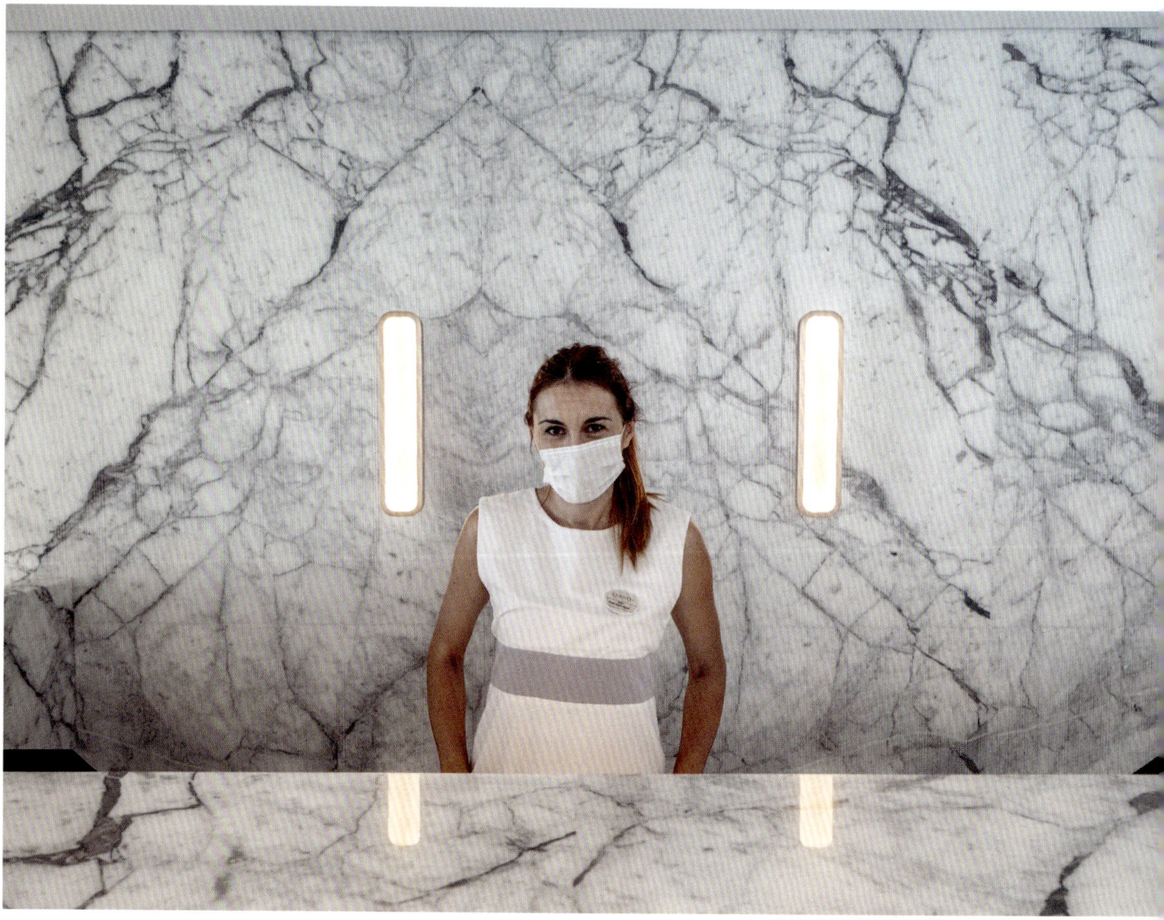

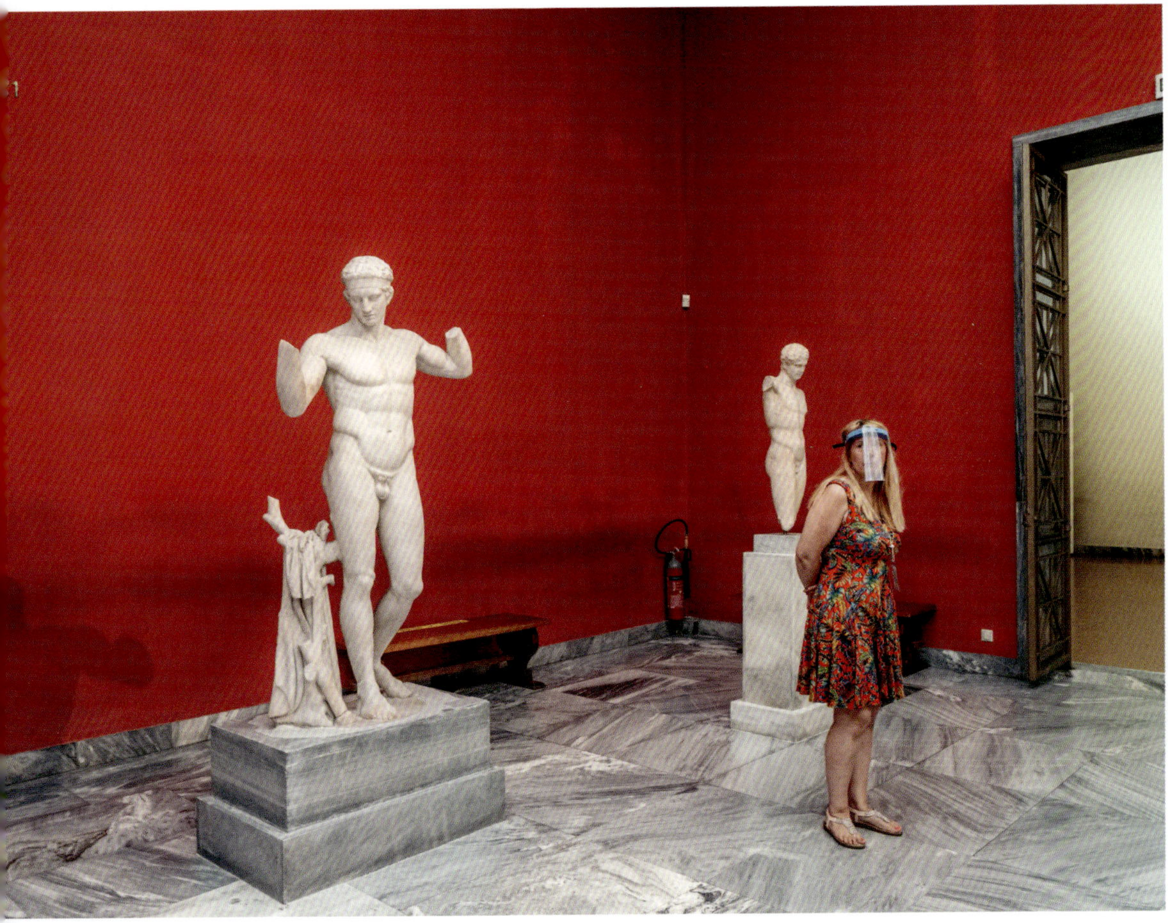

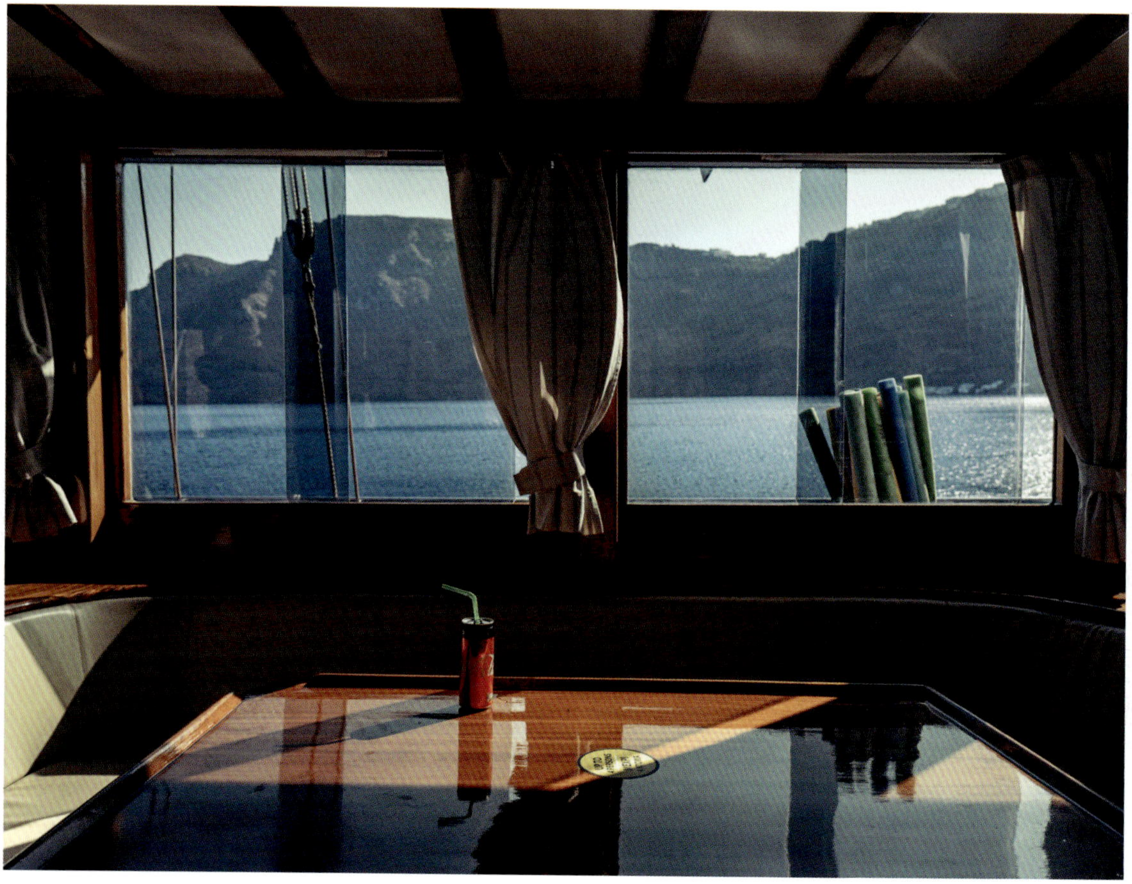

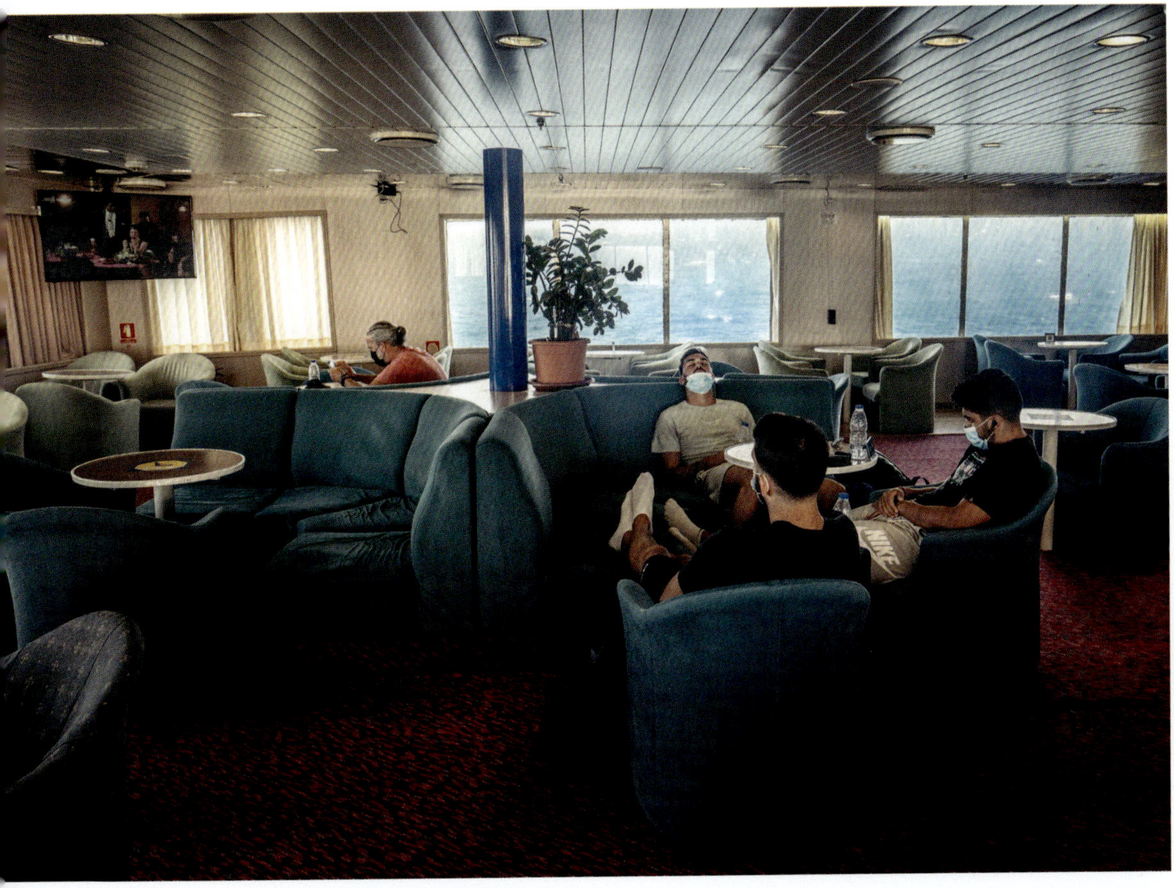
NIKE

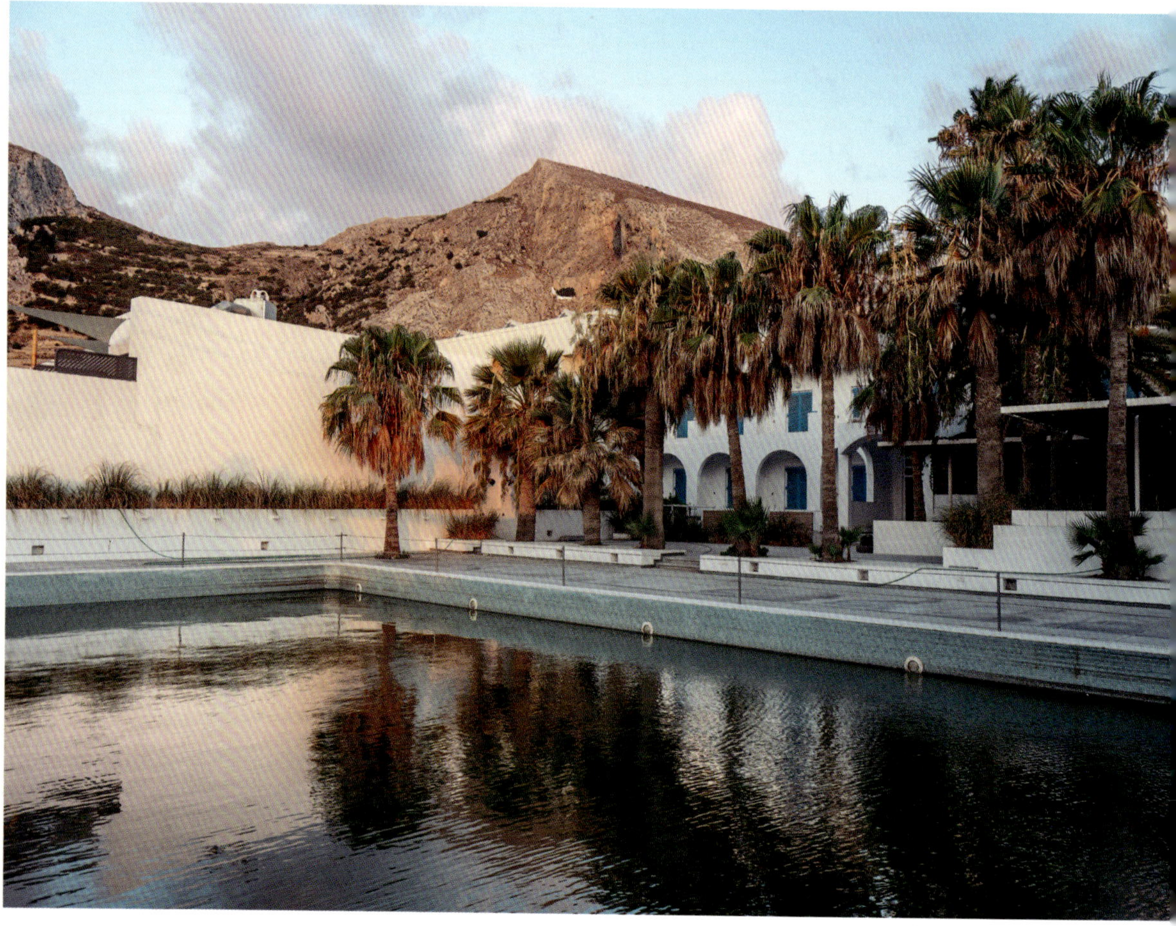

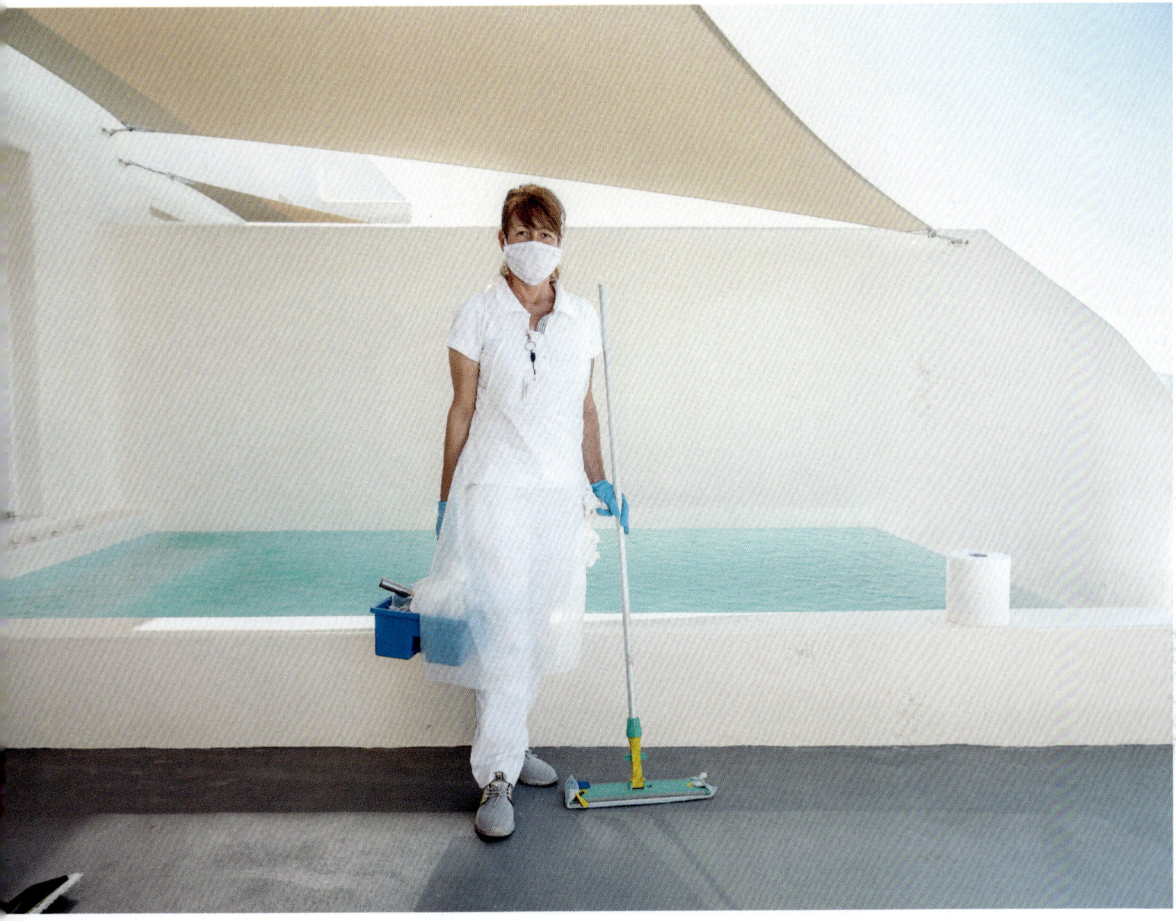

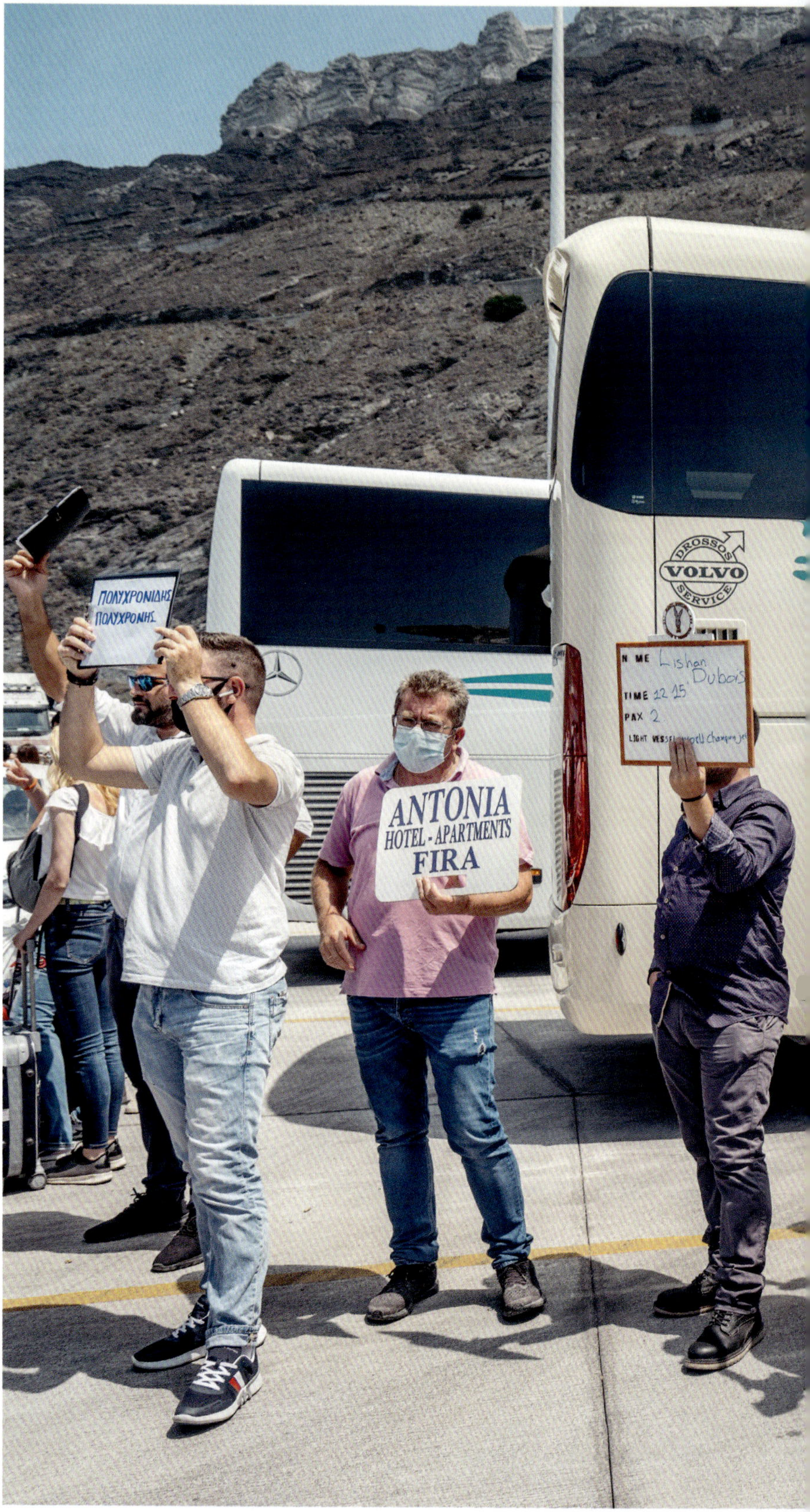
ΠΟΛΥΧΡΟΝΙΔΗΣ
ΠΟΛΥΧΡΟΝΗΣ
ANTONIA
HOTEL - APARTMENTS
FIRA
DROSSOS
VOLVO
SERVICE
TIME 12 15'
PAX 2

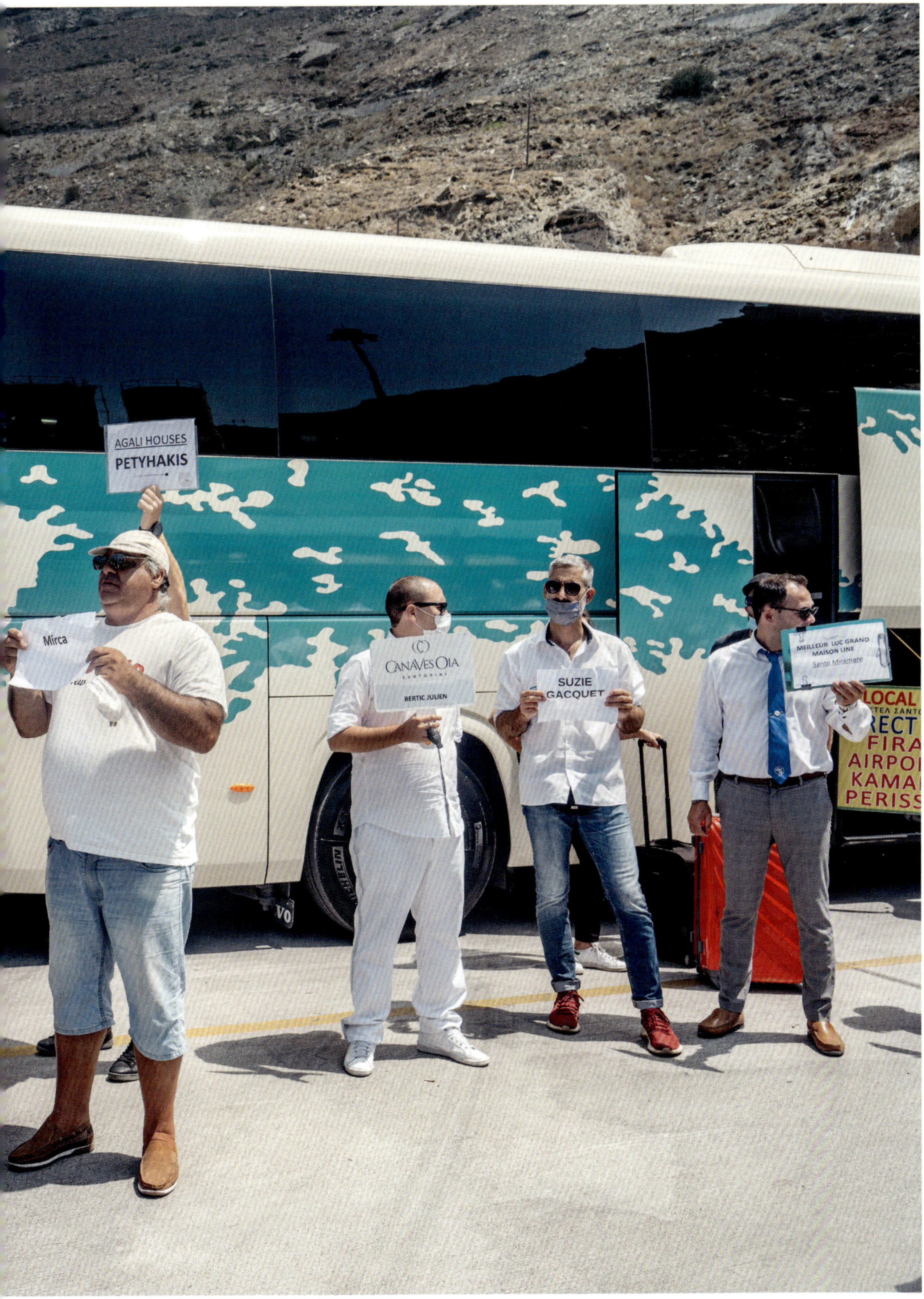
AGALI HOUSES
PETYHAKIS
Mirca
CANAVES OIA
SANTORINI
BERTIC JULIEN
SUZIE
GACQUET
MEILLEUR LUC GRAND
MAISON LINE
Santo Miramare
LOCAL
FIRA

Luana Rigolli, Italy
Empty Billboards

We are constantly bombarded by advertisements on the web, in magazines, on TV and even in the street. The COVID-19 epidemic in Italy and the ensuing lockdown have also changed the marketing strategies of big companies, which used to place huge banners on advertising spaces on the facades of city buildings undergoing renovation. Astonishingly, these spaces are left blank, empty, without any sort of communication, amplifying the emptiness left by the absence of tourists and visitors who used to fill the streets of Italy's popular towns.

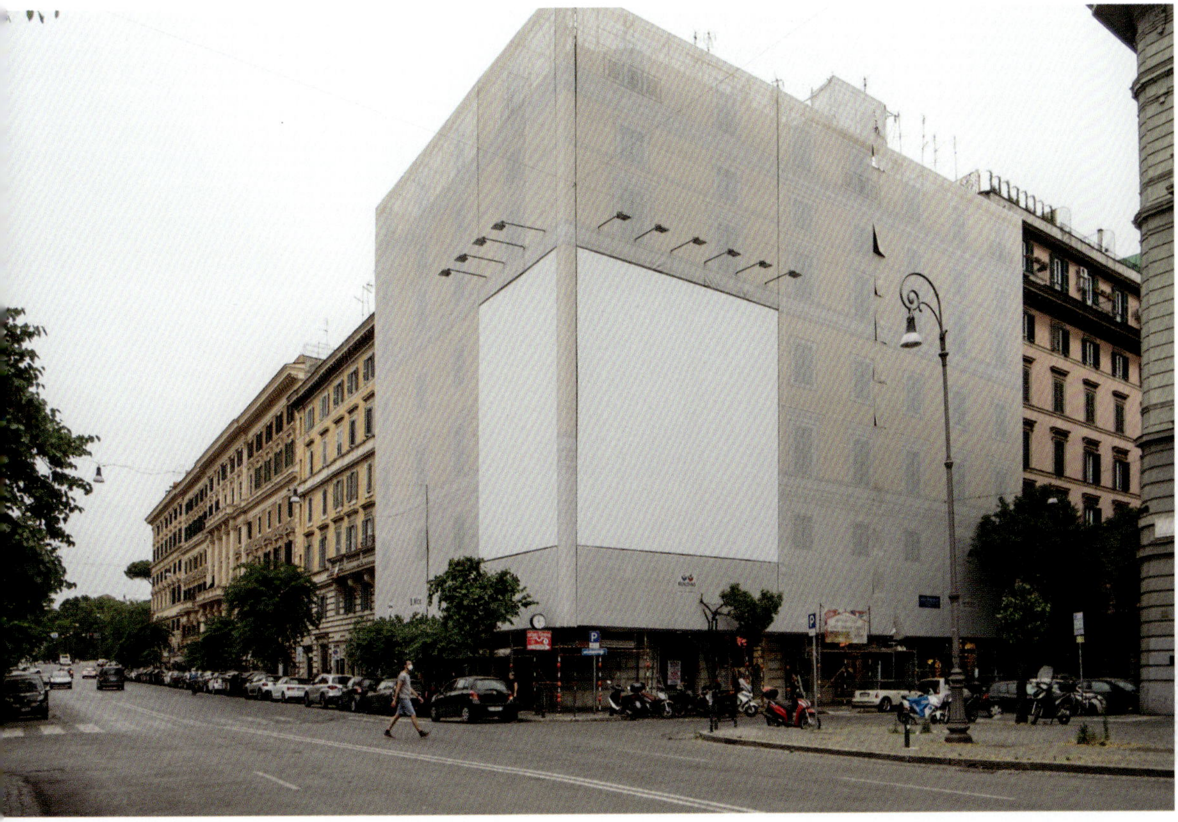

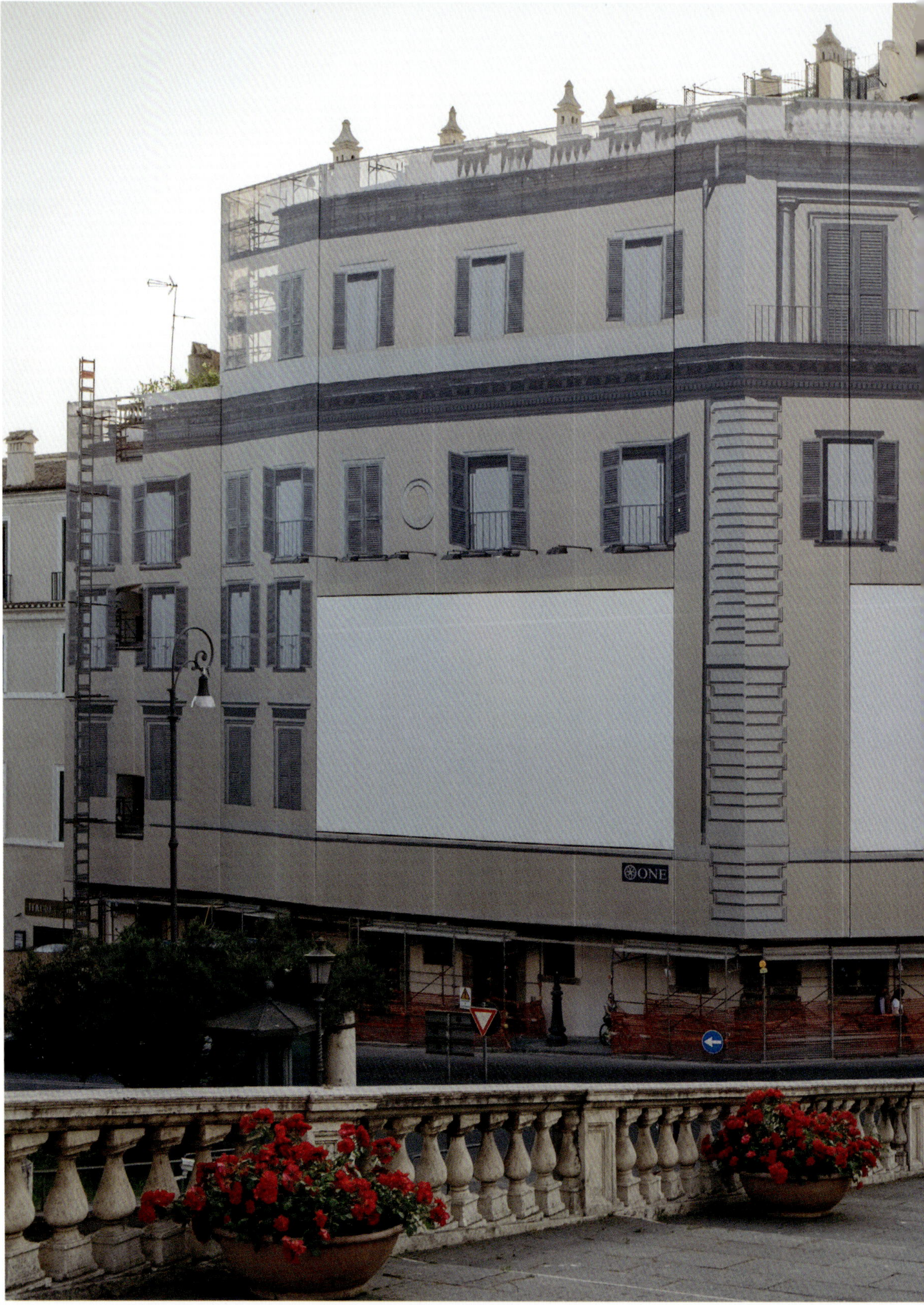
ONE

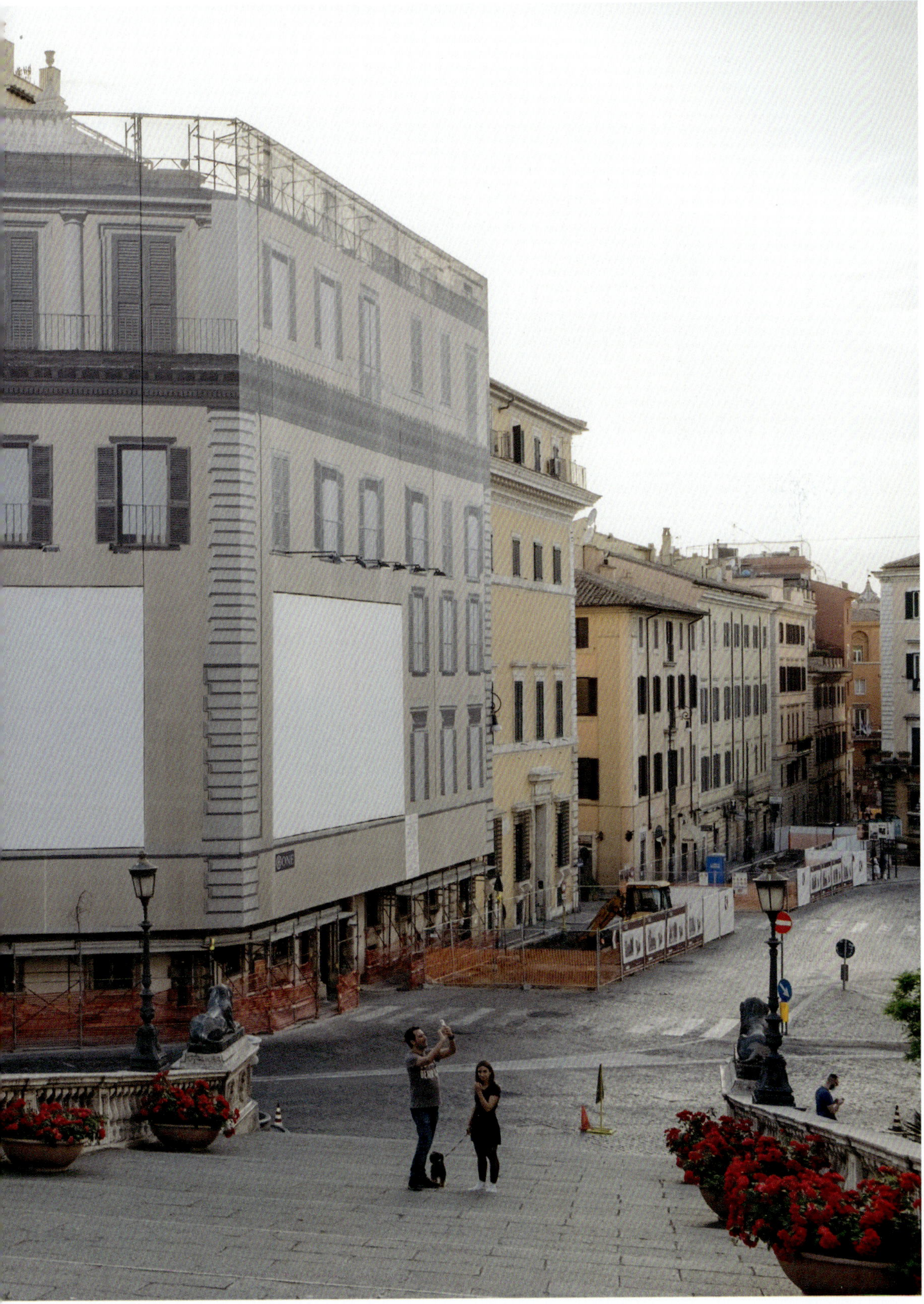

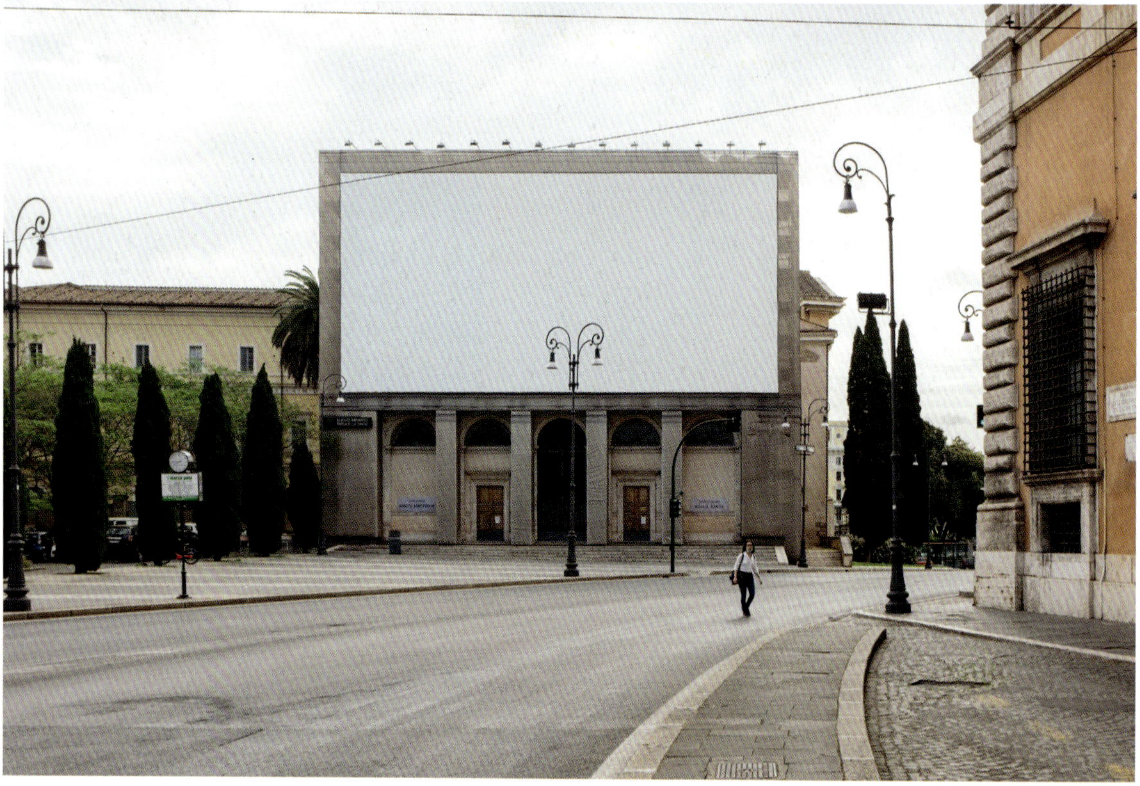

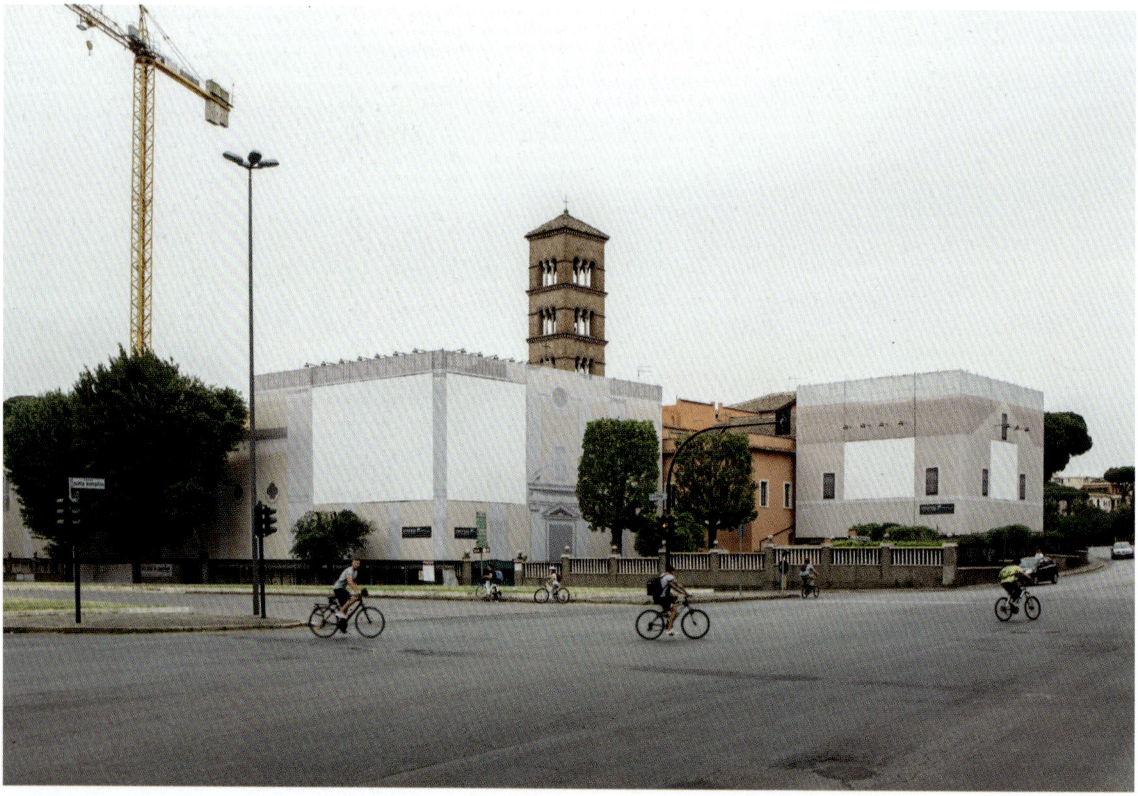

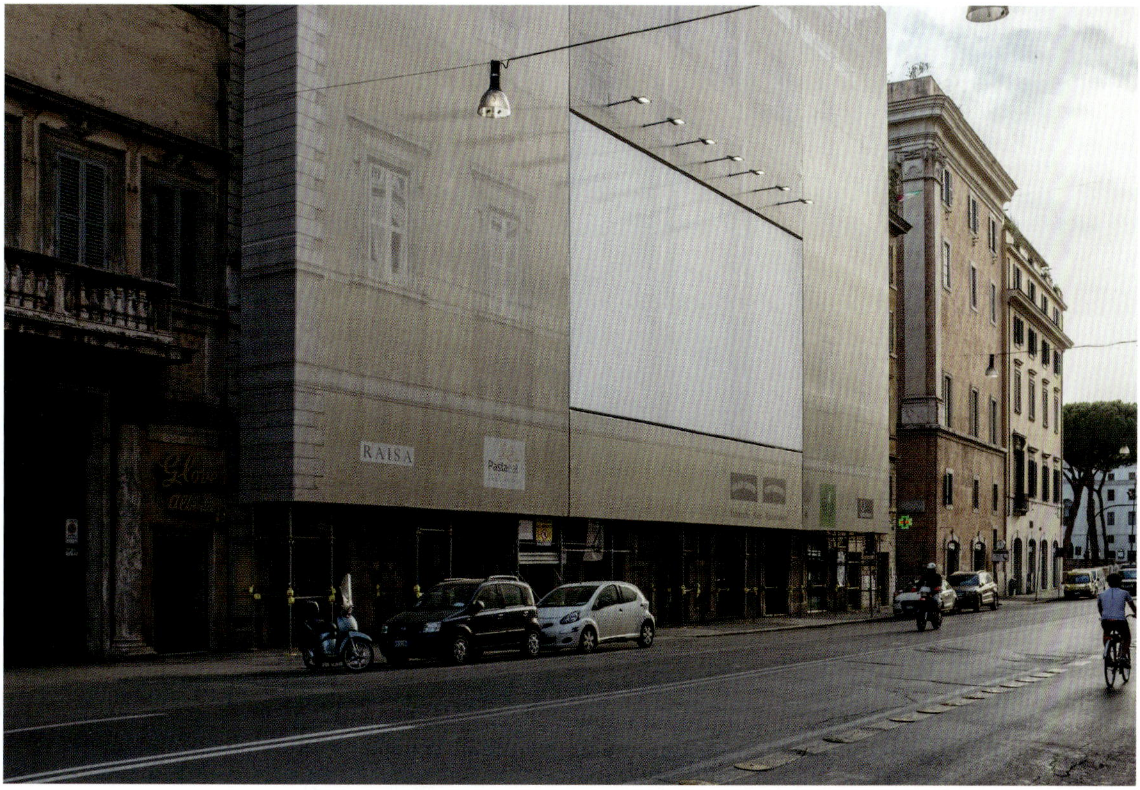
RAISA

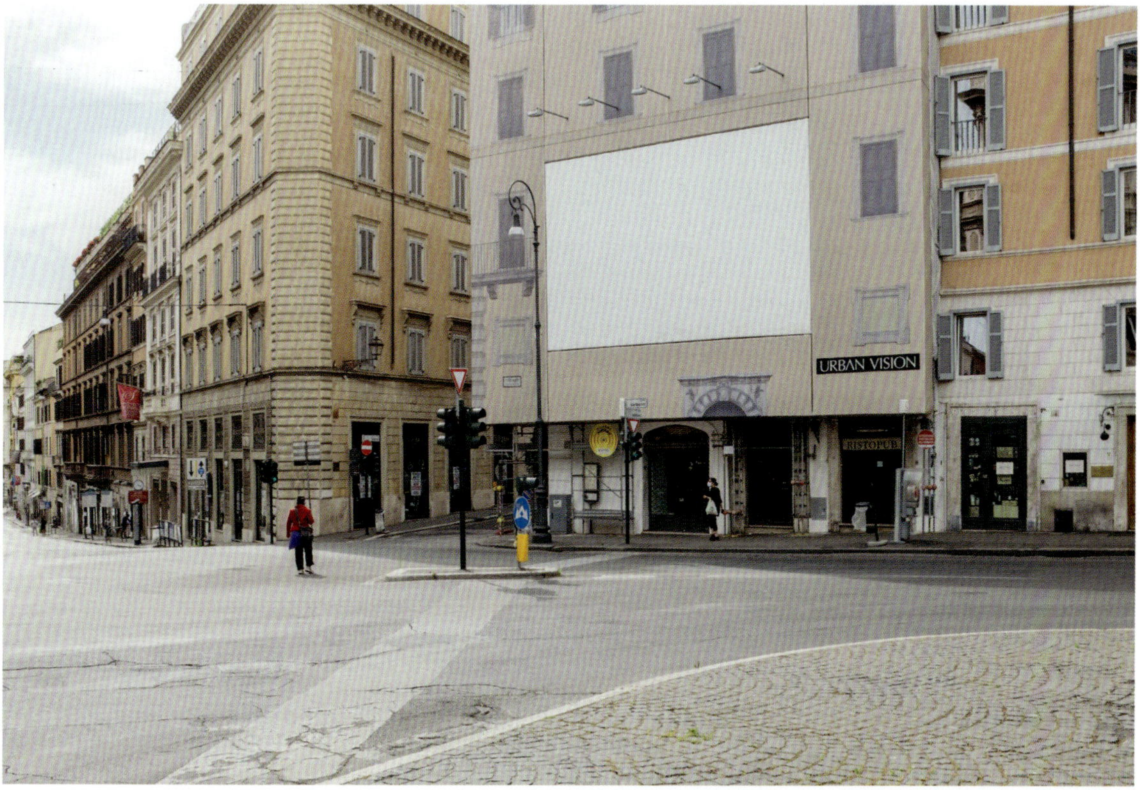
URBAN VISION

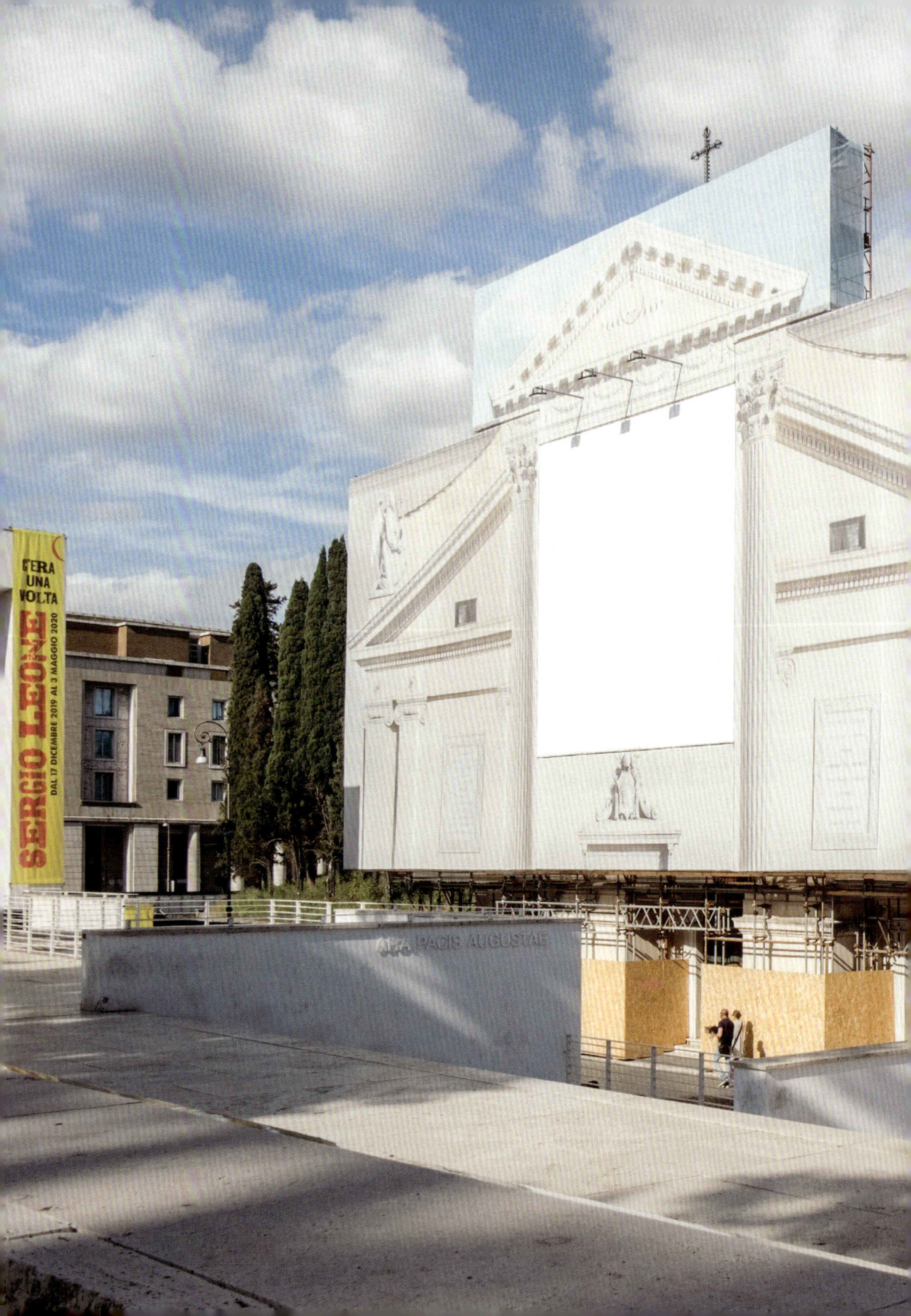
C'ERA
UNA
VOLTA
SERGIO LEONE
DAL 17 DICEMBRE 2019 AL 3 MAGGIO 2020
ARA PACIS AUGUSTAE

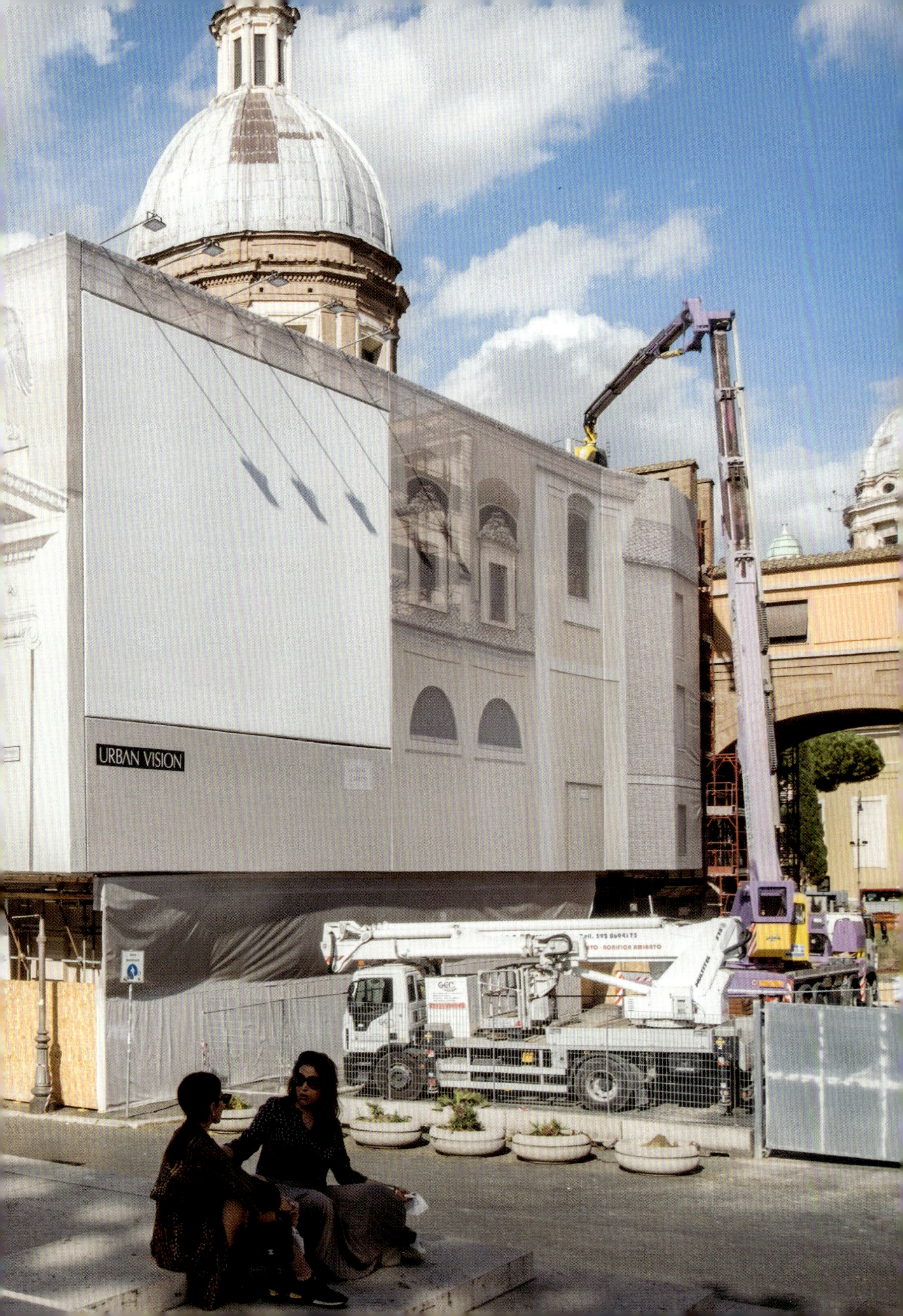
URBAN VISION

Gabriele Galimberti, Italy
Support Local Business

Massimo Razzi

Let me introduce Donatella Ficini: her family from Altopascio went to sell bread in Turin and there she became famous; there are also Silvia and Riccardo Tortoli, *pizzicagnoli* (delicatessen & cheesemongers) in Florence in Borgo San Frediano; Davide Viganò keeps his "vegetable garden" in the heart of Brera, in Milan, and Rahman Sohel runs a mini-market in Piazza Nazario Sauro, in Florence. These are the proud little shopkeepers who, at the time of COVID-19, raised their heads and found in their neighbourhood a commercial and social role that was perhaps deemed lost.
Gabriele Galimberti went to look for them in Turin and Milan, as well as at his home in Florence, and portrayed them like this: strutting, at the entrance to their shop or inside, in front of their fully stocked counter, wearing the face mask that marks these sad days, but aware that they are deeply part of a community of people. Not only part, perhaps, but almost sentinels and defenders of a space that in these months has remained open. Because, without them, we couldn't carry out eating and living as we did. Because they had the task of keeping alive a light in the streets that plunged into darkness even during the day. Not only a light, but also a rediscovery because Galimberti explains to us that the queues in front of the supermarkets are long and tiring and that's why people, whenever possible, returned to their local shopkeeper, from whom, until recently, one used to go shopping only to avoid a last minute shortage of bread or tomatoes.
Even in front of the local *pizzicagnolo* there's a queue. But it seems more human and bearable. On the door, directing the traffic, there isn't a young boy who says "next one goes ahead", but (behind the mask) a familiar face and a friendly voice that may call you by your name: "Come on, Mrs. Maria... It's your turn, Mr. Massimo, please stand there on the right". Someone who knows you and, if he sees Mrs. Pina, who is 94 years old, lets her in first after a brief consultation with the line of people you all know.
A community, in short, with its choreographer directing the dances

from the door of his shop. Thus, bakers, *pizzicagnoli*, fishmongers and greengrocers form a gallery of colourful and strong-rooted images. It feels like being inside Guttuso's Vucciria, the depiction of a street food market in which every person, whether selling or buying, has a role and a story. This way, Galimberti wanted to pay homage to the rediscovery of the local shopkeeper's role. And he tells us what Filippo, a greengrocer in Florence, explained to him: "When the big supermarkets came into town years ago, we small traders were almost wiped out, it was very difficult to fight against the competition. People prefer to shop where they can find everything, often to the detriment of product quality. With this crisis, many people now no longer want to go to places that are very busy. At small traders like us, the queues move much faster and people can establish a relationship of trust with the owners. We guarantee the origin of our products ourselves and people appreciate that, especially at this time of fear and emergency".

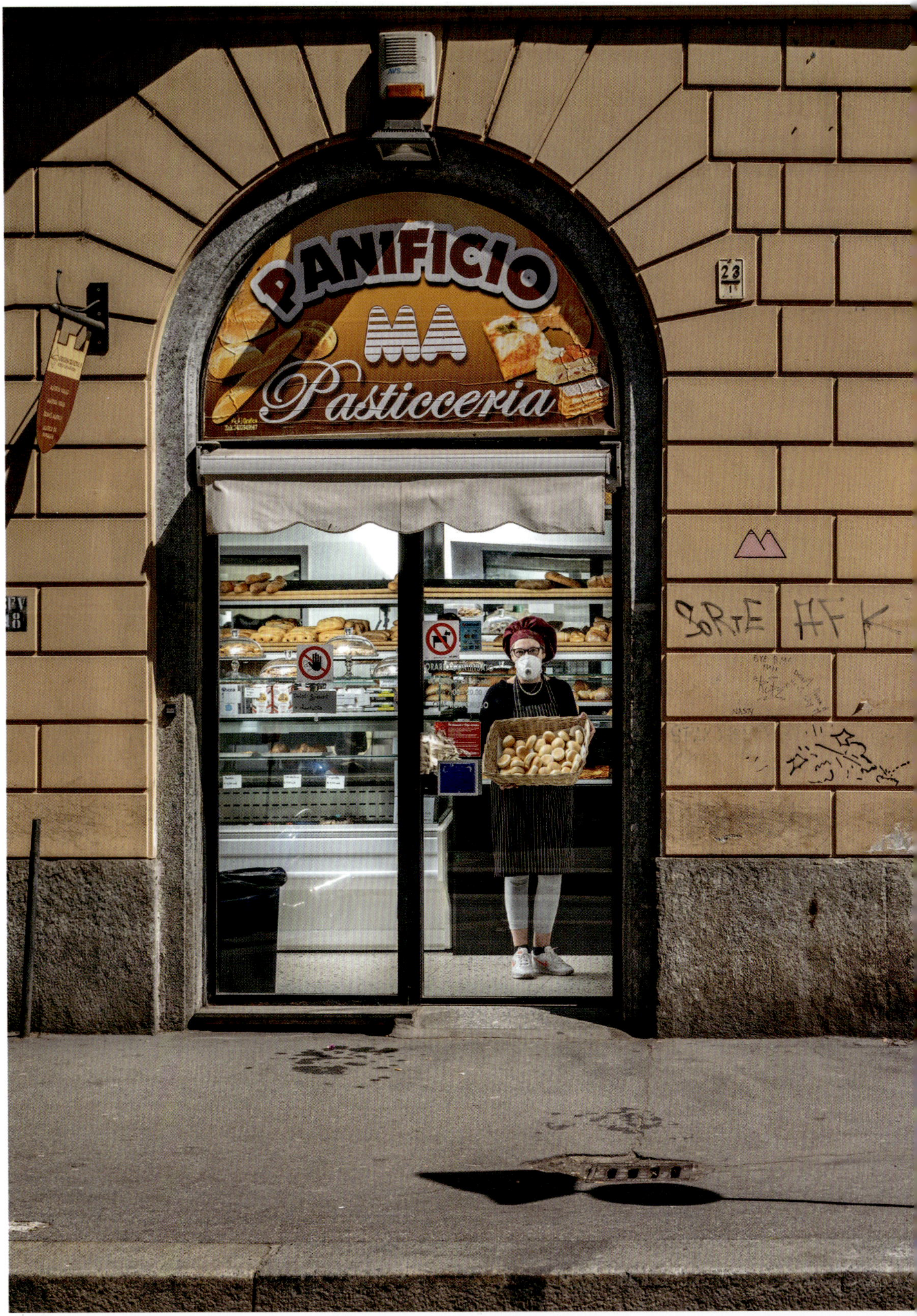
PANIFICIO
MA
Pasticceria
23

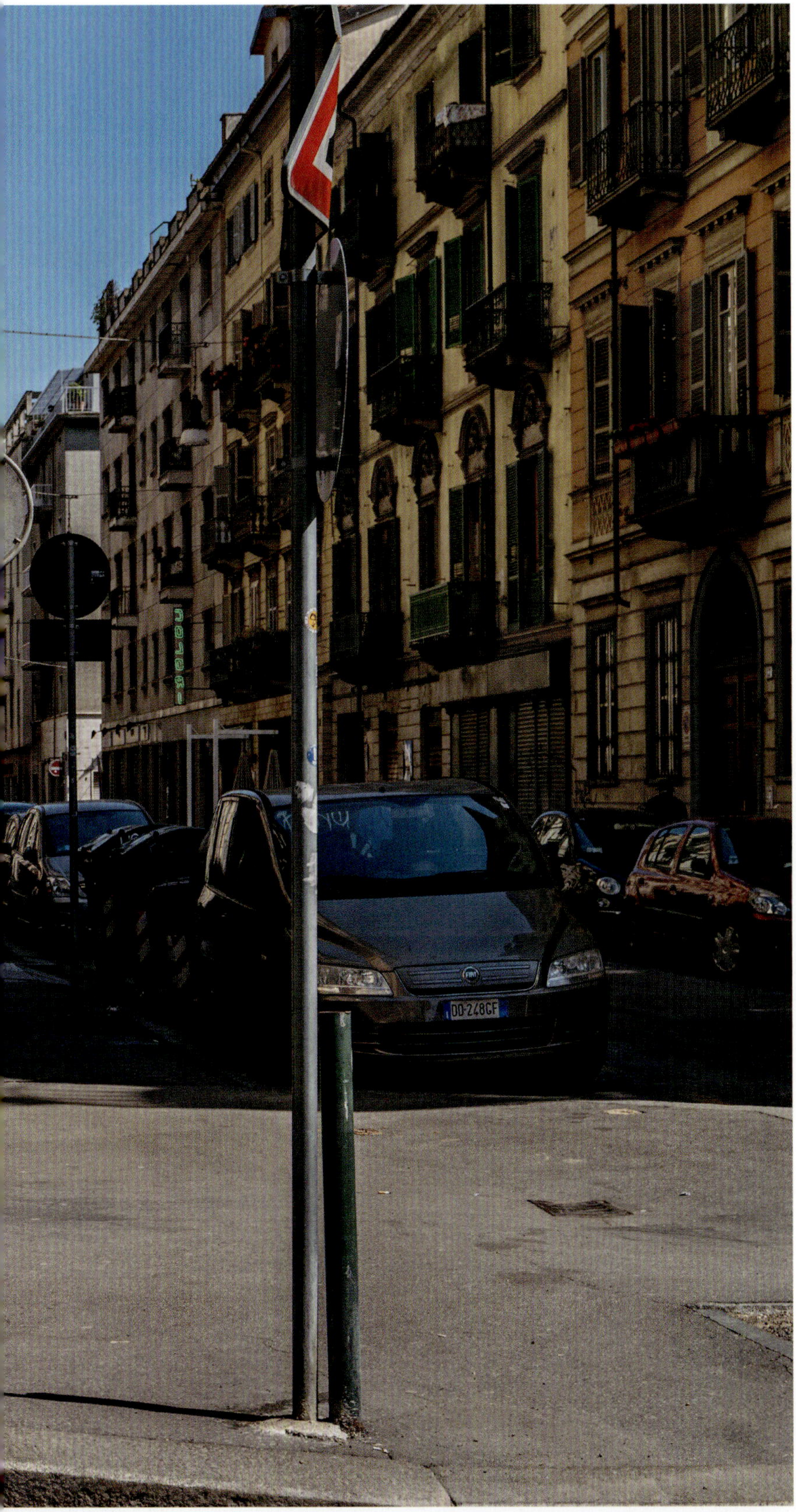
DD-248CF

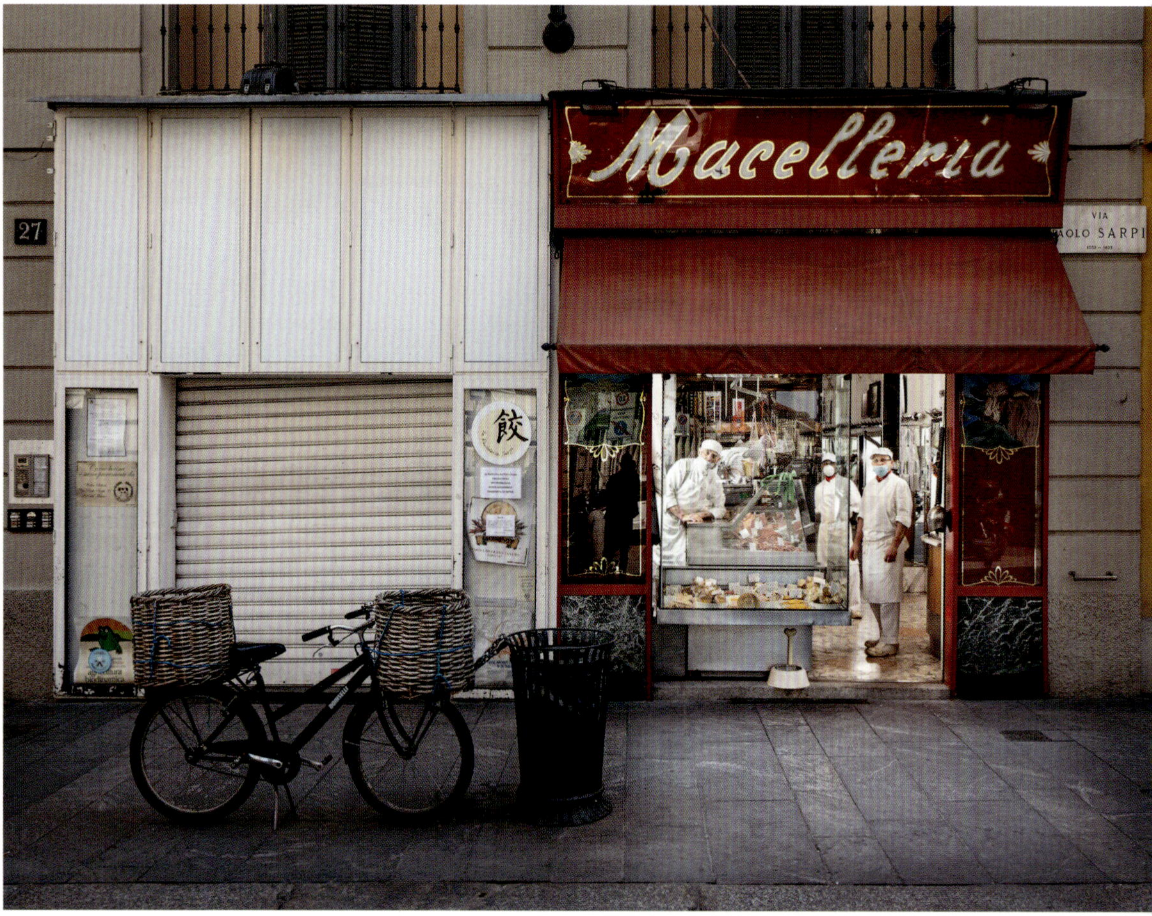
Macelleria
27
餃
VIA

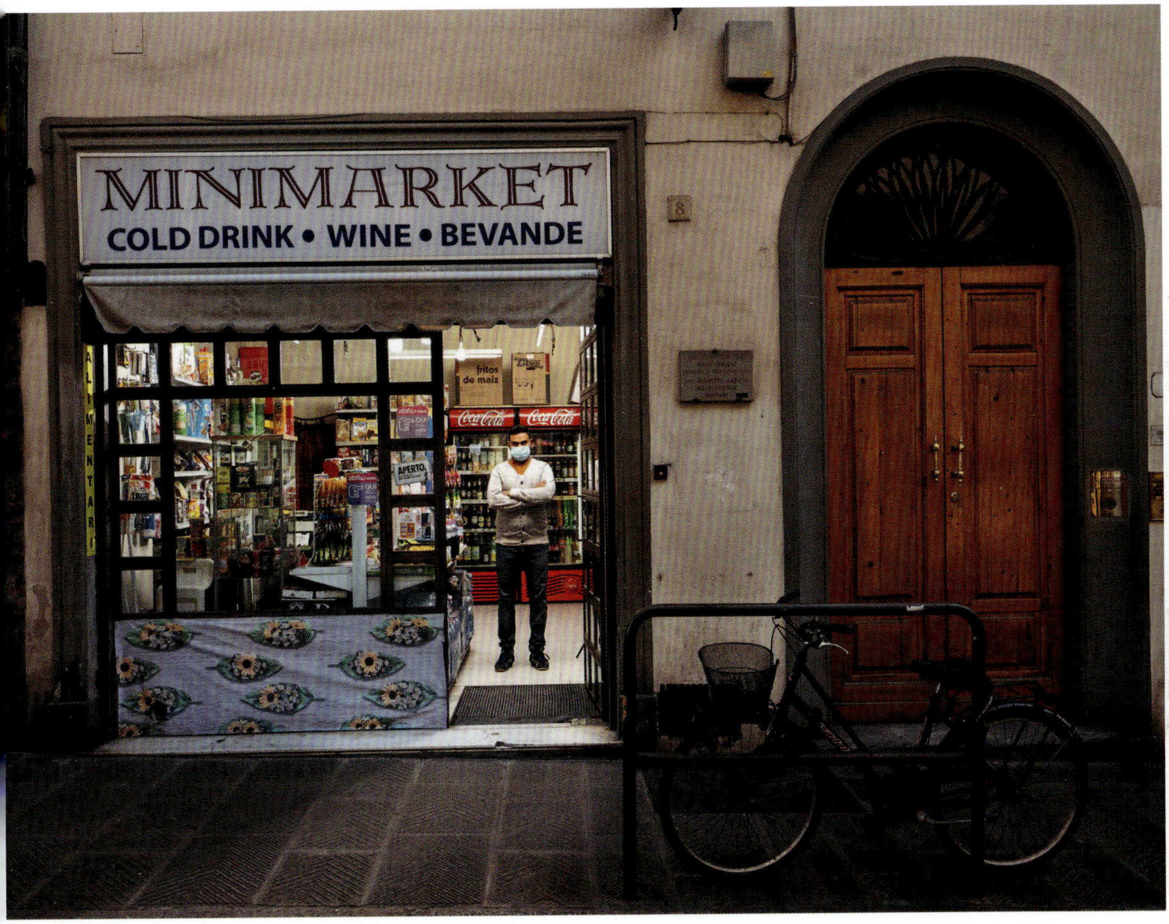
MINIMARKET
COLD DRINK • WINE • BEVANDE

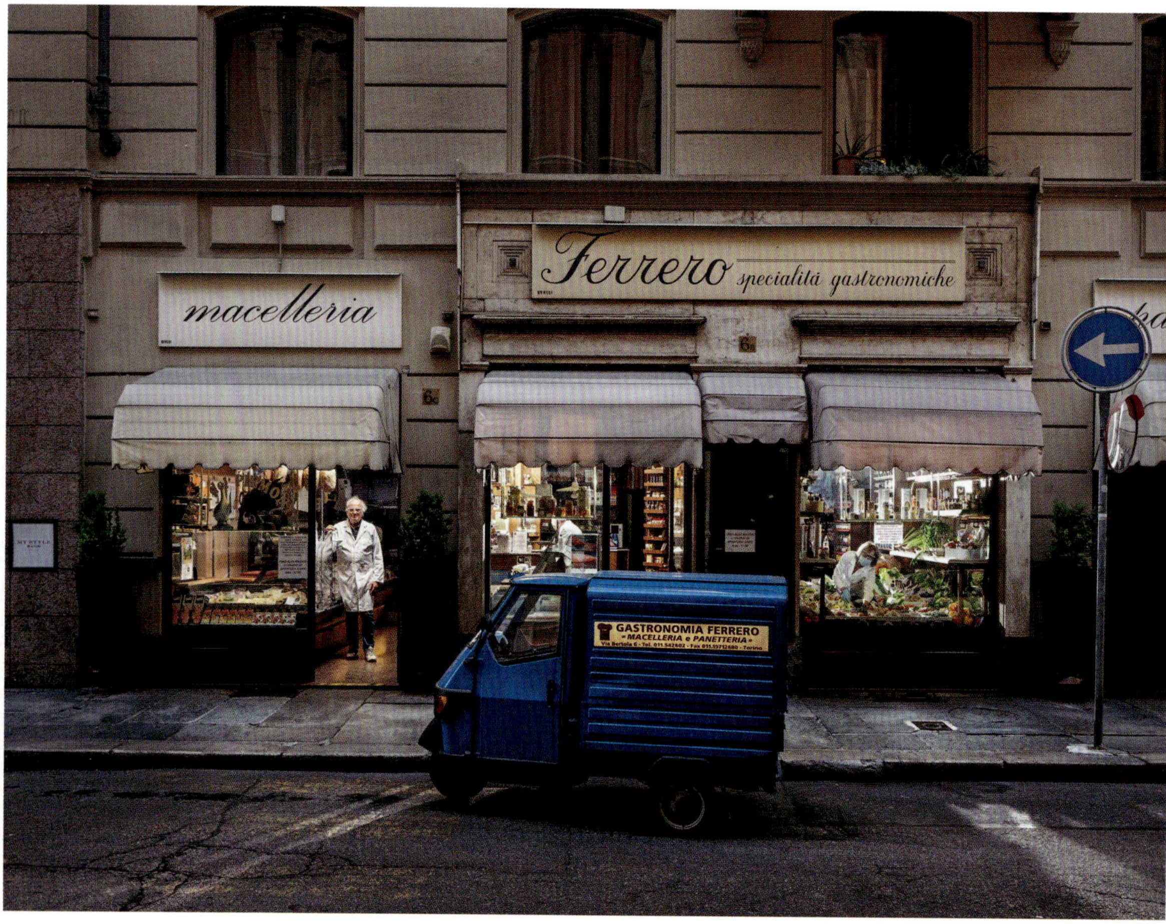
macelleria
Ferrero specialità gastronomiche
GASTRONOMIA FERRERO
» MACELLERIA e PANETTERIA «

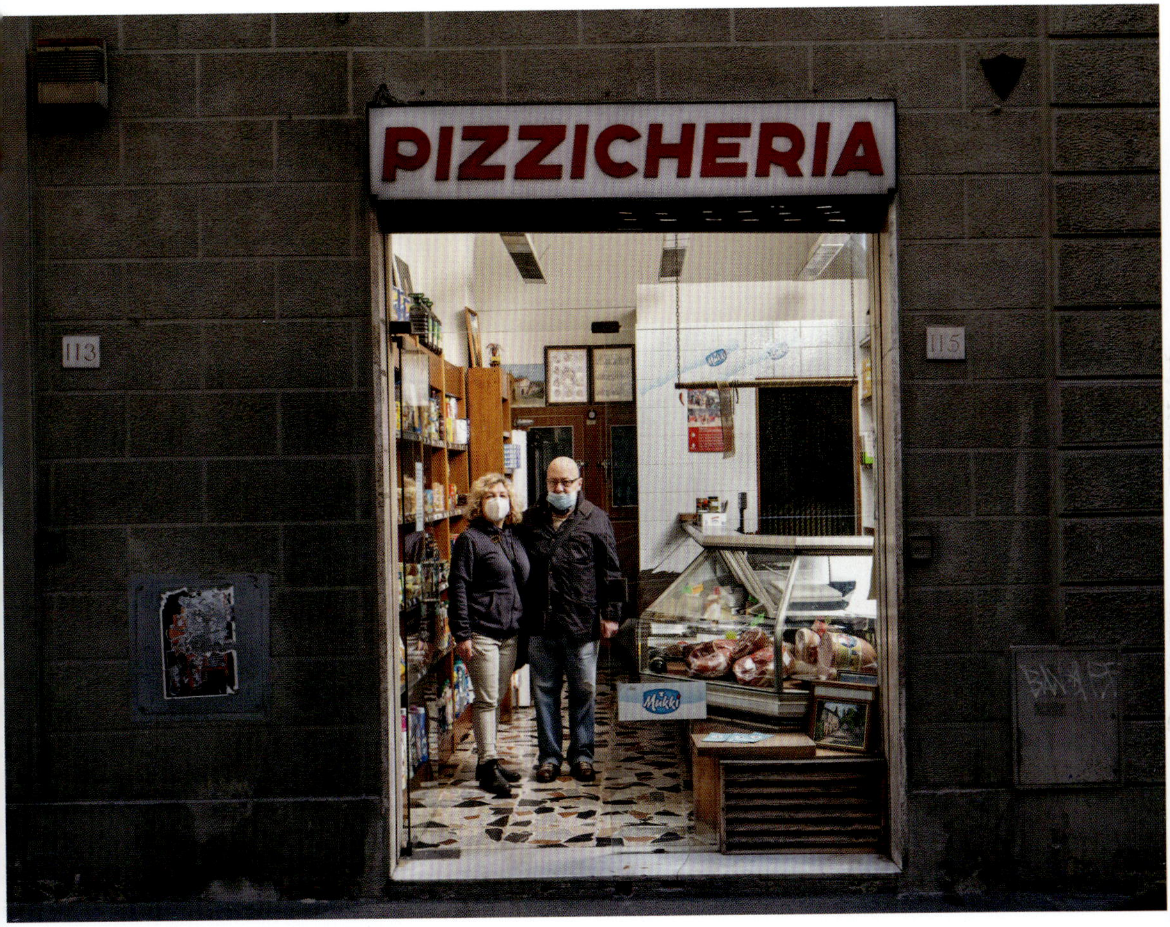
PIZZICHERIA
113
115
Mukki

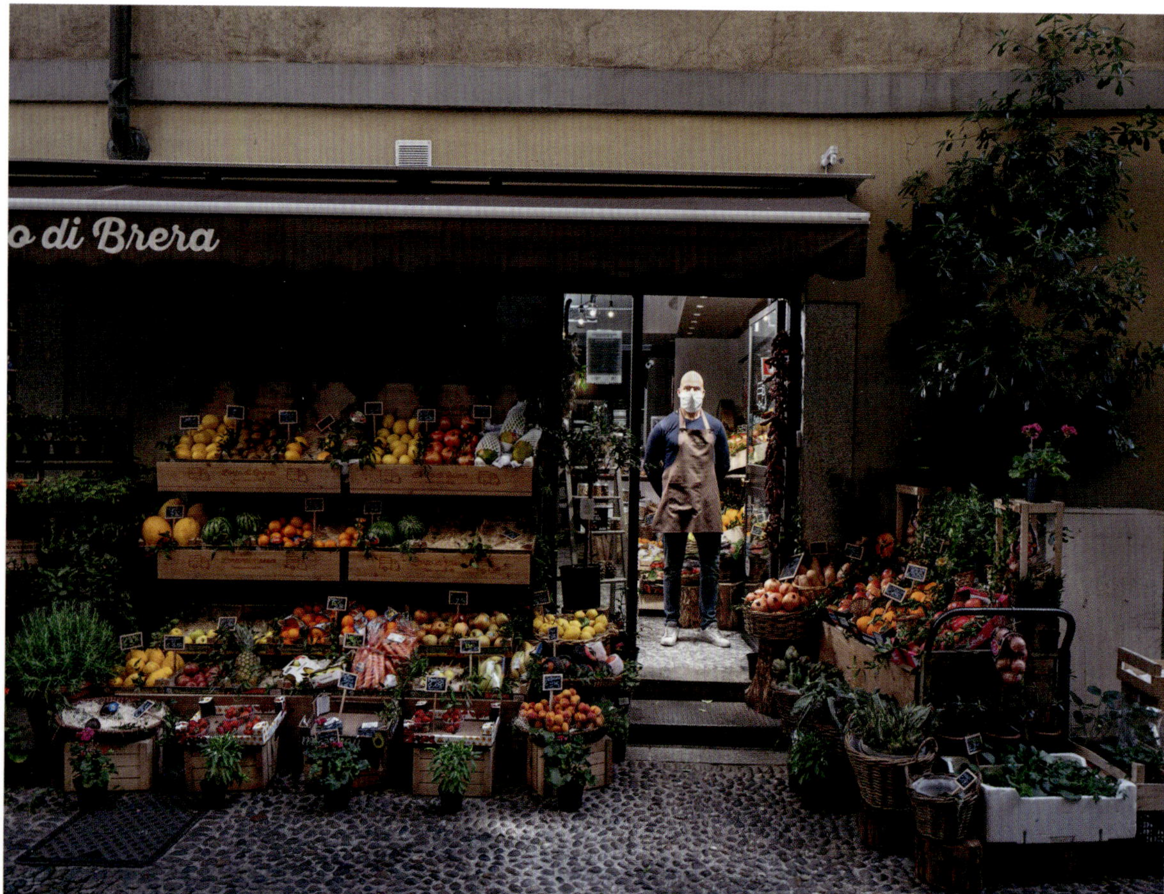
o di Brera

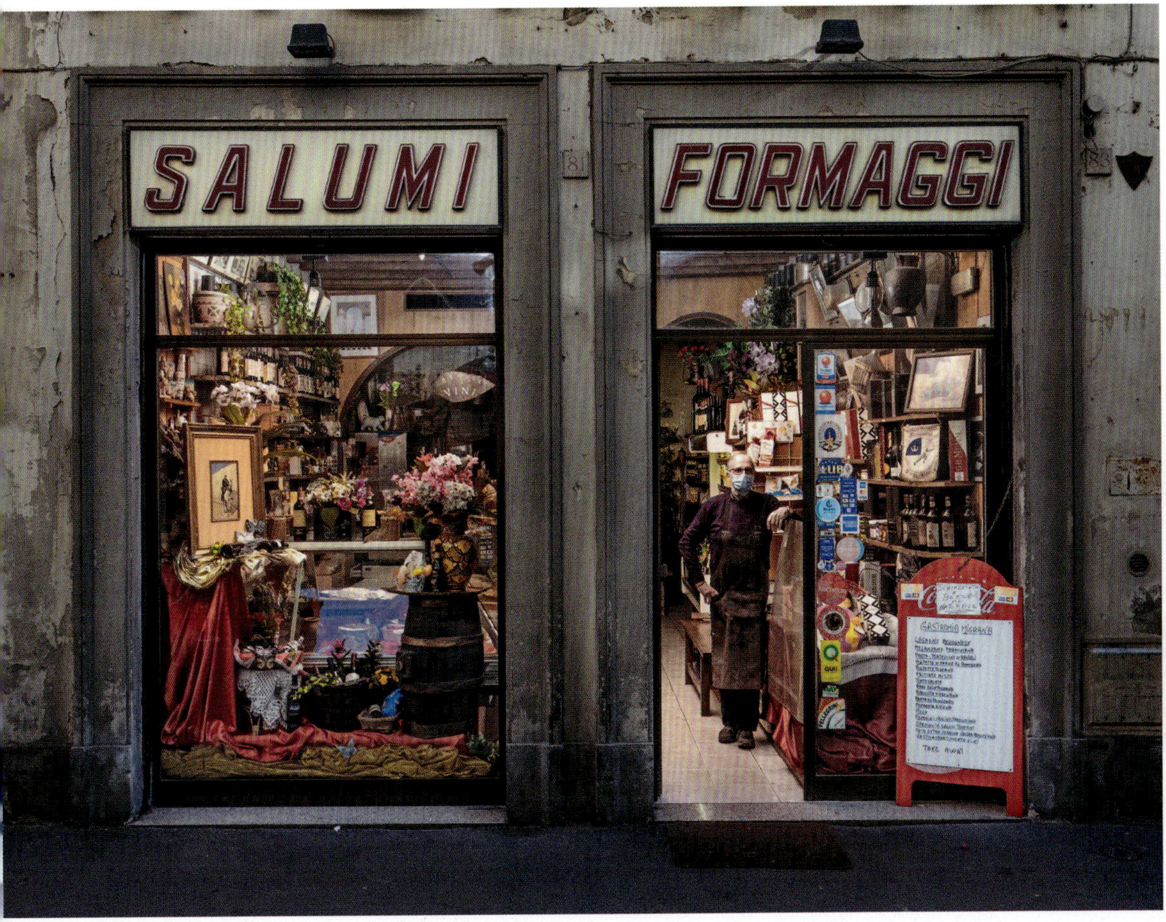
SALUMI
FORMAGGI

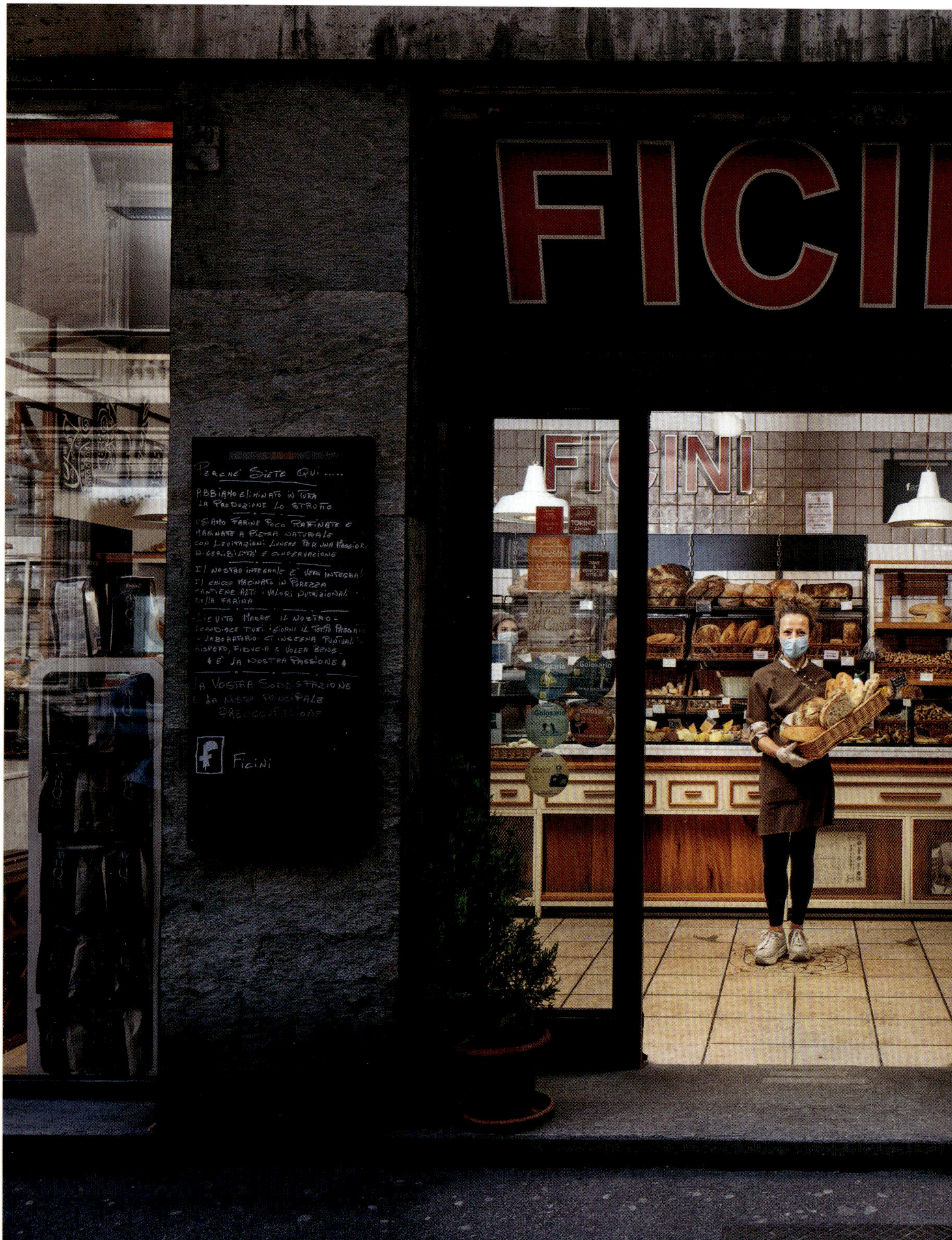
FICINI
PERCHÉ SIETE QUI.....
ABBIAMO ELIMINATO IN TUTTA
LA PRODUZIONE LO STRUTTO
IL NOSTRO INTEGRALE È VERO INTEGRALE
È LA NOSTRA PASSIONE
Ficini
FICINI

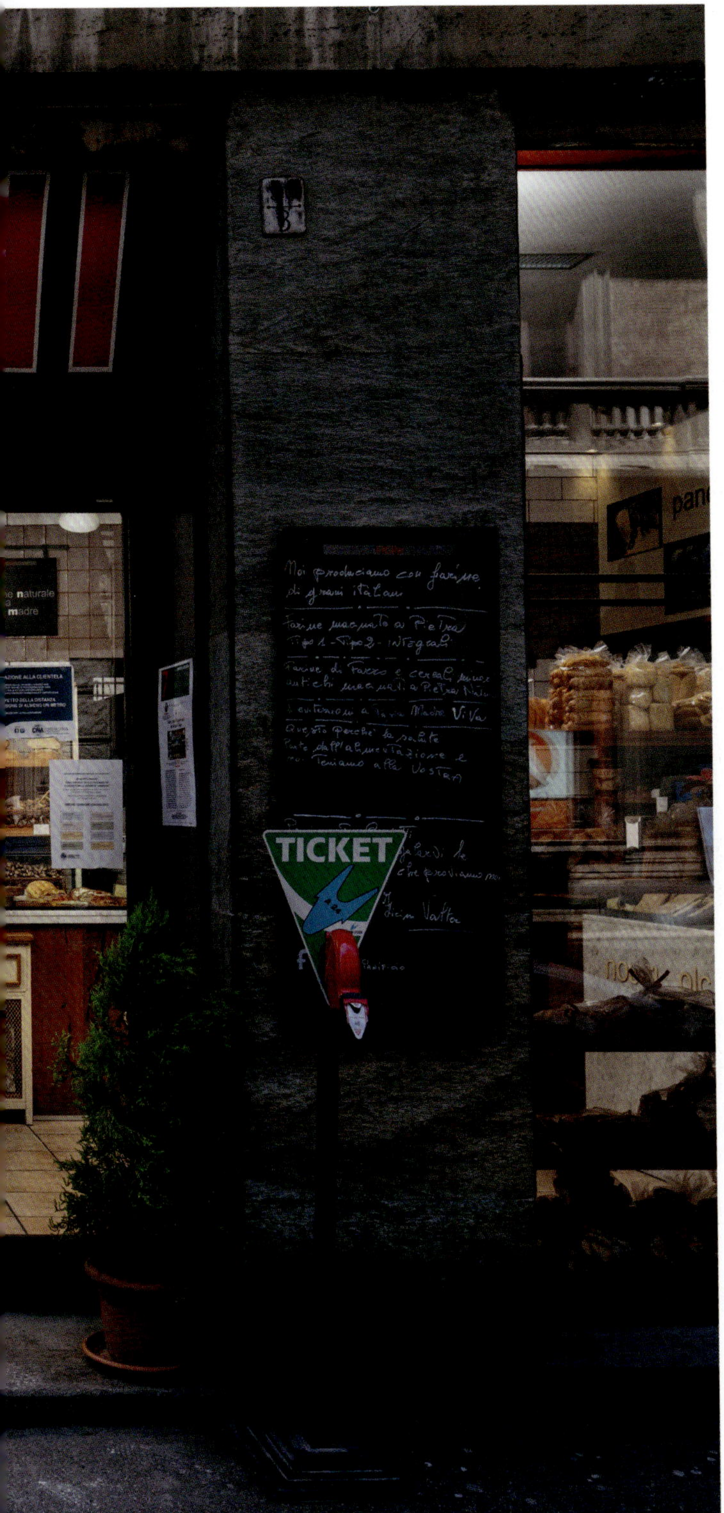
Noi produciamo con farine di grani italiani
Farine macinate a Pietra
Tipo 1 - Tipo 2 - Integrali
Questo perché la salute
TICKET
pane

04. The Economic Effects
Captions

Mattia Balsamini, Italy

Boxes filled with masks almost ready to be shipped. Siom Termoplast, Fiume Veneto (Pordenone). 10 April 2020.
(Page 251)

Phases of the preparation and mixing of the disinfectant gel. Politecnico di Milano.
The hospital's chemistry department started producing a sanitising gel, according to the recipe of the World Health Organisation,for the emergency caused by the COVID-19 pandemic and distributed free of charge to health organisations, to the Civil Protection of Lombardy and also to the Milanese prisons of San Vittore, Opera and Bollate.
20 April 2020.
(Page 252)

The cutting process of each individual mask produced with non-woven fabric. Prada production plant in Montone (Perugia).
9 April 2020.
(Page 253)

Inside the lab where different types of filters and materials are being tested to study the filtering capabilities, particularly of face masks. Politecnico di Milano. The hospital's lab are used for all types of analysis necessary to certify individual protection devices that companies wish to donate or place on the market. 20 April 2020.
(Page 254, top)

Quality control and finishing of the face masks. Prada production plant in Montone (Perugia). Prada, one of the leading brands in the fashion and luxury sector worldwide, has decided to make its contribution by converting the factory from the production of trousers to that of 110,000 masks for the medical staff of Tuscany. 9 April 2020.
(Page 254, bottom)

Steps of 3D printing and 3D scanning of the mockups. Siom Termoplast, Fiume Veneto (Pordenone). The company, specialised in plastic material printing engineered, developed and printed a face mask which filter can be easily replaced. The production capacity is 7,000 pieces per week and the goal is to produce a total of 20,000 pieces that will be entirely donated to the Civil Protection and to the municipality of Fiume Veneto.
10 April 2020.
(Page 255, top)

Assembly line of cardiosurgery circuits. Inside Eurosets in Medolla (Modena) which produces extracorporeal pulmonary appliances. The only Italian company to manufacture these appliances that reproduce the work of pulmonary alveolus and artificially generates the carbon dioxide-oxygen exchange, putting the lungs to complete rest, when the pulmonary ventilator are no longer enough. Eurosets went from producing 300 to 1,200 oxygenators in a month. Almost all 130 employees moved to its production line.
16 April 2020.
(Page 255, bottom)

A worker spraying disinfectant in different areas of the factory to avoid spreading of the virus – Faber, in Cividale del Friuli (Udine), has been very thorough in enforcing safety measures to avoid the spread, from workers distancing to providing individual safety measures such as face masks and tapping pens for digital devices. 24 April 2020.
(Page 256)

Torbole, Lago di Garda. Seatex, owned by Luca Gavioli, is a small company that normally repairs sails for windsurfing, kitesurfing and boats. Gavioli thought of turning mono-film into antivirus visors.
It has provided some samples to the Red Cross and to some companies that consider that protection system very practical. The material used is the mono-film that is usually used for sails, very light in weight and thickness, to which the support is applied in order to be worn on the garment. Luca Gavioli has made several of them and has put them on trial, but now, in order to start a small production to be distributed to retirement homes, RSAs or hospitals, he must wait for the Ministry's approval. 22 April 2020.
(Page 257)

Assembly line of cardiosurgery circuits inside Eurosets in Medolla (Modena) which produces extracorporeal pulmonary appliances. 16 April 2020.
(Page 258)

Density tests of the disinfectant at ICR, Industrie Cosmetiche Riunite (united cosmetic industries). 16 April 2020.
(Page 259)

TerraProject, Italy

The photographs were taken between May and June 2020.

Florence. Alessio Tizzanini at the entrance of Battistero, he works here since 2 years. The first day of reopening was May 22. For 2 weeks the entrance was free, in 24 hours the reservation agenda was completelly booked. (Page 261)

Florence. Opera del Duomo di Firenze. Inside the Battistero. All the restoration construction sites are stopped.
(Pages 262-263)

Rome. A family biking around the closed Colosseum. In 2018 the Roman amphitheatre welcomed a record: 7.6 million visitors — an average of around 21,000 people a day — making it the most visited monument in the world.
(Pages 264-265)

Florence. The entrance of Battistero. For security reasons the complex is able to host 300 people per day instead of 3,000. They calculate a loss of 20 million euros.
(Page 266)

Fiumicino. Veronica Panetta, 28-year-old, works for a security company operating in the Fiumicino International Airport.
(Page 267)

Rome. Caterina Zavoni, 33, has been working at the Hotel Quirinale since 2013. During lockdown the hotel has been opened but had no clients for 3 months. The first visitors arrived at the beginning of June. The hotel is part of Federalberghi, the main Italian association of hotels, which includes 27,000 of the 33,000 hotels present in Italy. To date, only 40% of the hotels are open. In big tourist cities the number is even lower.
(Page 268)

Florence. The Loggia dei Lanzi in Piazza della Signoria.
(Page 269)

Venice. A boat is navigating Canal Grande seen from the Rialto Bridge. The contraction of international tourism will reverberate above all on the art cities, such as Venice and Florence.
(Pages 270–271)

Daniel Etter, Germany

Nosa Aikpitanyi, a cleaner at an emergency ward at the Uniklinik Bonn, poses for a portrait in Bonn. Aikpitanyi, originally from Nigeria, has been cleaning the emergency ward for more than decade. 5 May 2020.
(Page 273)

Police officer G. poses for a portrait in Berlin. 28 May 2020.
(Page 274)

Corpse washer Nadine Eicher poses for a portrait in Berlin. The ritualistic washing before burial is essential for practicing Muslims. 23 April 2020.
(Page 275)

Head butcher Silke Kulschewski poses for a portrait in Wahlsdorf-Liepe. Meat processing facilities have been responsible for some of the worst COVID-19 outbreaks in Germany and the US. 20 May 2020.
(Page 276)

Care worker Miroslawa Thomale with Kayra, one of the children with severe disabilities she works with in Berlin. For parents of children with severe disabilities, it is increasingly hard to find people to help them take care of their children since the demanding nature of the job and the low pay. 10 June 2020.
(Page 277)

Firefighters André Weinand, Santiago Pantaleon and Andreas Krämer pose for a portrait in Bonn. They are based at the Uniklinik and also handle emergency helicopter landings. 8 May 2020.
(Page 278)

Kindergartener Myriam Peker poses for a portrait with some of the children in her care in Berlin. During the lockdown measures kindergarten had to keep working to take care of children of people in essential jobs. 26 May 2020.
(Page 279)

Paramedics Florian Pützstück and Carmen Jänicke pose for a portrait at the Uniklinik in Bonn. Despite seeing an influx of COVID-19 patients, the feared surge of patients on intensive care has not happened at the Uniklinik until this point. 5 May 2020.
(Page 280)

Farmer and shepherd Johann Nesges poses for a portrait in one of his stables in Wahlsdorf-Liepe. During the peak of the first wave of the pandemic, prices for sheep skin and wool dropped near zero since the supply chain to processing countries like Turkey broke down. 5 May 2020.
(Page 281)

Lou Lou D'Aki, Greece

The photographs were taken in August 2020.

Morning view over an empty beach at Rhodes.
(Page 283)

Desi, from Bulgaria, wears a mask at the reception desk at Canaves Oia Suites – a five star hotel where she has worked since 2010. She says that the main difference from other years is that, this year, the bookings are received last minute. And that there are no American guests.
(Page 284)

A museum guard at the National Archeological Museum in Athens wears an obligatory face mask while guarding one of the exhibition halls.
(Page 285)

When Caldera's sunset tour leaves the Old port in Fira, the ship is generally filled with tourists who want to spend the afternoon cruising around Santorini and to see the sun set. This season the number of sold tour tickets were down 96%. Each person boarding the ship got its temperature taken, face masks were obligatory and the tables were marked with stickers indicating the number of people allowed.
(Page 286)

Some people napping on a ferry crossing from Santorini to Rhodes island. This year, the common spaces of the ferry have stickers on tables and chairs telling passengers where they are not allowed to sit. Everyone on the ferry has to wear a face mask and keep a distance and the ferry capacity accepts a reduced number of passengers.
(Page 287)

View over a closed up hotel at Kamari beach, Santorini. This year, due to COVID-19, the beginning of the touristic season in Greece was postponed 3-4 months and some hotel owners decided not to open up their hotels, bars and restaurant for the remaining 3 months of the season.
(Page 288)

Ivanka from Bulgaria poses for a portrait, wearing the obligatory PPE, before cleaning a room at Canaves Oia Suites where she has worked as a housekeeper for the last 14 years. New government regulations require hotels to skip housekeeping service altogether due to the pandemic but since this is out of the question in a luxury hotel.
(Page 289)

Tour guides at Fira port, Santorini with signs and face masks. This year there are no cruise ships coming into Santorini where tourism has decreased drastically.
(Pages 290–291)

Luana Rigolli, Italy

The photographs were taken between May 2020 and January 2021.

Via Cola di Rienzo, Rome.
16 May 2020.
(Page 293)

Empty billboard space in front of the Campidoglio, Rome.
10 May 2020.
(Pages 294–295)

Empty billboard space in front of Basilica di San Giovanni in Laterano, Rome.
11 May 2020.
(Page 296, top)

Piazzale Numa Pompilio, Rome.
16 May 2020.
(Page 296, bottom)

Via del Plebiscito, Rome.
10 May 2020.
(Page 297, top)

Piazza Barberini, Rome.
10 May 2020.
(Page 297, bottom)

Empty billboard space on Lungotevere in Augusta, Rome.
12 May 2020.
(Pages 298–299)

Gabriele Galimberti, Italy

The photographs were taken between March and April 2020.

Rosa Casorelli, Ma Panificio, Turin.
(Pages 302–303)

Walter Sirtori, Enzo Strecaprete, Bilip Don, Macelleria Sirtori, Via Paolo Sarpi, Milan.
(Page 304)

Rahman Sohel, Minimarket, Piazza Nazario Sauro, Florence.
(Page 305)

Ezio Ferrero, Gastronomia Ferrero, Via Bertola, Turin.
(Page 306)

Silvia and Riccardo Tortoli, Pizzicheria Borgo San Frediano, Florence.
(Page 307)

Davide Viganò, L'orto di Brera, Milan.
(Page 308)

Coppini Paolo, Migrana (Salumi e formaggi), Borgo San Frediano, Florence.
(Page 309)

Donatella Ficini, Ficini Bakery, Via Berthollet, Turin.
(Pages 310–311)

05.

A Wounded Society

Gideon Mendel, United Kingdom
2 Meters: Masked Portraits on Ridley Road

These portraits were made on Ridley Road Food Market during the time of the coronavirus pandemic and lockdown. The red markings on the road were painted by Hackney Council to indicate the two metres of social distance that is advised for shoppers.

On a shopping trip shortly after the imposition of lockdown, I came across a team of workers painting red lines all the way down Ridley Road. They were starting at dusk, and told me that they had to work through the night to complete the task. I was intrigued by this new addition to the iconography of the street and returning to see how they might be working in practice I developed this idea of making portraits to include both masks and these new lines of separation.

This market has been an East London institution since the late 1880s, encapsulating the area's rich history of immigration and diversity. The market's traders and customers have shifted with the decades to draw many different communities. Besides having exotic produce from around the world it is also known as one of the cheapest markets in London. The market stalls and food shops that line the street attract shoppers from a wide variety of cultural backgrounds, both recent immigrants and many whose families have been in the UK for generations. The area has also been facing the twin challenges of rapid gentrification and local issues of deprivation accentuated by the government's austerity policies.

I have made the photographs with a constant, unchanging frame, capturing the different communities that rub up against each other in this space, hoping to give a sense of something uniquely local and global at the same time. In my experience of making these images, most of the people I approached were keen to be photographed, feeling that they wanted to advocate mask-wearing. Although much of their faces are hidden I found a quality to their gaze that reaches beyond the mask to portray a sense of resilience and strength in these difficult times.

They have widely different reasons for choosing to wear a mask. Some feel they are protecting others, some are fearful of contracting the virus themselves. But they are all united by the act of wearing a mask.

Masks can signify many things today — anxiety, isolation, social responsibility, fear or safety. Normally they are about blocking off from other people, creating distance and disguising identity. But in our "new normal" this material barrier has become a unifier, holding us together.

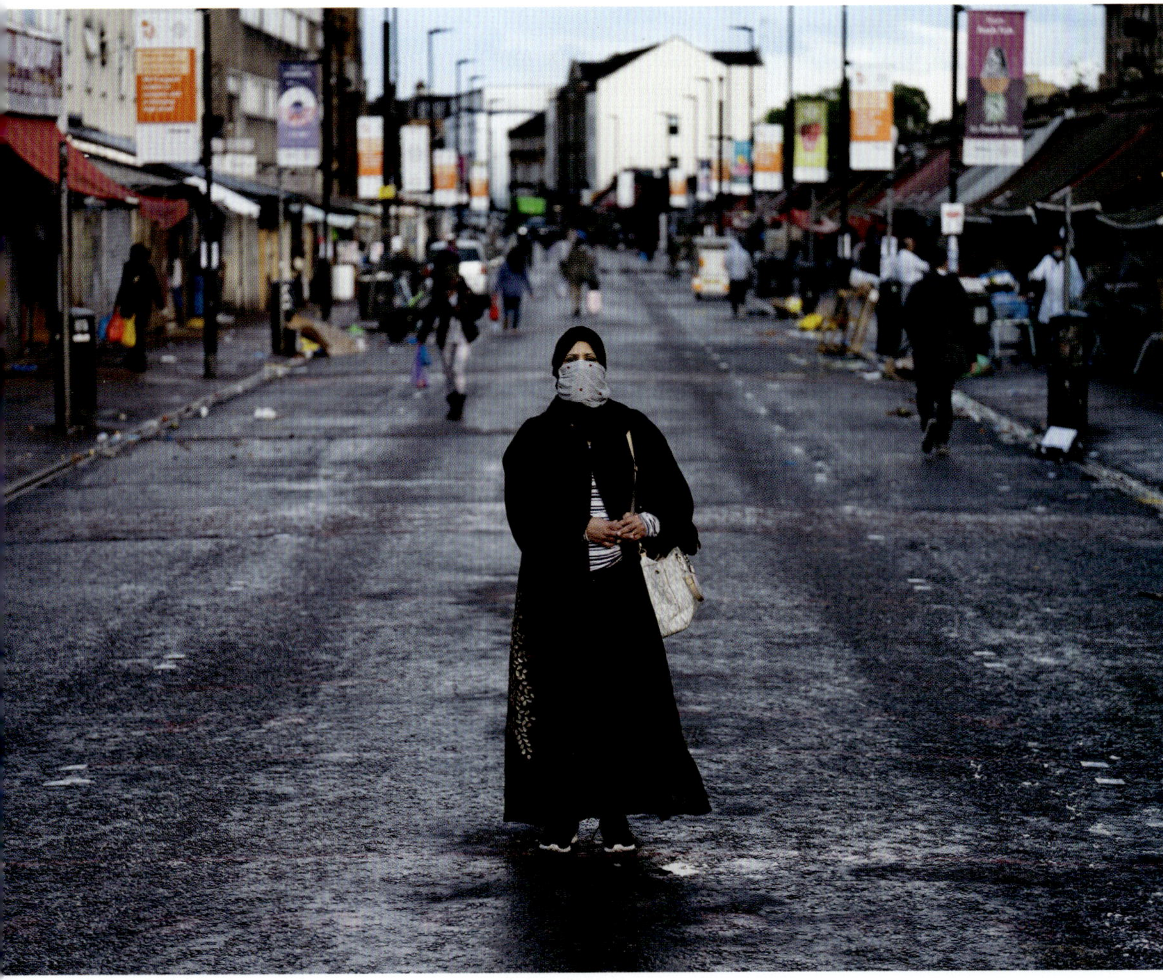

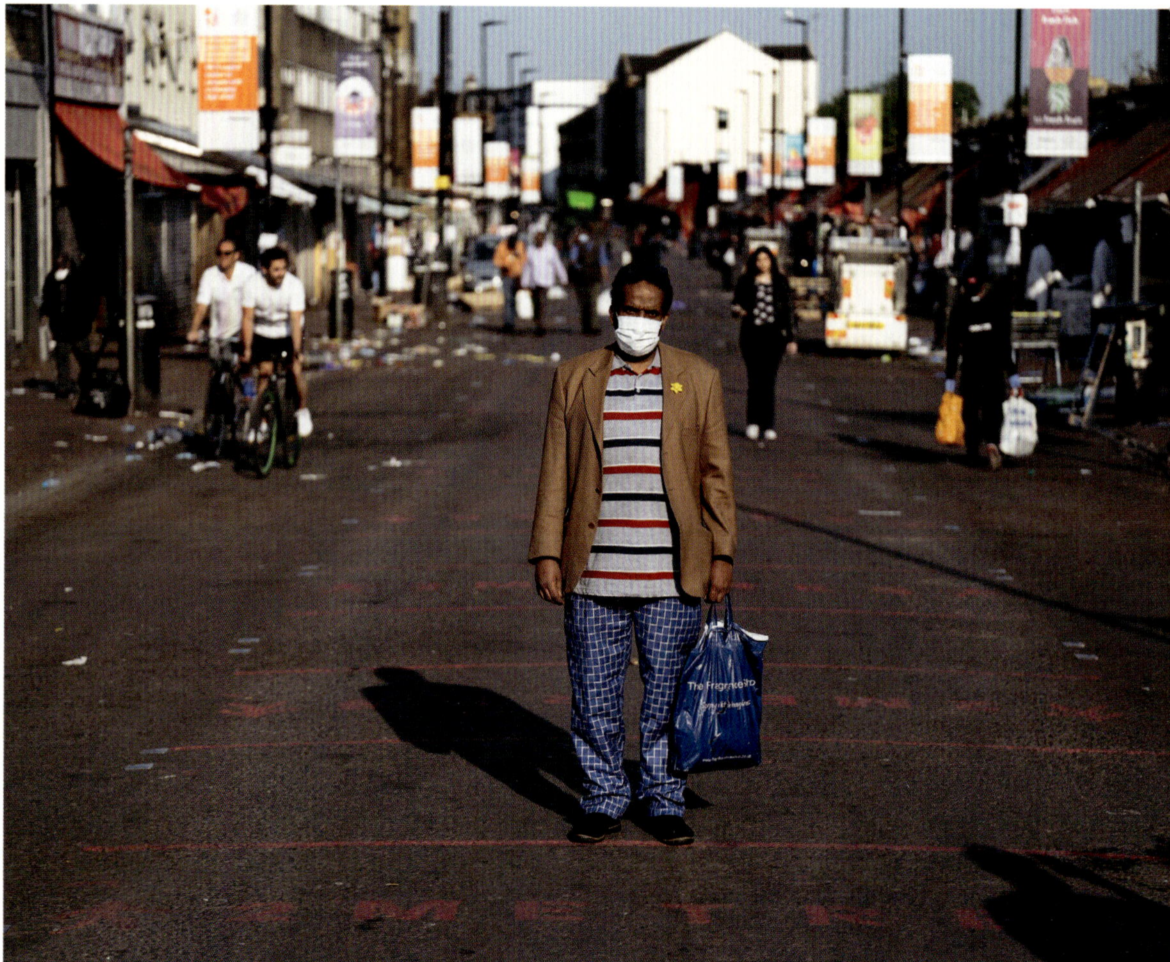

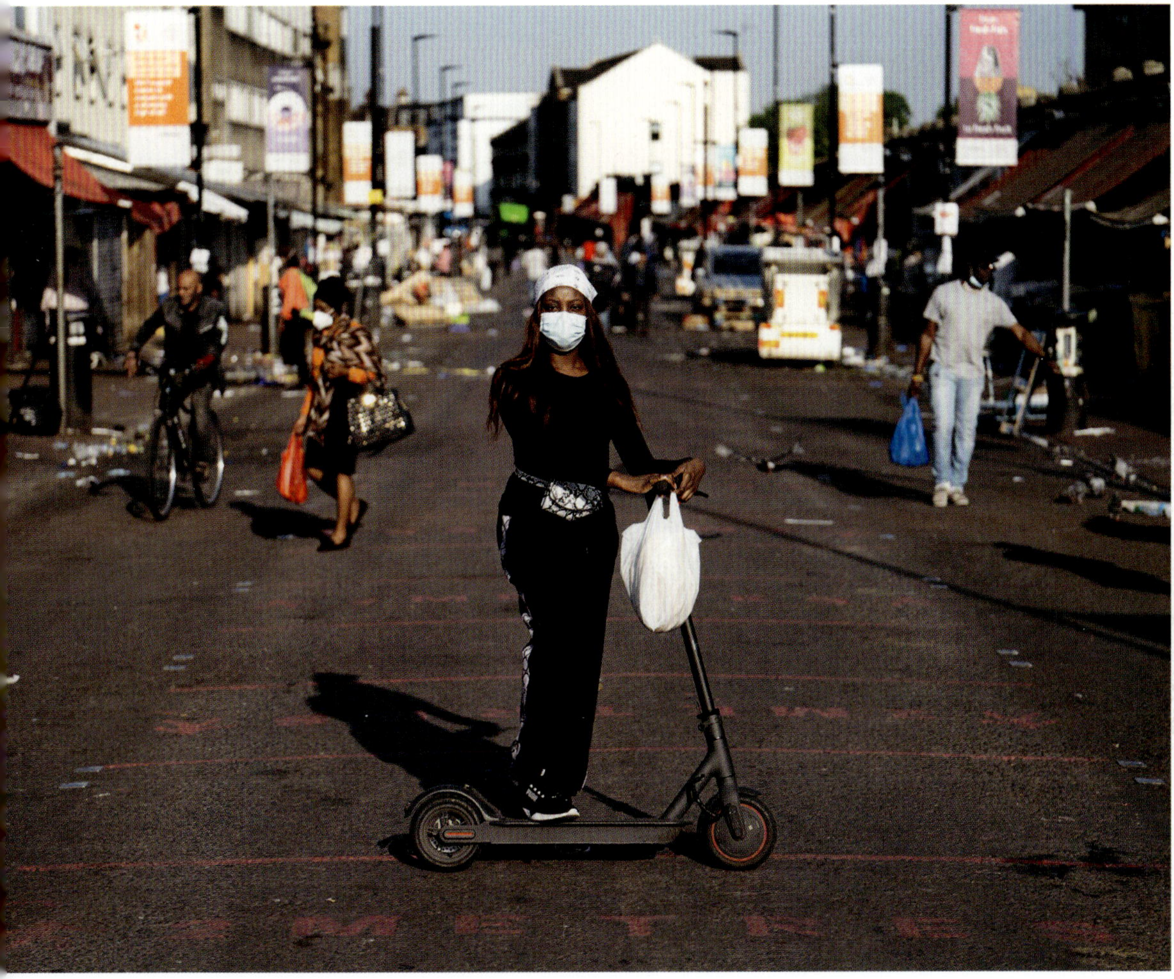

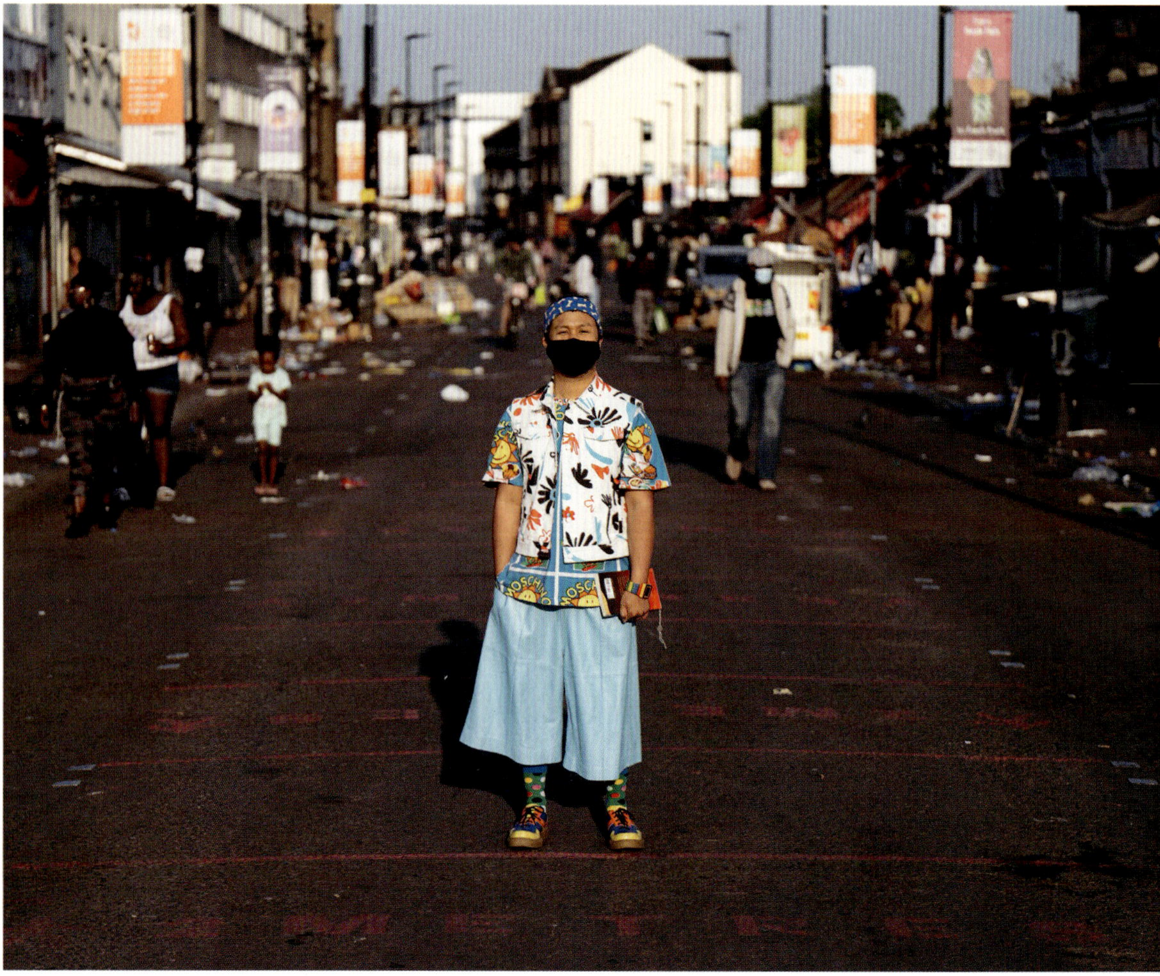
MOSCHINO

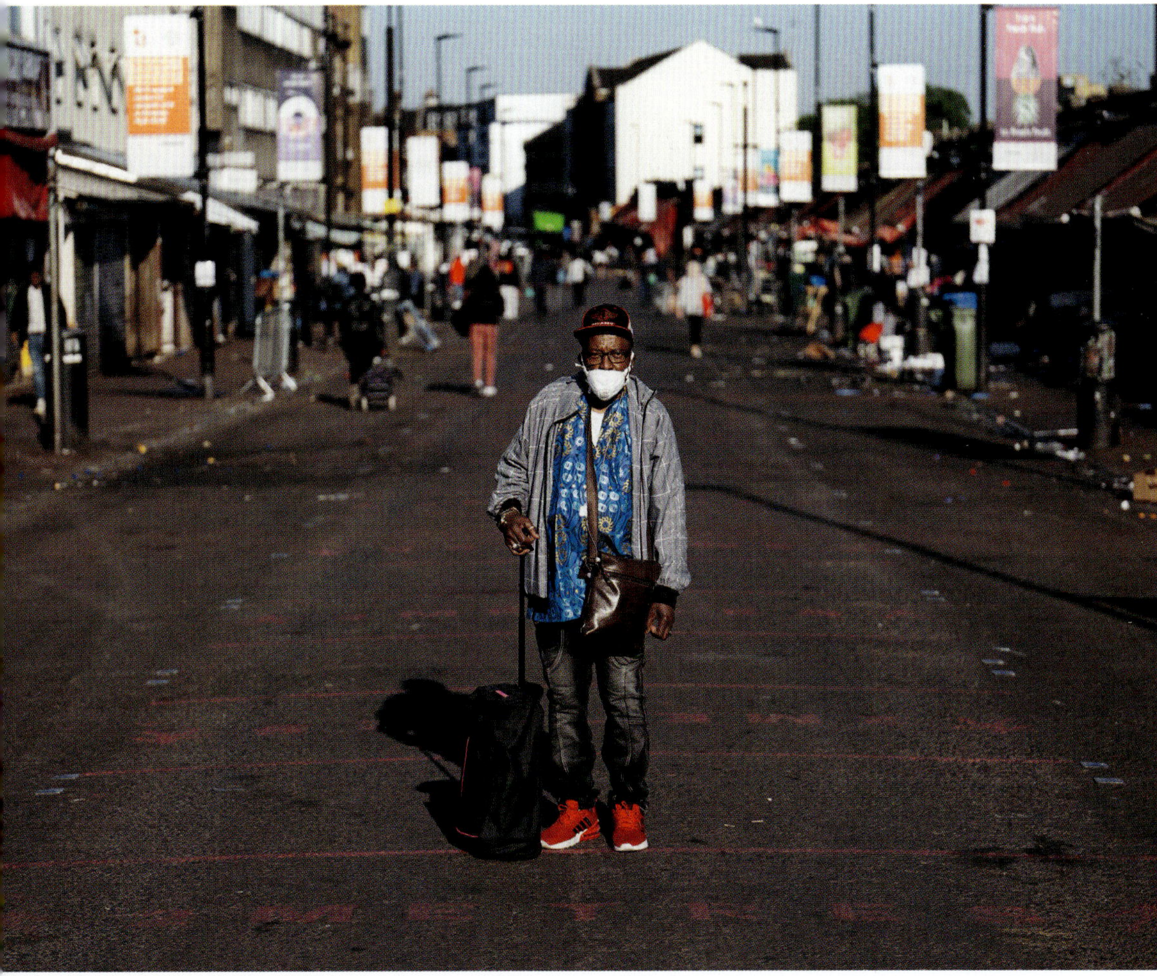

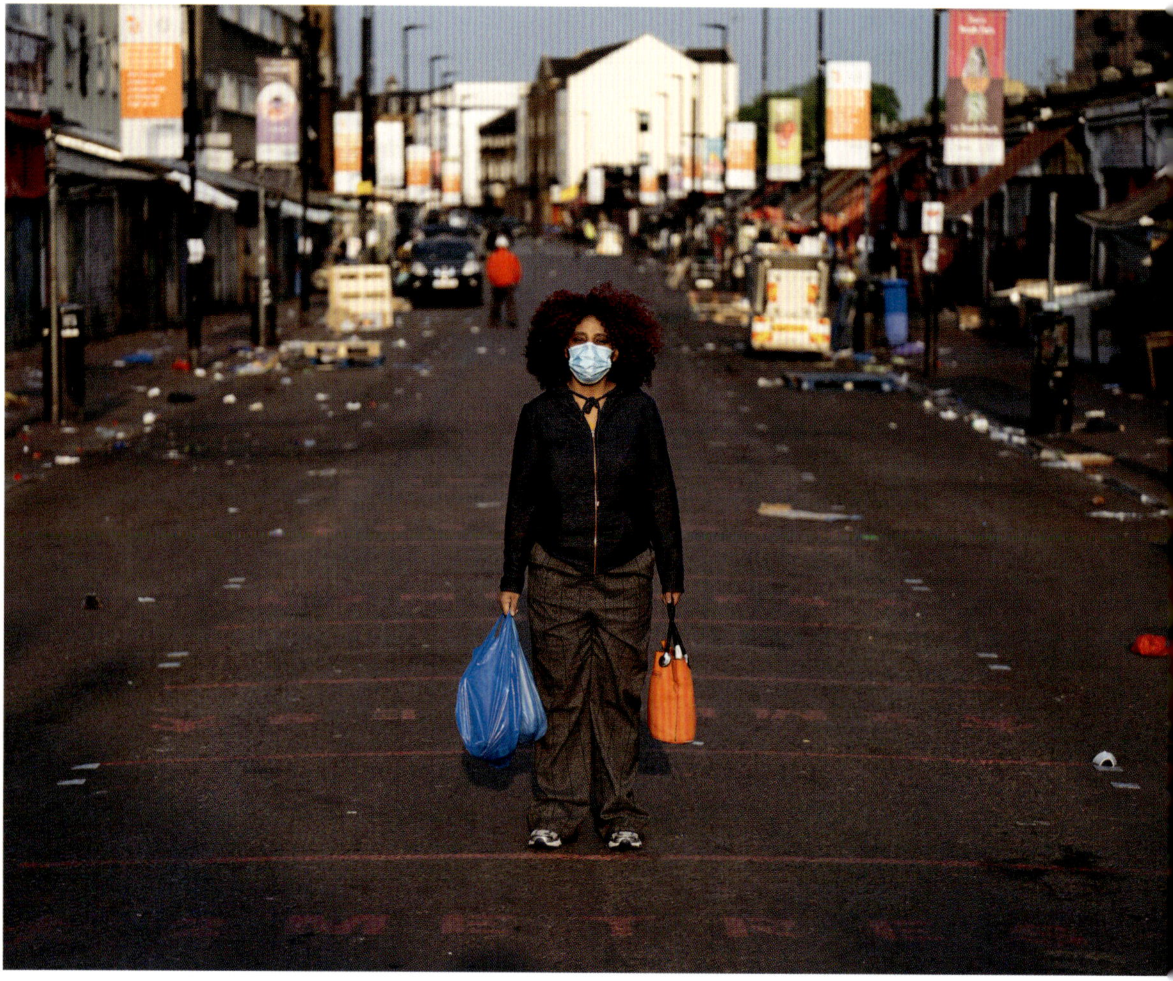

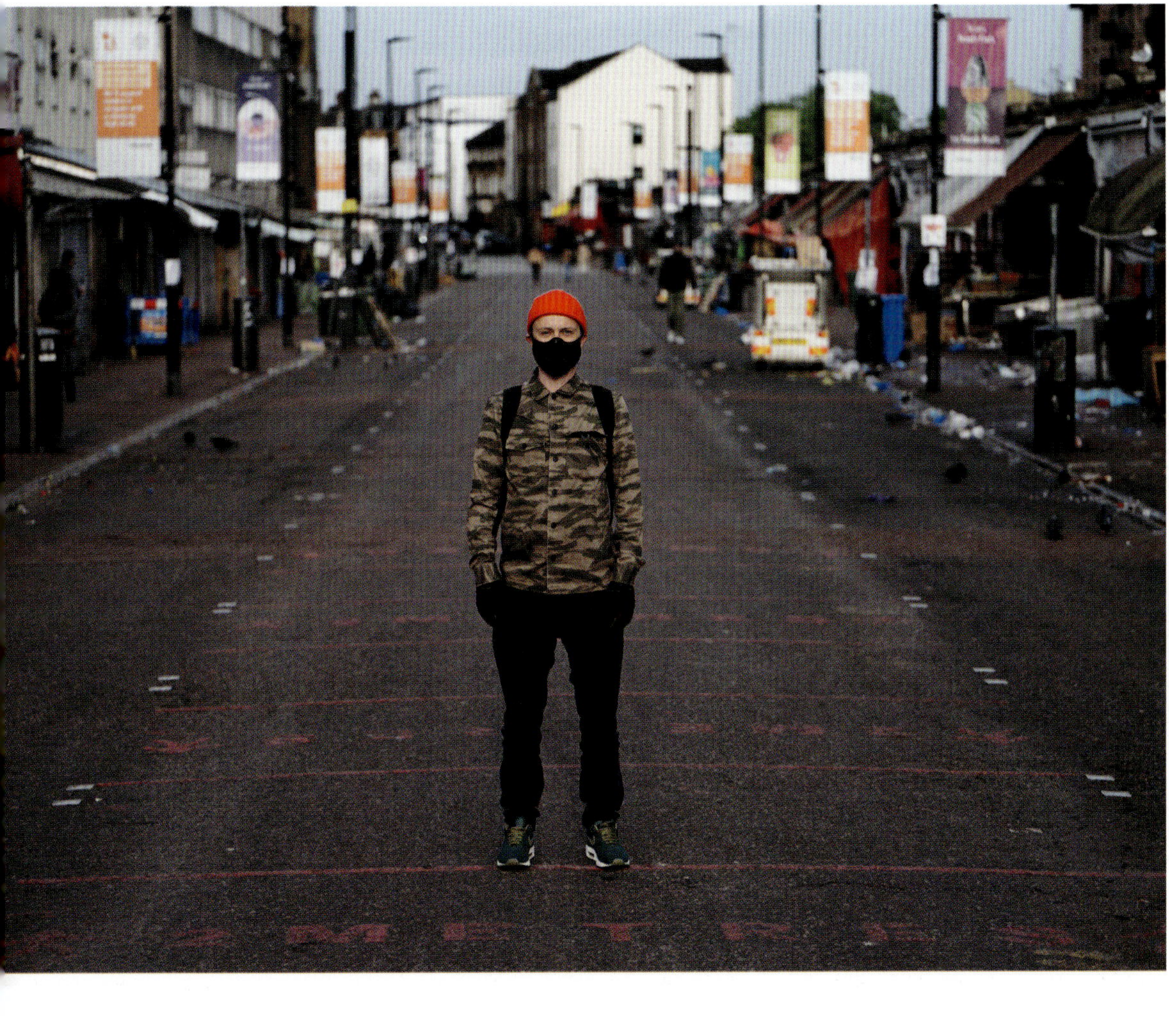

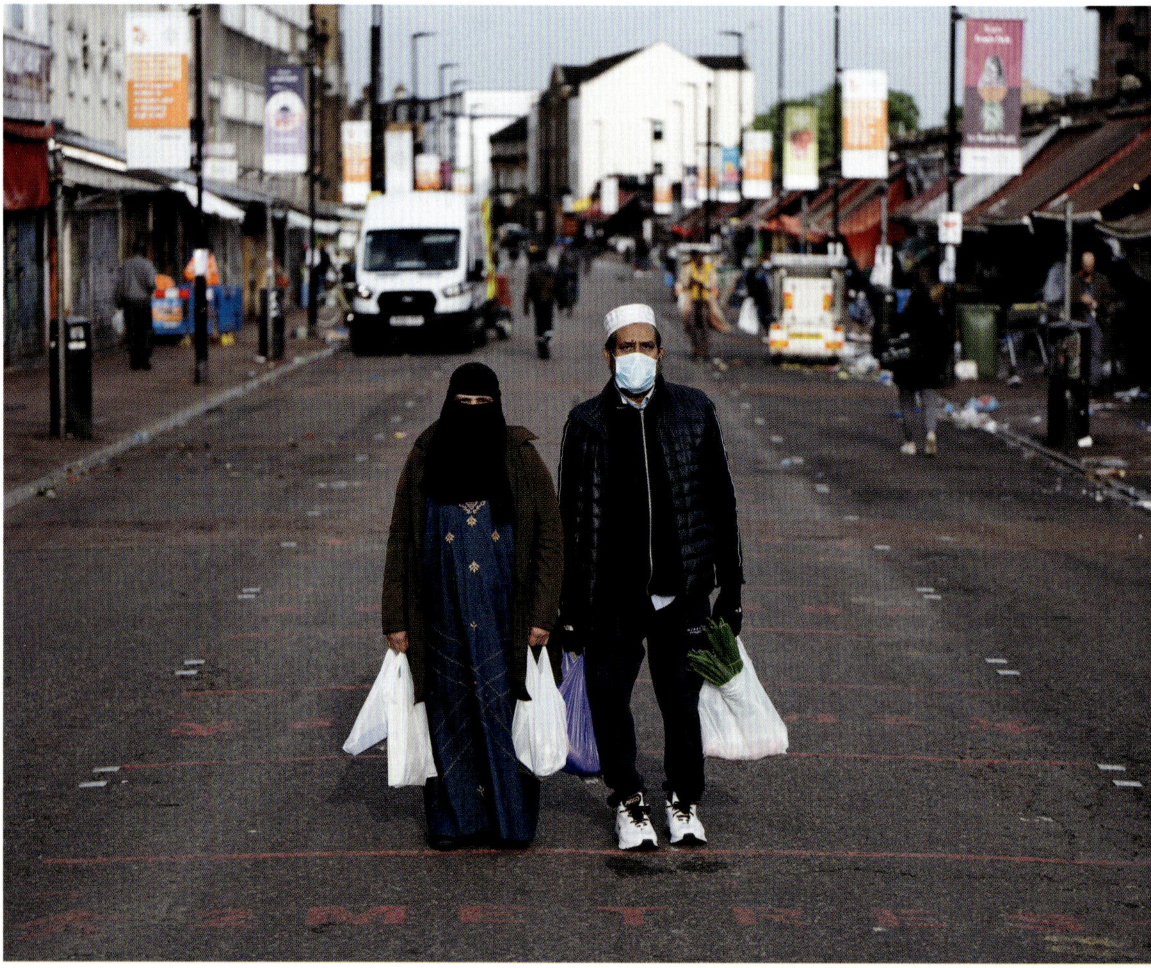

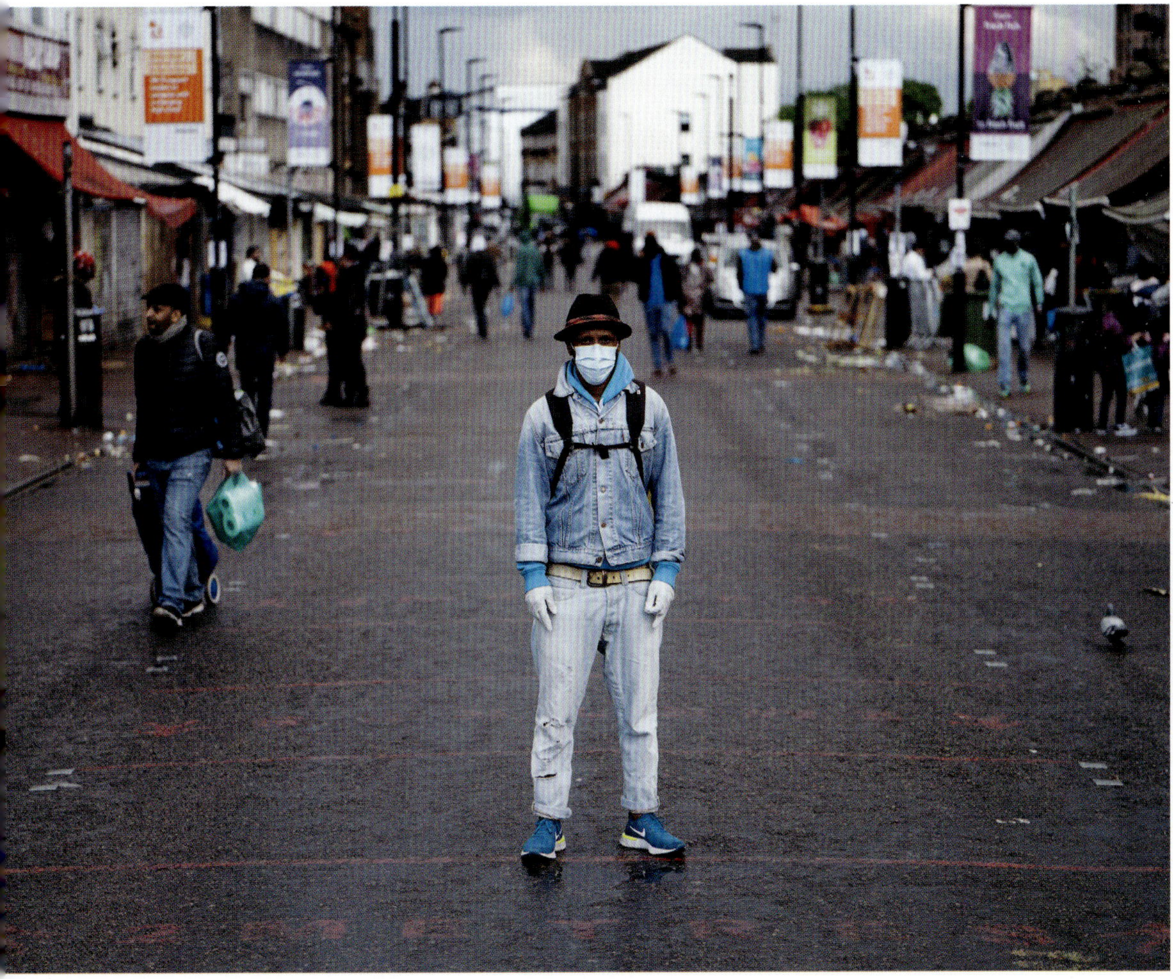

Nanna Heitmann, Russia
Pandemic of Social Inequality

After six weeks of a country in lockdown, people are running out of money. Almost half of the population has no savings or just enough to survive for one month. The official unemployment rate in Russia is now 1.4 million people, twice as much as in early April.
Those people who already live under precarious conditions are the ones hit harder by the pandemic. I visited different charities to see how the lockdown affected Moscow's most vulnerable. Miloserdie, a Russian Orthodox charity usually feeds around 50 people a day. These days, just in the morning hours more than 150 people already streamed into the tents for some instant food and tea. Moscow's government so-called "social adaptation centres" don't have enough capacity to feed and accommodate all the people arriving now, those who are left without a home. Lana Zhurkina's charity Dom Druzey (House of friends) opened four new hostels in Moscow to host people who otherwise cannot quarantine themselves. A lot of people are being sent from the social adaptation centres to the hostels. Because of the high infection rates hospitals have to release their patients as soon as they don't have any life-threatening symptoms anymore. Old people, released from the hospital, are struggling alone in their home still weak and sick. Or, as I myself witnessed, a Veterans' Home refused to take back their resident without a negative test result. Lana Zhurkina refers that sometimes the ambulance brings homeless people to their hostel and only later warns them that the patient was tested positive for COVID-19. When they cannot go into quarantine, homeless people continue to walk around the city, infectious.
In addition, among the most vulnerable elements in society, women have to deal with the alarming issue of violence at home. Domestic violence has been a serious problem in Russia before and has grown worse. According to the UN, 14,000 Russian women die every year from the violence of their acquaintances. 940 is the number of similar deaths in the United States, where twice as many people live.
"In Russia, since April 10, the number of domestic violence cases has increased by at least 250%", the Kremlin's human rights commissioner, Tatiana Moskalkova, reports.
The coronavirus crisis is more serious on a worldwide scale so it is probably just the beginning of a newer, bigger crisis that will increase the number of vulnerable people in the coming months.

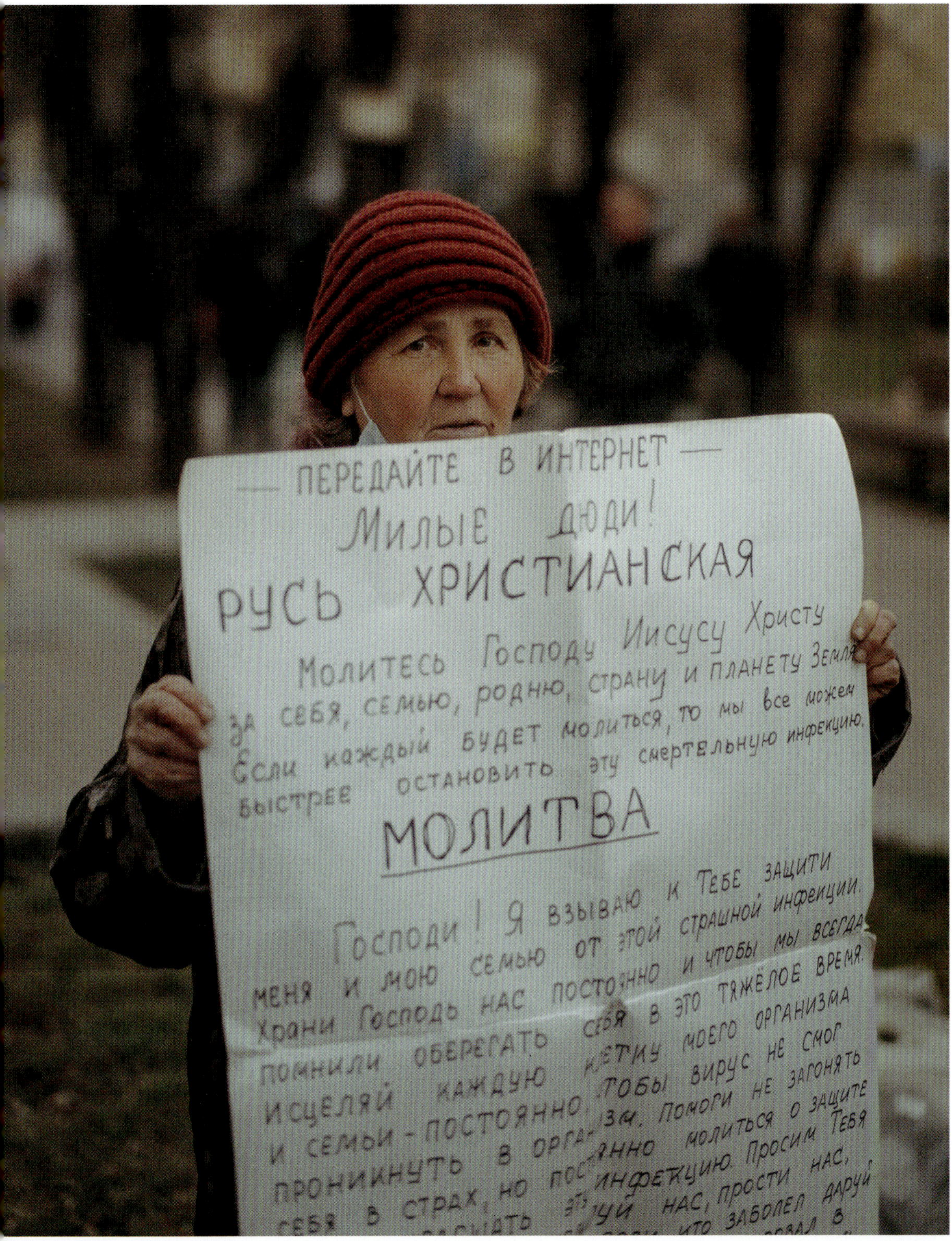
— ПЕРЕДАЙТЕ В ИНТЕРНЕТ —
Милые люди!
РУСЬ ХРИСТИАНСКАЯ
Молитесь Господу Иисусу Христу
за себя, семью, родню, страну и планету Земля
Если каждый будет молиться, то мы все можем
быстрее остановить эту смертельную инфекцию.
МОЛИТВА
Господи! Я взываю к Тебе защити
меня и мою семью от этой страшной инфекции.
Храни Господь нас постоянно и чтобы мы всегда
помнили оберегать себя в это тяжёлое время.
Исцеляй каждую клетку моего организма
и семьи - постоянно. Чтобы вирус не смог
проникнуть в организм. Помоги не загонять
себя в страх, но постоянно молиться о защите

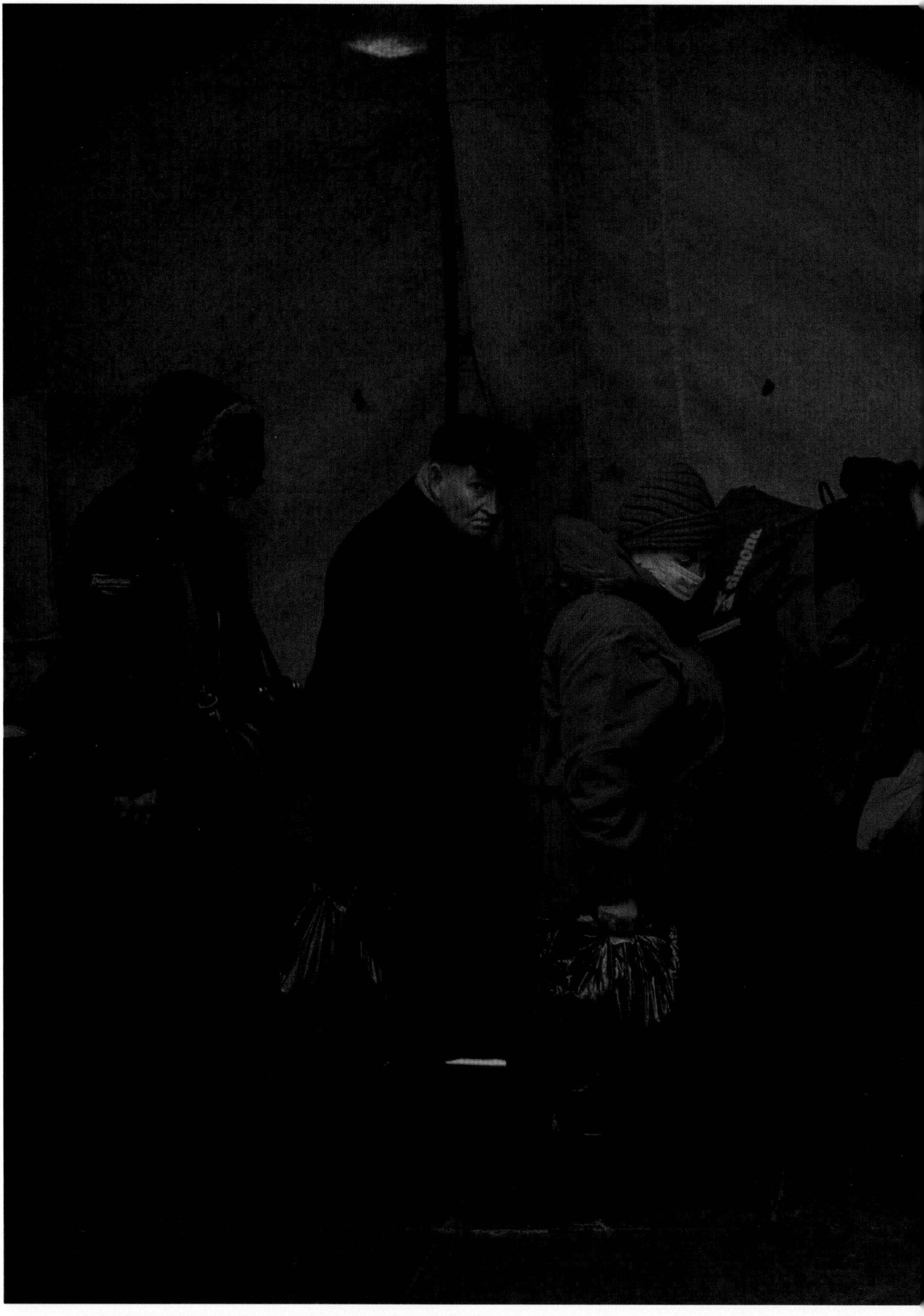

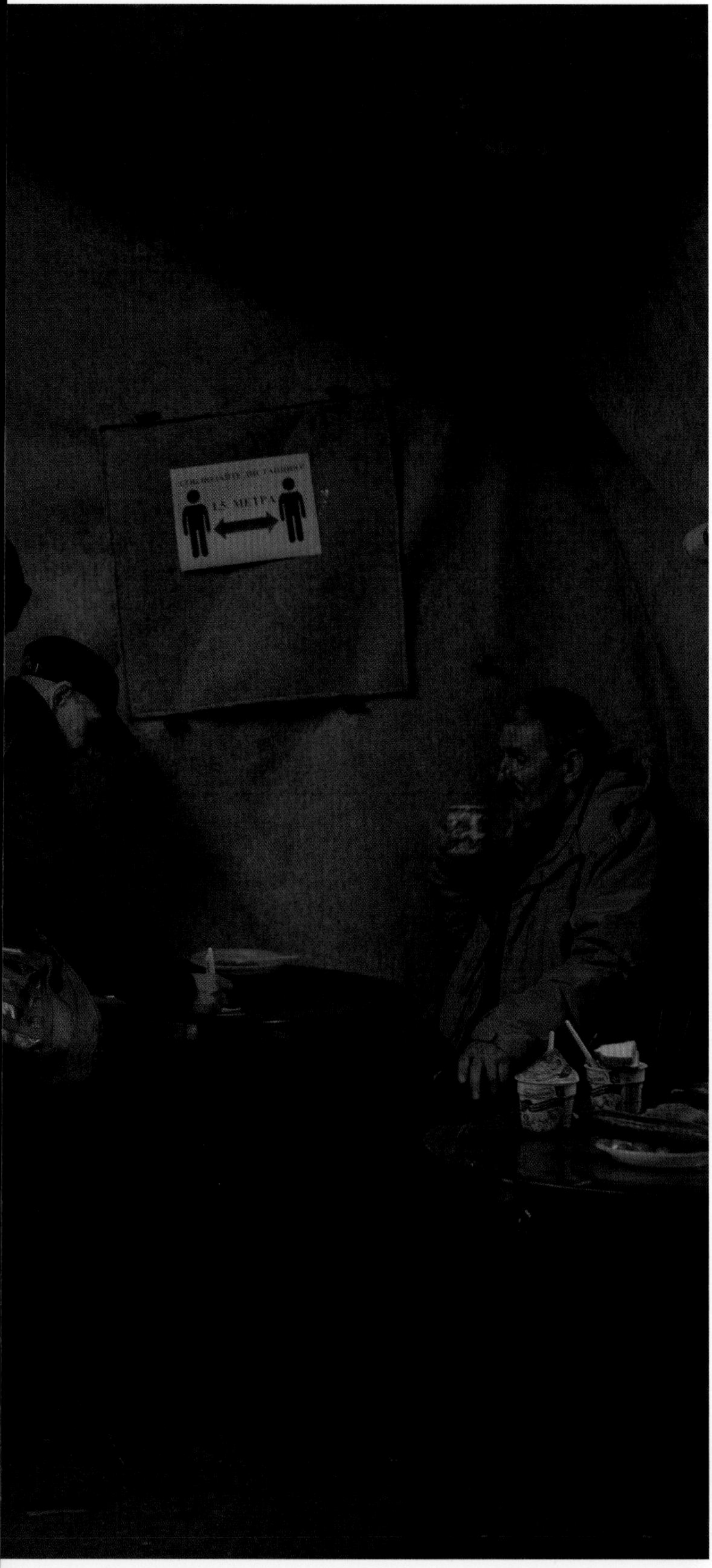

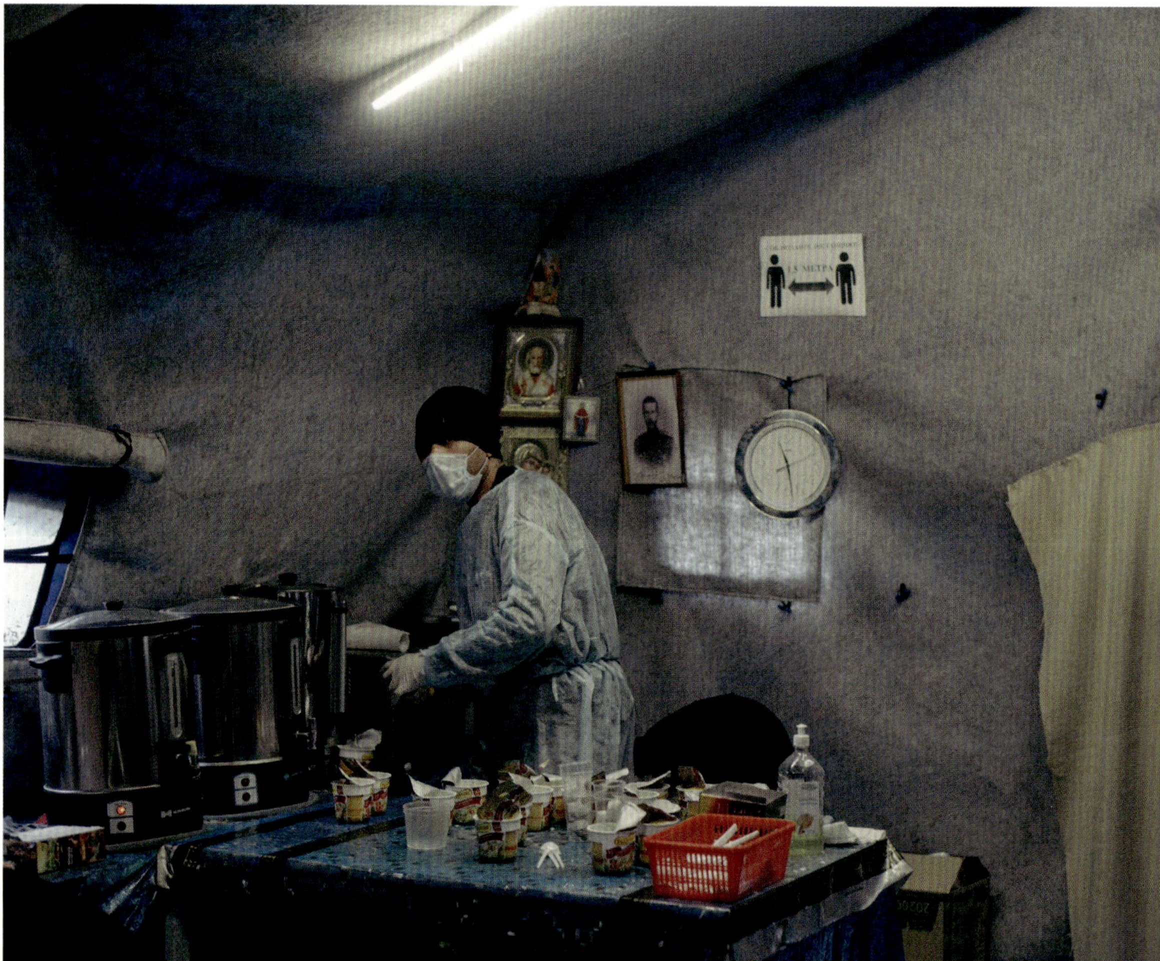

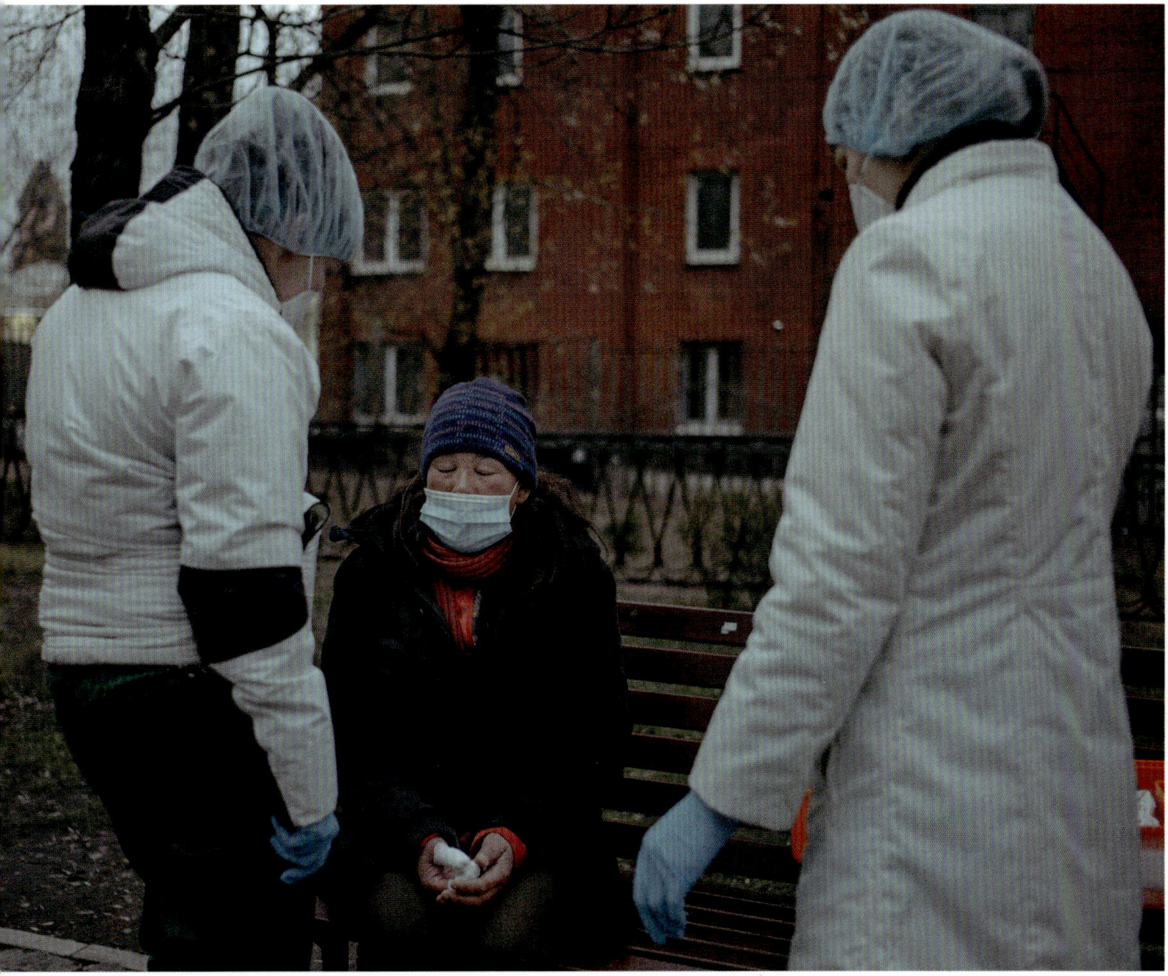

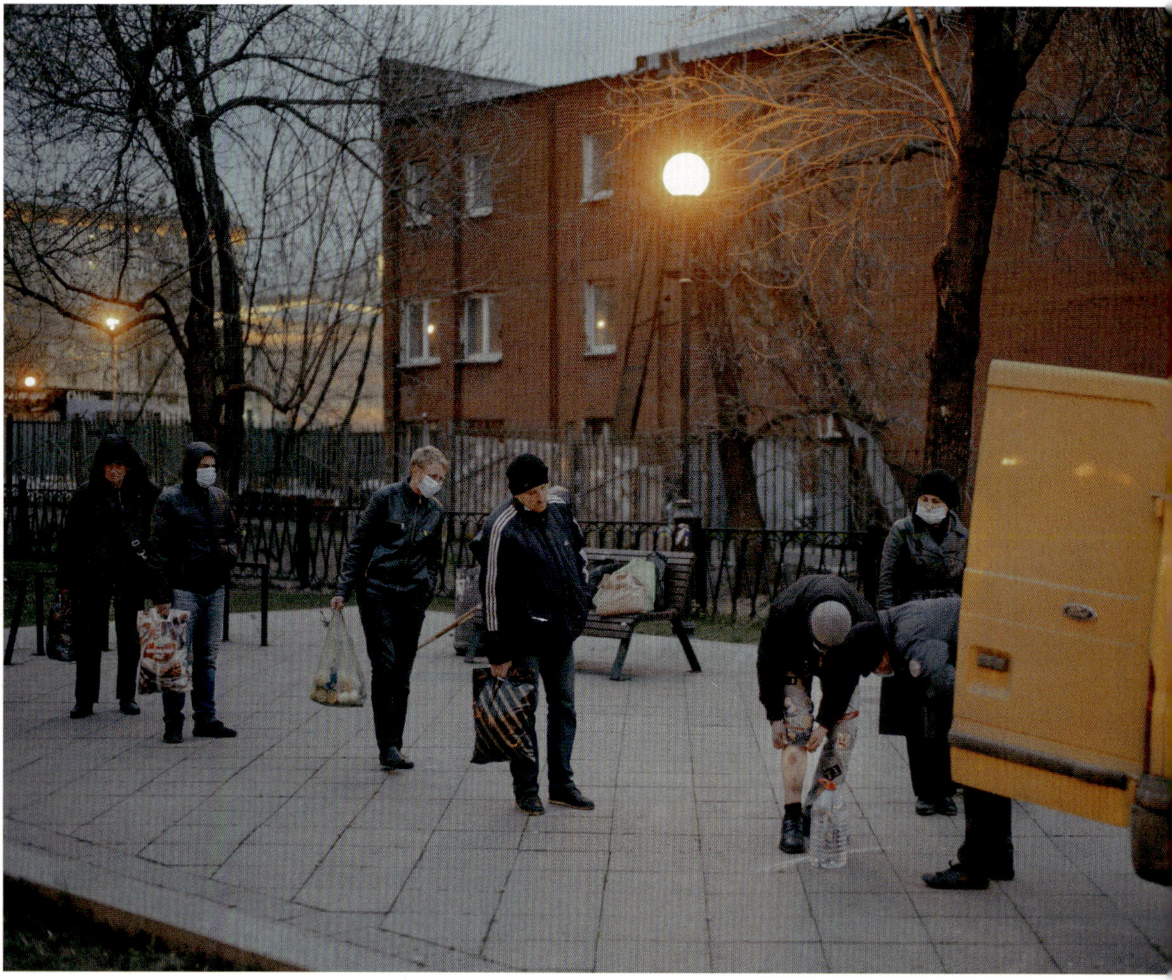

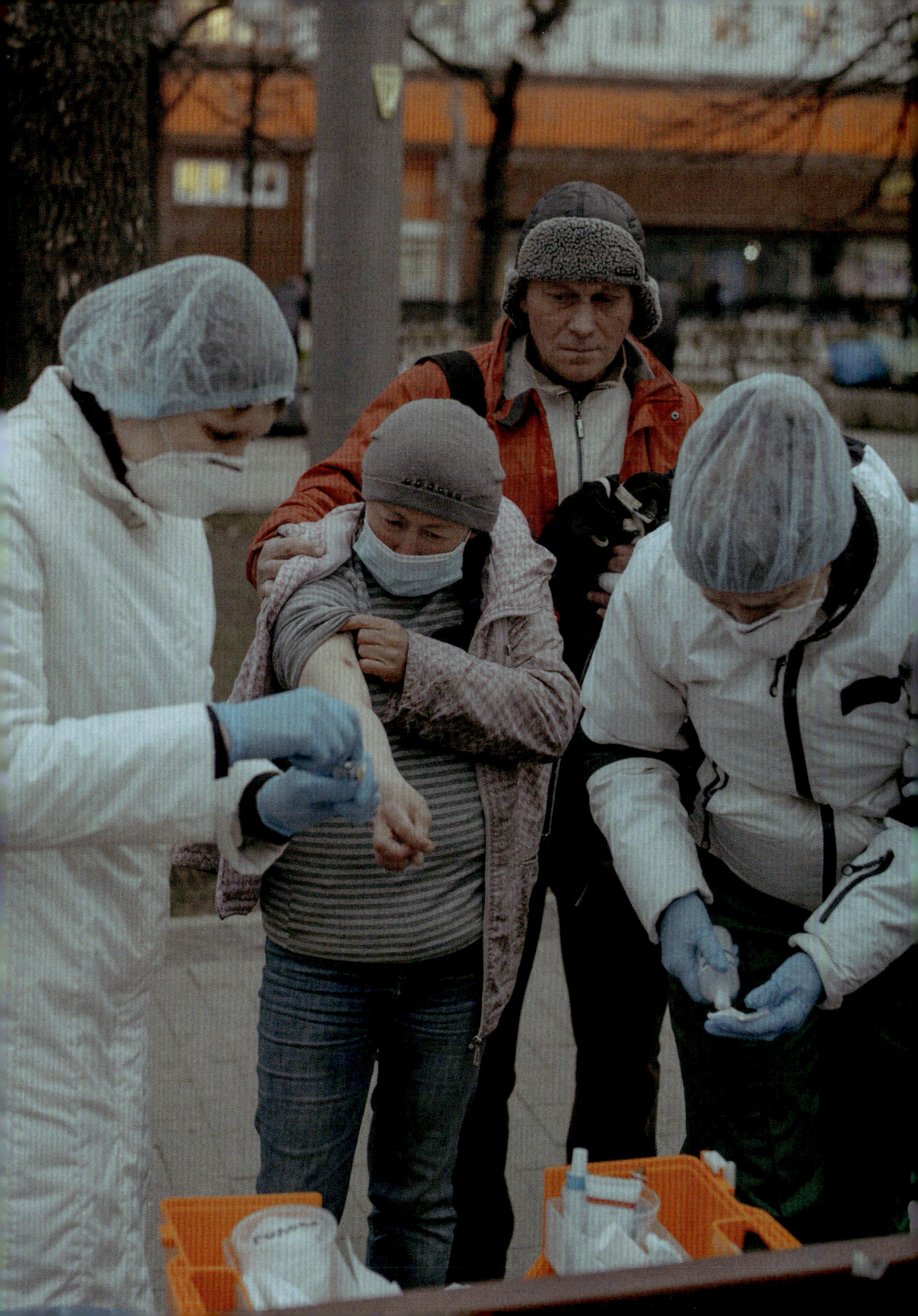

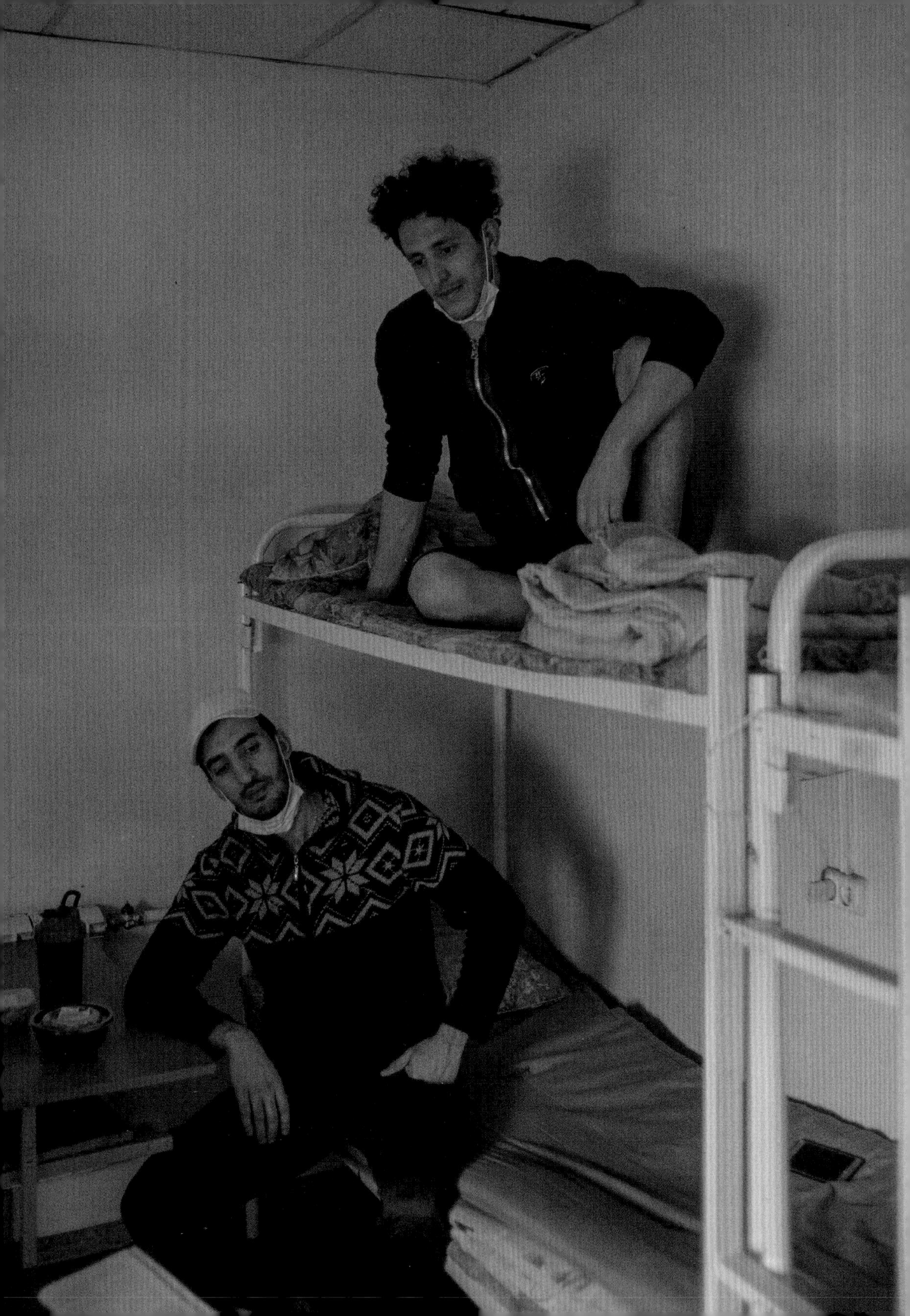

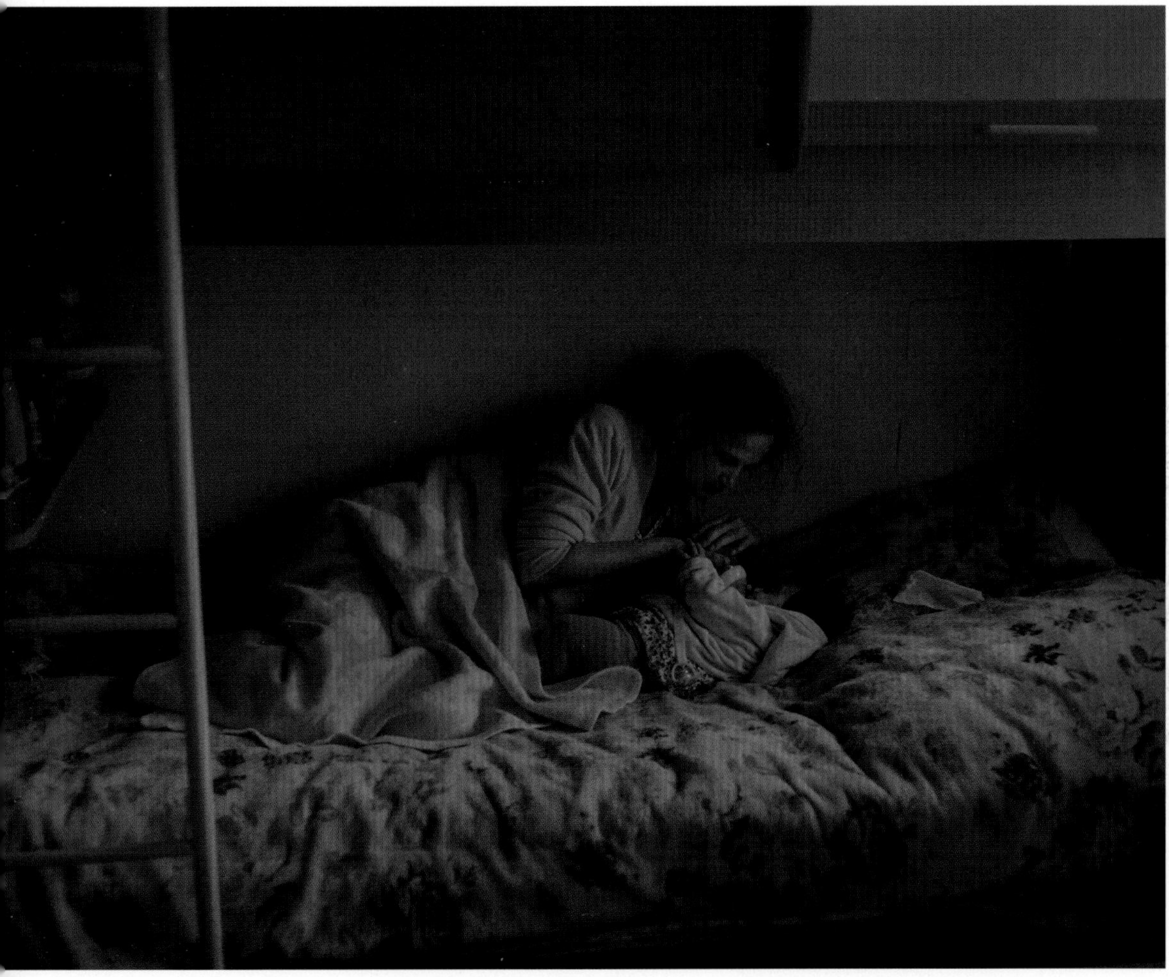

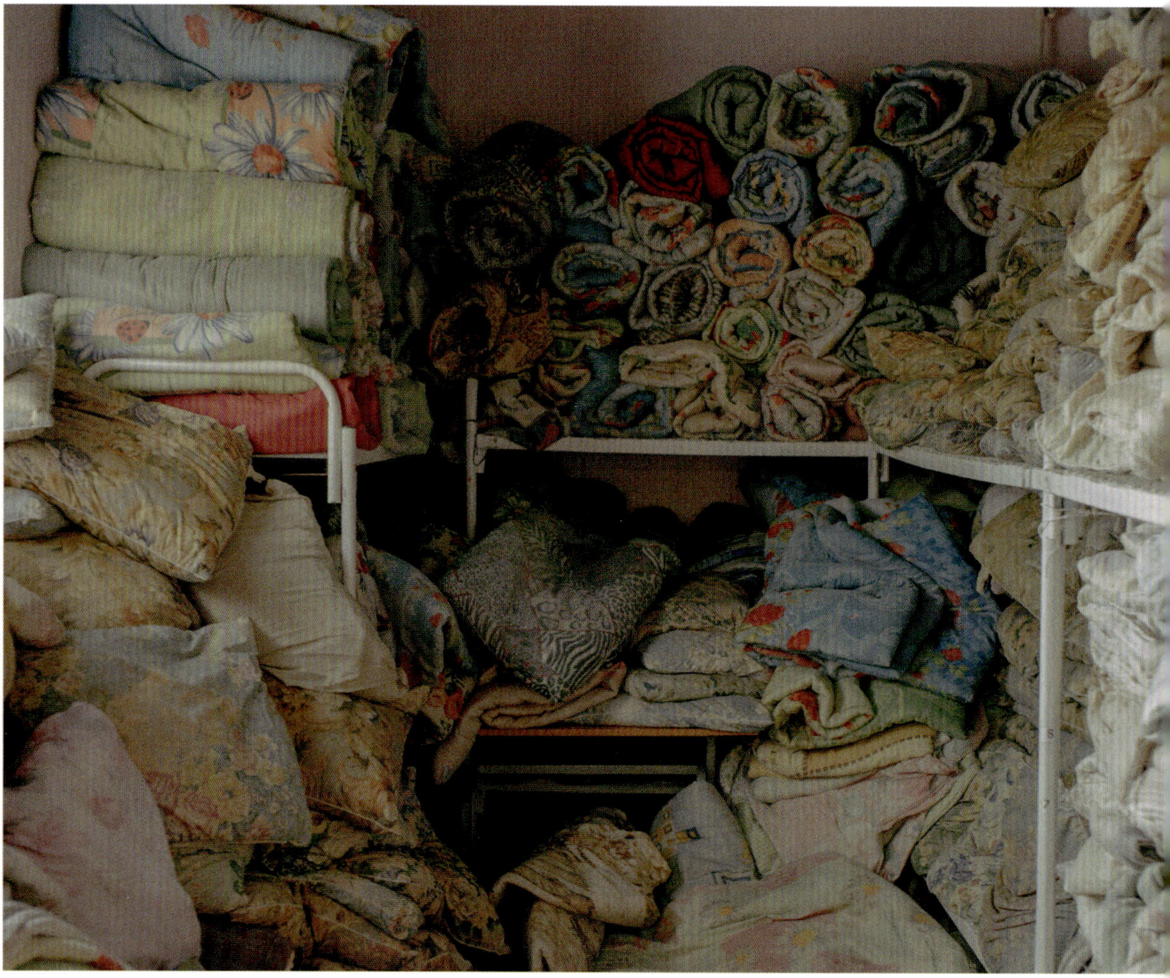

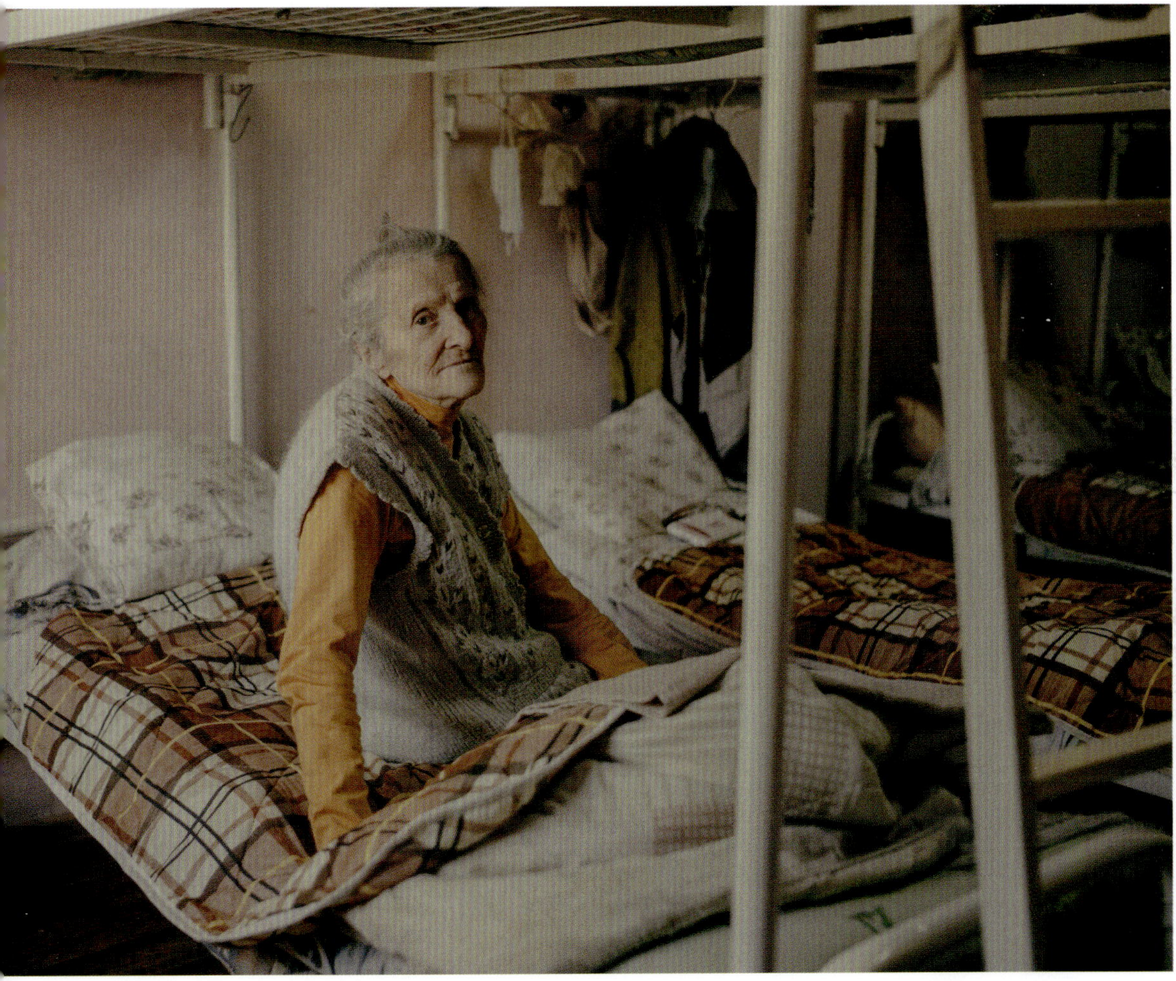

Nicoló Lanfranchi, Brazil
We Are Not All on the Same Boat

Massimo Razzi

"It was said that COVID-19 is a democratic virus because it also affects rich people and rulers like Bolsonaro and Johnson. But it was in Brazil that I witnessed and was able to document that this is not the case." Nicoló Lanfranchi, a photographer from Milan who has been living in Berlin for years, happened to be in Brazil, in Rio de Janeiro, when the first lockdown measures were implemented in Italy: "I had recently arrived in Brazil to shoot a documentary on popular herbal medicine, when the pandemic rose within a couple of weeks while President Bolsonaro kept downplaying it, arguing with the governors of the different states who had to deal with dramatic situations".
Lanfranchi's photos tell the story of life at the time of the lockdown in some poor areas of Rio like Cidade de Deus and, in particular, Cruzada São Sebastião. The latter is a vertical "favela", meaning that it is located within one of the richest neighbourhoods of Brazil called Leblon — an enlightened urban planning initiative that turned into a disaster due to the inability of the institutions to help those who live there and to create the necessary socio-economic fabric. It was built in 1955 by the famous bishop Helder Camara, a great defender of human rights and poor people.
Brazil has split in half on the Covid issue. Bolsonaro's delusional statements referred to it as a mild flu and the president even made a joke about the fact that the health of the Brazilian people deserves to be studied, because some people are capable of diving into a sewer without anything happening to them. The governors of São Paulo and Rio, on the other hand, realised how serious the situation was (Brazil reached almost 5 million infected and almost 150,000 dead out of a population of 209 million inhabitants by September 2020), and tried to do something about it, asking for benefits for the poorest population. Only very limited funds were granted and, while the rich or those who had a stable job could get by even staying at home, maybe working remotely, the poor could not make it. Because the poor, in Brazil and elsewhere, survive thanks to a street economy that consists of going out of the house every day to earn a living through odd jobs and small businesses. This was not possible during the lockdown and many were forced to go out anyway and risk their lives.
In his images there are many funerals of people who died of COVID-19. "In Rio they built a vertical cemetery", says Lanfranchi. "They say it was already planned but for many it was a measure to deal with the high number of deaths." Funerals are attended by very few people and there are mostly just gravediggers wearing protective overalls and masks as they lower coffins into graves.

While photographing in a cemetery he meets Henrique burying his 82-year-old mother. And here, Lanfranchi tells us a sad and terrible story that concerns him personally: "During my Brazilian lockdown, my father, Piero, who was 72 years old, died of Covid. He lived in Voghera, went to the hospital to have a cast removed and contracted the virus. I could not move from Rio, I could not reach him. He left like many others in Italy, without solace and without a funeral". Nicoló told Henrique about his concern for his hospitalised father, as if to somehow justify his presence in that private moment. "I attended his mother's funeral with my father in mind. Before saying goodbye, Henrique thanked me for being with him at that last good-bye."
Lanfranchi's photos, with their hard, strong, but not lively colours are deeply incisive. They tell us many human stories: protests against Bolsonaro, volunteers who bring bags of basic necessities to the favela for those who are in need, and people who live of what the streets can offer. But there are also Bolsonaro supporters who march on the streets, full of arrogance in spite of the ban on gatherings. And there is the legendary Copacabana beach, emptied by the pandemic. It's the upside down world at the time of COVID-19: a world we didn't think we'd have to get used to.

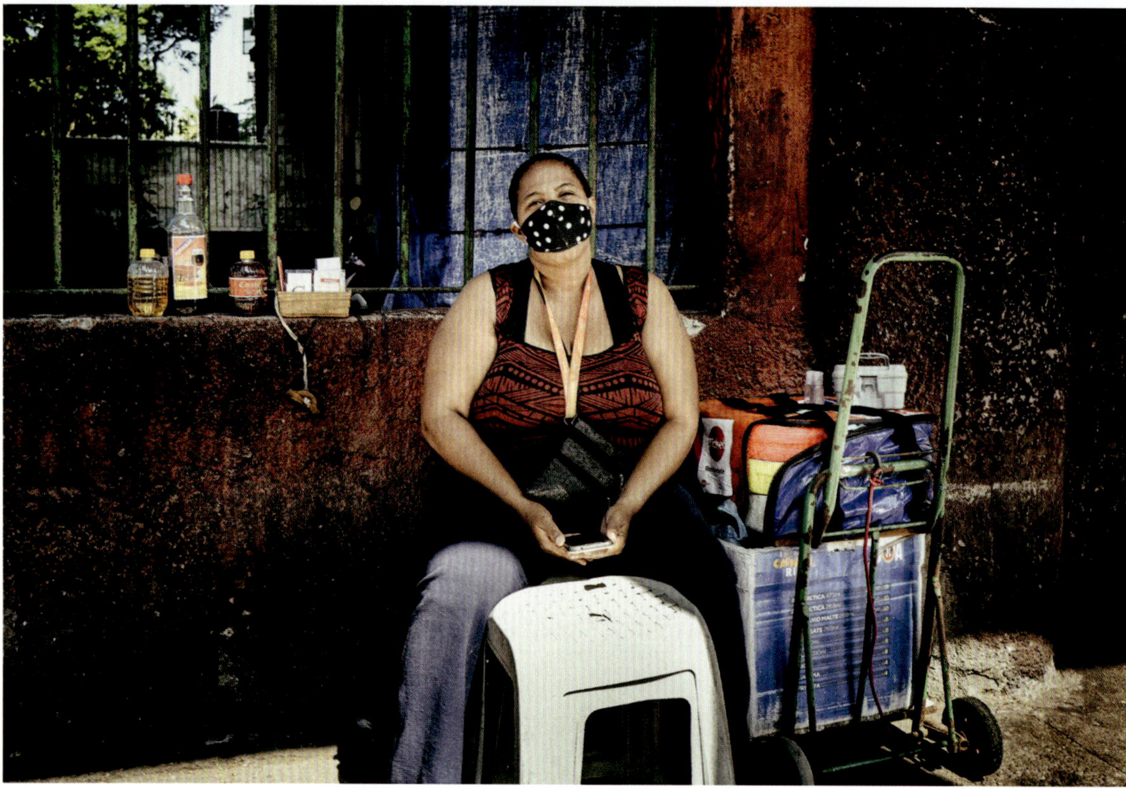

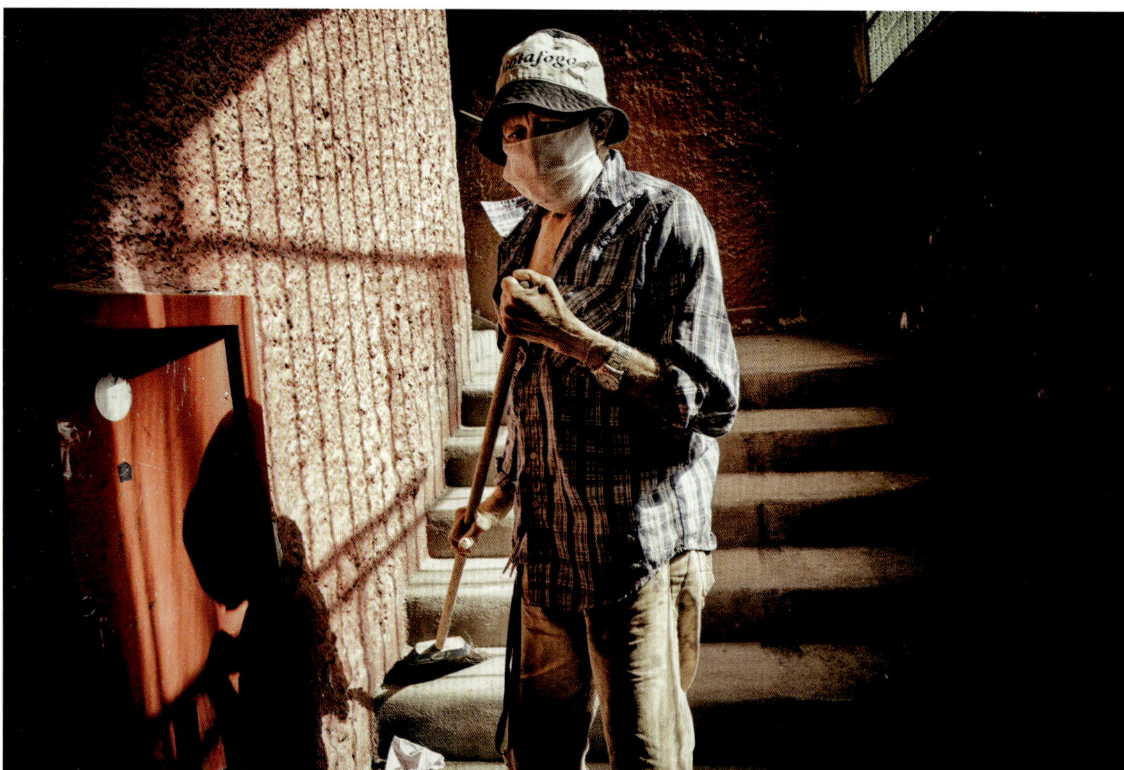

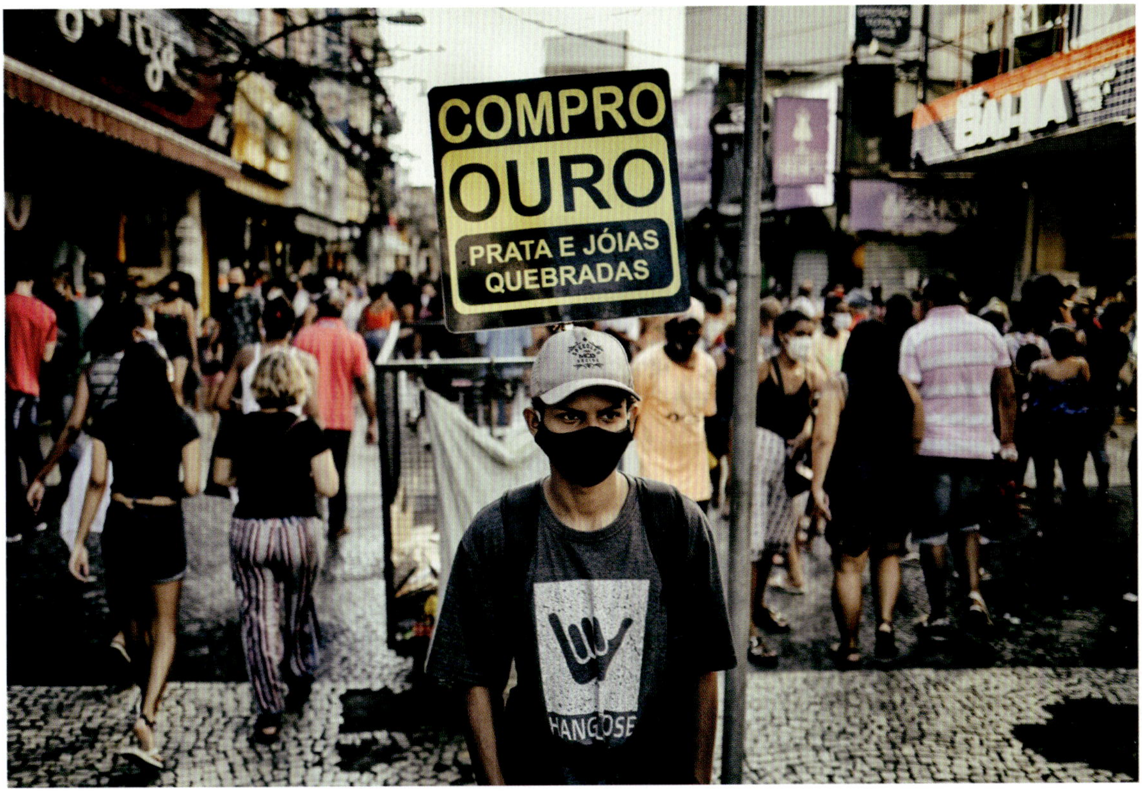
COMPRO
OURO
PRATA E JÓIAS
QUEBRADAS
BAHIA
HANG LOSE

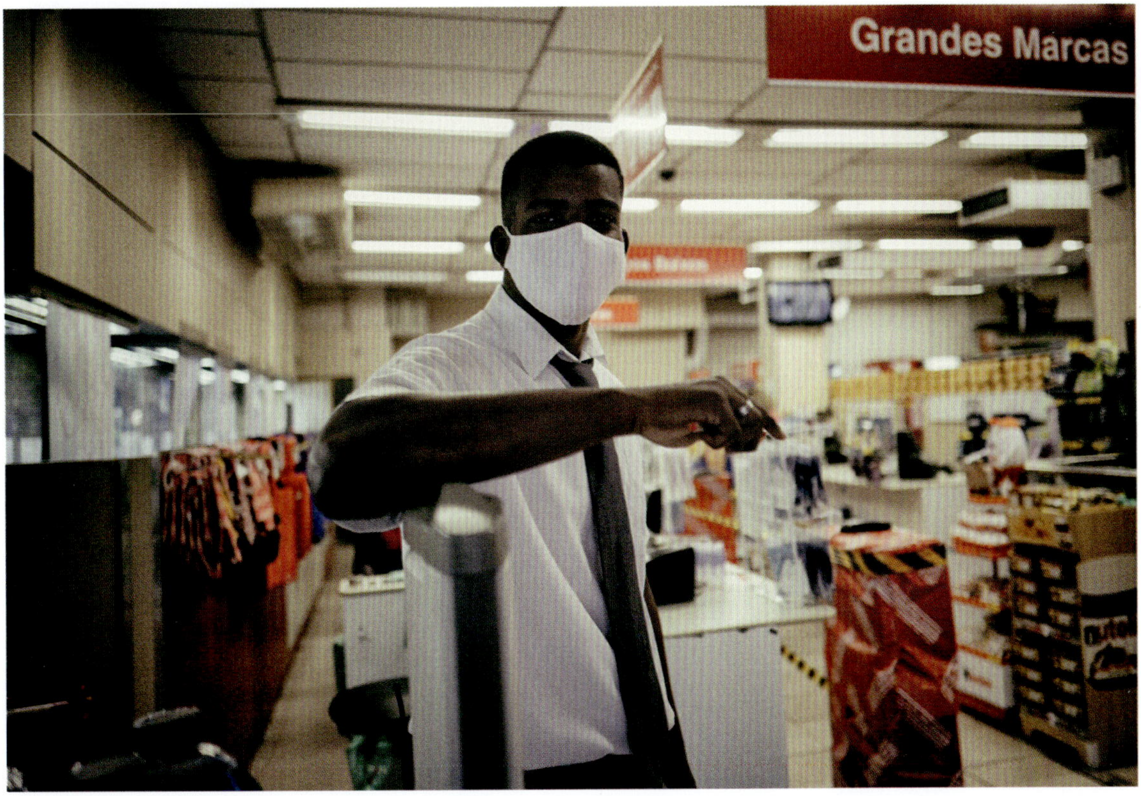
Grandes Marcas

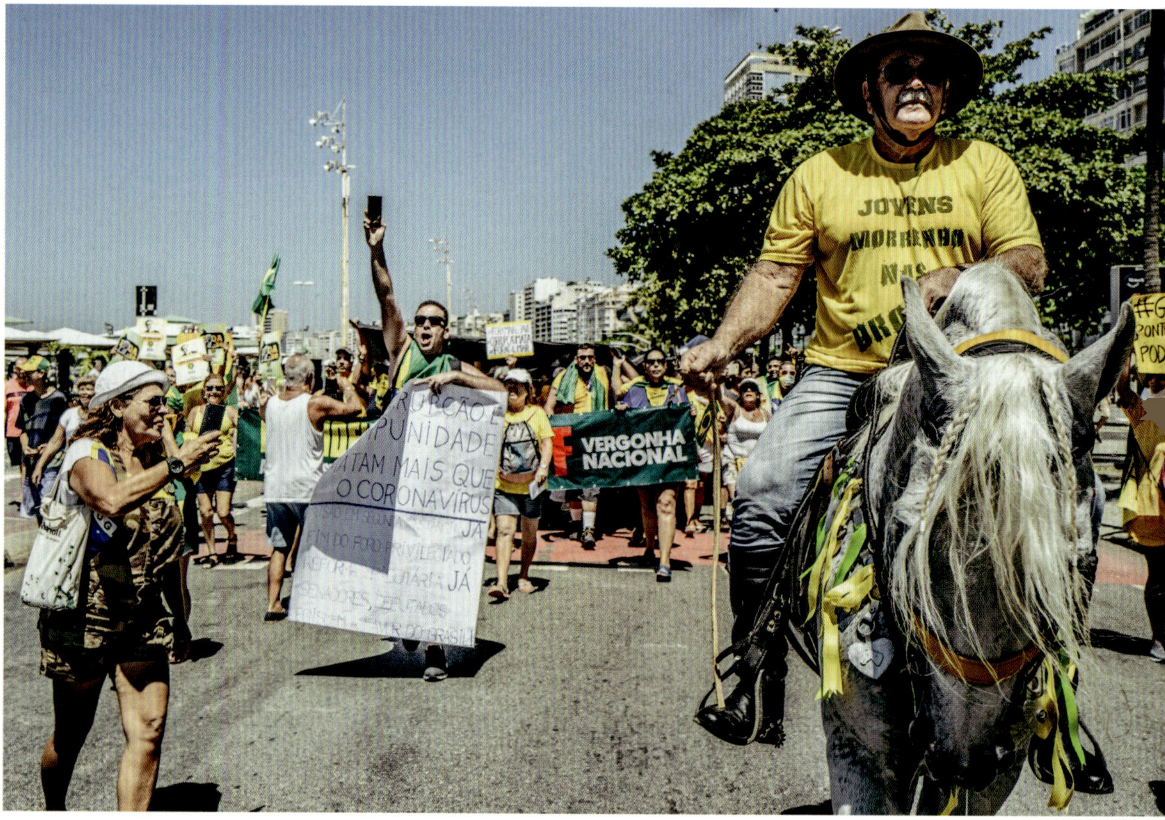

MAIS QUE
O CORONAVÍRUS
VERGONHA
NACIONAL
JOVENS

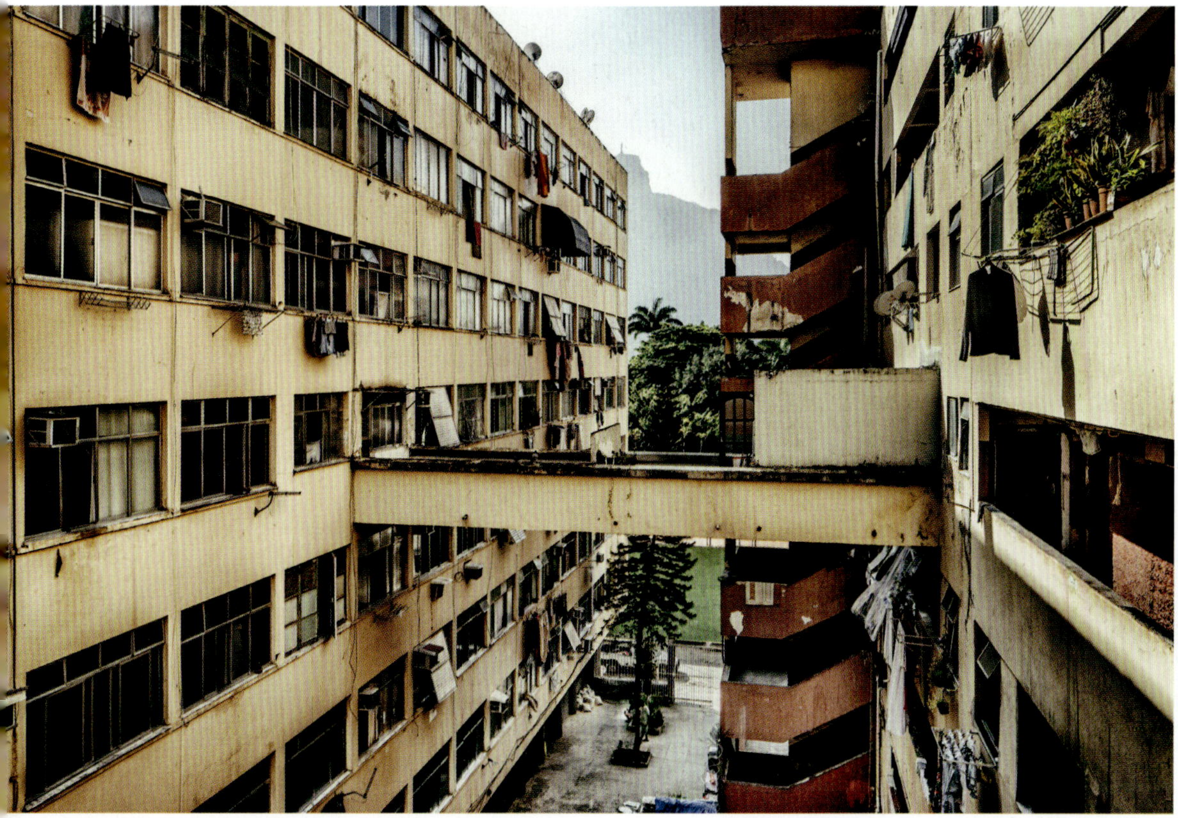

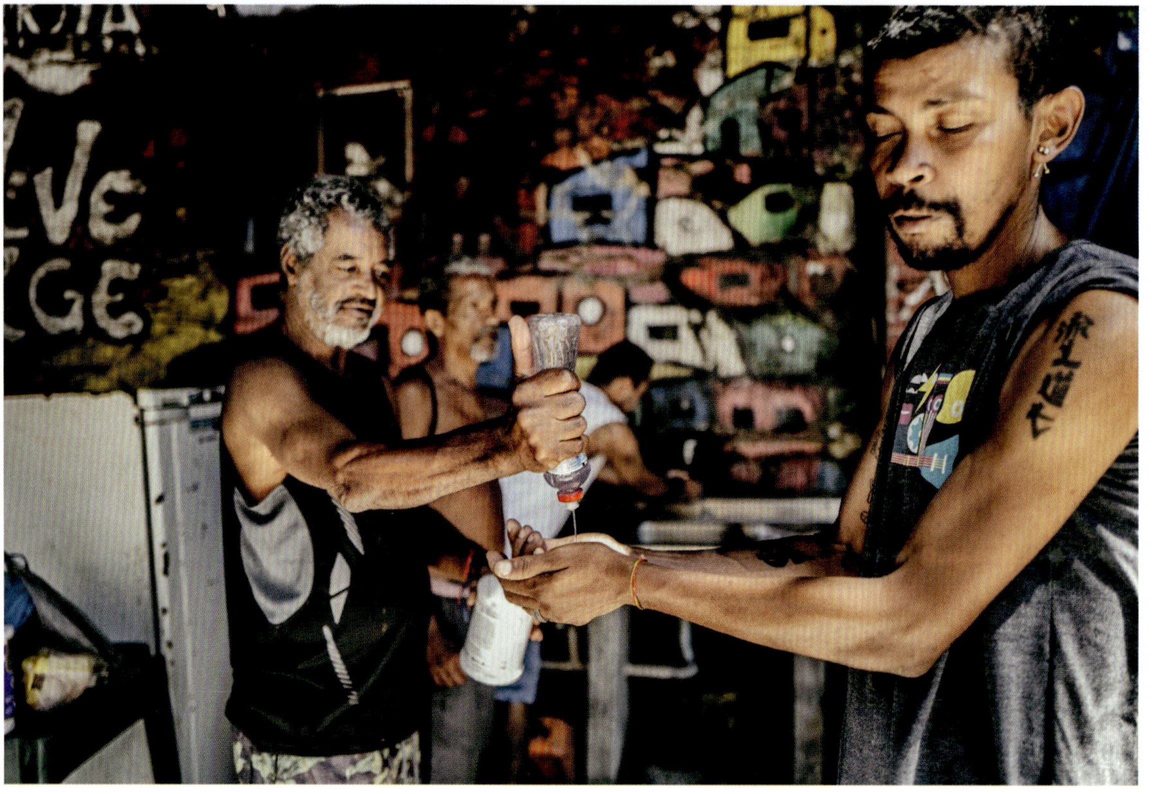

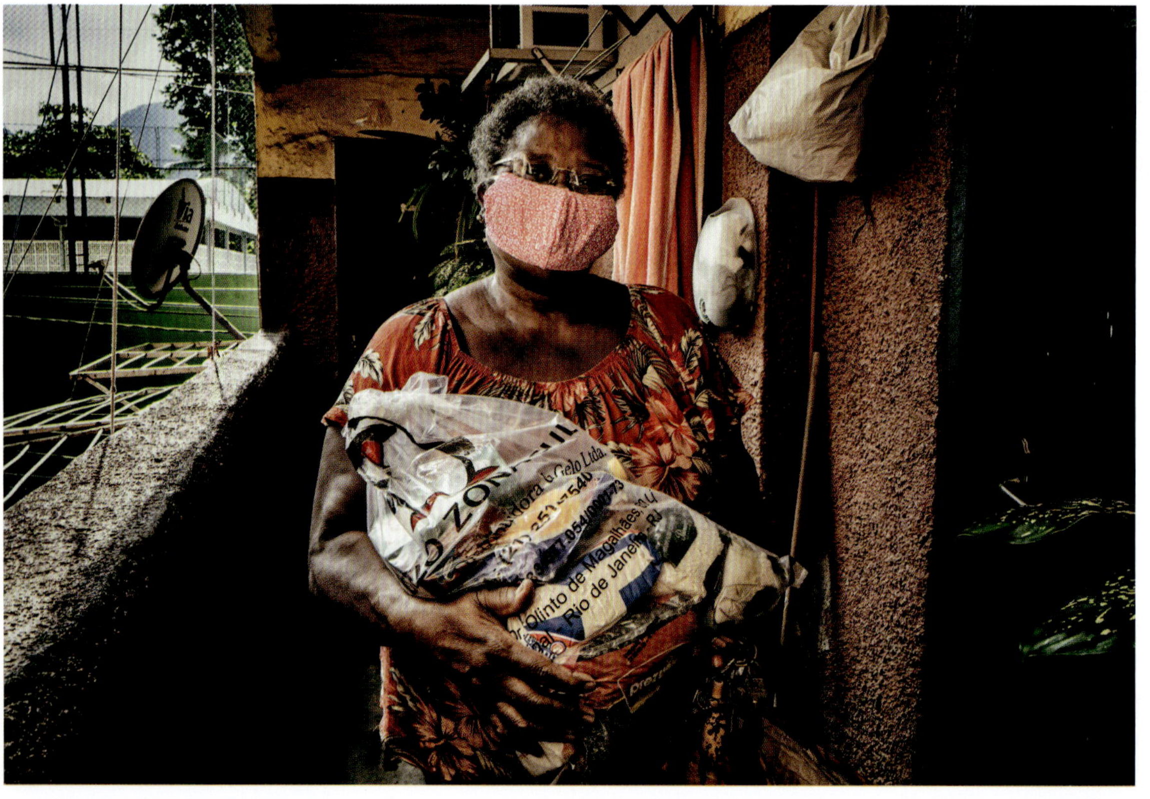
Gelo Ltda.
Olinto de Magalhães

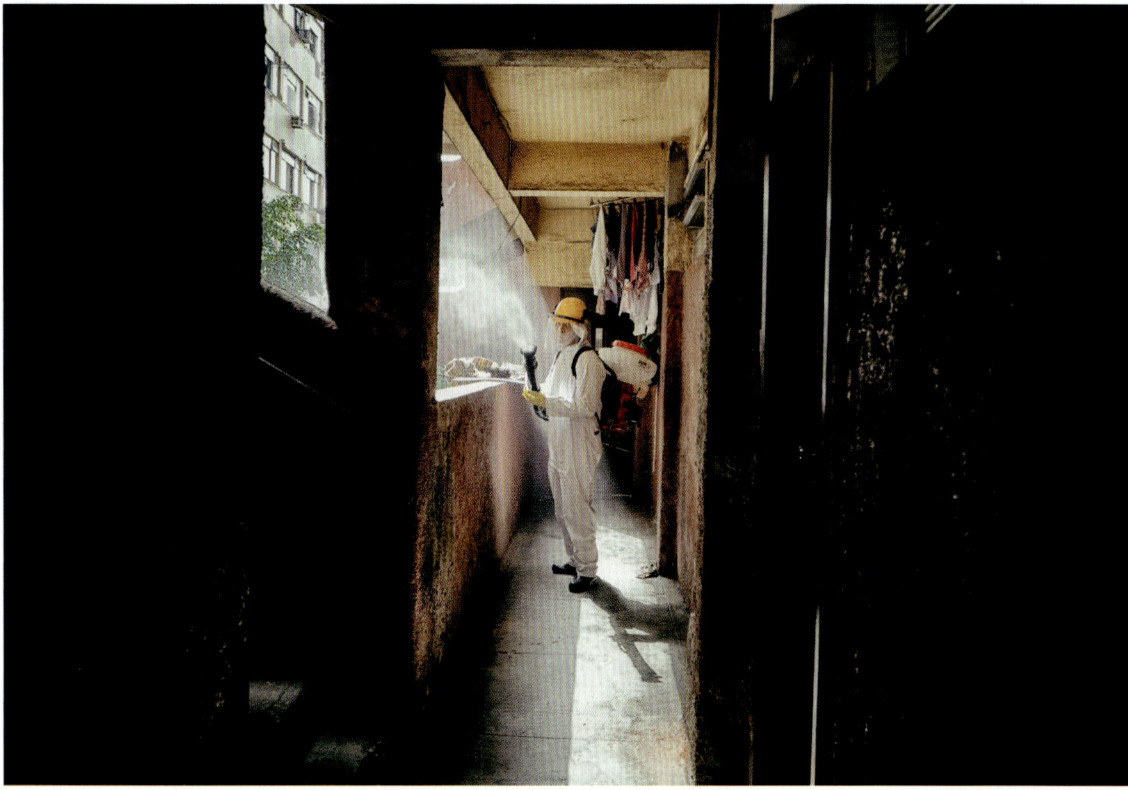

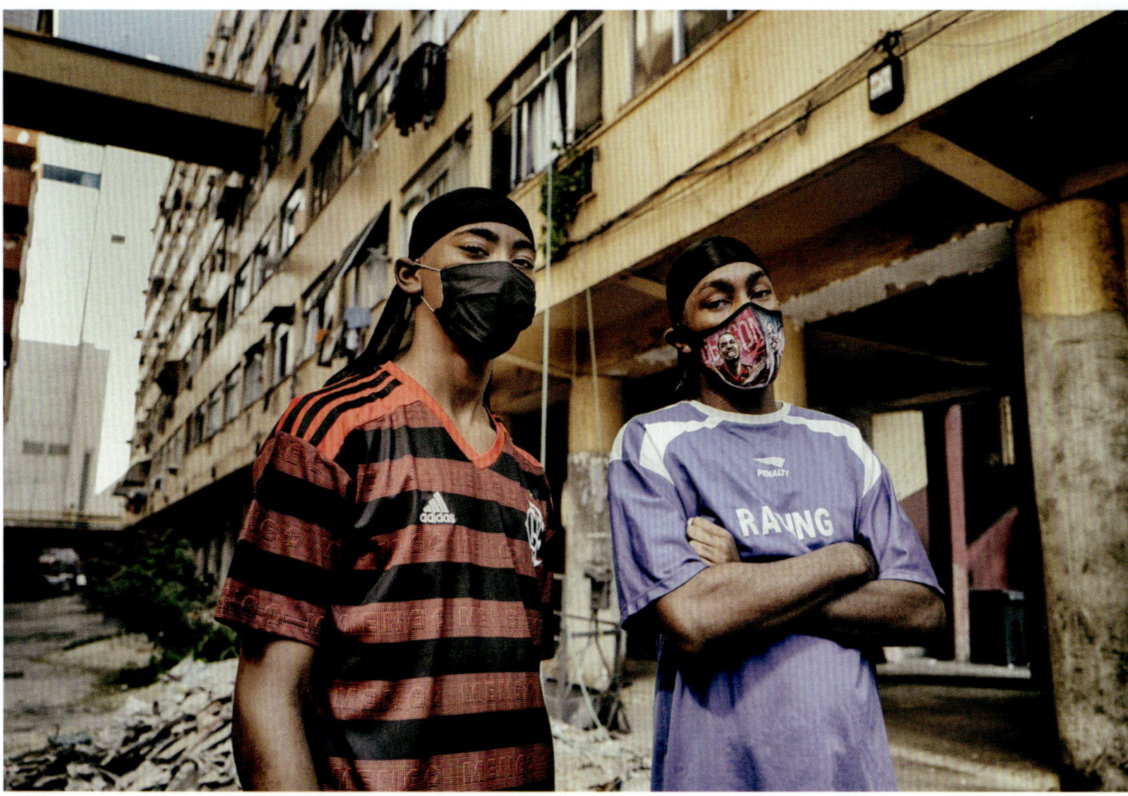
adidas
PENALTY

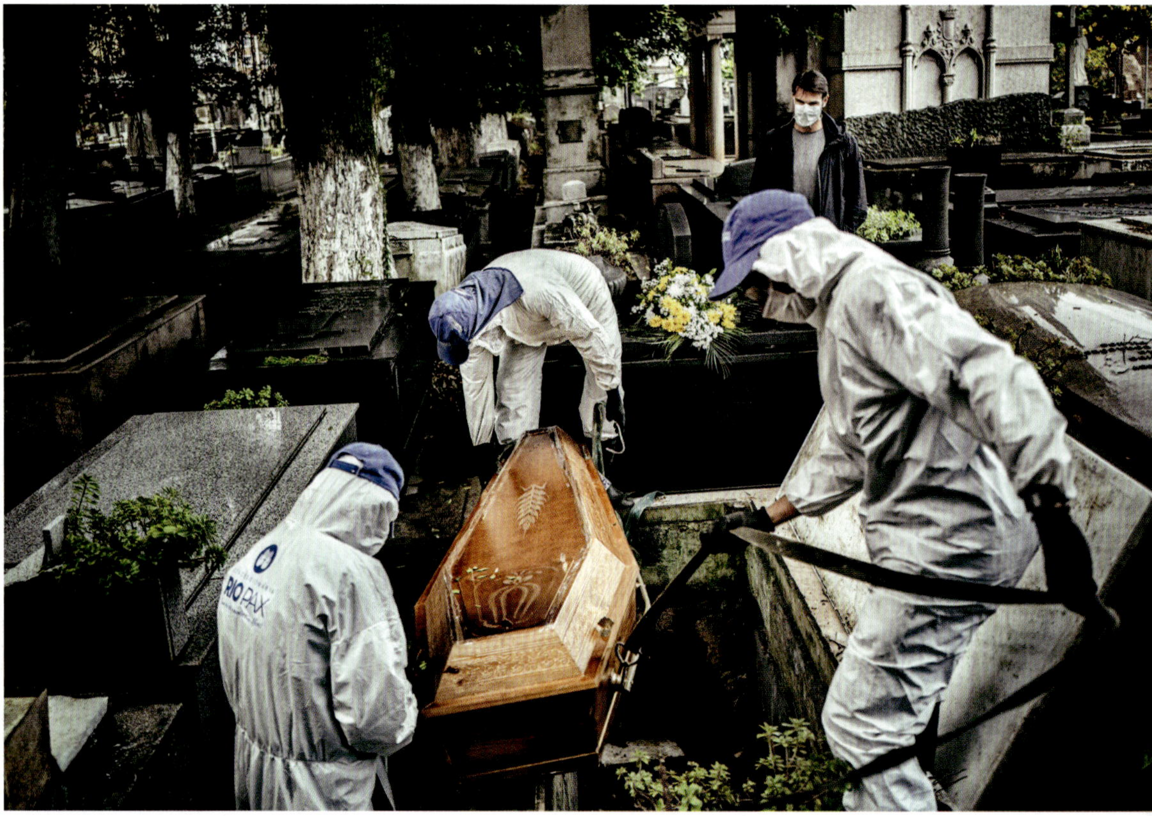
RIO PAX

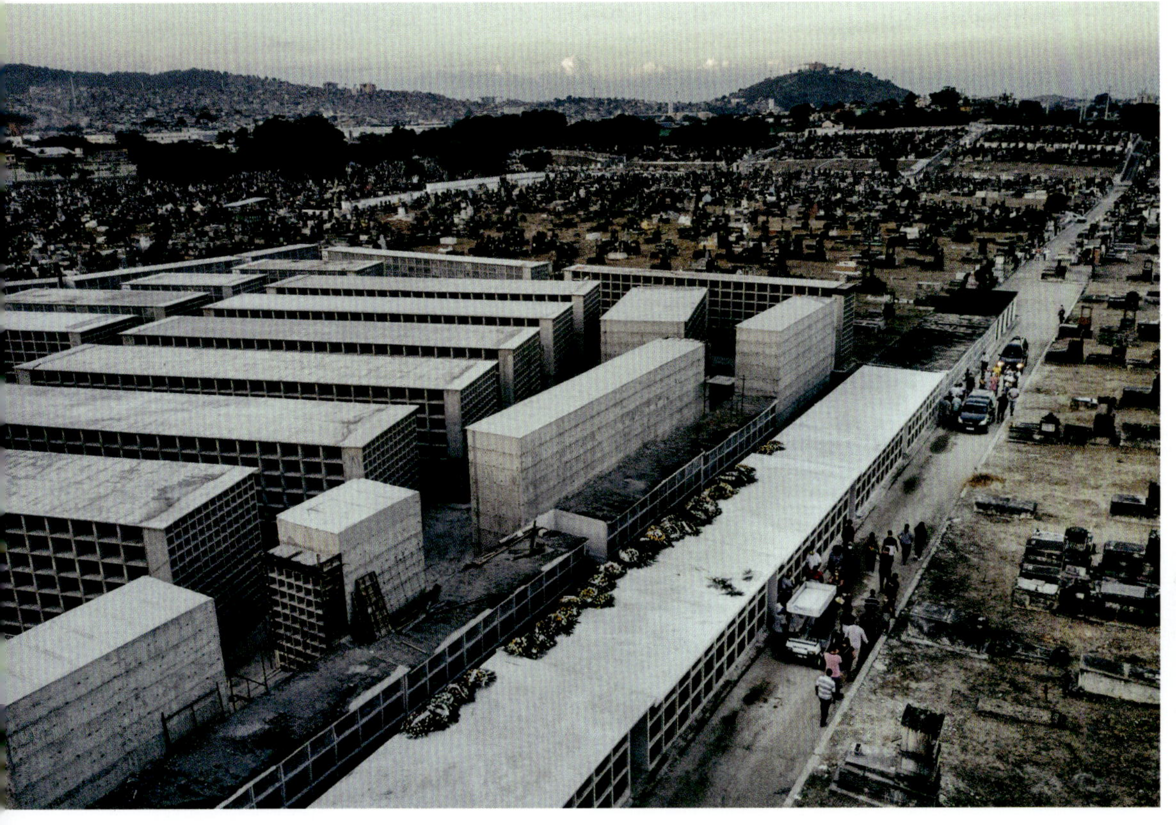

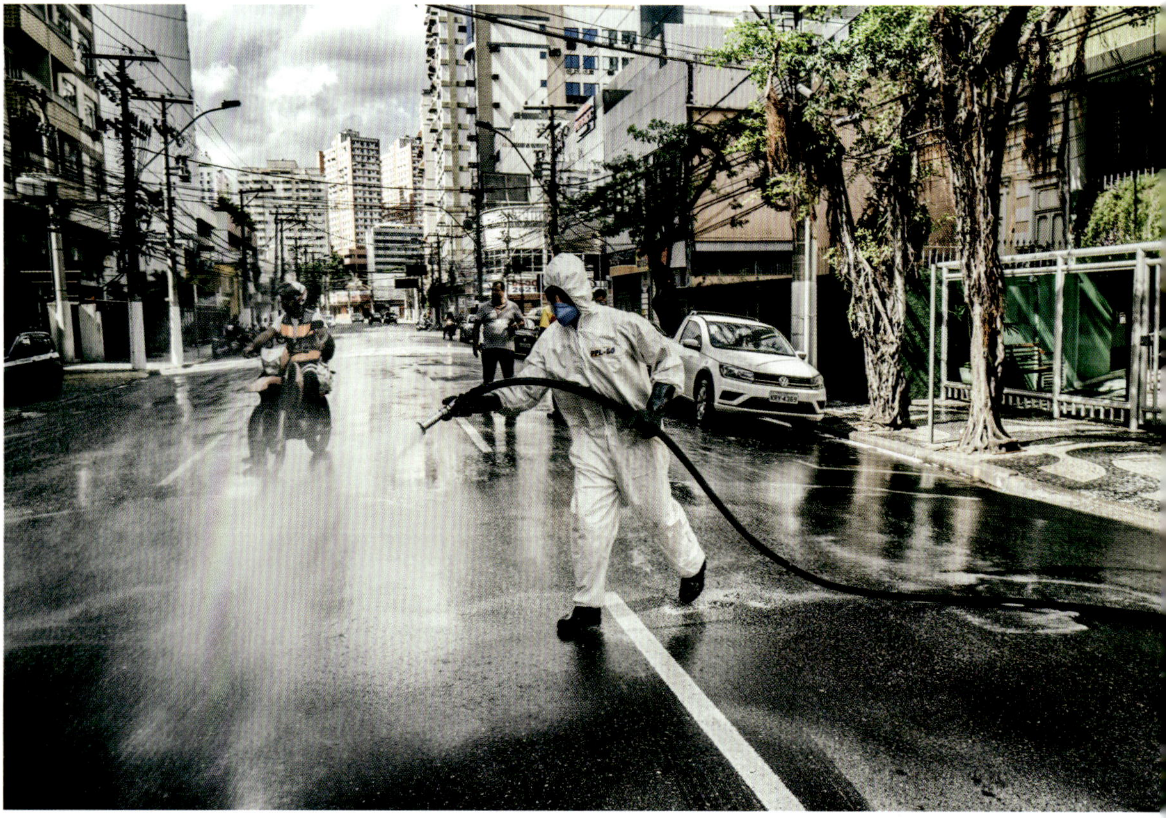

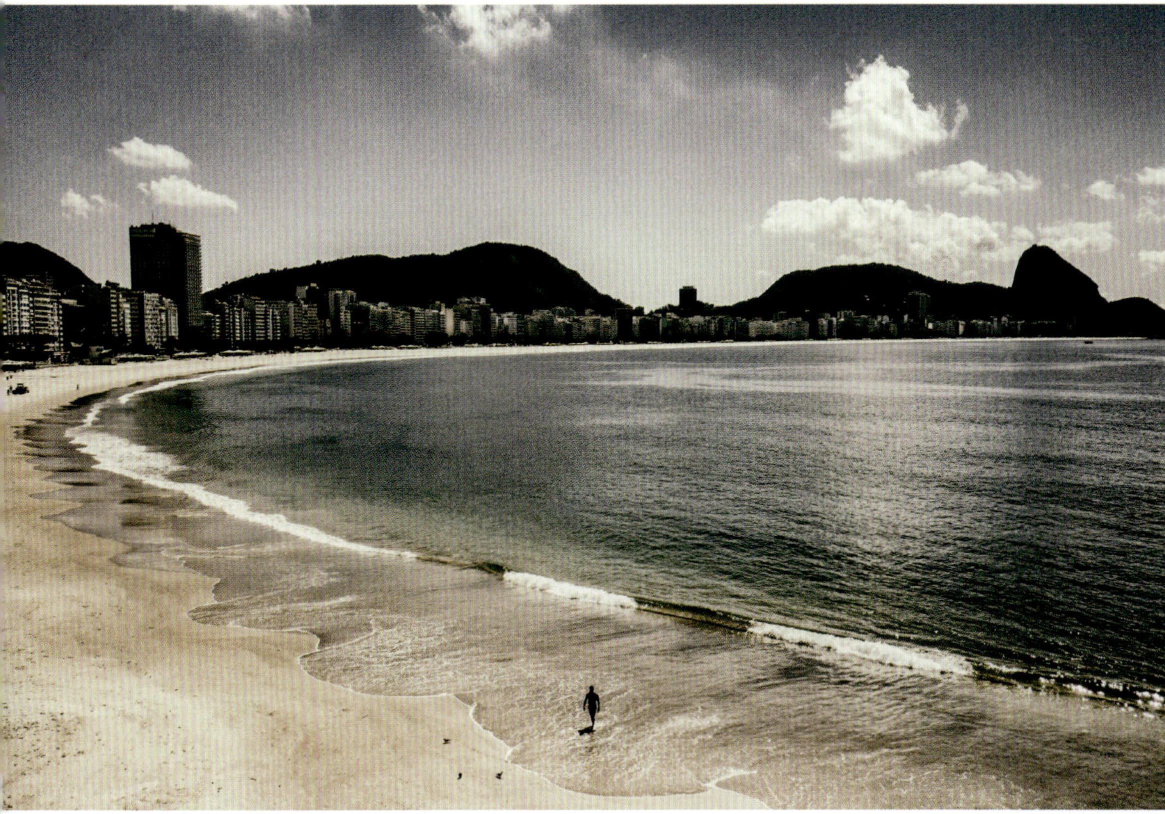

Farshid Tighehsaz, Iran
Death Has a New Name

According to the World Health Organisation (WHO), prior to the COVID-19 pandemic, in January 2020: "Depression is a common illness worldwide, with more than 264 million people affected. At its worst, depression can lead to suicide. Close to 800,000 people die due to suicide every year. Suicide is the second leading cause of death in 15- to 29-year-olds". With the matter of the current pandemic, our lives changed dramatically, contributing to a pervasive sense of uncertainty, loss, and isolation. These factors combined to increase anxiety and depression worldwide. This makes depression the most destructive threat on Earth for mankind.
Unfortunately, despite this ongoing human catastrophe, our modern world and the media have no attention to that monster that is growing every day and becoming an anonymous beast. The world is very unkind to depression and depressed people — it humiliates them. The modern world only promotes happiness without creating happiness. Undoubtedly, that traumatic condition is the most damaging in closed and critical societies. Iran was the second country to declare deaths due to the virus, within 50 days after China, on February 18 2020. By mid-year according to official statistics, Iran was hit with more than one million and a half total cases and more than sixty thousand deaths. However, unofficial statistics show four times more. When the coronavirus outbreak arrived in Iran, life was on a vague path long before that. The country had been plagued by multiple crises and complexity for decades. The geopolitical and economic crisis due to sanctions created a lifetime of fear because of the theocratic regime; in addition, we must include the continuous hostile threats with the US. While the death toll was rising every day, the situation became alarming: that of a society moving towards a social catastrophe. These events brought about an experience of psychological trauma, whose effects also reshape social behaviour. There is a transformation happening in the psychological dimension of everyday life and its relationship with the environment: an invisible mutation that hides behind masks and gloves. The pandemic became an excuse for the government to justify death and depression. Where human rights are political, health is also a political issue. Where you can be arrested, imprisoned and even executed for any ridiculous reason, how hopeful can life be? Where there is no value in human life, what difference is there between life and death?
In this situation, I am not sure about anything except my feelings. This is the exact point from which I try to photograph what I feel and how the world presents itself to me. Documenting those feelings and events gives me a certain hold on life conditions here. What I feel is real. It hurts me, it gives me insomnia. It throws me into depression. I feel the rope around my neck all the time. It kills me slowly. I can't breathe.

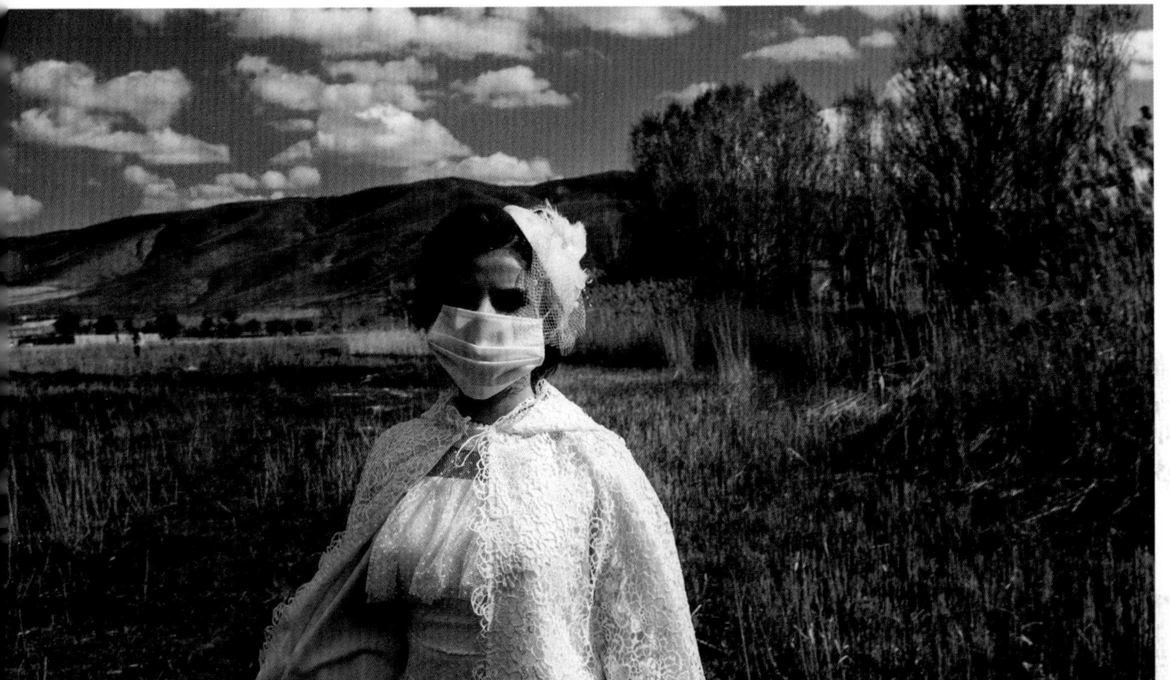

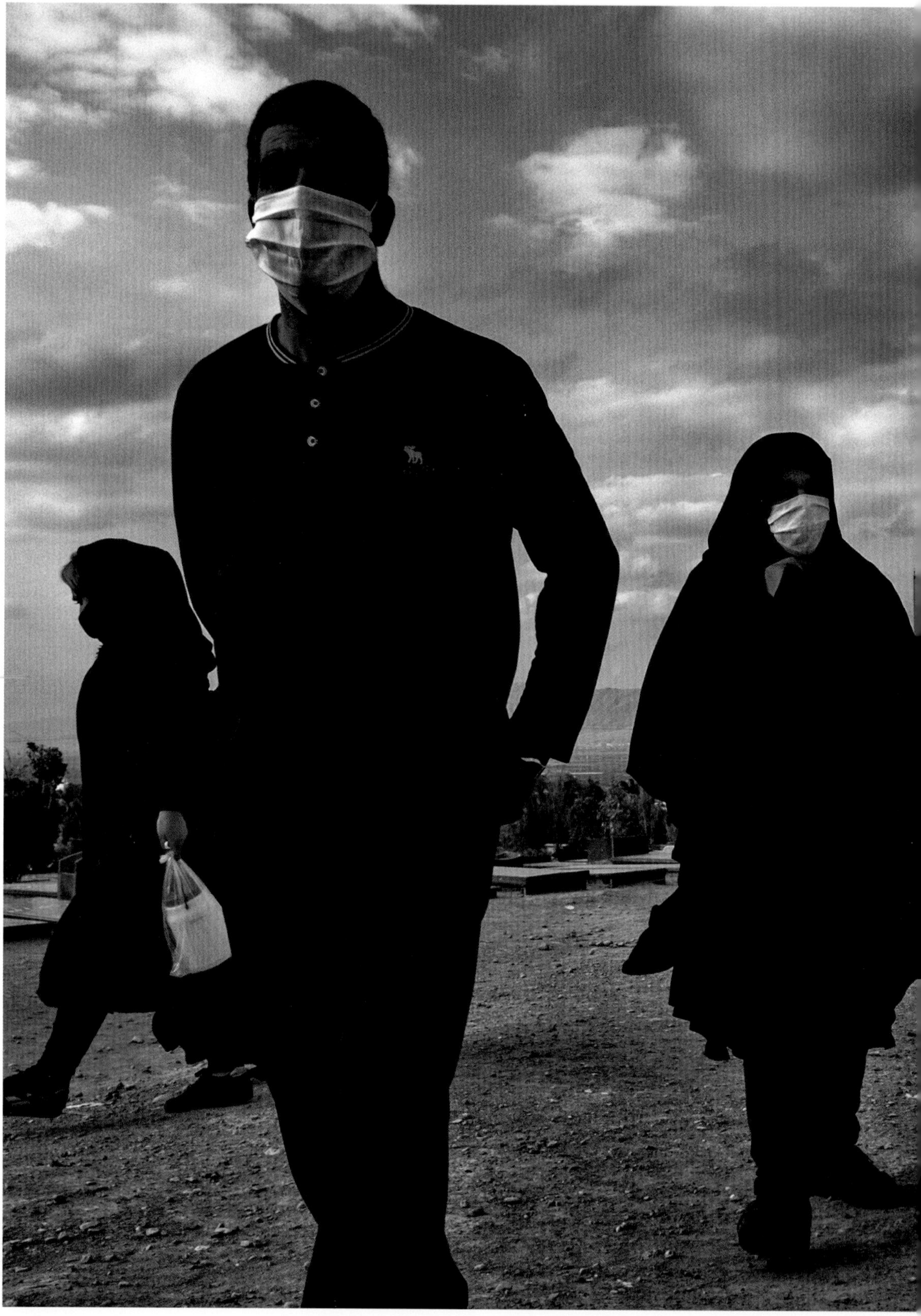

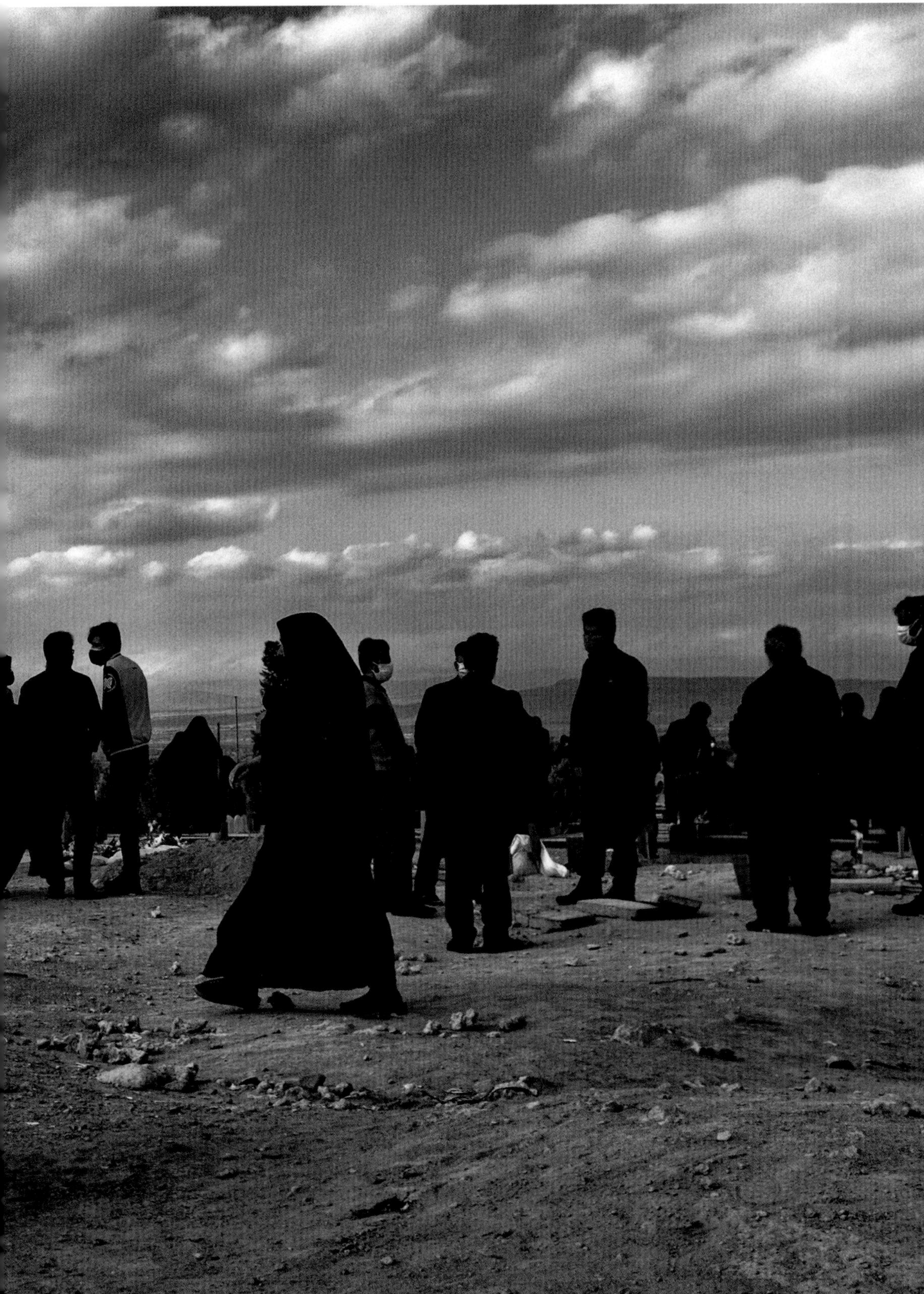

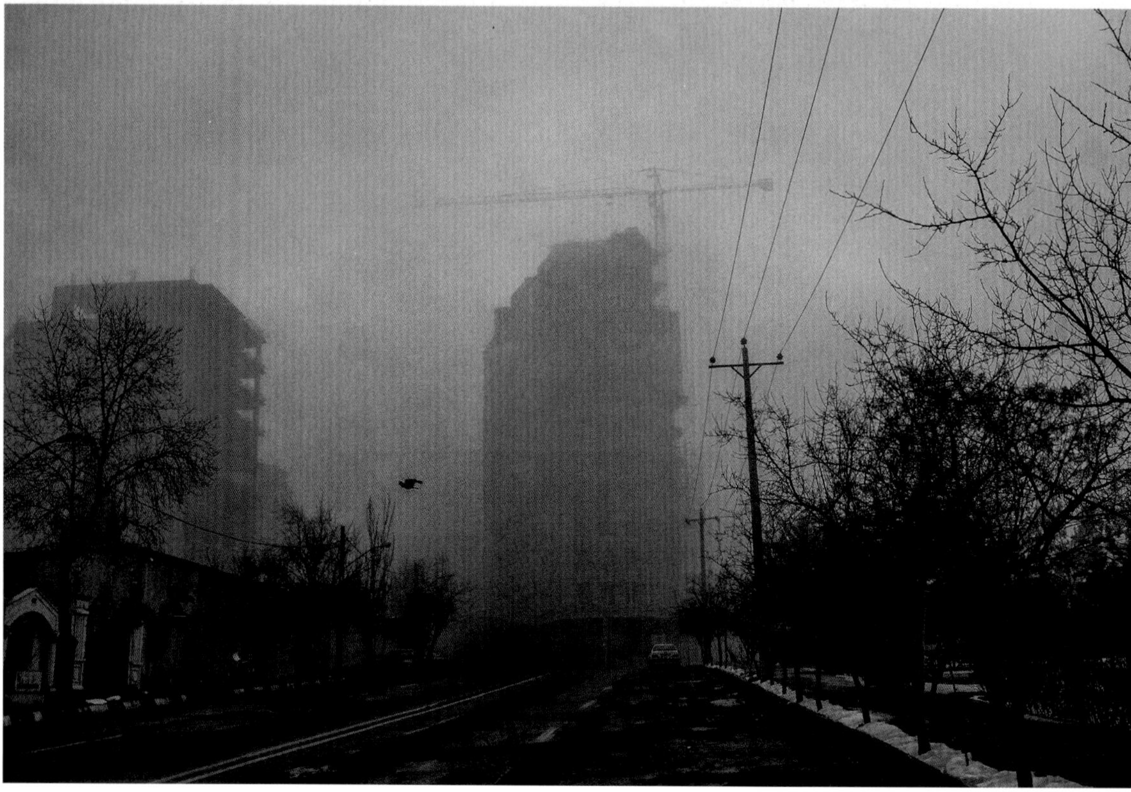

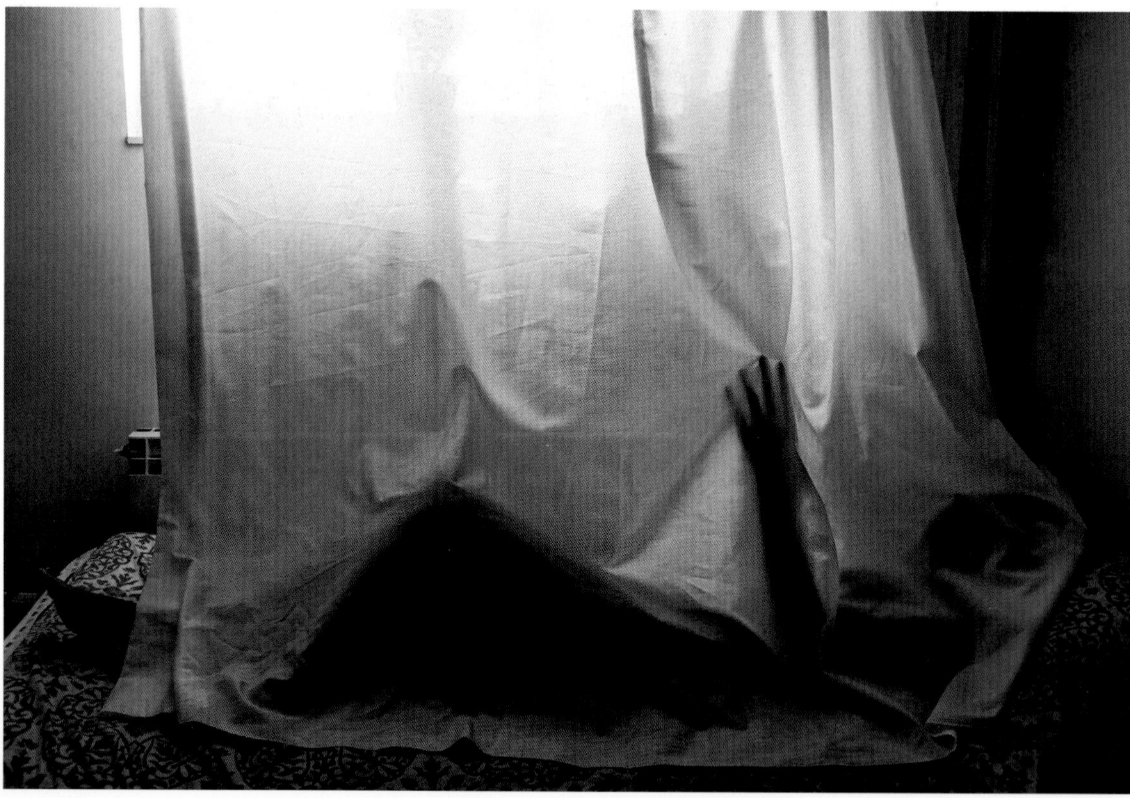

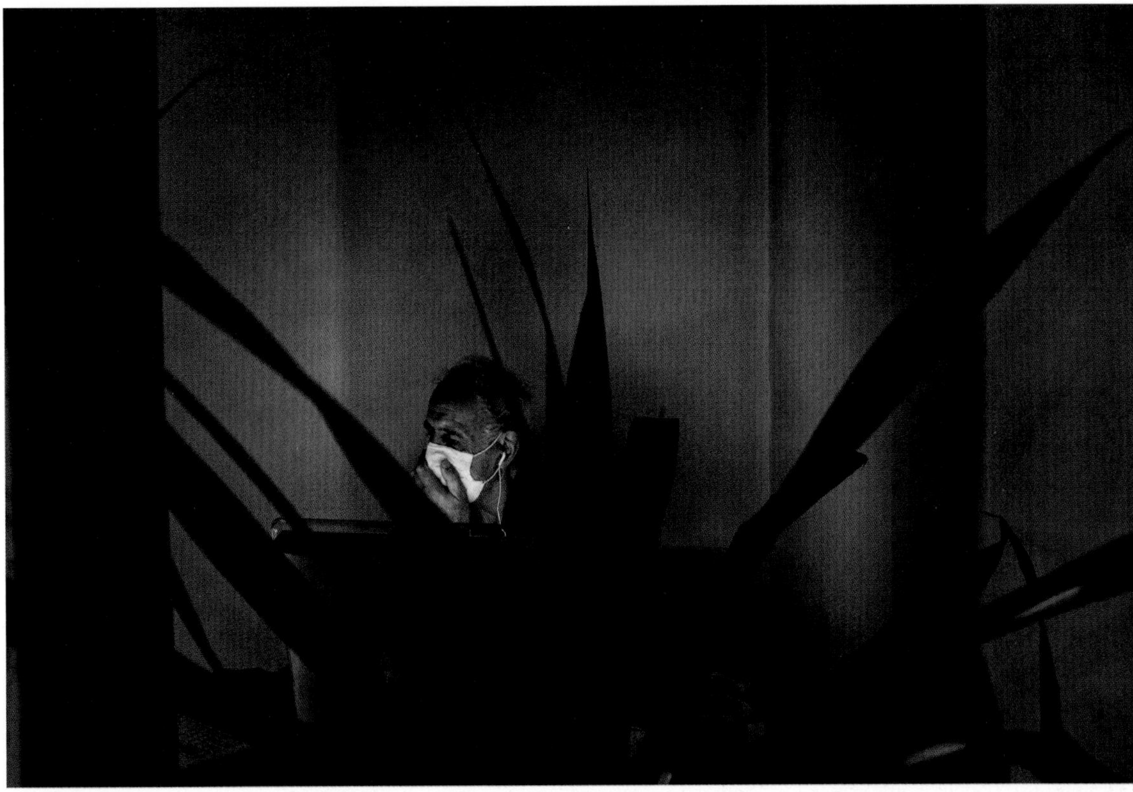

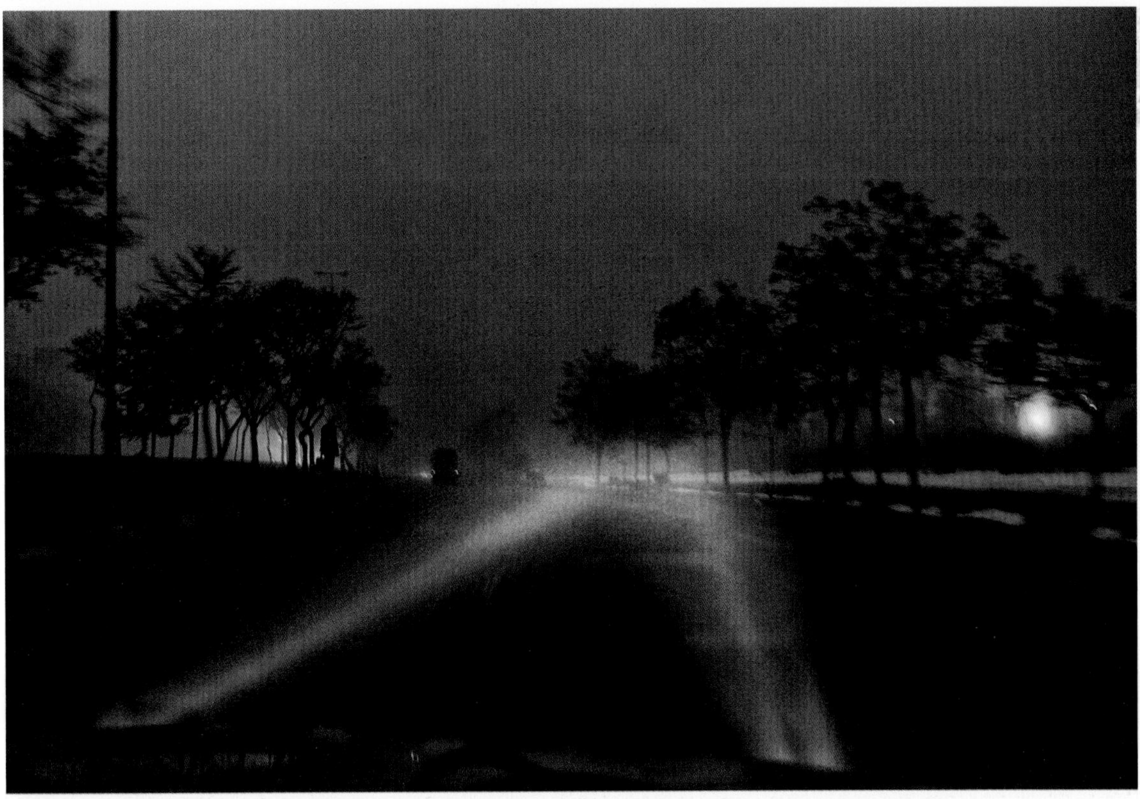

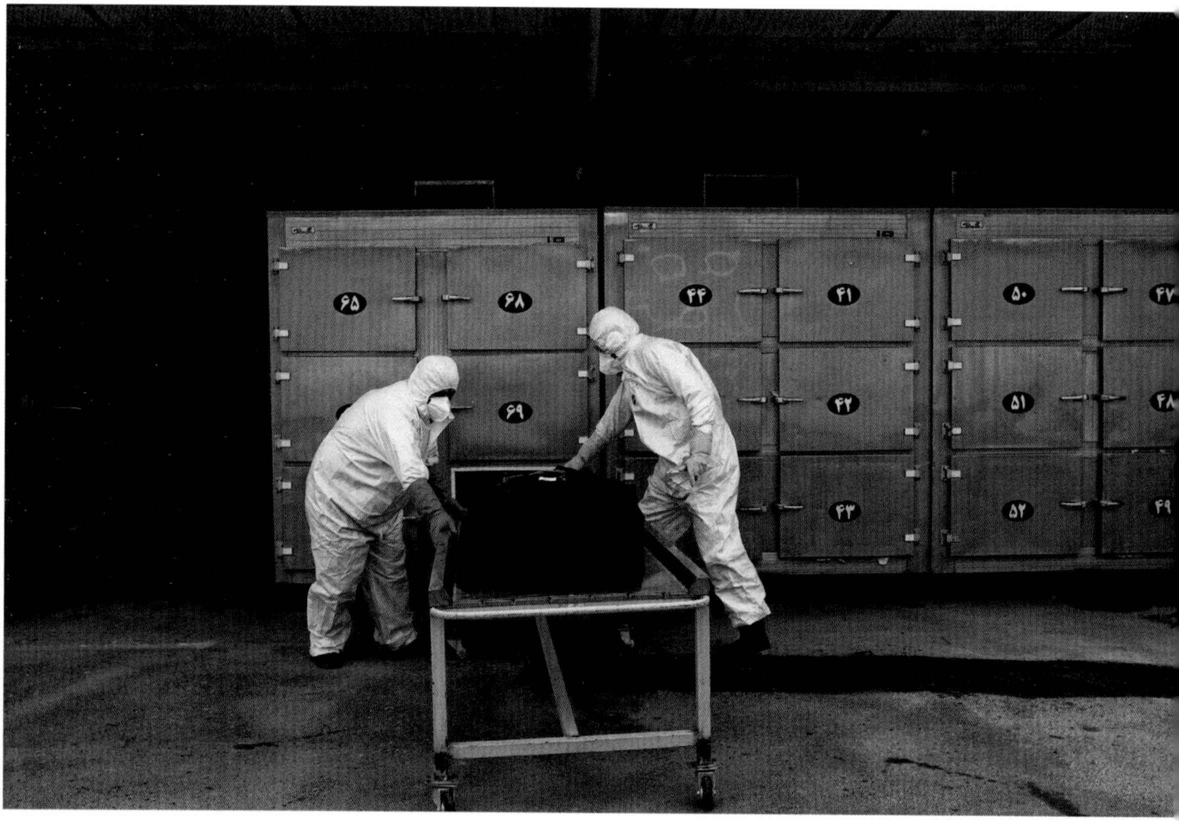
۶۵
۶۸
۶۹
۴۴
۴۱
۴۲
۴۳
۵۰
۵۱
۵۲

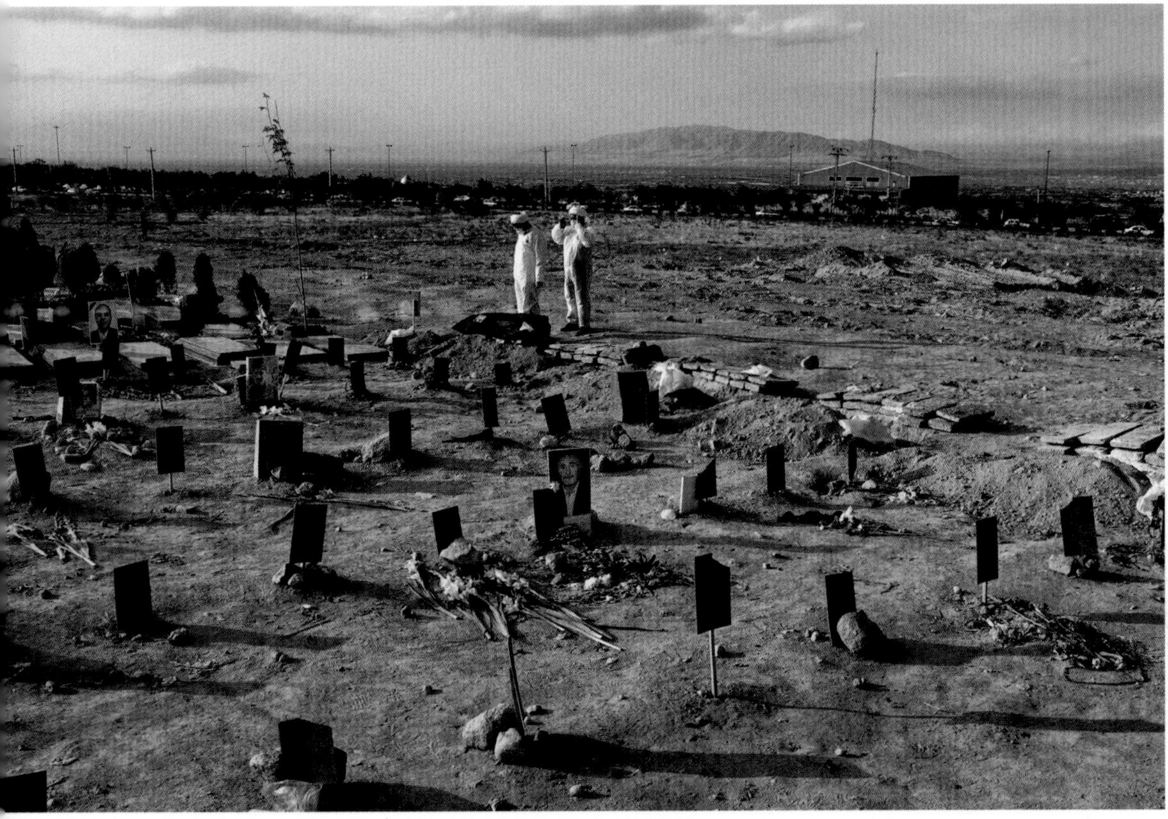

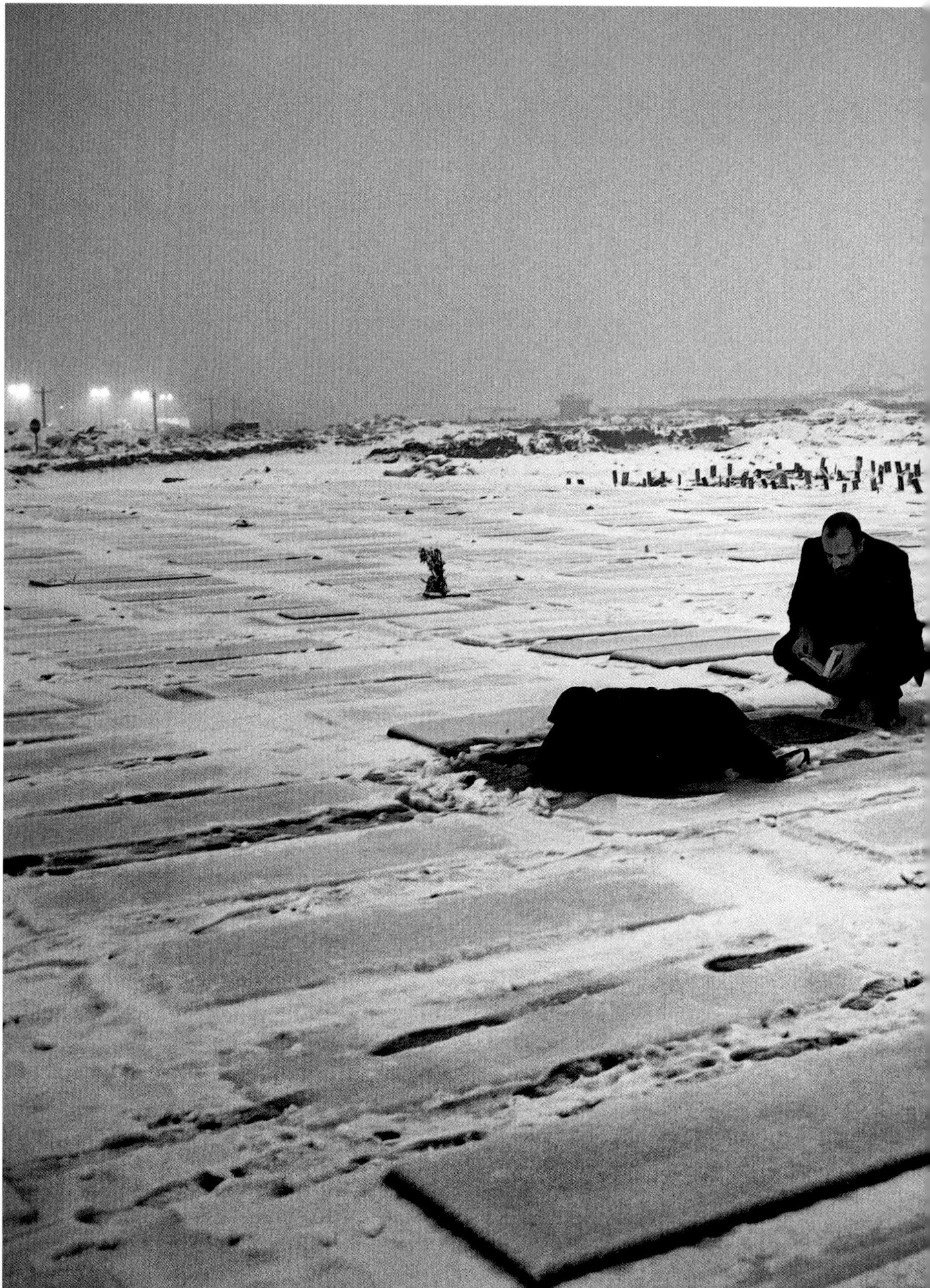

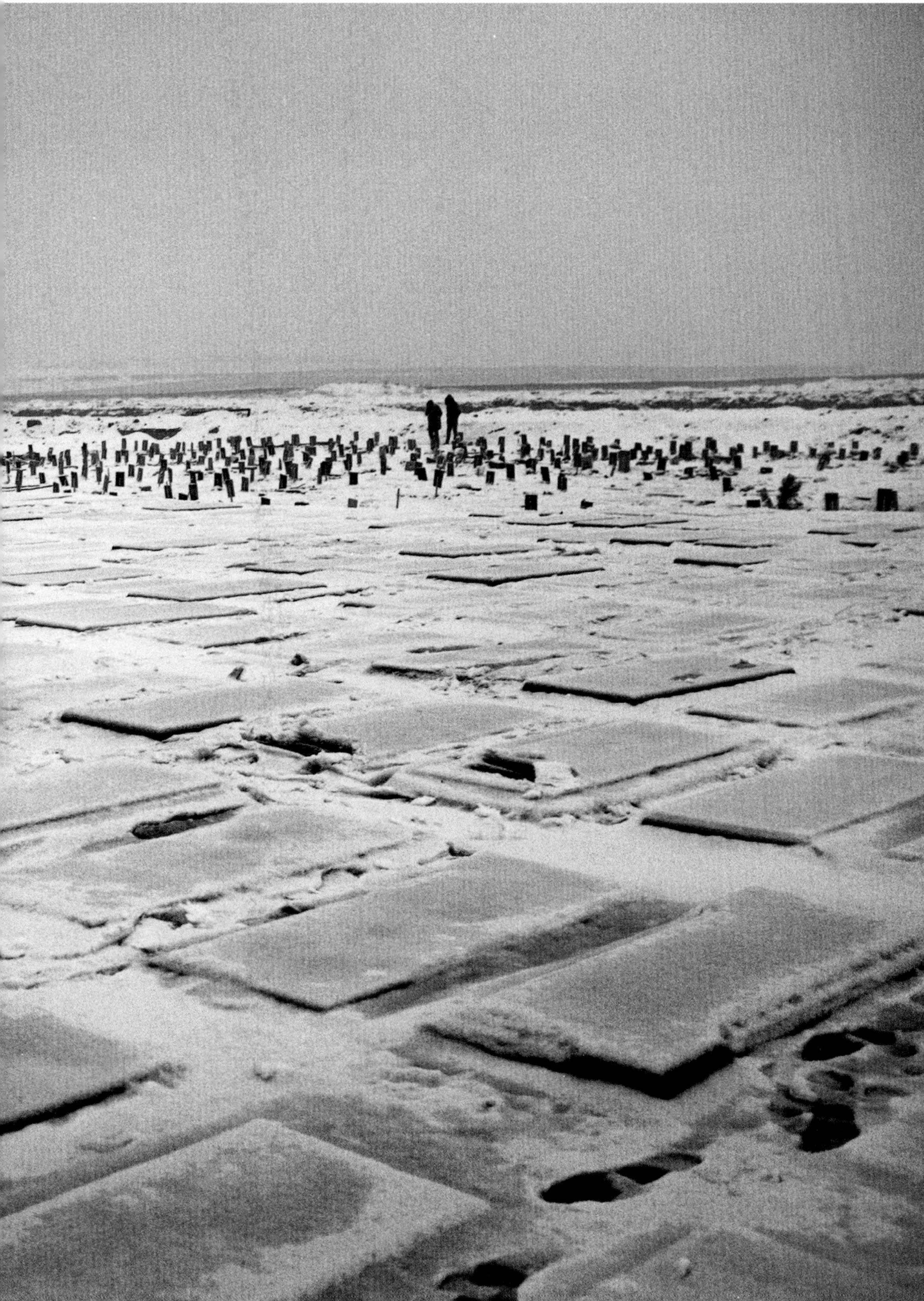

Michele Spatari, South Africa
No Place Like Hope

Marco Longari

It went from the surprise that sprung from a distant observation to a disillusioned denial; it became slowly part of a new normal, and finally hit the mark with the power of surging numbers and the inevitable toll of deaths. Predictably, the pandemic reached South Africa: its coming has blurred racial and economic divides and put strain to deep running fault lines, contradictions etched into its people consciousness.

At the beginning of March 2020, amid raging numbers in China and in Europe, South Africa discovered that Patient Zero was among its population, and a scramble to contain the panic and the rush to supplies was finally met by an inevitable lockdown.

Deserted streets, panic buying and curfew. The humming of the South African Army patrol vehicles and the familiar blue lights of the police filled the streets of Johannesburg. From deep into their recessed dwellings and into the overcrowded buildings and the shacks of the informal settlements, residents learned the reverse irony of "physical distancing": a defiance to the law of physics, a surreal reality for those to whom the simple notion of "space" sounds unmeasurable.

But the measure of it has been imposed with sticks and whips. With rubber bullets shot at close range. During night raids where residents have been woken from their provisional beds in overcrowded rooms. Life at the margin of the society has been reduced to a matter of square meter occupancy.

South Africa saw its numbers climbing, masks on noses and hands in gloves, peeking over the shoulders and making peace with a new reality: the people, its most vulnerable people, were starving. The lockdown left an economy already in survival mode, on its knees: the hand-to-mouth feeding scheme that has most of their able men and women leaving the inner city and the townships looking for wages that would feed their families revealed its bare teeth, its limits and its failure.

As kilometres long lines have recalled in the memory of South Africans the queues that marked the passage from the horror of Apartheid into the new democracy, the private sector and few public actions have tried to patch the emergency. The livelihood of thousands of families were now on the line. A food line.

A relatively young population is put to test, its resilience proofed against underlying HIV and TB conditions, adding insult to injury in an explosive mix of racial tensions, exacerbating economic disparities and feeble governance. Stay at home, they said.

In South Africa it's a thread that pulls memories from the past. Apartheid, dispossession, segregation. As the Army's presence on the streets melts away, a nation is relieved from an unnecessary burden: now will be the time to steer the republic towards its recovery. Before it will be time to mourn its dead.

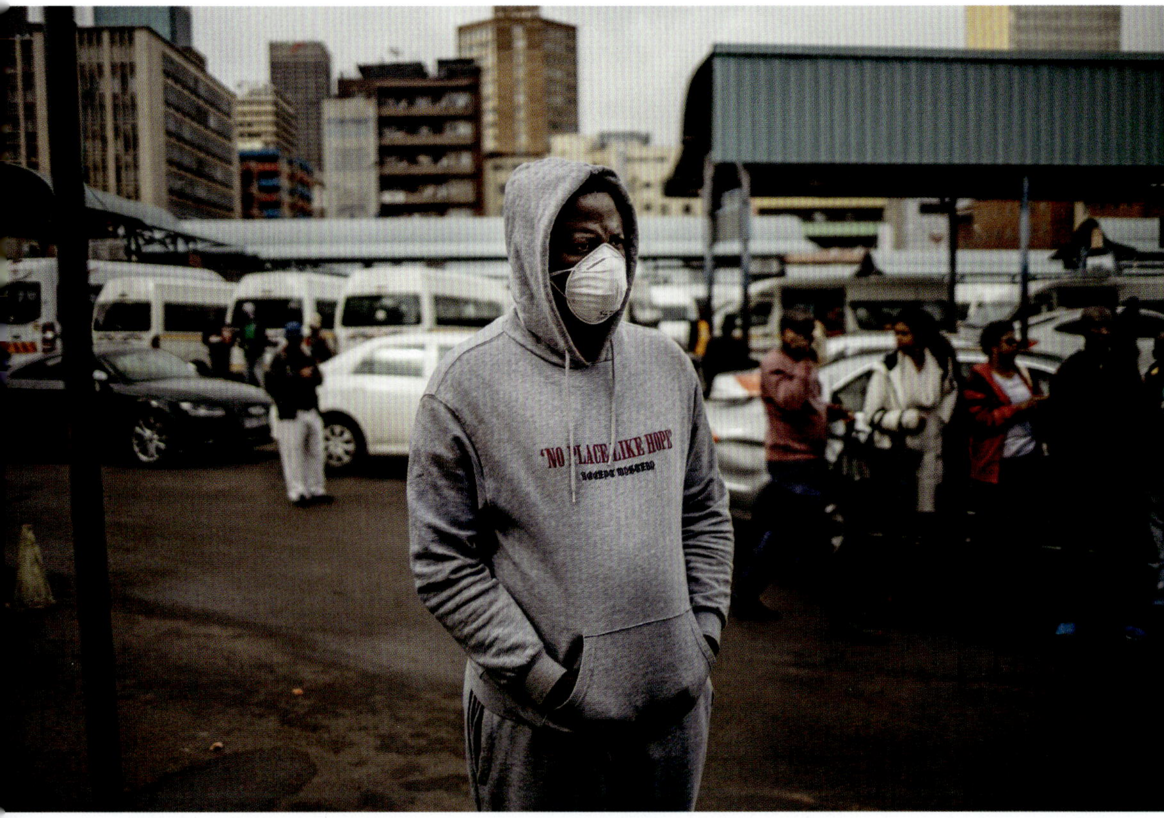

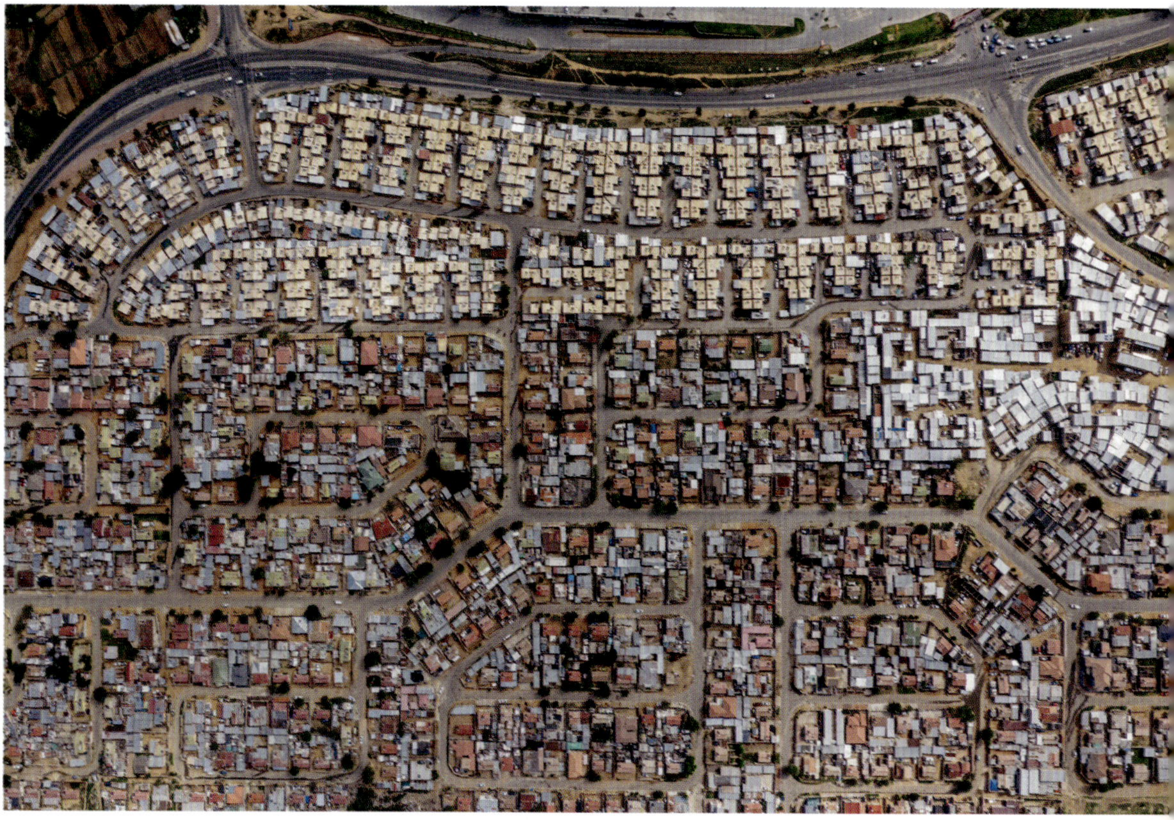

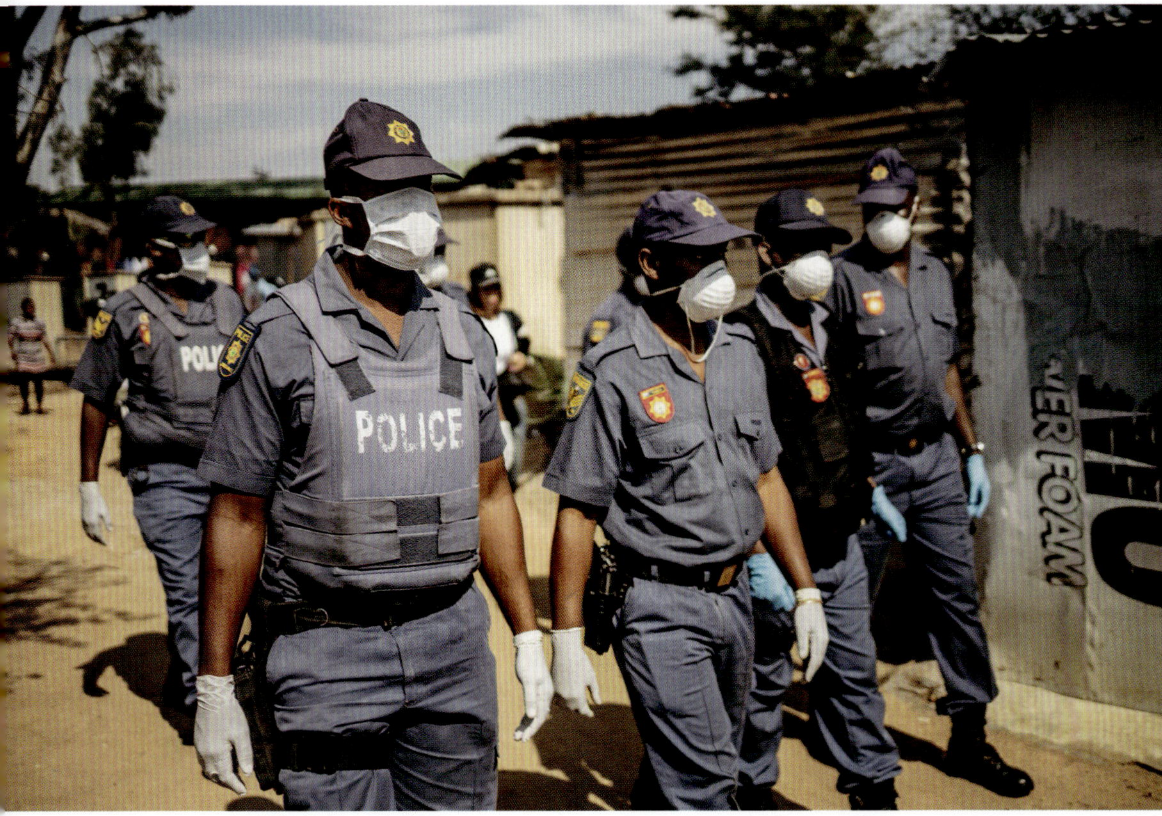
POLICE

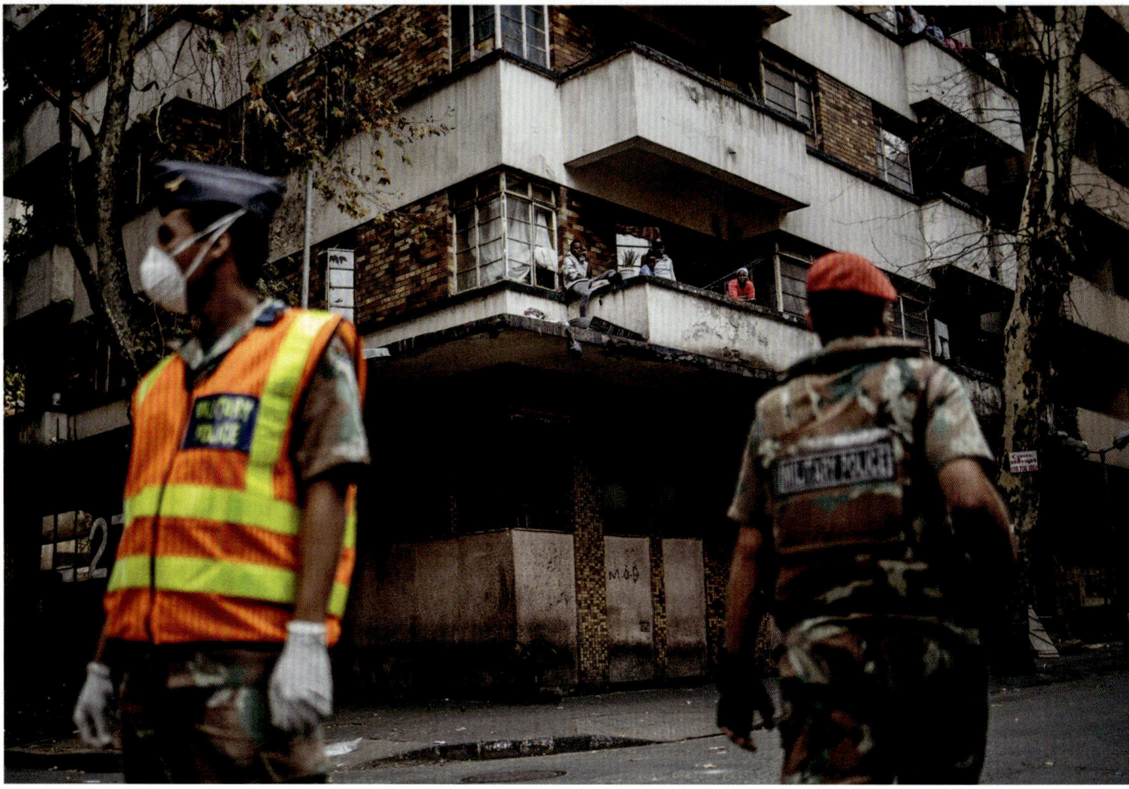
MILITARY POLICE

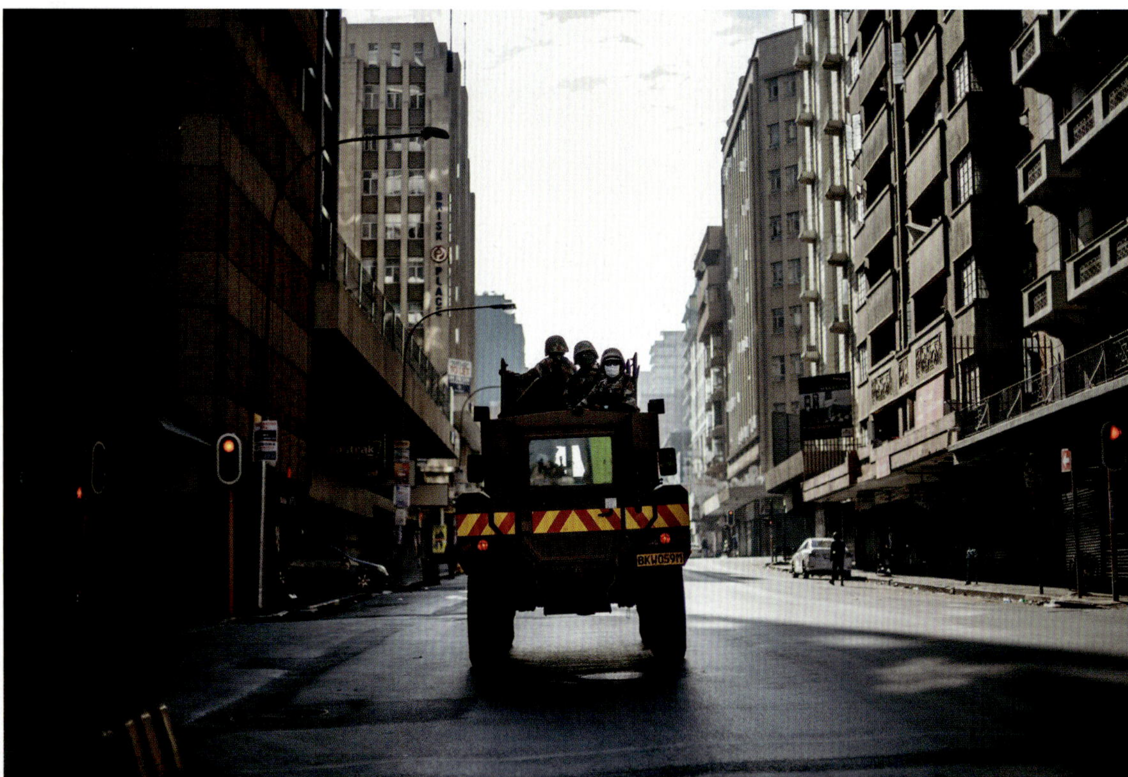
BRISK PLACE

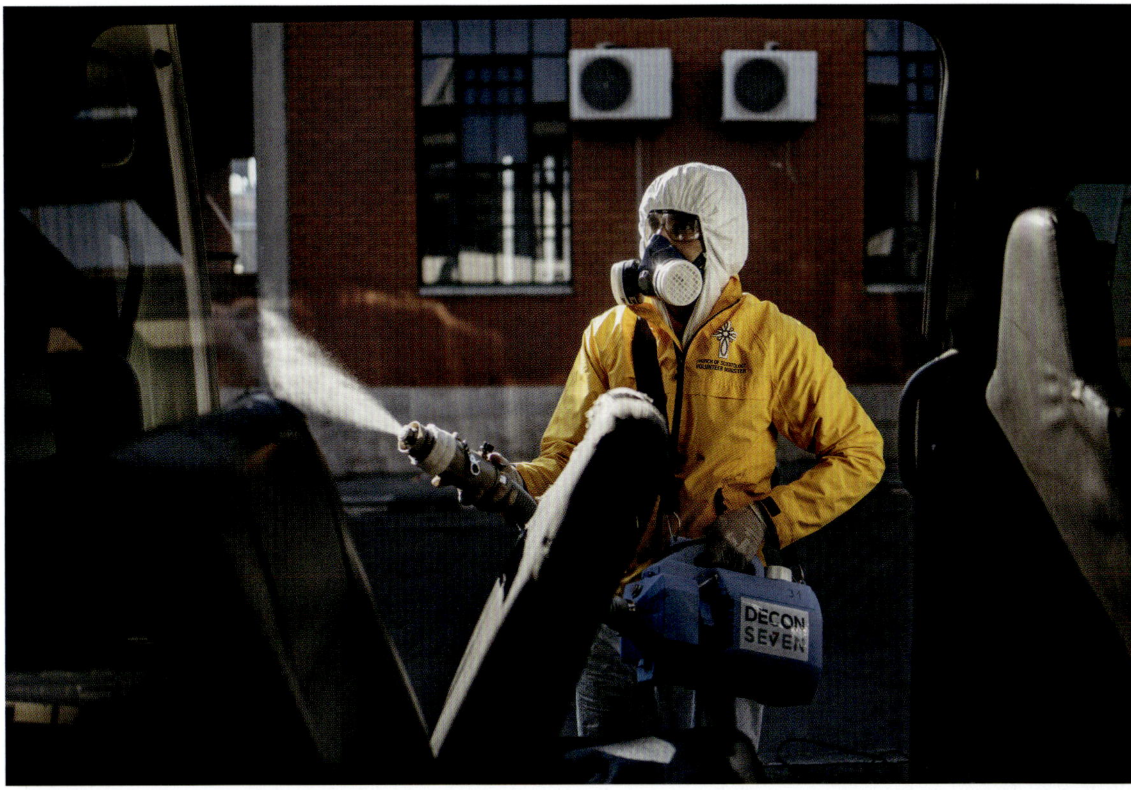
DECON
SEVEN

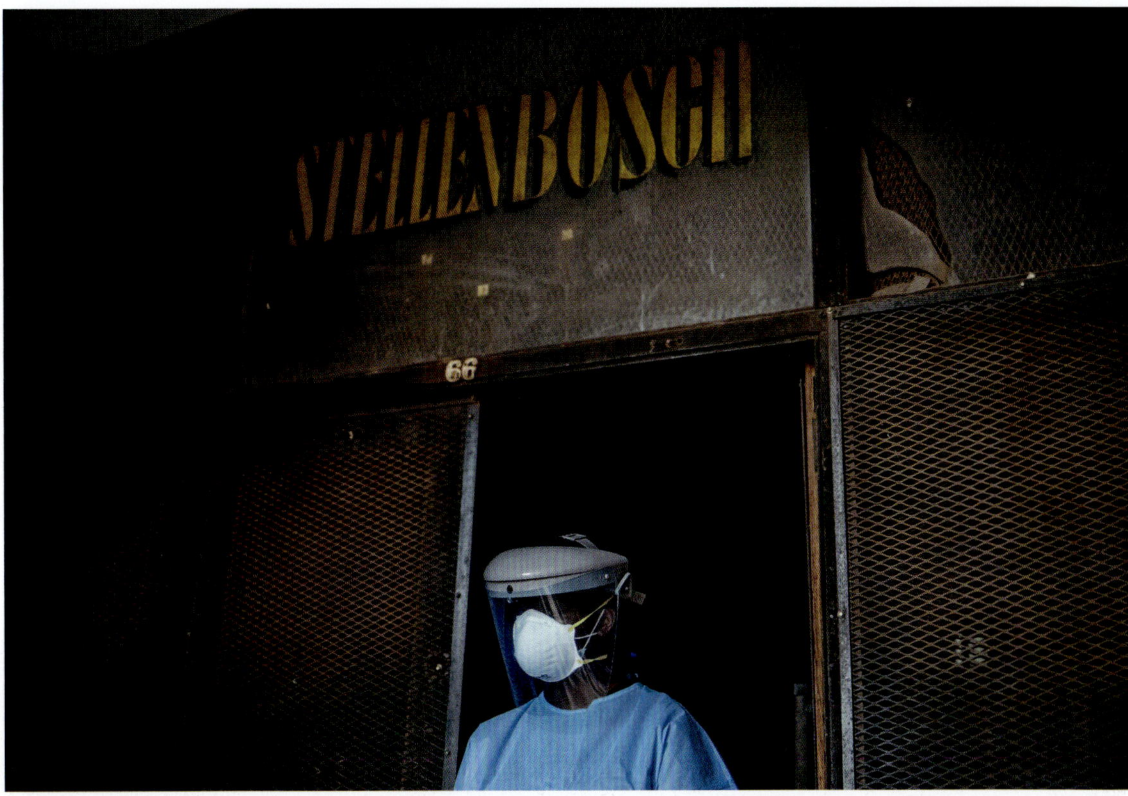
STELLENBOSCH
66

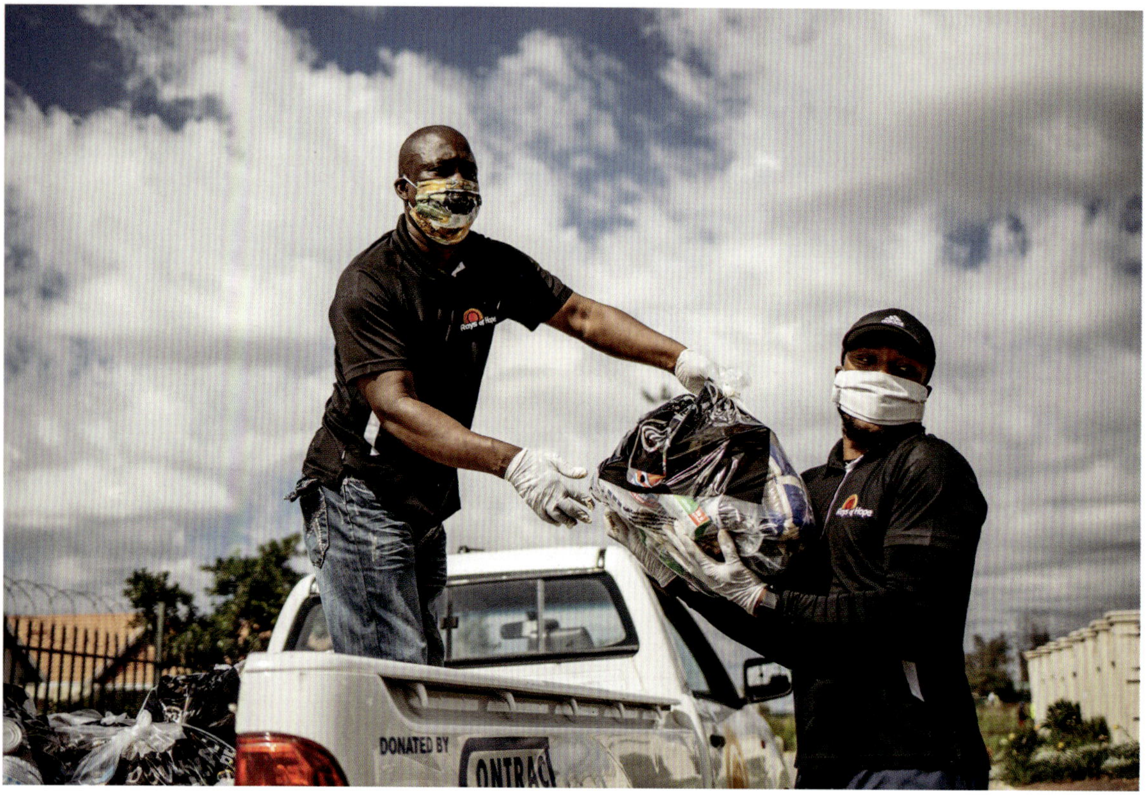
DONATED BY

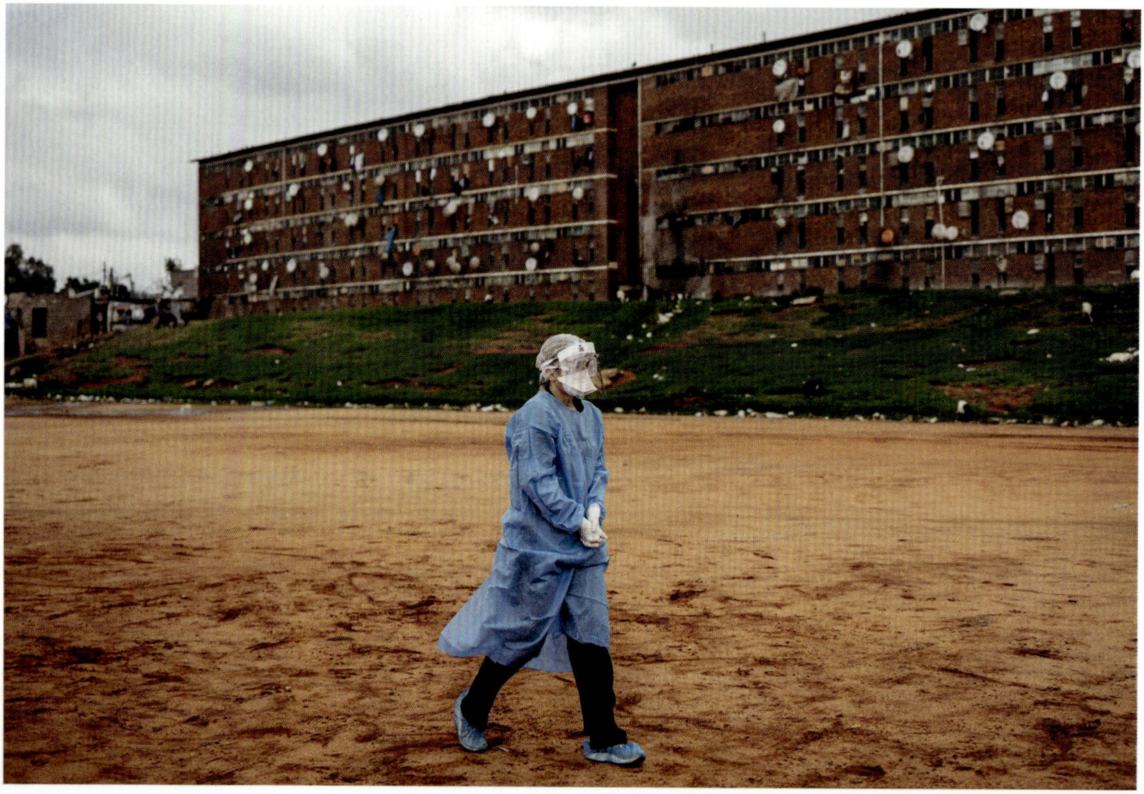

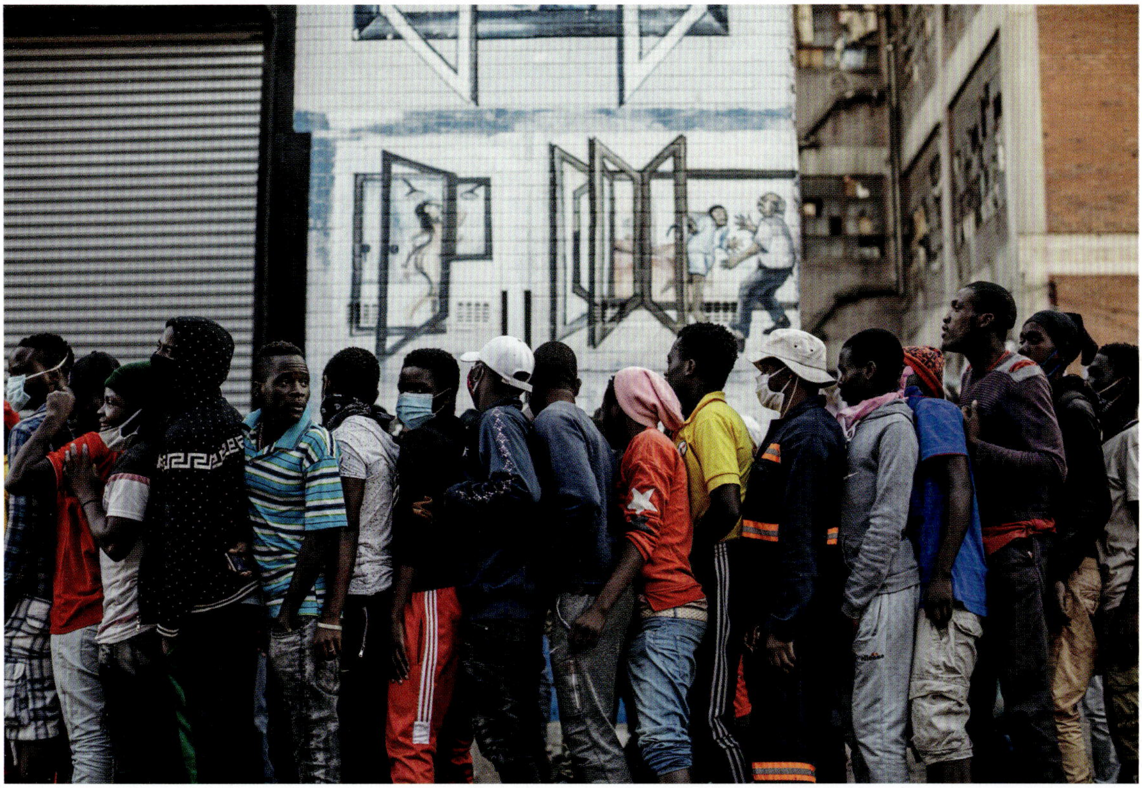

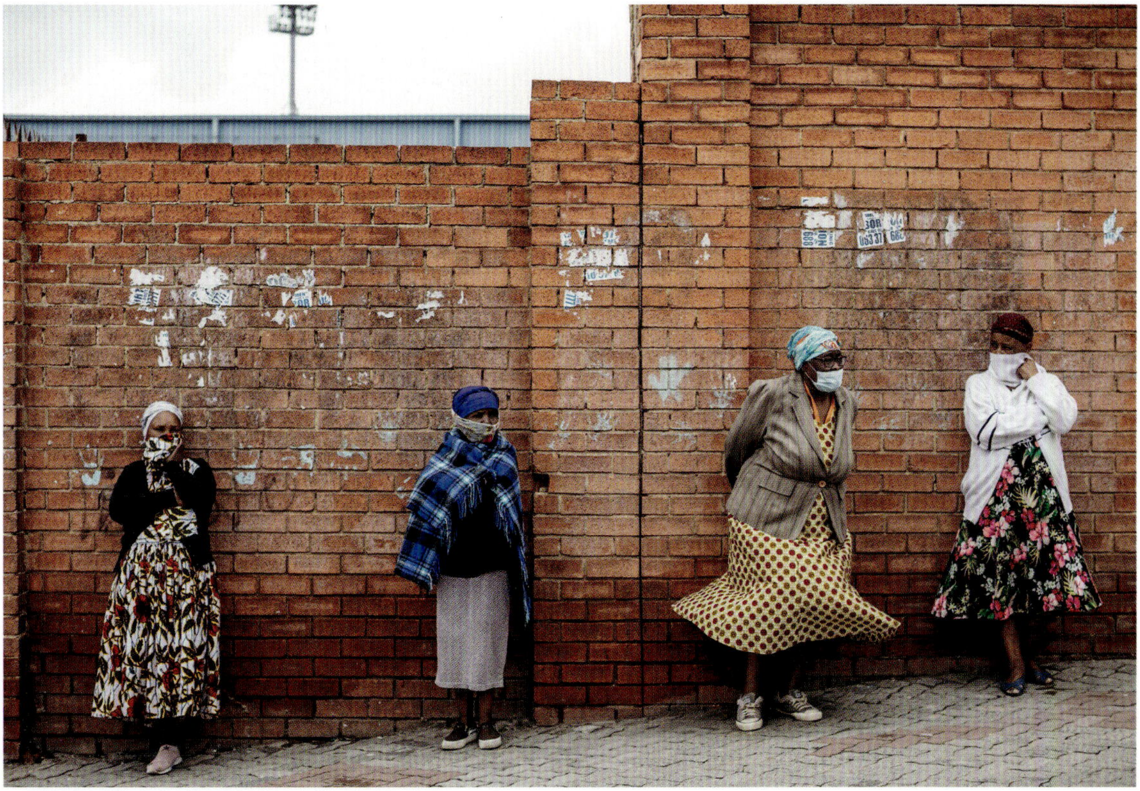

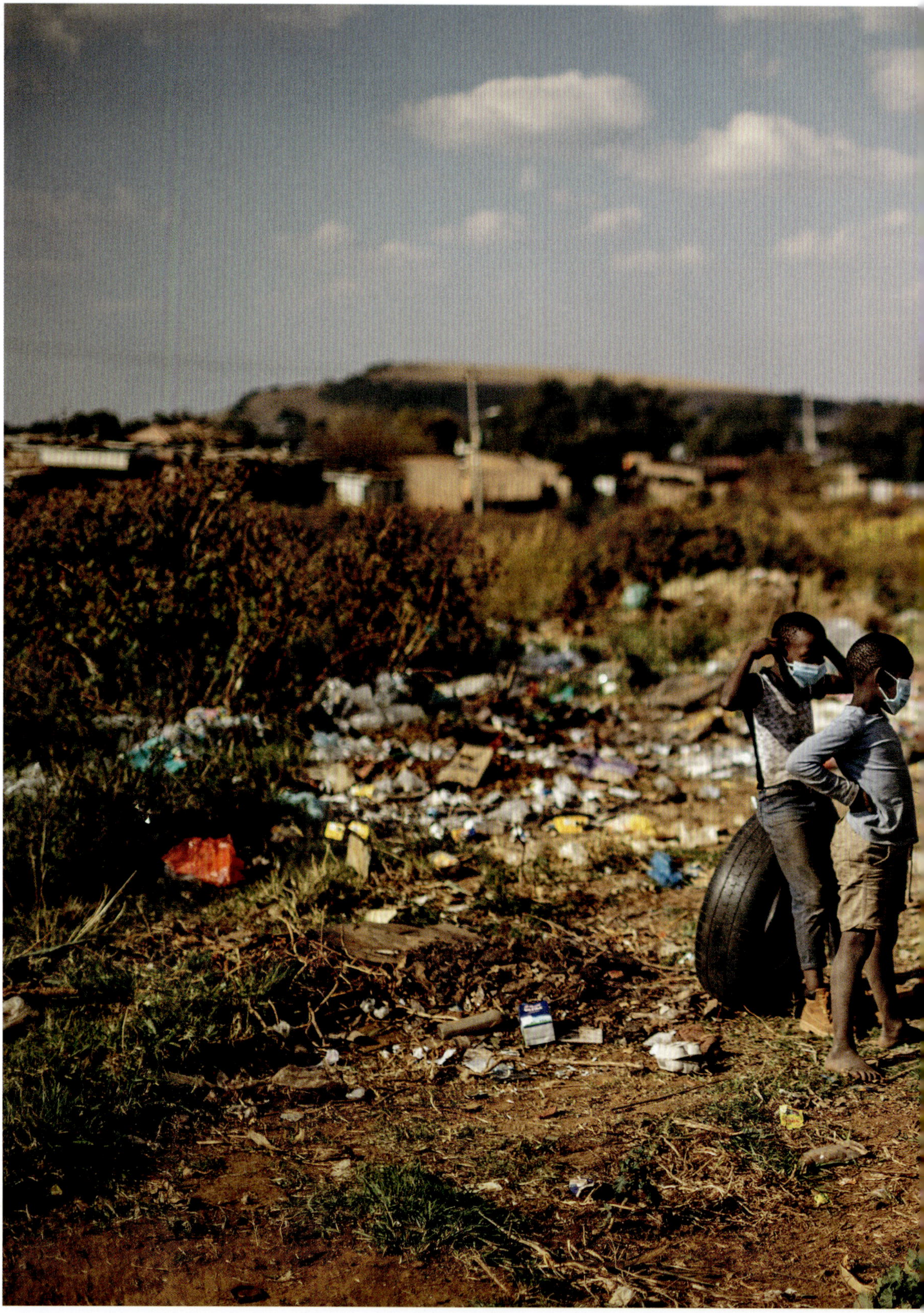

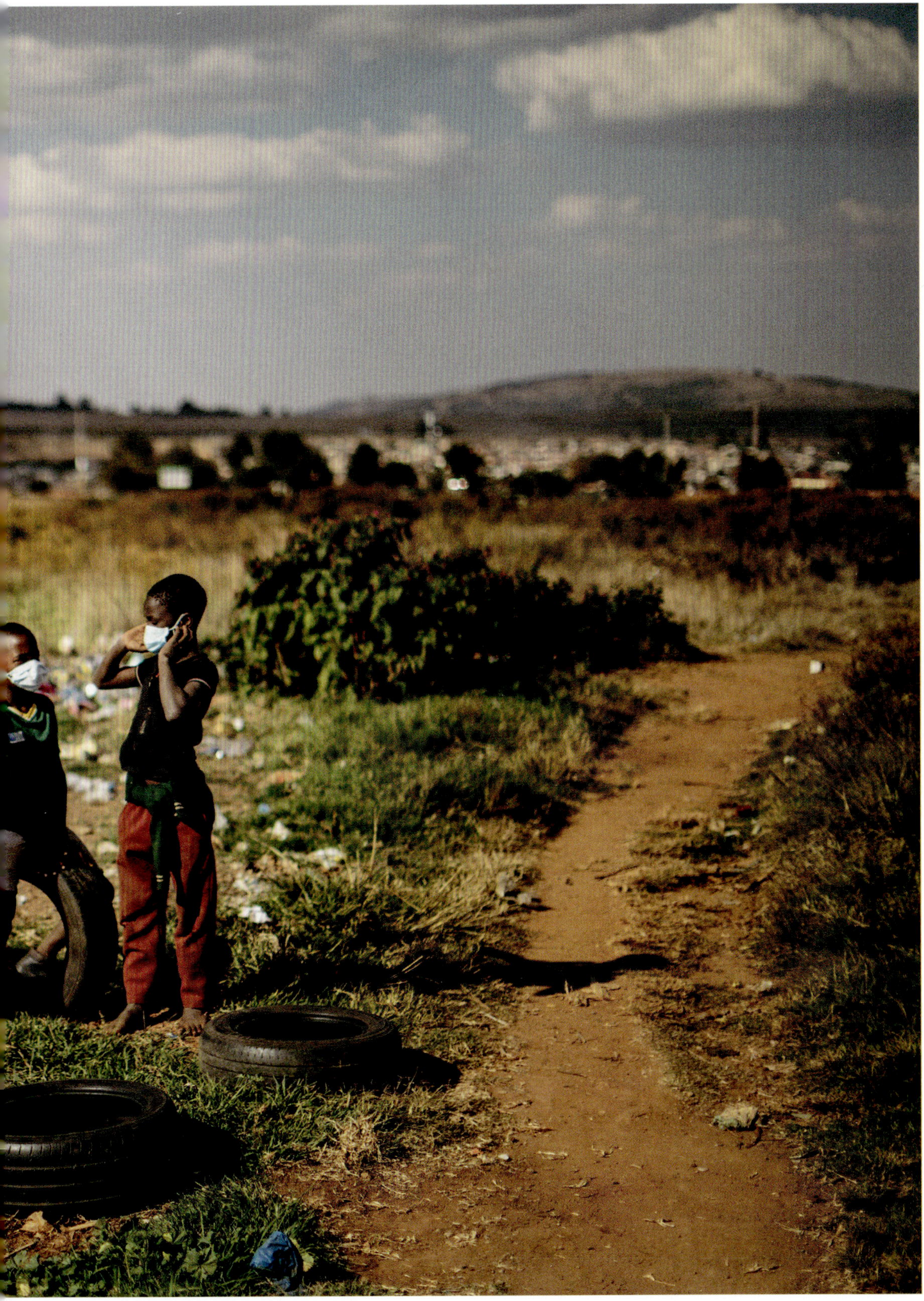

Colin Dutton, Italy
Threshold

There's no doubt that the lockdown will have had an effect on the well-being and development of children around the world and some, unfortunately, will have suffered more than others. I made these photographs in the north of Italy during the height of the coronavirus lockdown in the Spring of 2020. They are children of different ages photographed on the threshold of their home; a threshold representing the physical and psychological space to which they were confined for more than two months during one of the strictest lockdowns in Europe.
The word "threshold" can also be defined as an event that provokes change and I wanted to document this point of change in the lives of these children. For me, they are images of isolation but also of stillness, of non-action: waiting for the return of possibility. I gave each child a print so that in the future they can remember who they were, and where they were when it happened.
The series was shot in a small provincial town and as such there are some kids living in large houses out in the countryside and others in small apartments in the town centre. Having space will have helped to some degree during those months of quarantine. The effects of social isolation, however, will have been felt equally among them all.

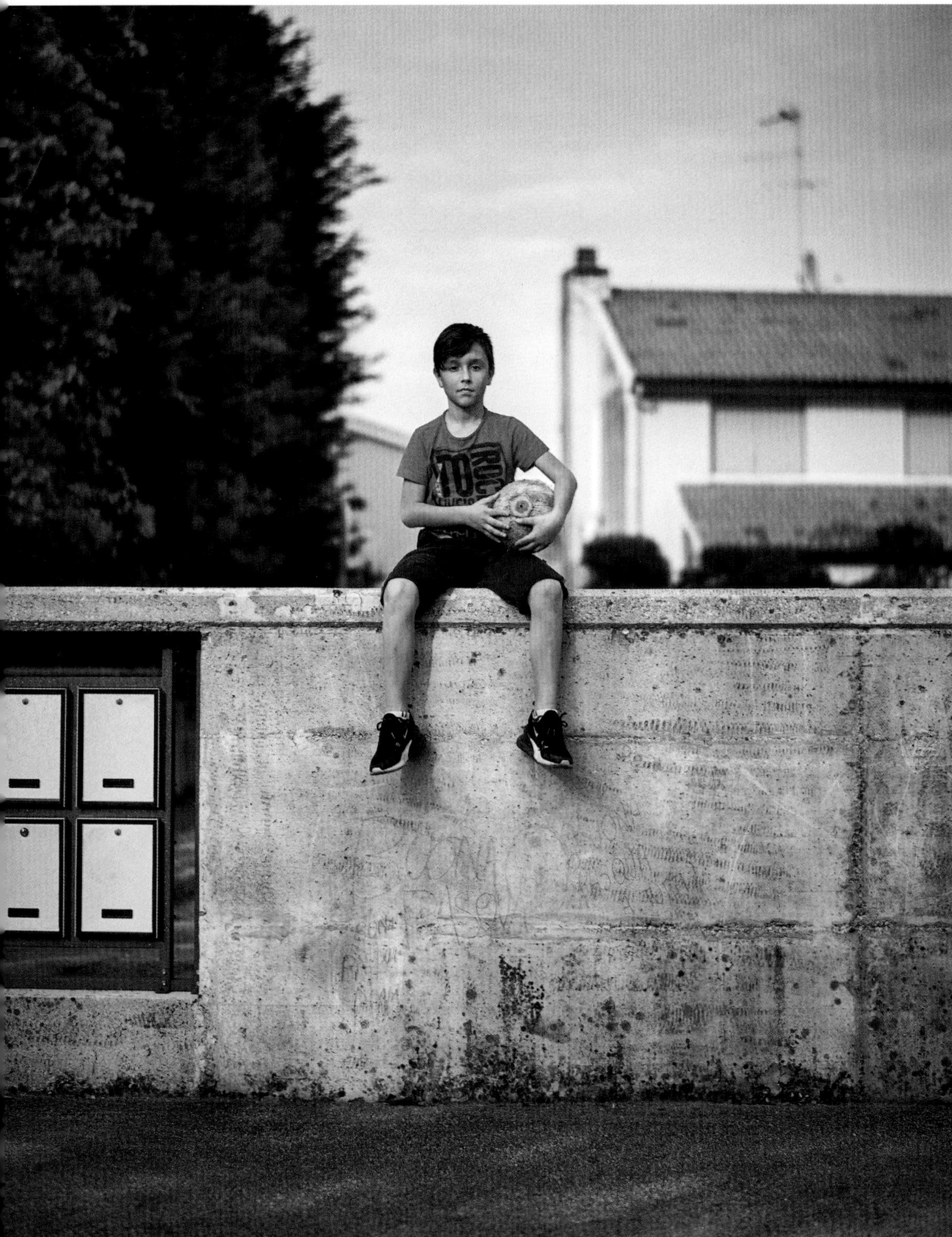

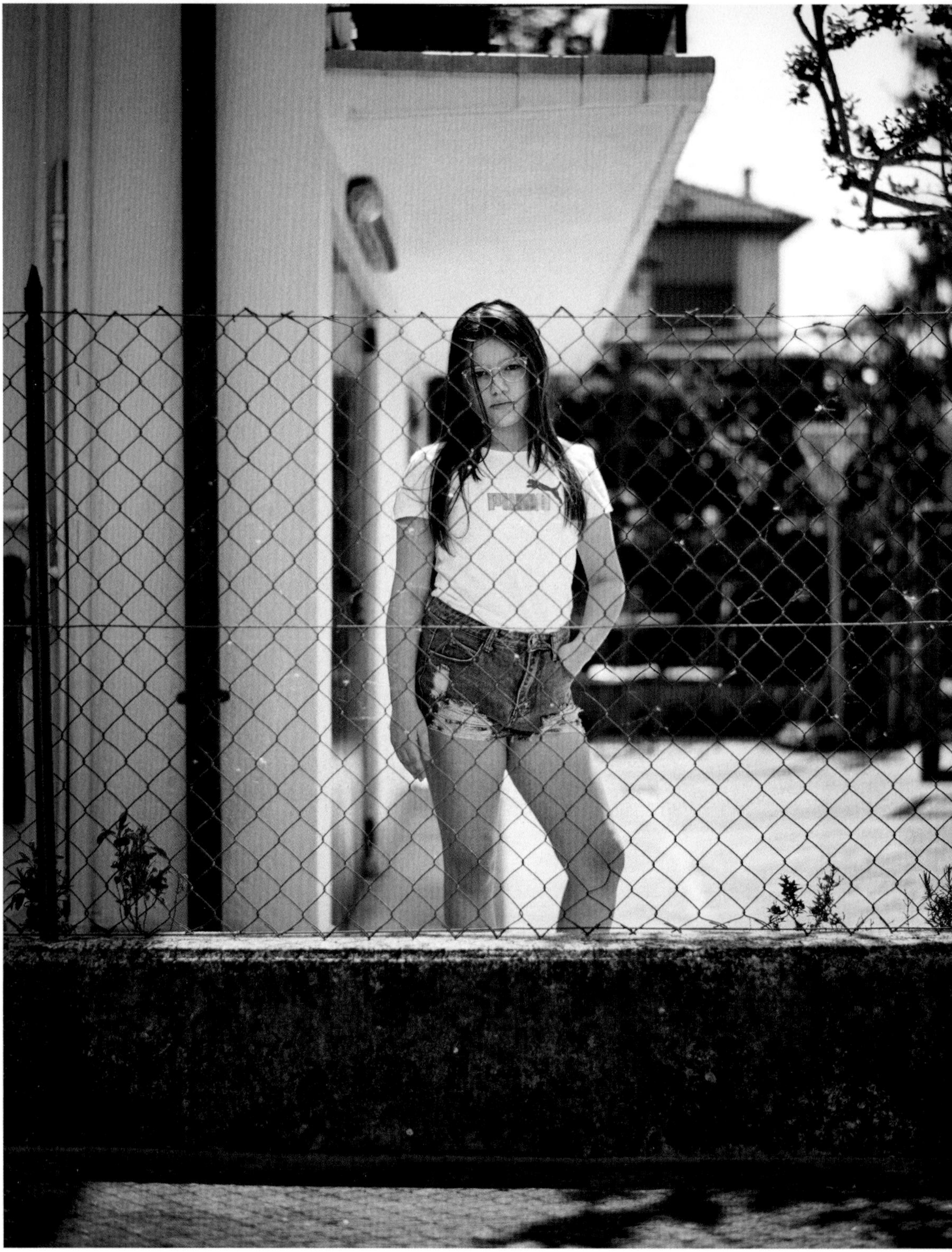
PUMA

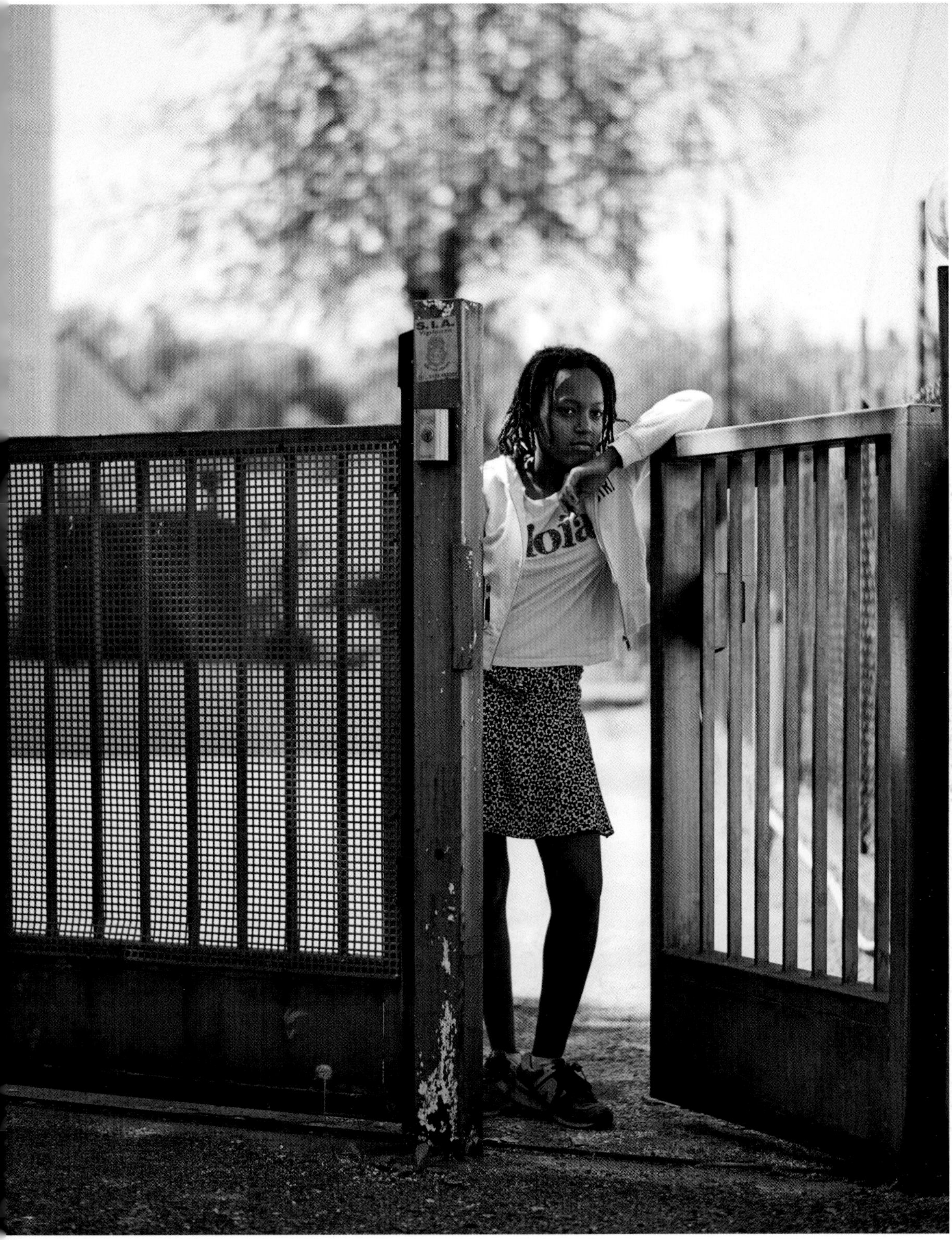
S.I.A.

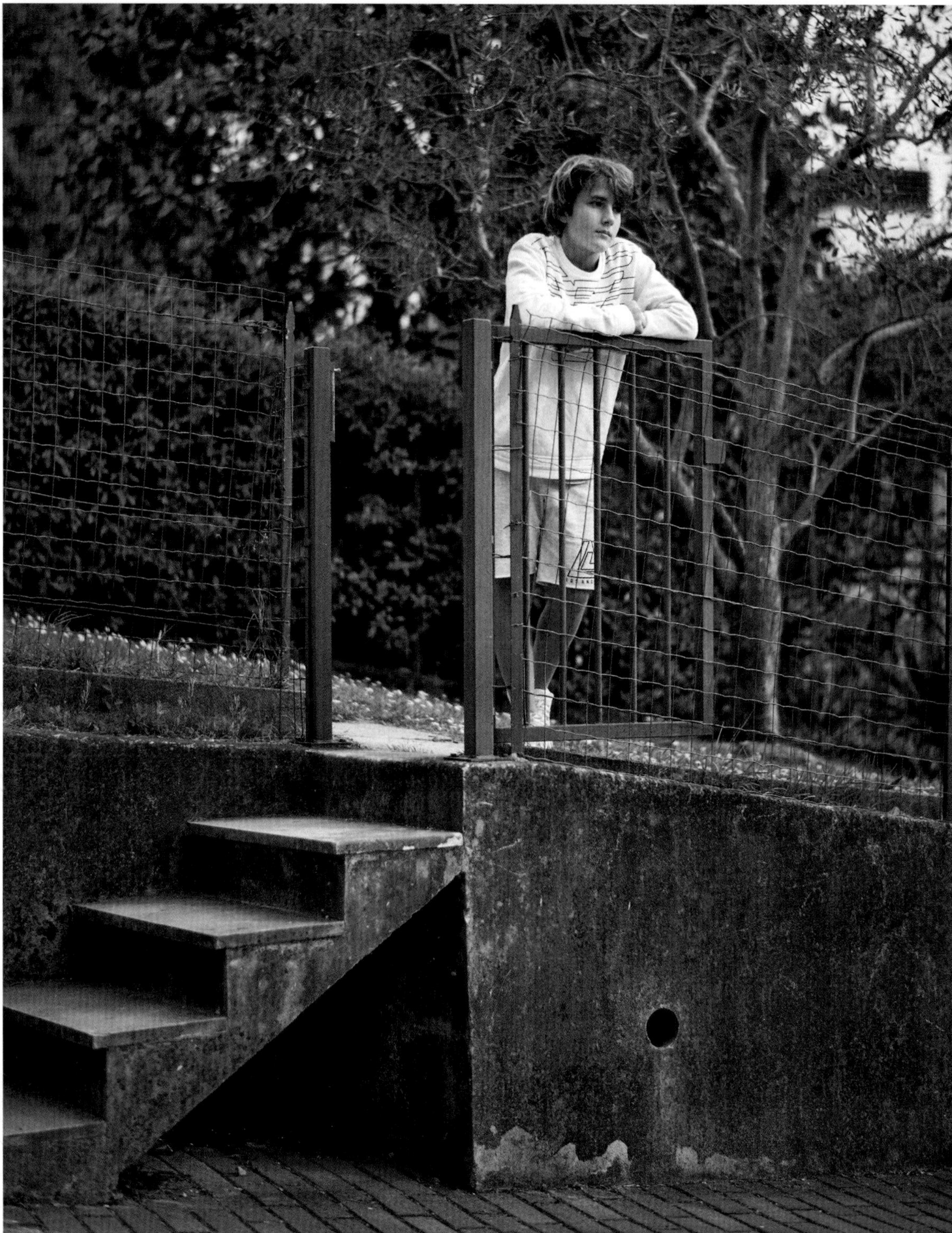

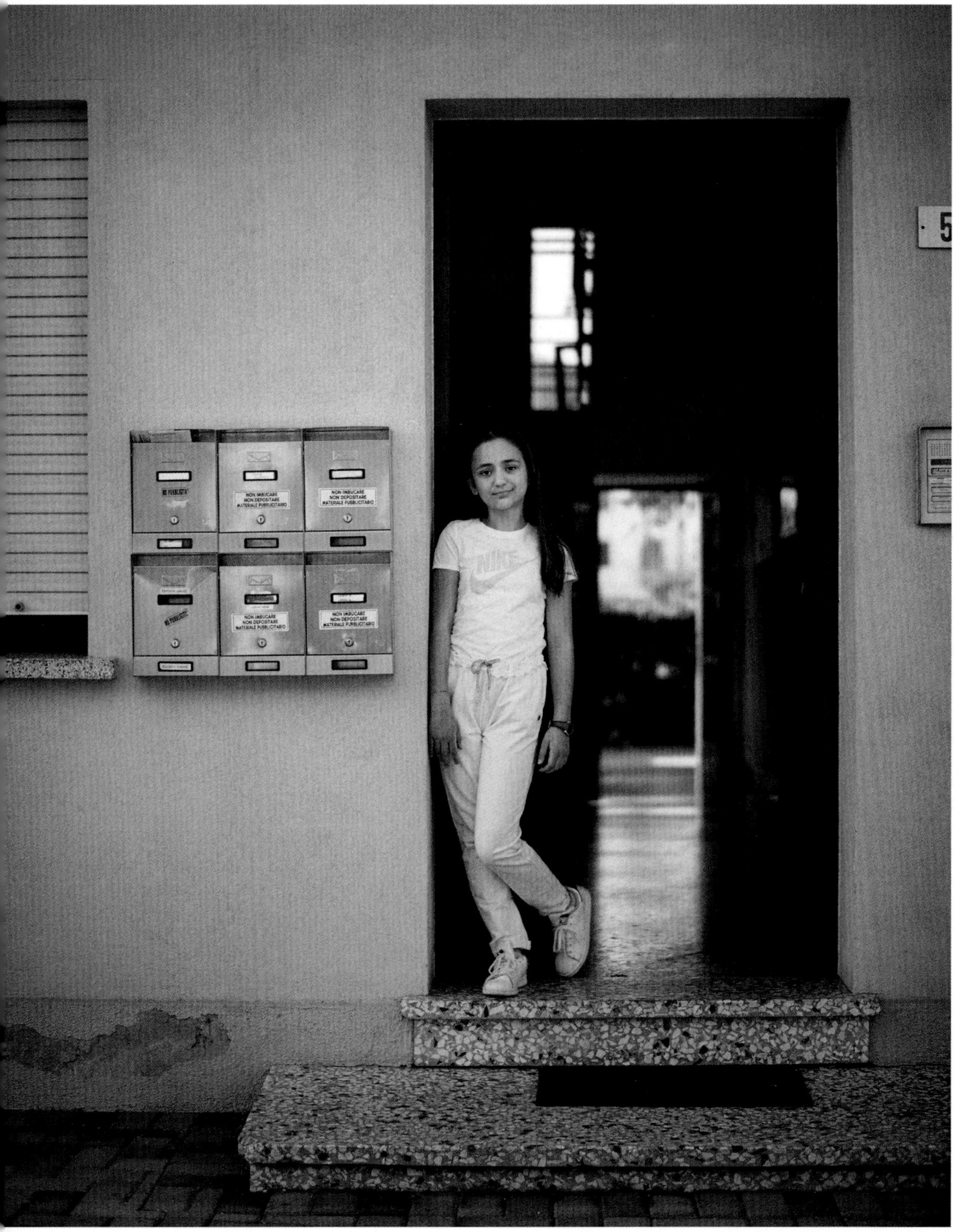
NON IMBUCARE
NON DEPOSITARE
MATERIALE PUBBLICITARIO
NIKE

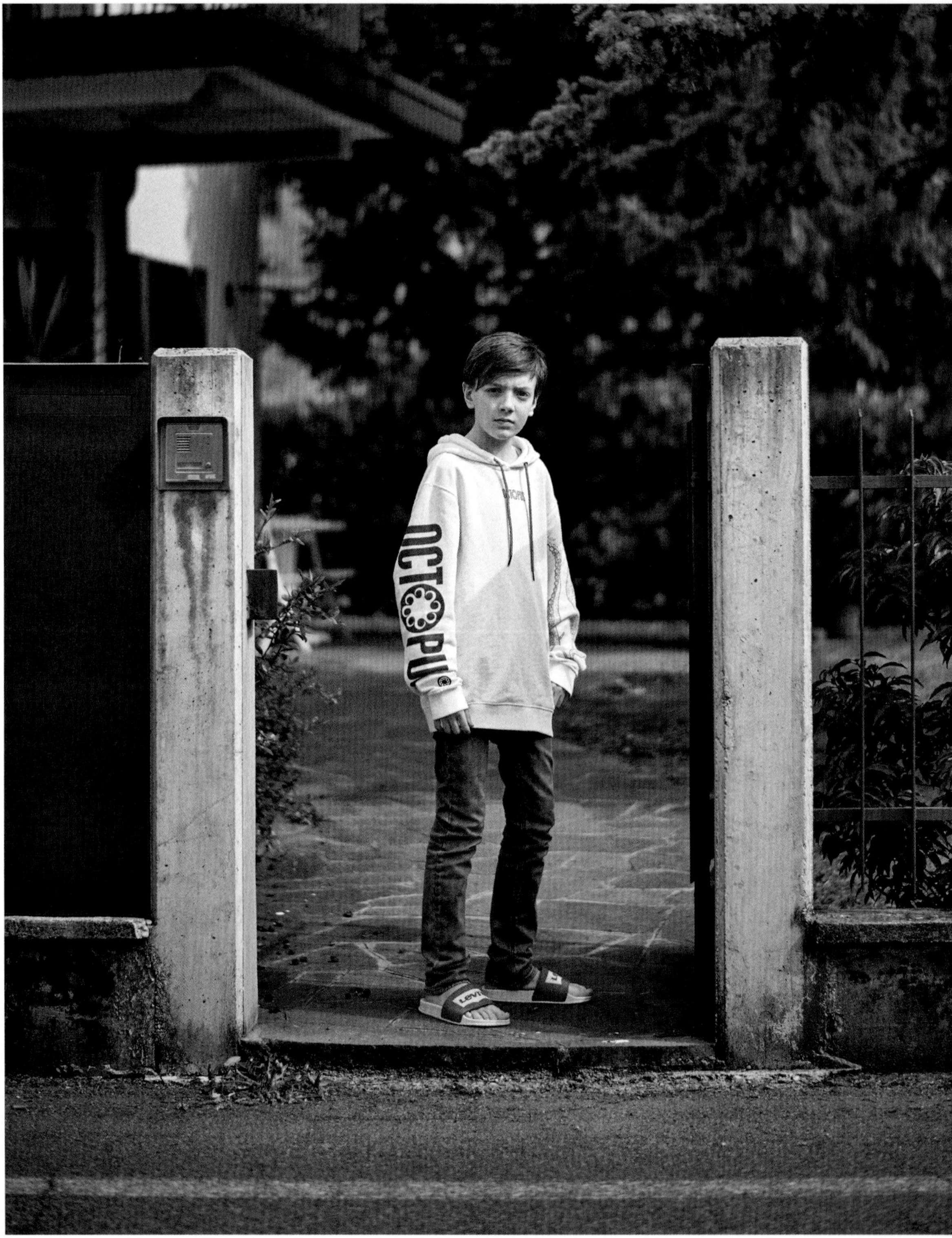

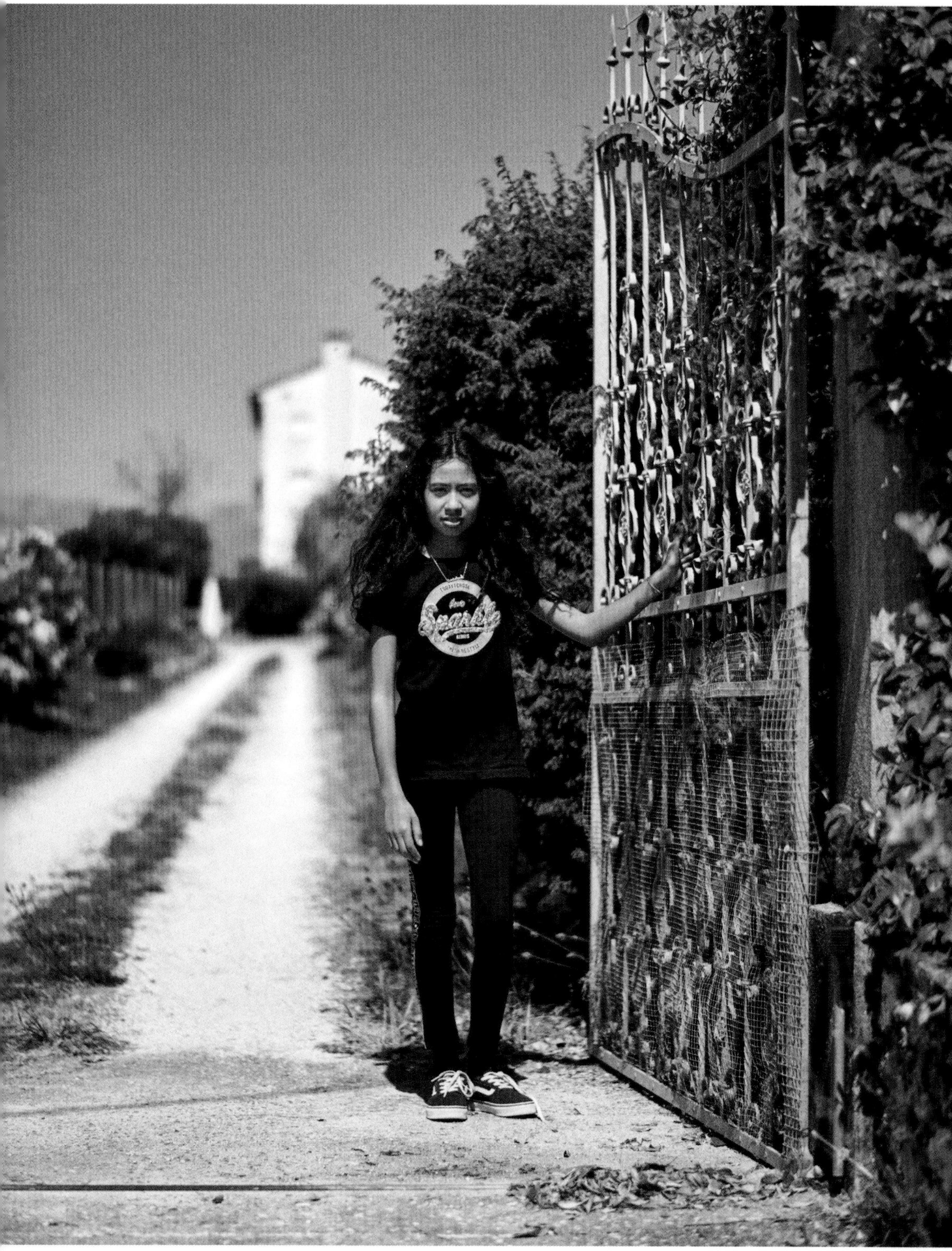

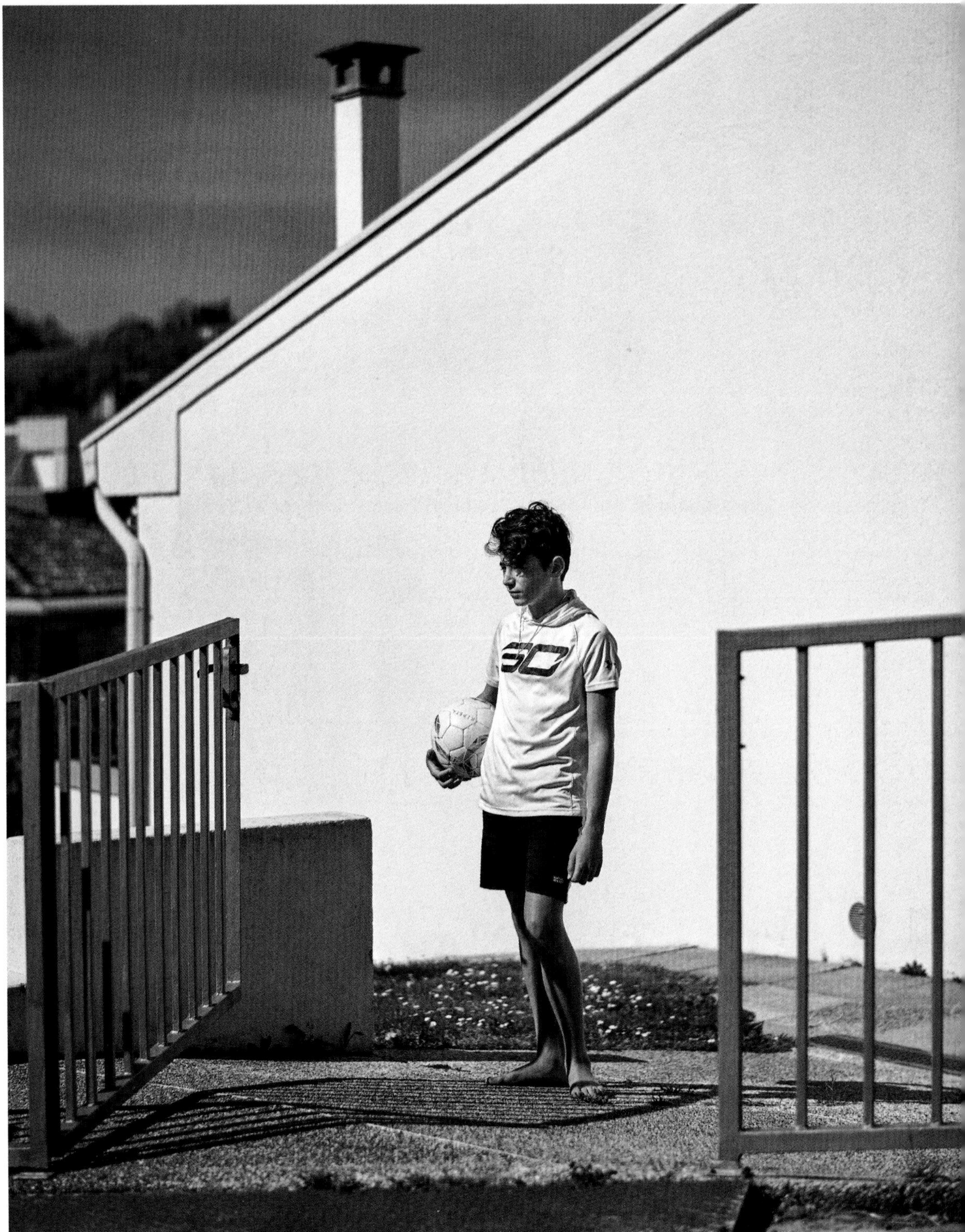

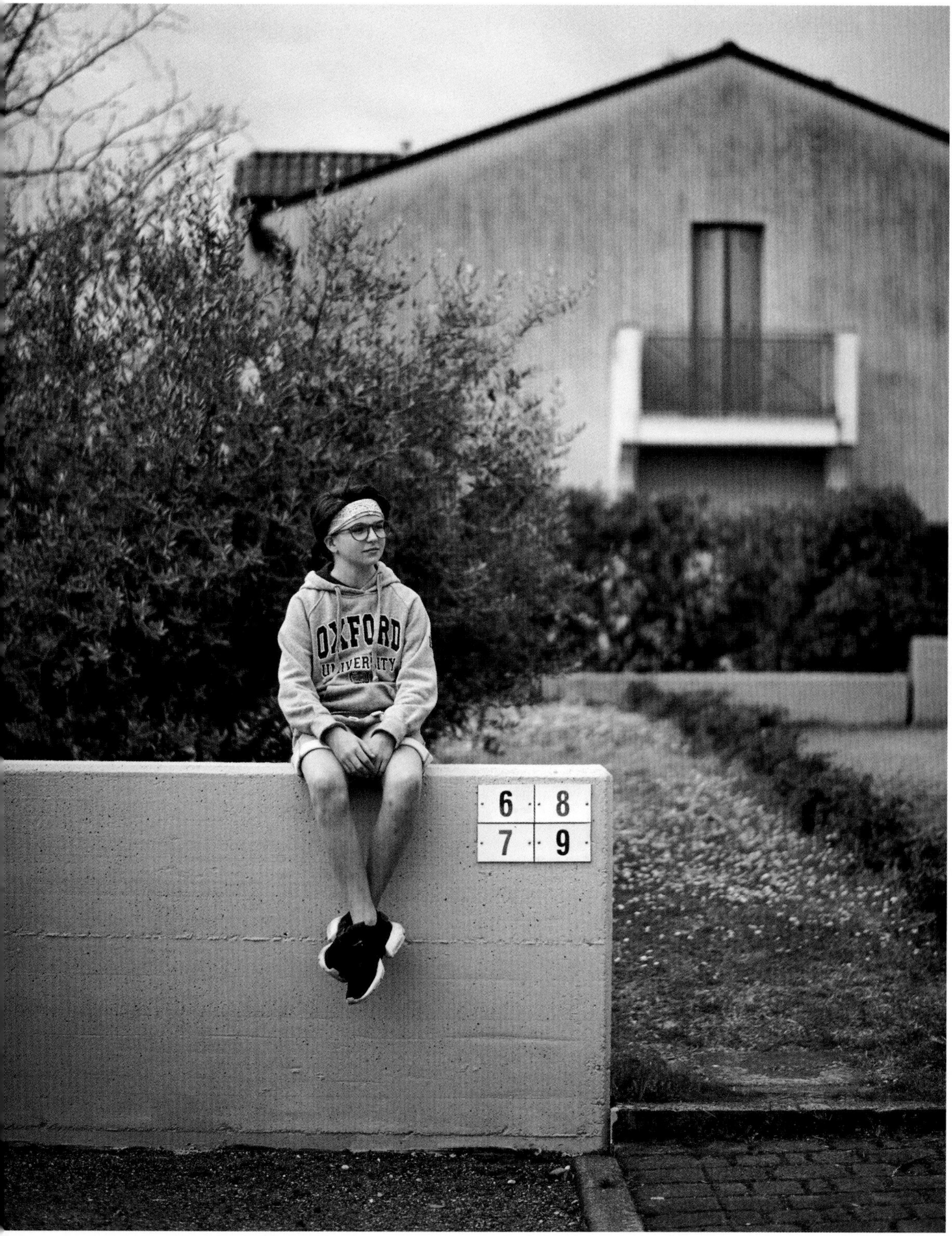
OXFORD
UNIVERSITY
6 8
7 9

05. A Wounded Society
Captions

Gideon Mendel, United Kingdom

The photographs were taken at Ridley Road Market in Hackney, London, between April and May 2020.

Ibtisaam Ali, accountant
I am a single parent and I have my three children and two grandchildren living at home along with my disabled brother. He has been happy because we're spending a lot more time together. I left my job a month before the lockdown and I now have been approved for universal credit, but my financial situation is hard with five people to support. My one son is a key worker for Sainsbury and he helps. I'm making masks for everybody now. I bought the fabrics on Holloway Road for one pound per metre. The elastic came from when I used to make clothes. It's very expensive to buy masks now. I don't want to buy masks every day to throw away. I am almost 50 and I am used to staying at home but it's hard for my family because they're young and they are just starting their lives, I am Muslim so I am used to covering my face in public, but wearing a mask is different because it's tighter than the loose veil I normally wear. It covers your chin and it makes it hard to breathe.
(Page 319)

Hamed Ali, carer
I work as a carer in Dalson, Monday to Friday. It has been hard because there are fewer carers working. I feel very worried about going outside sometimes. I wear a mask because I feel that anxiety, I don't like it but I have no choice. I need to protect myself and others.
(Page 320)

Fatima Farif, student
This situation now is difficult, I miss being outside and exploring London, I like taking the underground. I'm studying Business and Accounting and the course has moved online since this pandemic. It's not been too bad but I miss going to campus. I take wearing a mask outside very seriously because I have a condition called sickle cell anemia, which means that I am part of he vulnerable group. Because of this, I have been really worried about going outside. I go out only to buy food and nothing else.
(Page 321)

Manny Wongkaew, creative director, stylist and lecturer at UAL (University of the Arts London)
This is a big shift in my life. Normally I am always out and come home just to sleep. Now I am home all the time and it has opened me up to my local community. I have been walking on the canal as my daily exercise. I wake up, shower and then I'm ready to work. I finish work. I'm home all the time. Life is much simpler. I don't miss commuting at all. I'm a creative director and I teach. The classroom is now online. This can be an exciting opportunity for engaging and sharing ideas, but it is also hard. I miss physically creating something.
I support wearing masks to protect myself and protect people in our community.
(Page 322)

Helbing Cabral De Almada, retired
This situation is really hard for me because I'm an outgoing person; I like to be outside so staying home every day is hard. Wearing a mask is not easy but it's for our own good. I go on walks sometimes and to get food but that's it. At home I live with my daughter and my partner. We're all self-isolating together.
(Page 323)

Julliet Makhapila, community educator and poet
It's terrible to see that so many people are losing their lives through this pandemic. It makes you realise life is short. But it is also a good reminder that we are all connected to each other. We need to learn to share more in this world. The little things in life are the most beautiful of all: smiling every day and loving our neighbours. COVID-19 also reminds us that social inequality is very real. I am constantly worried about shops closing or not having any food. COVID-19 has also made certain products become very expensive and that impacts people who have less money. Today was my first time wearing a mask. I think if you have a good quality mask it tricks your mind into thinking you're going to be okay. For me, having one is just a comfort. I don't believe it really makes a difference and I think the biggest practice is having good hygiene. Also washing hands, social distancing and self-isolating.
I worry that masks could bring about more crime, because it conceals people's identities. But I understand we need to follow guidelines given by our government.
(Page 324)

Adam Hammond, IT manager
My girlfriend moved here from Croatia about three weeks before the lockdown. Previously we'd not spent more than two weeks together, even though we've known each other for twelve years. It's been really great, actually. Having been stuck together now for six or seven weeks, she feels like this is home. It's been really nice to have her here. The situation hasn't really affected me financially because I can work from home. In a way it's made it quite easy to work and live with other people in the flat because we all are very busy, working eight hours a day. And then we look forward to cooking and drinking and hanging out all together after. I'm getting kind of comfortable with it I guess, which is a strange thing, isn't it?
(Page 325)

Ambia Rahman and Khalisur Rahman, housewife and retired chef
Ambia: This situation stops you from doing anything. We've been spending time inside the house and we live with our two grown up children so it feels crowded. You feel like you want to go out, but you know you can't. I have a garden and I feel lucky about that. We sit out there when the sun is out. Sometimes my husband and I go for a walk. I feel if people are wearing masks it's okay but there are so many people that are not wearing any.
This situation is not coming to an end soon. We want it to come to an end so that we can go back to how life was before. And that's why people need to wear masks and wear gloves. They need to be cautious so this can end faster.
(Page 326)

Abdalla Elbiiman, shop assistant
My work situation has not changed too much so that's okay. I am still able to work in the shop. Work is busier than usual so it keeps my mind occupied. I find wearing a mask too much, it doesn't feel natural and is uncomfortable on my face. But I wear it so I am safe and other people feel safe.
We do what we can.
(Page 327)

Nanna Heitmann, Russia

Lubov is from Wolgograd and says she came to Moscow 10 days ago. She is holding a poster with a prayer against the coronavirus. She says she will be standing with it in front of the Duma the next day. Park near Kurskiy train station, Moscow, April 2020.
(Page 329)

At the tent of the Russian Orthodox charity Miloserdi that feeds homeless people every day. Because of new hygienic rules only a few people at once are let into the tent. So many people have to wait in front until their turn. Moscow, May 2020.
(Pages 330-331)

In the tents of the charity Miloserdi a volunteer prepares food for people in need. Usually they feed around 50 people a day. Since the outbreak started already more than 100 people came to eat at Miloserdi only in the morning hours. Moscow, April 2020.
(Page 332)

A woman recently lost her work in a greenhouse in Dagestan and is stranded now in Moscow, homeless with a high fever and a cough. Lana and Marian, doctors from Dom Druzey, a charity that helps homeless people, provide basic medical care. April 2020.
(Page 333)

People left without a home wait in a line to receive medical treatment or medicine. Doctors notice a rise of pneumonia cases among homeless people. Park near Kurskiy train station, Moscow, April 2020.
(Page 334)

Lana and her colleague from Dom Druzey (House of friends) treat a homeless couple in the park. Lana tells me that cases of pneumonia among homeless people have risen but they will never know if it was Covid. Park near Kurskiy train station, Moscow, April 2020.
(Page 335)

Areski and Mokrane are both students from Algeria who were studying Russian in St. Petersburg. They came to Moscow in the hope the Algerian embassy would organise a flight back home without any results. Now they are stranded in the quarantine hostel of the charity Dom Druzey. May 2020.
(Page 336)

Natascha and her daughter Uliana in the Mother's House of the Russian Orthodox charity Miloserdi. Natascha has been living here since February. She says that the father of her child was abusive to her. As most women in the shelter she is waiting until quarantine is over to be able to prepare documents and start a normal life. Moscow, May 2020.
(Page 337)

Storage in the newly opened guesthouse, a shelter organised by the charity Dom Druzey. Moscow, May 2020.
(Page 338)

Claudia Ignatovna, 80-year-old, just moved into the new opened hostel of the charity Dom Druzhey. She is tired of being moved from one place to the other all the time. She worked as an engineer in the Soviet Union. As it happens often to elderly people in Moscow, where the cost of living is expensive, her niece betrayed her and took away her apartment so now she is homeless. May 2020.
(Page 339)

Nicoló Lanfranchi, Brazil

Luciana Machado, 41-year-old, alcohol and cigarette vendor on the sidewalk in front of the buildings. Cruzada São Sebastião, Leblon. 18 May 2020.
(Page 342, top)

An inhabitant of a building cleans the access stairs to the apartments of the Cruzada São Sebastião social housing complex, Leblon. 23 May 2020.
(Page 342, bottom)

Man with sign offering to buy gold on crowded street in the suburb Duque de Caxias, Rio de Janeiro, the day of the reopening of the shops. 25 May 2020.
(Page 343, top)

Andre Felipe, 26, at work in the Americanas market in Ipanema. 18 May 2020.
(Page 343, bottom)

Supporters of the Brazilian President Jair Bolsonaro during a protest in Copacabana, despite the ban on agglomeration.
27 March 2020.
(Page 344)

The courtyard between 2 of the 10 buildings in Cruzada São Sebastião social housing in Leblon. 18 May 2020.
(Page 345)

A check point at the entrance of the favela Dona Marta, Rio de Janeiro, where people washing their hands, leaving and entering the favela. 27 March 2020.
(Page 346, top)

An inhabitant of a building with a "cesta basica" (bag of basic necessities such as rice, beans, sugar...) just received from a group of volunteers working for a local NGO, in front of her apartment in the Cruzada São Sebastião social housing complex, Leblon. 23 May 2020.
(Page 346, bottom)

Disinfection of the buildings in the Cruzada São Sebastião social housing complex, Leblon. 18 May 2020.
(Page 347, top)

Kauan Alves, 17-year-old, and Alexandre Silva, 19. Alexandre is a student. "I take the pandemic seriously, I only go out if there is a need". He lives with his mother (48) and grandmother (64) who still work as cook and street sweeper. "Racism, inequality? It's not something born now, so I can't feel anger. It is dissatisfaction. I continue on my way." Cruzada São Sebastião, Leblon. 18 May 2020.
(Page 347, bottom)

The funeral of Elizabeth Baez, 82-year-old, died with COVID-19. In the presence of her only son, while her husband is also hospitalised in the intensive care unit, also with COVID-19. Cemetery of São João Batista, Rio de Janeiro. 08 April 2020.
(Page 348)

The new vertical section where the body of the COVID-19 victims are now buried in Inhaúma cemetery, Rio de Janeiro. 18 May 2020.
(Page 349)

Street cleaners at work, in the city of Niterói. 27 March 2020.
(Page 350)

The empty beach in Copacabana during the lockdown. 27 March 2020.
(Page 351)

Farshid Tighehsaz, Iran

My sister Shadi posing for a picture on her wedding day in the suburb of Tabriz. She married in the first three months after the pandemic was officially announced. Her wedding day was very quiet and with no guest. She said: "I had no ever imagined that my wedding would be like this. Coronavirus truly changed normal life, it makes us alone and fearful". 6 May 2020.
(Page 353)

People came to the cemetery for their family member who died because of COVID-19. They are not allowed to approach the burial ground and they must assist from afar. 8 October 2020.
(Pages 354–355)

The view of a half-finished building abandoned due to the lockdown in the city of Tabriz. 25 February, 2020.
(Page 356, top)

Sima lies on her bed naked and covers her body with a curtain at at home in Tabriz, in self-quarantine. "Here I have to hide all my femininity and now I have to hide myself from this invisible enemy", she said. 24 July 2020.
(Page 356, bottom)

70-year-old Abbas is reading the news about Iran's political tensions with US in his laptop during self-quarantine. He was a political activist during Iran's revolution. That time he and his brother were imprisoned because of their activism. In recent years Abbas got hyperglycemia disease and he has to be under a strict diet and stress control. In the current pandemic time he has to be careful and stay at home in Tabriz, in self-quarantine. 22 November 2020.
(Page 357, top)

Unknown future. Tabriz, Iran. 25 February 2020.
(Page 357, bottom)

Two cemetery tecnicians carry the dead body for washing before burying. Approximately more than twenty COVID-19 case bodies are buried every day in Tabriz's public cemetery. 8 October 2020.
(Page 358)

Two clerics are praying for a dead person before burial in Tabriz's cemetery. According to official statistics more than 60 thousand people died in Iran because of COVID-19 till now. 8 October 2020.
(Page 359)

Mother and father came to their son's grave in Tabriz. He was 25 years old when he died because of coronavirus. 26 November 2020.
(Pages 360–361)

Michele Spatari, South Africa

A man over-watches a taxi sanitation at Wanderers taxi rank in Johannesburg Central Business District. March 2020.
(Page 363)

The deserted street of Alexandra township during the national lockdown imposed to stem the spread of COVID-19 coronavirus in Johannesburg. April 2020.
(Page 364)

Members of the South African Police Service (SAPS) patrols the densely populated Diesploot township in Johannesburg wearing face masks and gloves amid concerns over the spread of COVID-19 coronavirus. March 2020.
(Page 365)

A patrol of South African National Defence Forces Military Police walks in the streets of Hillbrow, Johannesburg, as residents look from the balconies. March 2020.
(Page 366, top)

A South African National Defence Force (SANDF) Armoured Personnel Carrier in the Johannesburg Central Business District during the first day of the national lockdown. March 2020.
(Page 366, bottom)

Steven Smith, a Scientology volunteer minister, sprays a taxi with disinfectant at the Bree taxi rank in Newtown, Johannesburg, during a sanitisation drive organised by the religious movement. May 2020.
(Page 367, top)

A Gauteng health Department Official gets ready for a door-to-door testing drive in Yeoville, Johannesburg. April 2020.
(Page 367, bottom)

Volunteers from the Rays of Hope NGO moves food parcels for a meal distribution in Alexandra, Johannesburg. April 2020.
(Page 368, top)

A doctor walks toward a patient during a COVID-19 coronavirus screening and testing drive in front of the Madala Hostel in Alexandra, Johannesburg. April 2020.
(Page 368, bottom)

Men queue for a food portion package during a distribution organised by a local Muslim organisation in the Kwa Mai Mai area of the Johannesburg Central Business District; May 2020. Over 50 people, residents of the same building and mostly migrants are currently unemployed because of the lockdown imposed by the South African authorities to curb the spread of COVID-19 coronavirus. Dozens of the foreign nationals are unable to feed themselves, as the only charity providing them with food has not brought any in several days.
(Page 368)

Johannesburg's Alexandra township residents queue to be tested at a COVID-19 coronavirus screening and testing drive-in. April 2020.
(Page 369)

Children play outside the Vlakfontein Clinic in Lenasia, south of Johannesburg. May 2020.
(Pages 370–371)

Colin Dutton, Italy

The photographs were taken in April and May 2020.

Alessandro, 11-year-old.
(Page 373)

Veronica, 10-year-old.
(Page 374)

Genet, 11-year-old.
(Page 375)

Giorgio, 13-year-old.
(Page 376)

Ilarja, 10-year-old.
(Page 377)

James, 13-year-old.
(Page 378)

Sabrina, 10-year-old.
(Page 379)

Alessandro, 12-year-old.
(Page 380)

Eugenia, 13-year-old.
(Page 381)

06.

A New Normal

Michele Borzoni, Italy
How to Social Distance

Giuseppe Smorto

Bans, forbidden seats, mandatory routes, all cities at the time of the pandemic are full of limits. Urban space has become a threatening place, full of dangers that frighten precisely because they are invisible.
The impact of social distancing does not only have to do with physical proximity and our sense of distrust, but also has important repercussions on how we experience the public space.
A collective condition is what stands out from Michele Borzoni's photos: in his work on "social distancing" he seems to look from above at supermarkets, schools and universities, outdoor masses and prayers on Fridays, kiosks and concerts, condominium meetings and railway stations. But his approach is not about detachment, it is instead the gaze of everyone, of what we have been and are in these months of sacrificed freedom and stifled passions. This made us more equal.
We even saw powerful personalities and unreachable footballers queuing up for groceries, a sign that the enemy is mutual, the meeting space has become threatening. No coincidence, Borzoni chose to set this work in Florence: because he too, like everyone else, got stuck due to the lockdown. But it is the most beautiful location: a city of art that has been on the move for centuries, with magnificent interiors and exteriors.
One may find resignation in these images, but the author sees a form of melancholy. "I would also call it nostalgia for the past times when we could meet without fear, nostalgia for a shared life. In addition, I find that there is also a certain obstinacy by the citizens, the desire to go back to our habits."
Yet the distance is evident, there is an explicitly cold vision of the scene, it somehow feels as if we were not part of it. But all of us certainly were part of it, and in a few years we could look at this photo and say: "That's how we were".
According to Borzoni, such a distance is "not only social, but above all physical". He wants to point out that in these photos there is nothing intimate – in fact the protagonists all seem to be alone. The luckiest ones speak from a distance or remotely.
Now that distancing has also become a family problem, because the enemy is also at home, we will have to think about narrating it.
But today, divided and distanced, we look in the direction of hope.

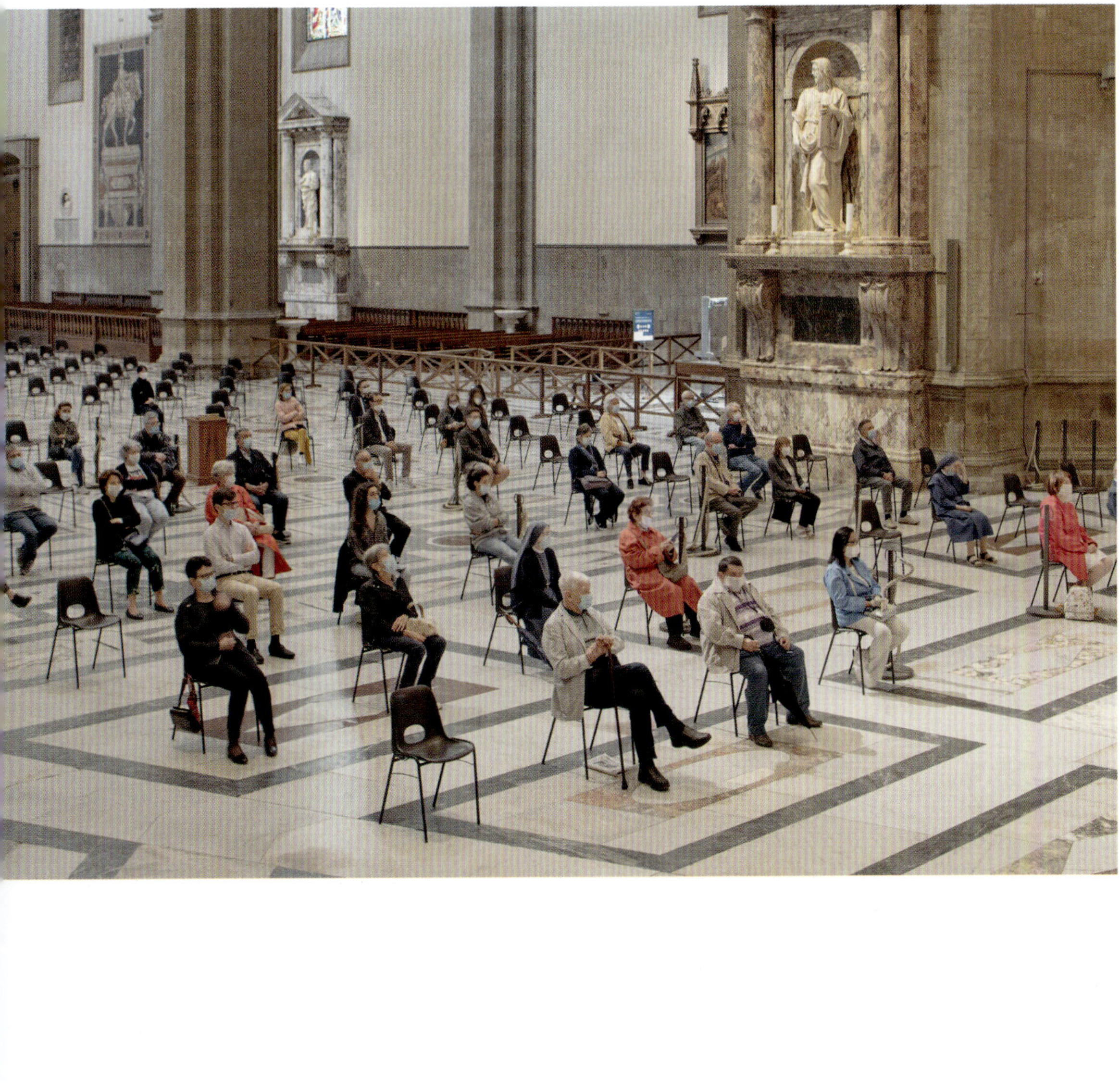

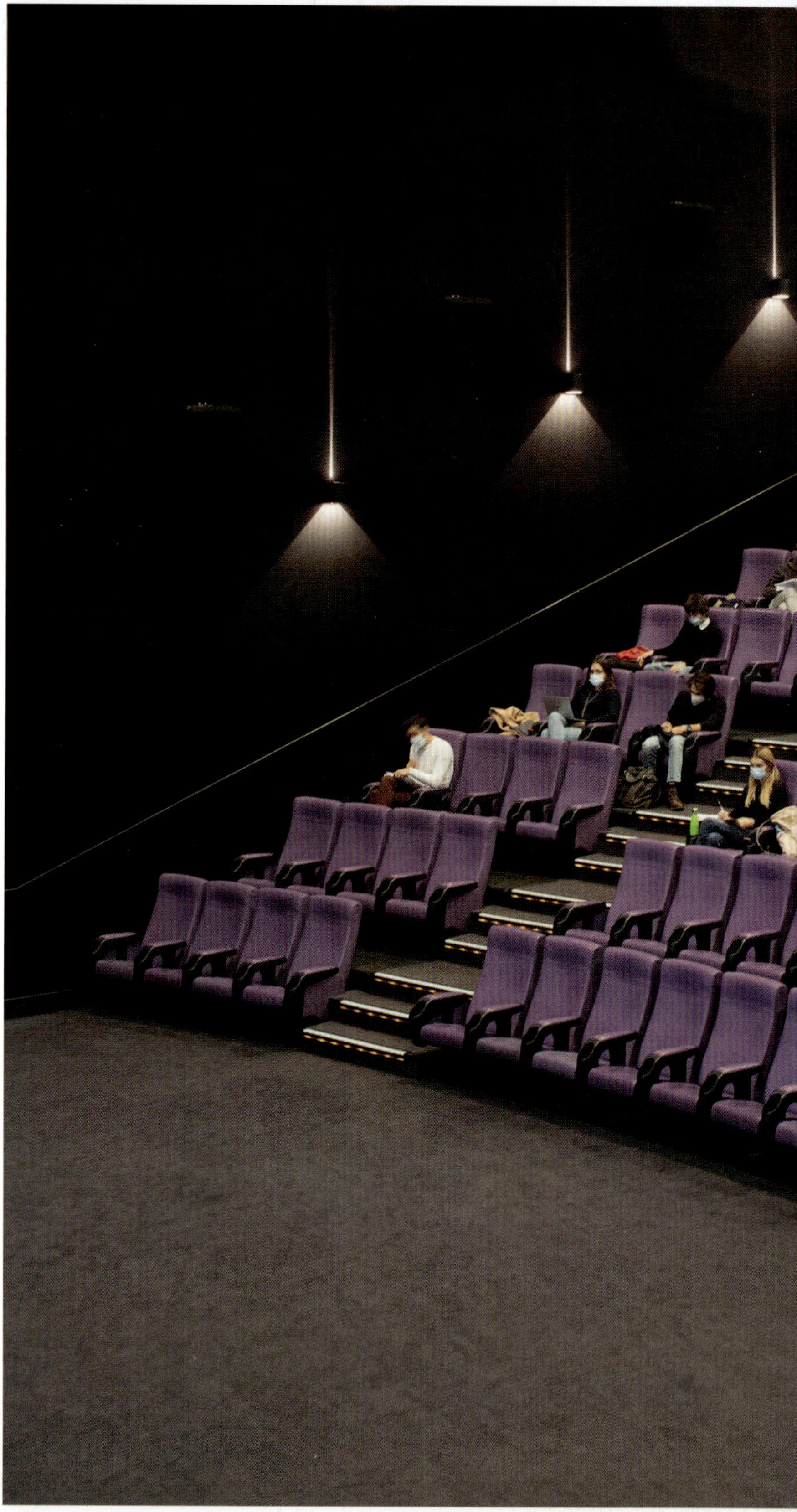

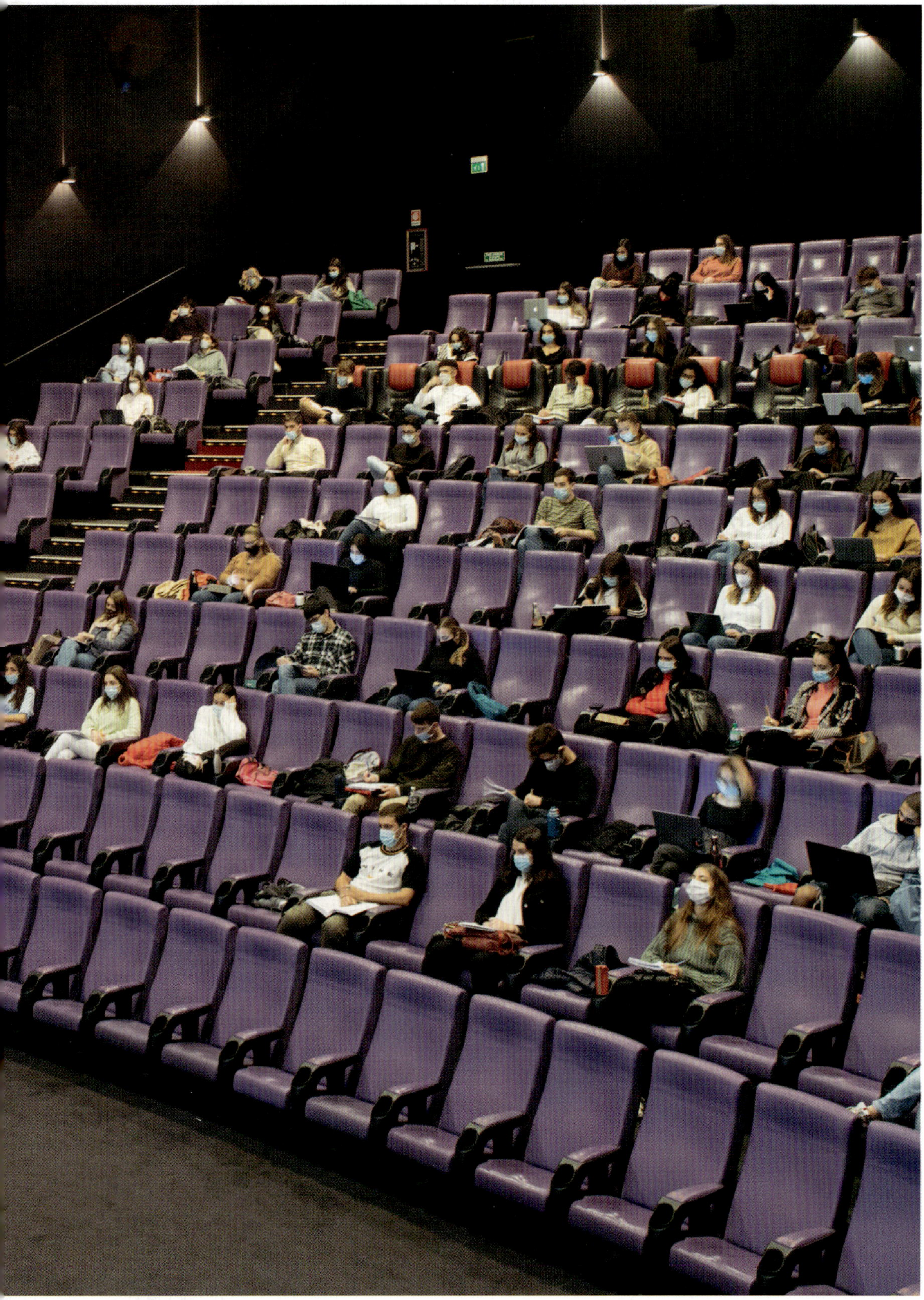

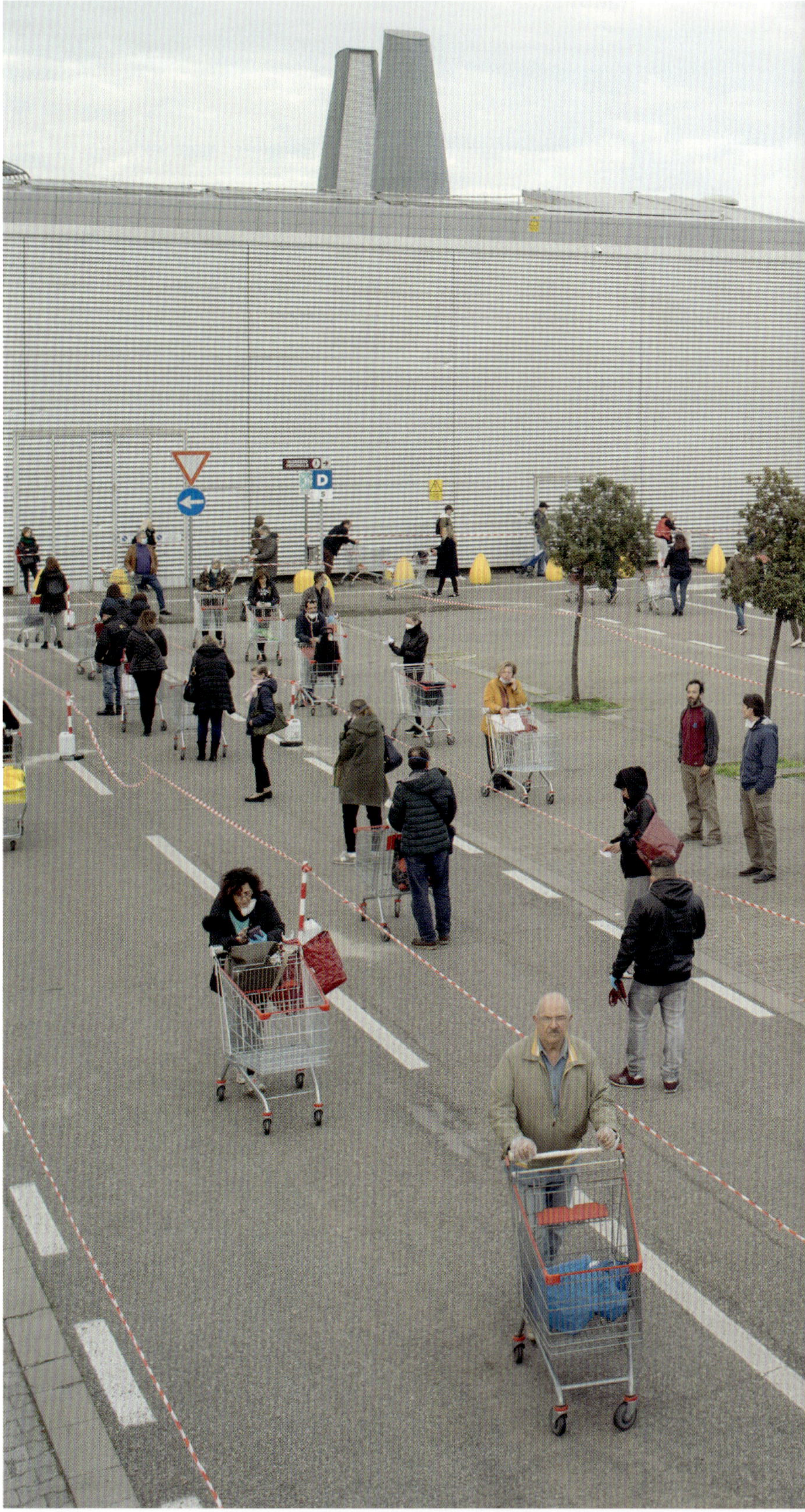

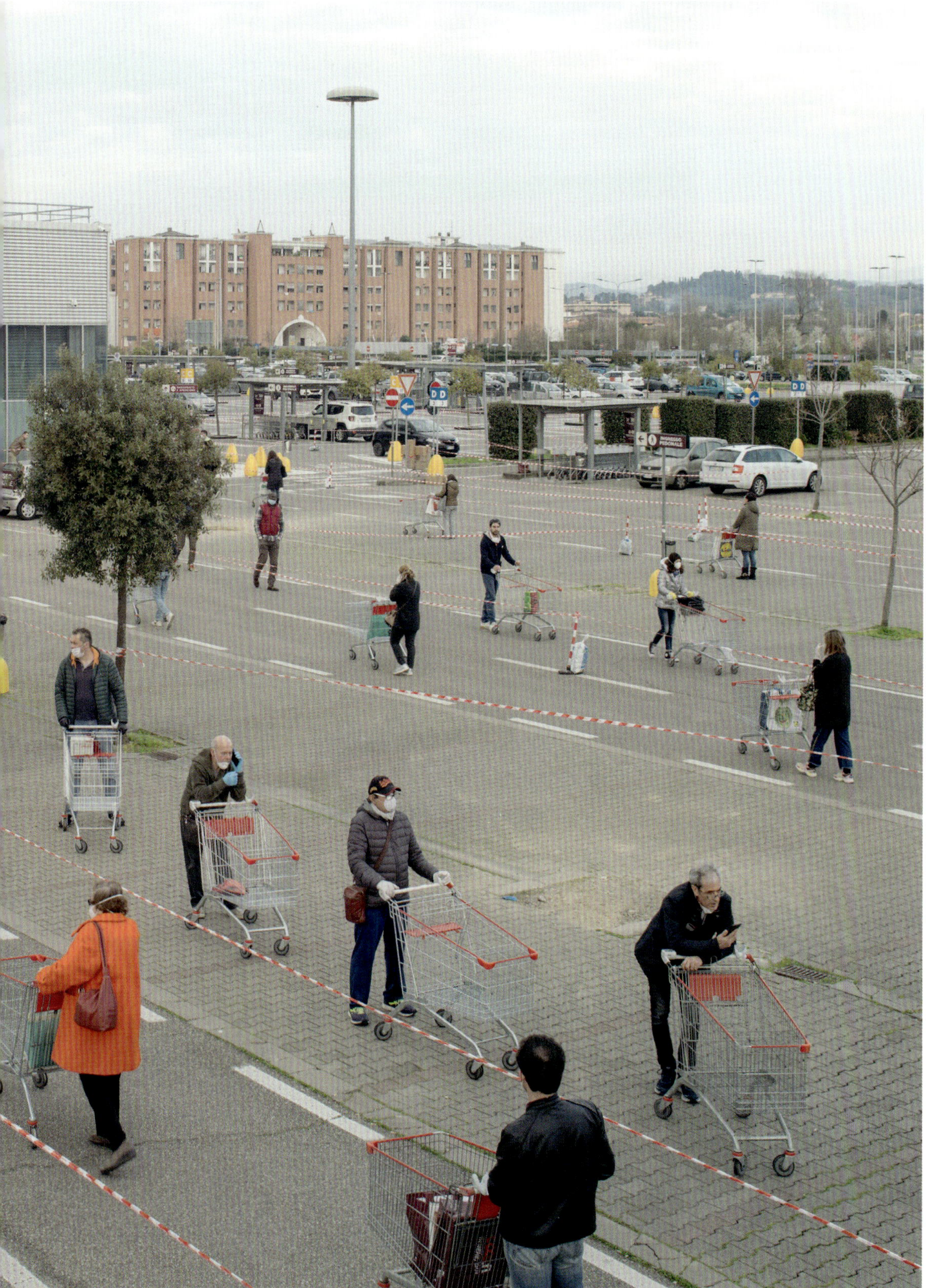

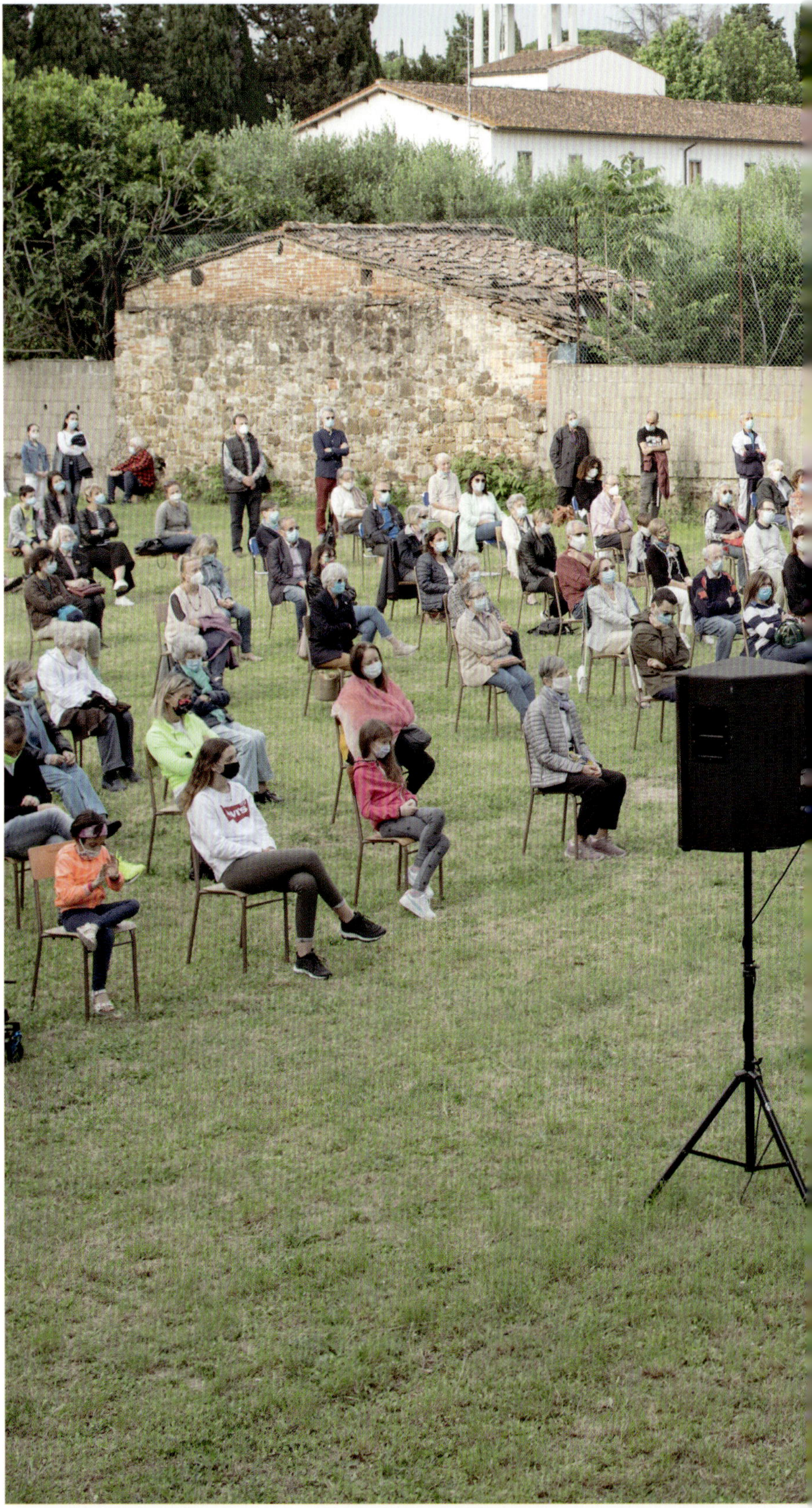

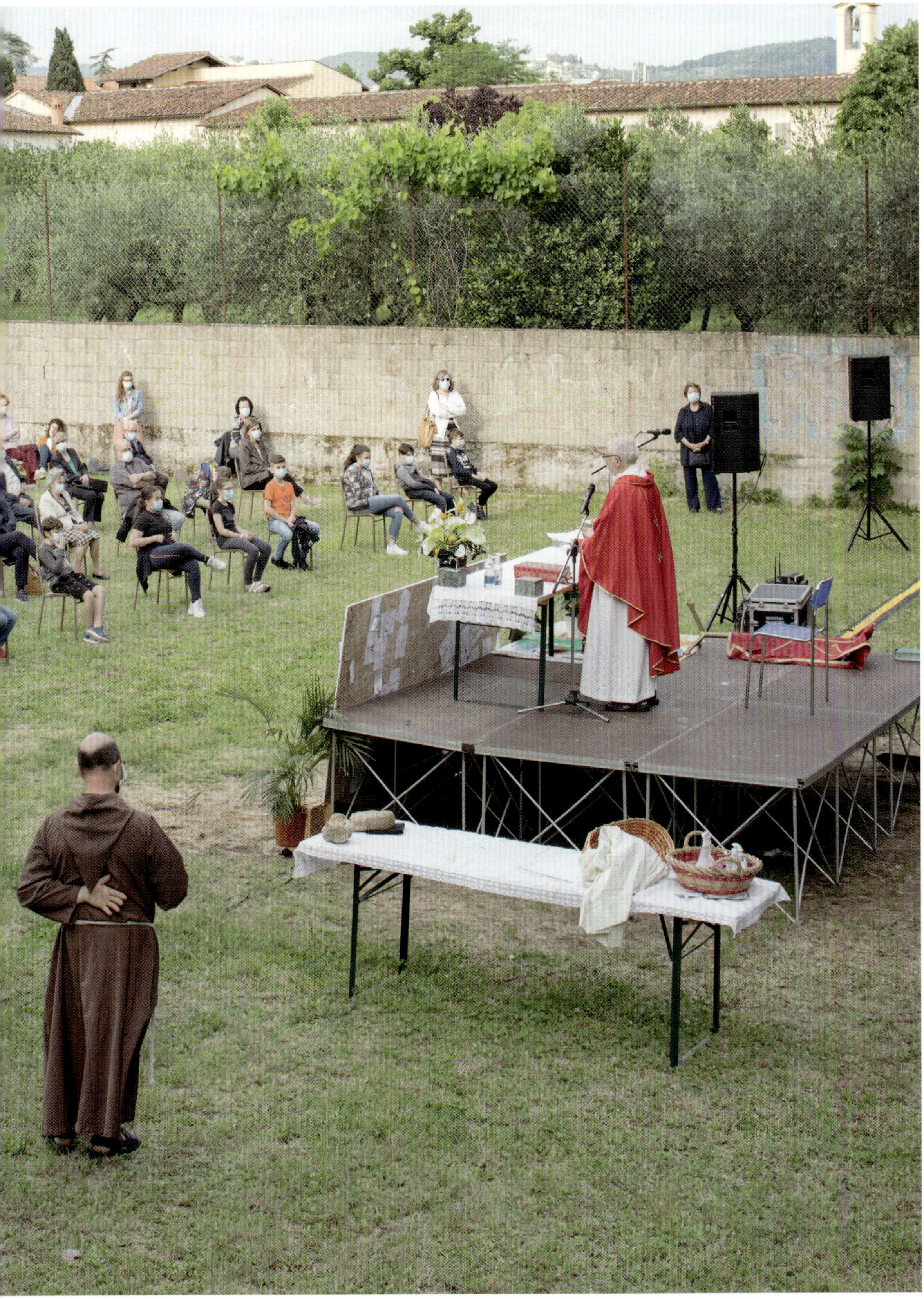

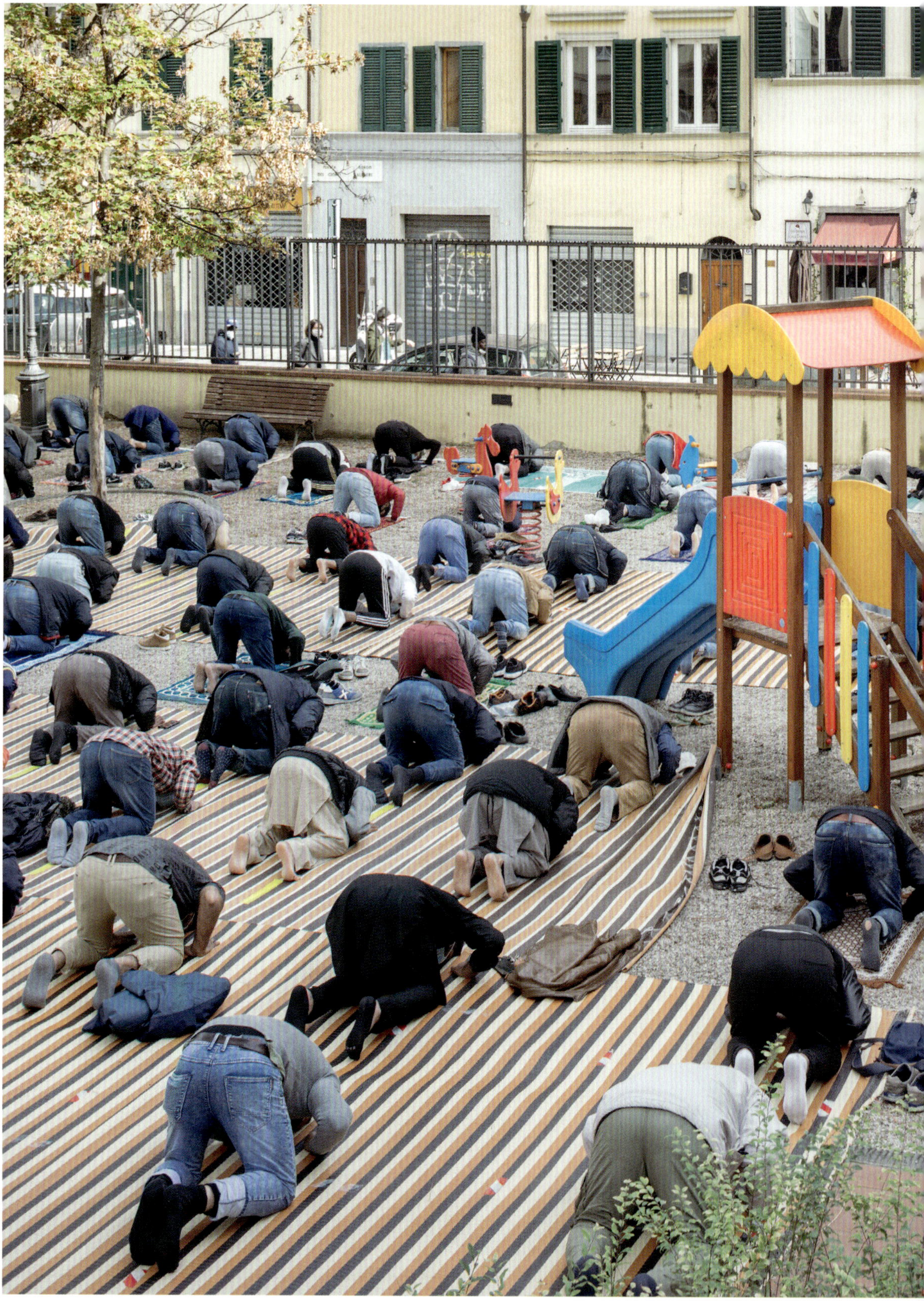

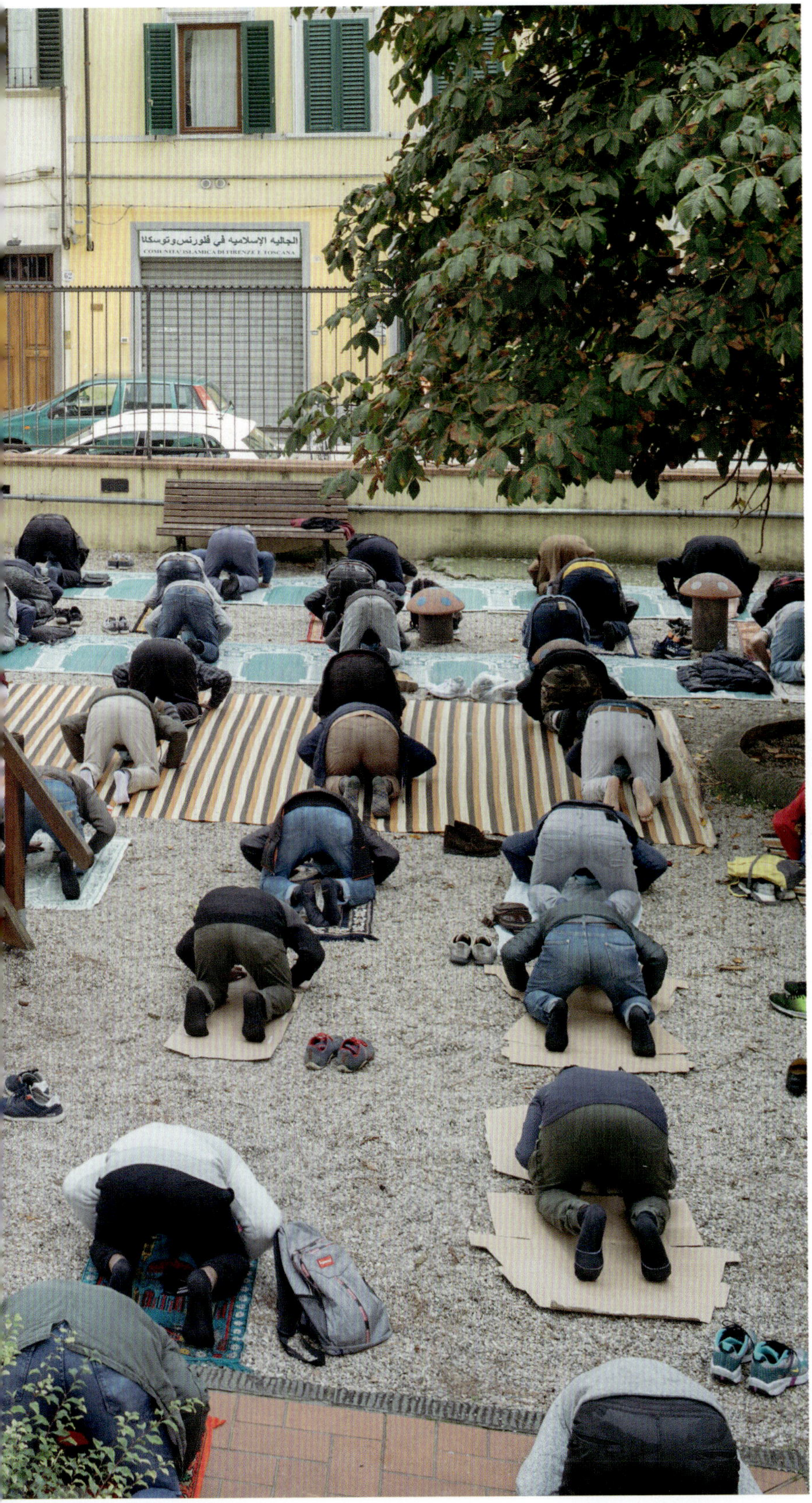
الجاليه الإسلاميه في فلورنس وتوسكانا
COMUNITA' ISLAMICA DI FIRENZE E TOSCANA

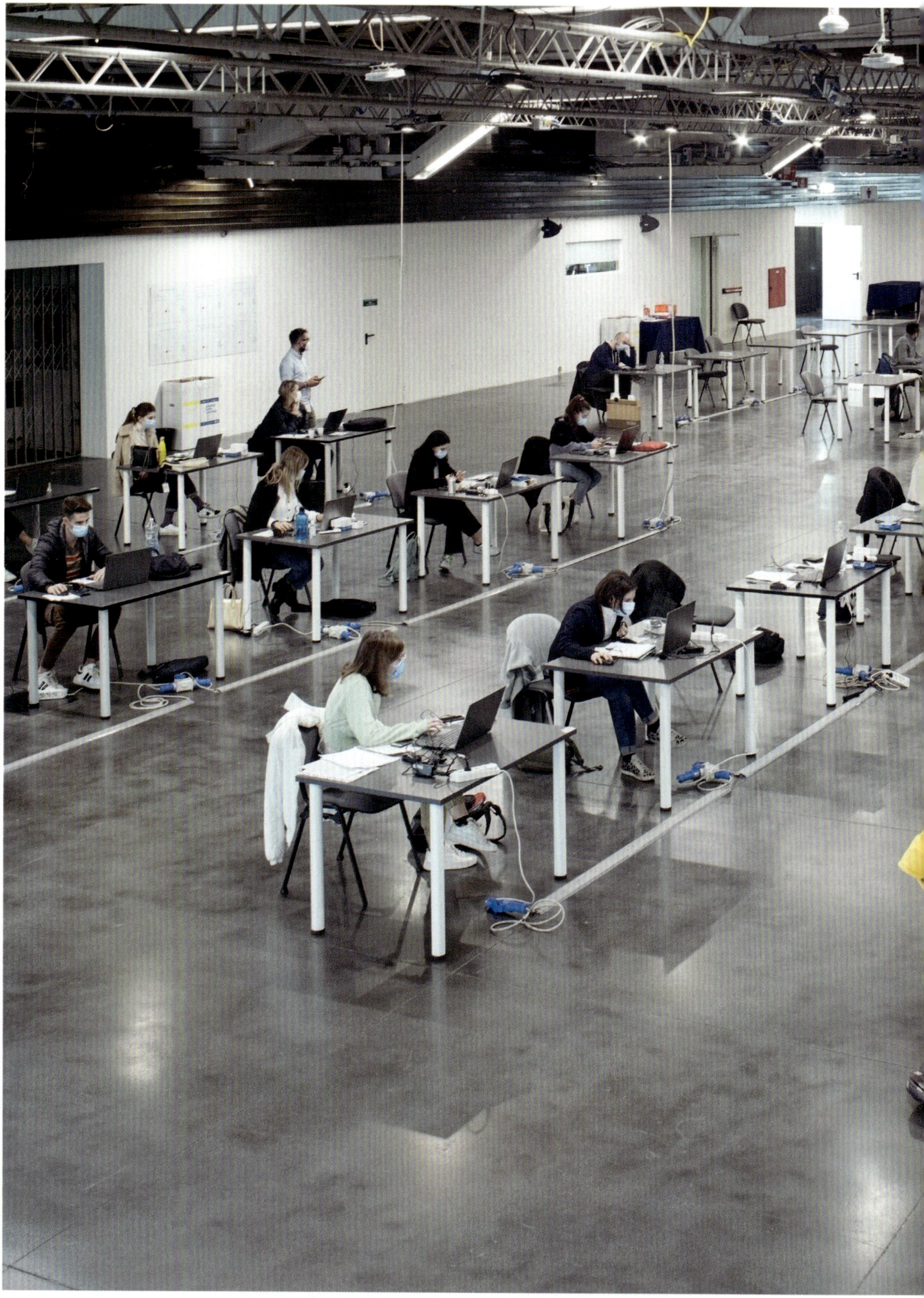

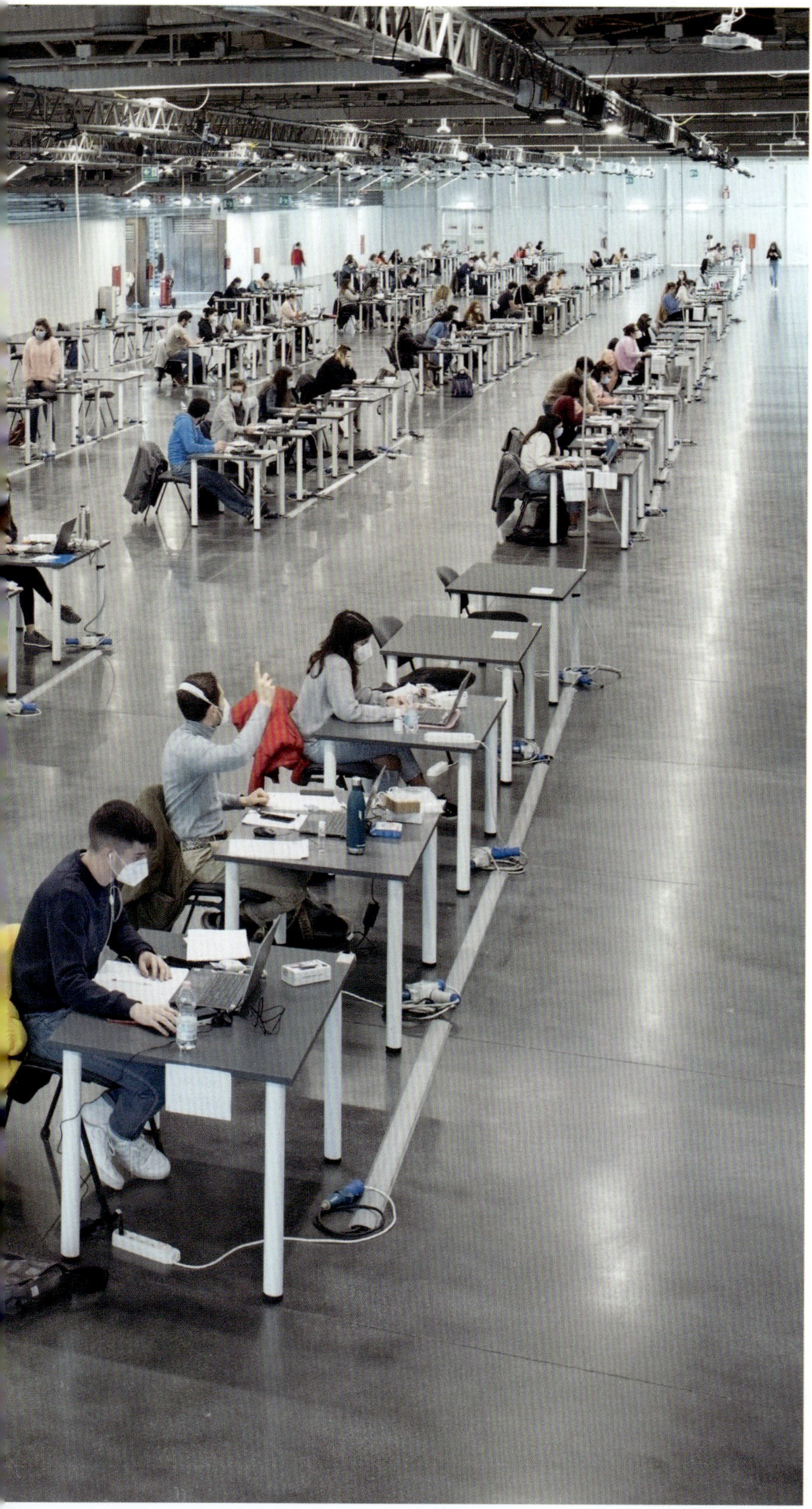

Davide Bertuccio, Italy
Where the Sea Fades

"I have been on board since January 25, 2020, I saw the ship stop and then leave again. I never got off. I have seen the world change from within. I don't know what the situation is outside, but here on board we do our best to contain the virus."
This is the testimony of a woman, employed by the MSC Grandiosa, the first ship in Europe to leave after the lockdown. It was October 6, 2020, nothing was going to change that much before then.
On August 16, 2020 (the day after the new Italian ministerial decree that allowed cruise travel to resume) the MSC wins its battle against the virus by sending the first ship into the water in record time. This result was possible thanks to the creation of a real social bubble, but above all, through this departure, new life was given to a movement that cost tourism several million euros in turnover throughout the Mediterranean.
On land, the beginning of a new normal had already occurred, but no tourist could imagine what the new prototype of a holiday onboard would be. Relentless checks punctuate the days: mandatory swabs to be carried out before boarding, hand sanitisation and masks even in outdoor play activities. Everything under control, leaving nothing to chance. The maximum number of passengers that can be accommodated onboard has been reduced from 5,000 to 1,500, but there has been an increase in national tourism, each blocked within its own borders to curb the spread of the virus.
Where the Sea Fades is a work of documentation of this new normal. Holidays have changed and with them our habits. We stand still and observe a world that remains the same, but changes in its intimacy. Time passes and life goes on, like the waves of the sea, which are hardly ever touched on a cruise.

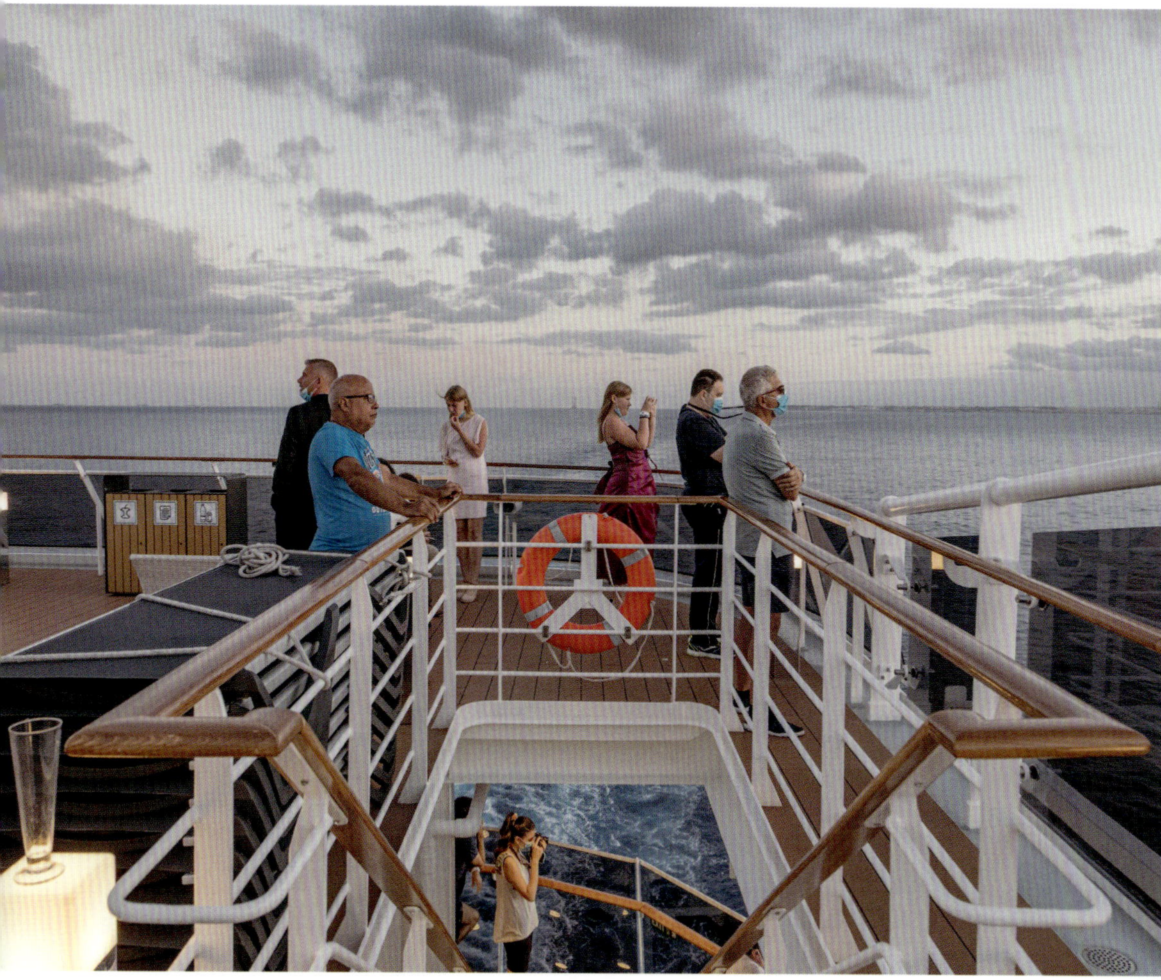

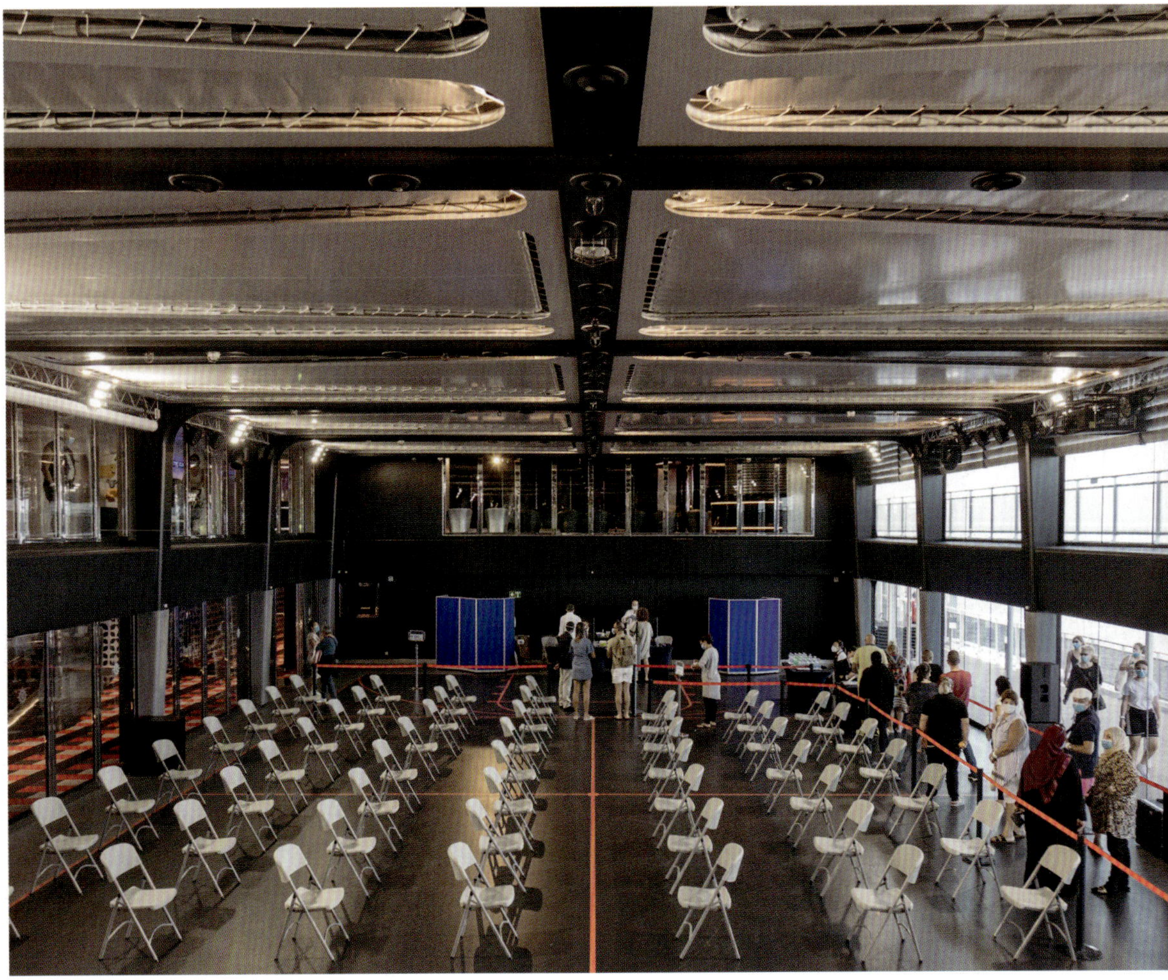

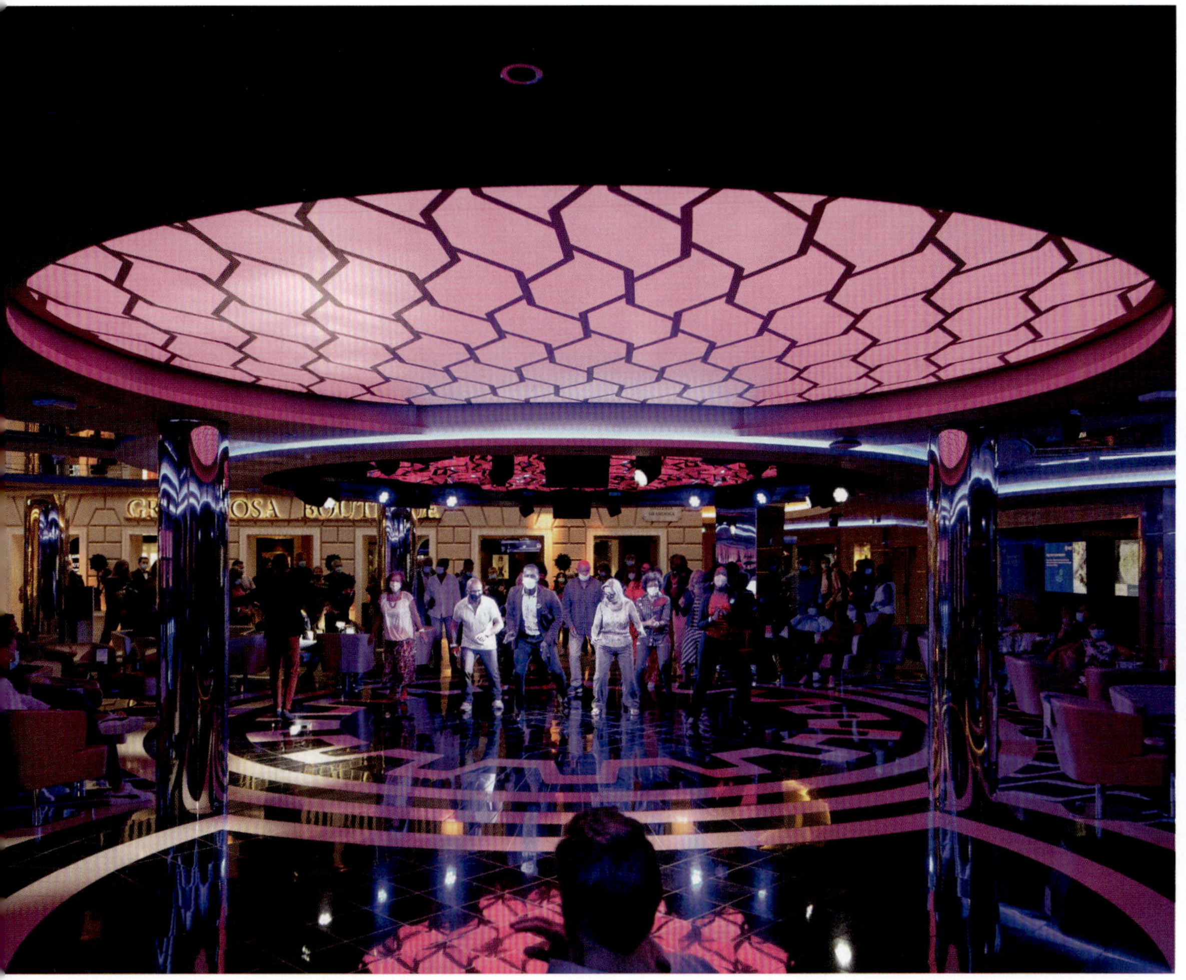

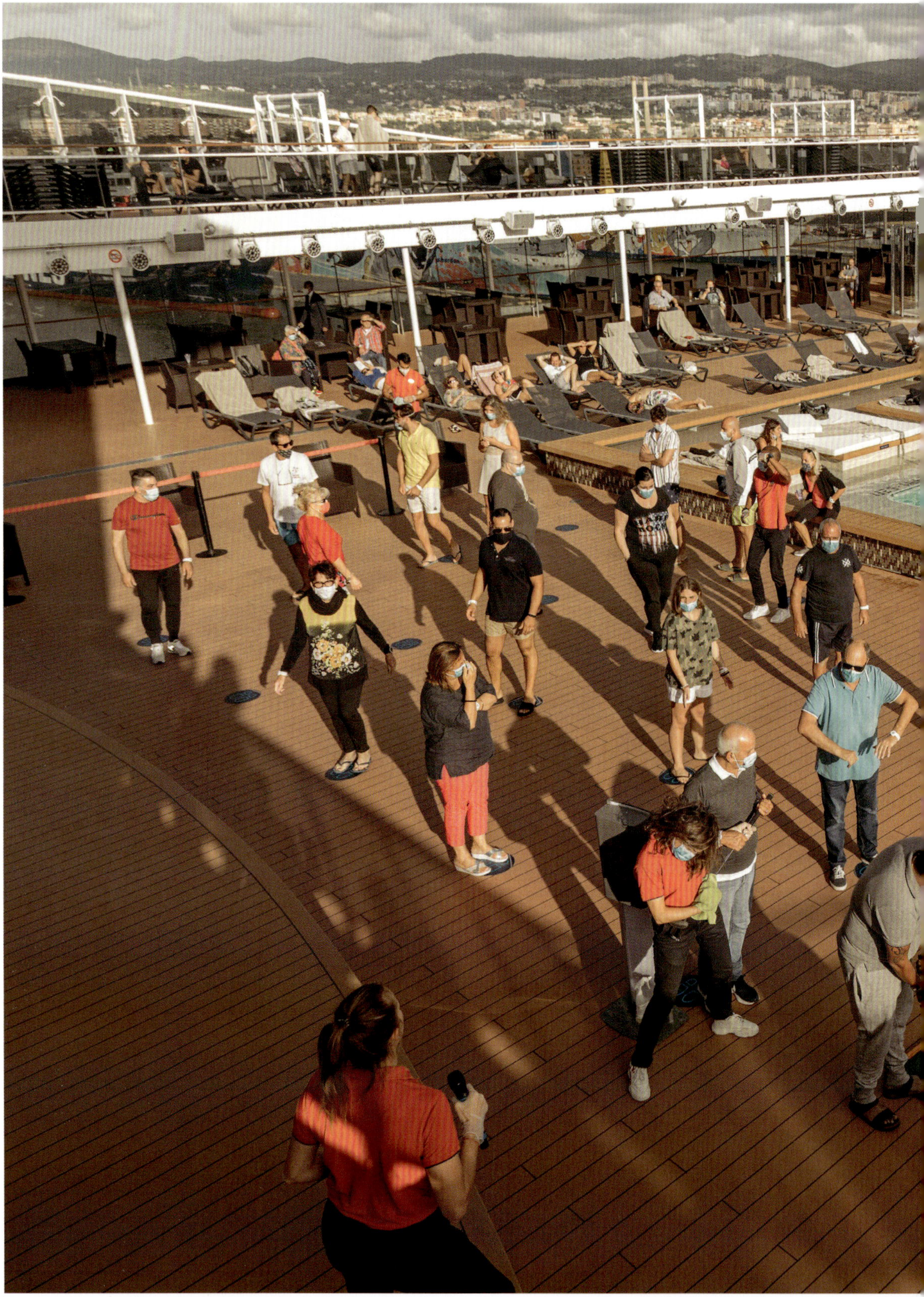

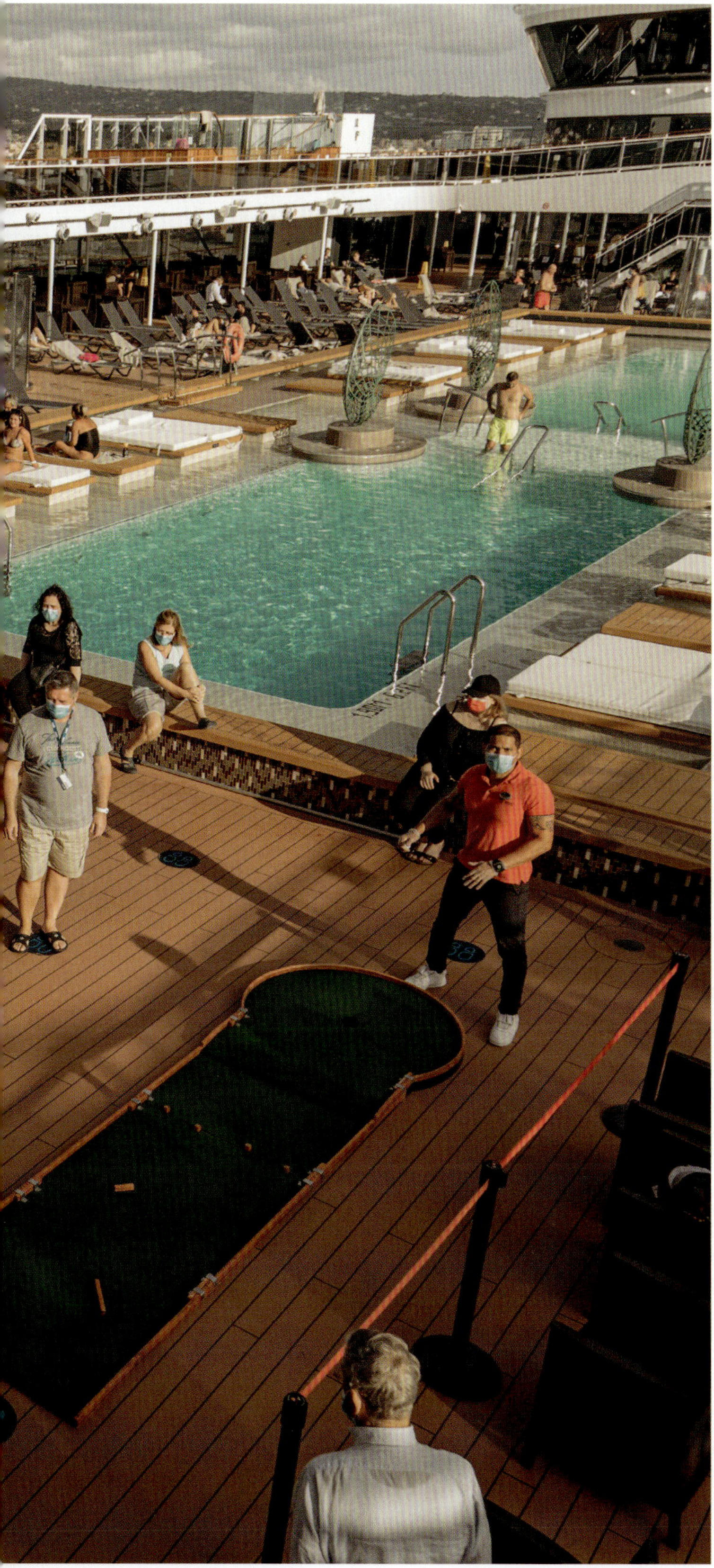

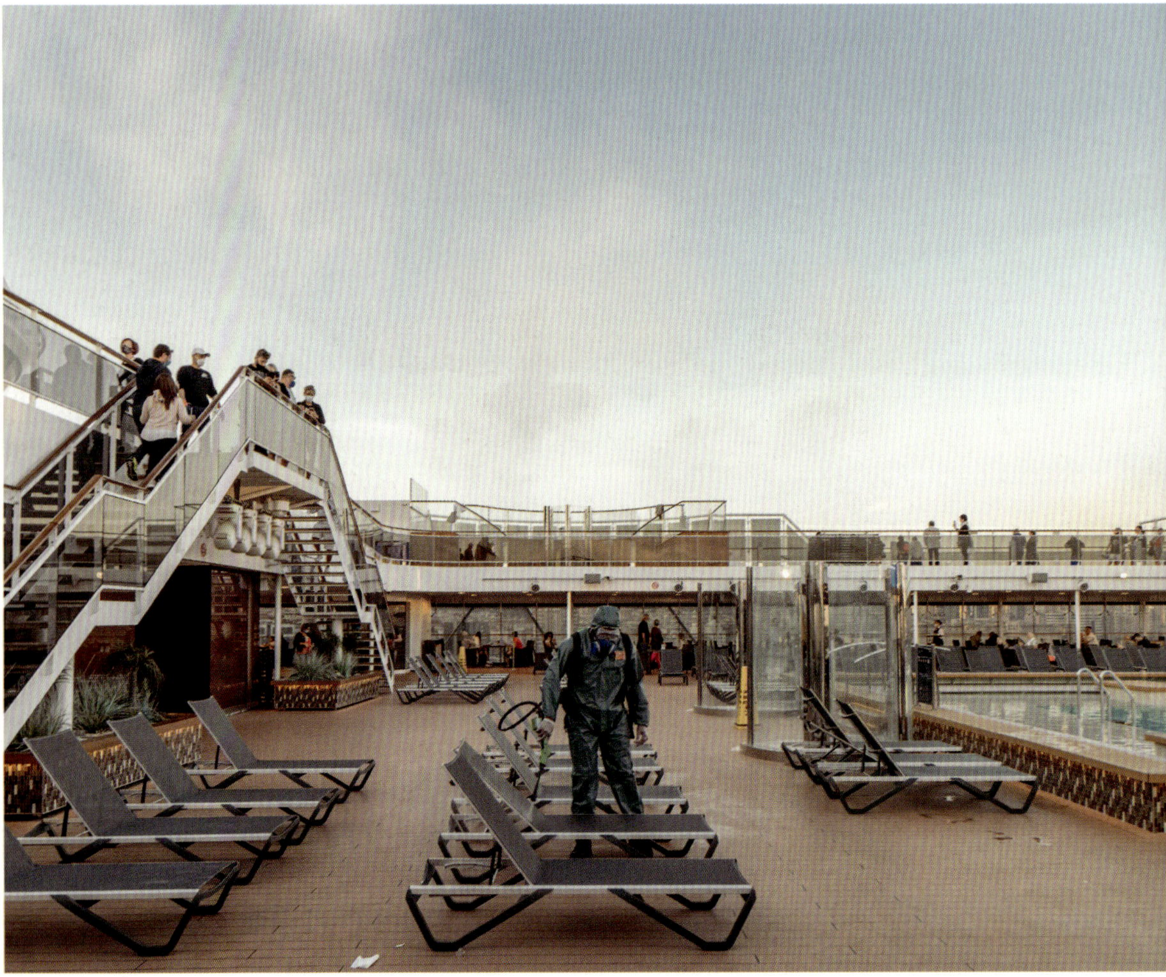

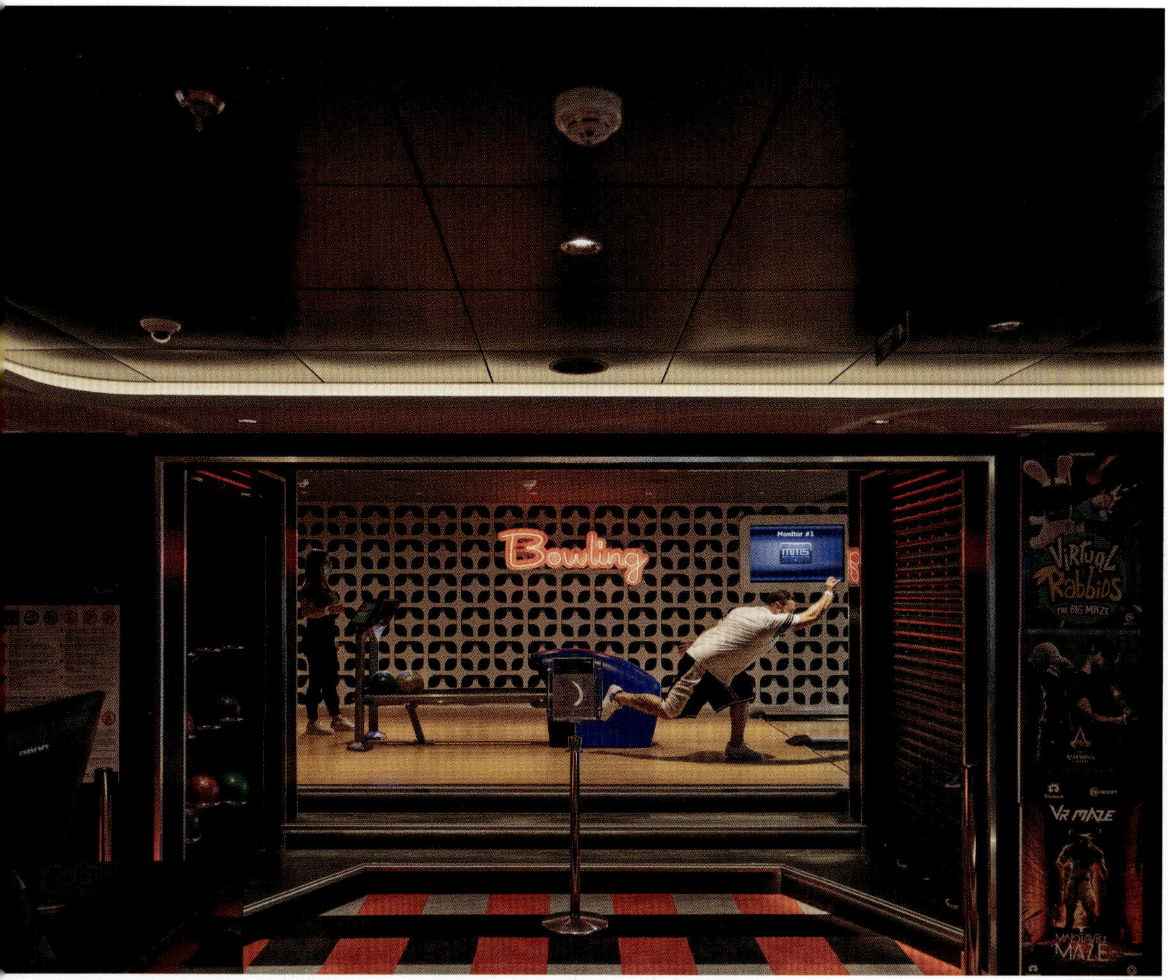
Bowling
Monitor #1
VIRTUAL Rabbids
THE BIG MAZE
VR MAZE

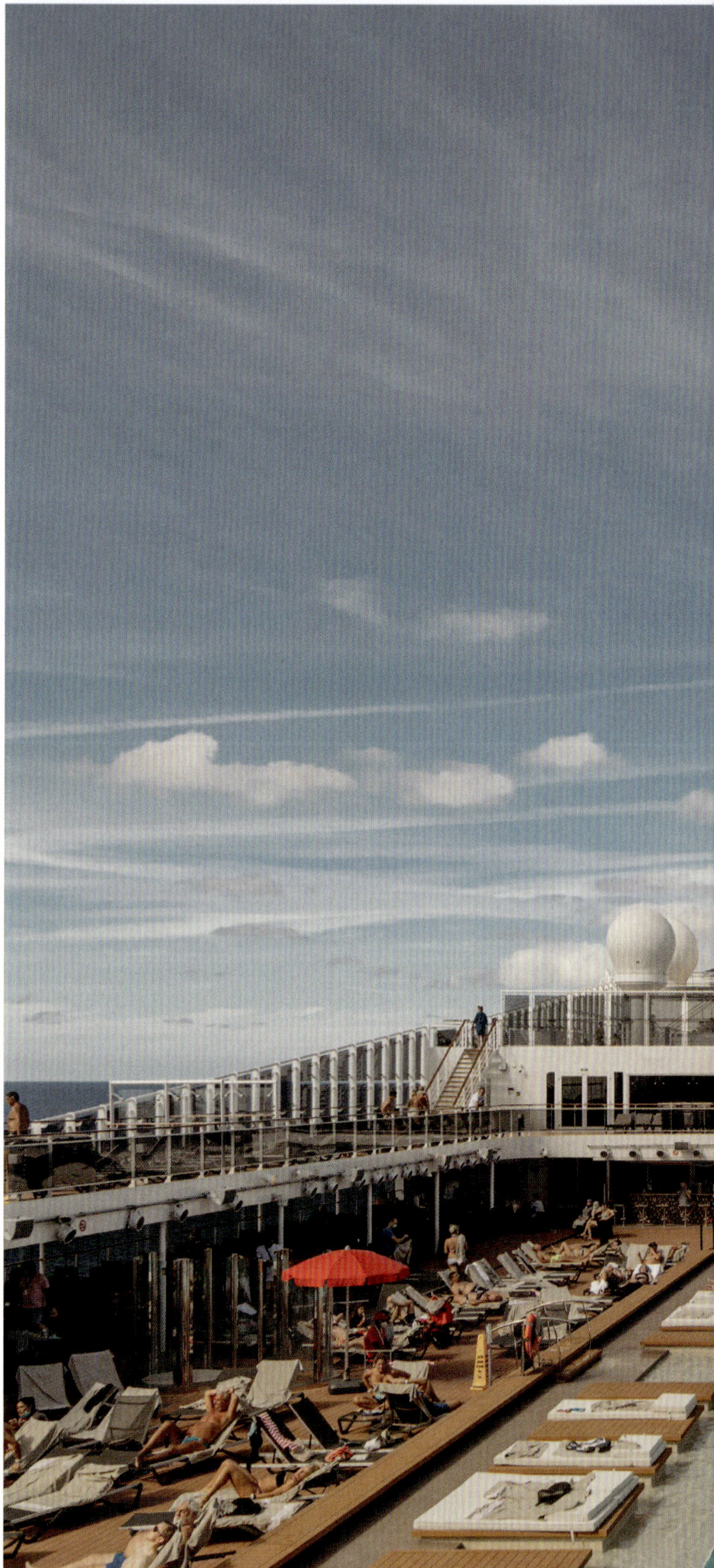

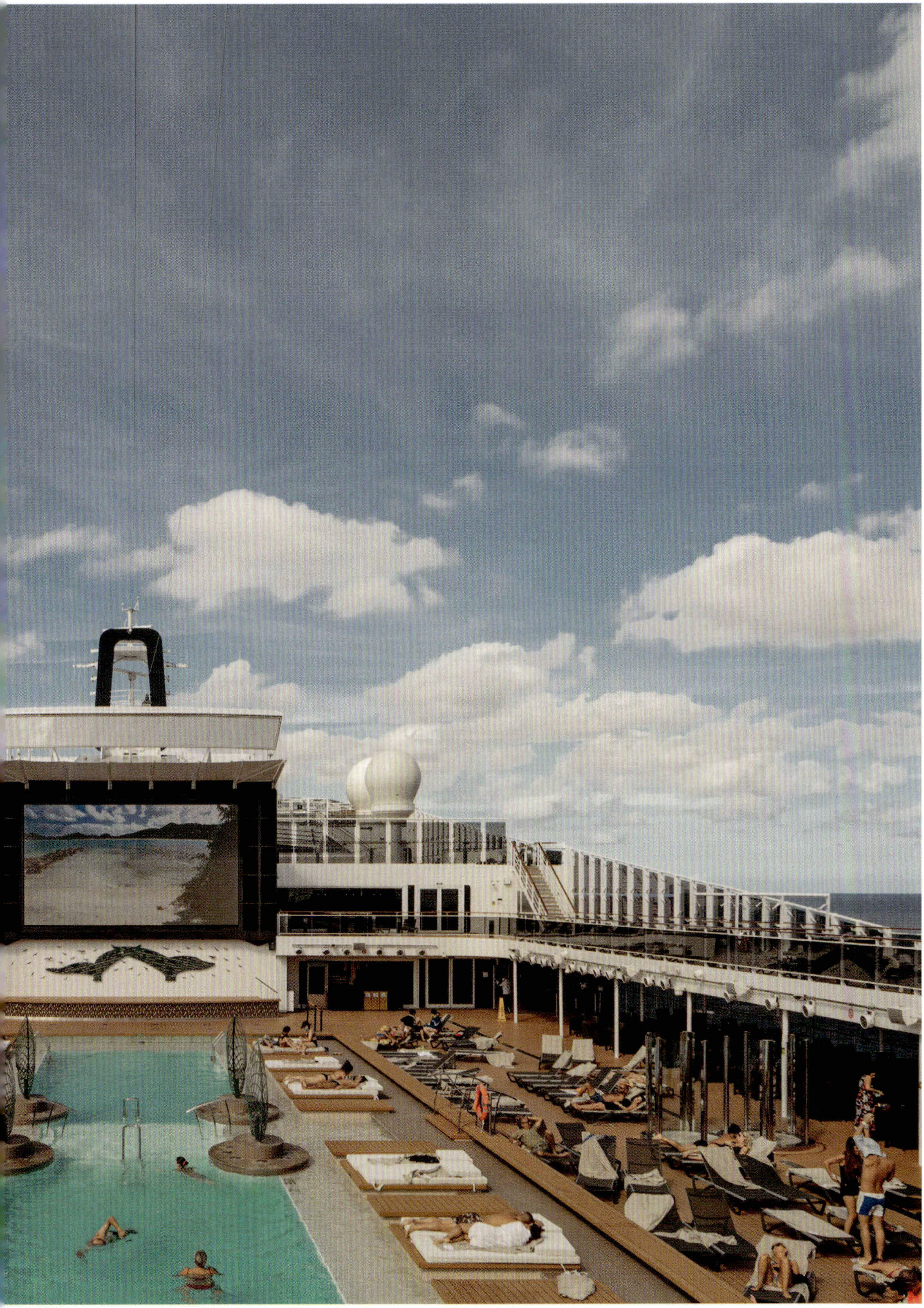

Anna Catalano, Italy
Every Room Becomes a Classroom

"We have decided to close out of caution, as the epidemiological situation is changing rapidly, and to suspend teaching activities outside the red zone until 15 March, starting tomorrow [...] As Minister of Education I hope that my pupils will obviously return to school as soon as possible and I am committed to ensuring that the essential public service, even if at a distance, is provided to all our students."

On March 4, the Minister of Education Lucia Azzolina expressed, with these words, a historic choice.

As the mother of Giulia, aged 6 and in her first year of primary school, I found myself immediately involved. What seemed like a small holiday had turned into something much more complex for all families with school-age children — we were publicly called upon to play a fundamental role in our children's education. Given this responsibility and motivated as a photographer by the need to understand the real impact of this step, I decided to follow the situation from the inside. To do so, I also narrated the situation in one secondary school institute and two high schools, in Calabria, where I was born and where I was working, moving between Distance Learning platforms and on-site lessons across the region in Paola, Catanzaro and Decollatura.

Only after obtaining the authorisation from the Ministry of Education, University and Research (MIUR) was I able to photograph the schools that were closed, to enter the homes of different families, to discover avant-garde institutes such as the scientific high school of Decollatura, a 4.0 school where Distance Learning was already a teaching tool implemented a long time ago and not a novel tool to be learnt in a few days.

What looked like a confused collage gradually took shape. I attended baccalaureate exams in the sole presence of the teachers and secondary school final exams at the children's homes, together with their parents. Dissertations and tests that had been carried out over a period that was overloaded with responsibility, while constantly sharing time and living space. I have seen grandparents acting as mums and dads, like Luigi, who bought a scanner to guarantee his only granddaughter the delivery of the papers for her high-school final exam. I was able to rediscover the importance of having friends with whom to share ambitions and dreams, as I watched Cristina and Sergio studying. I discovered that some thirteen-year-olds experienced gender equality as a topic to be informed about and to be discussed with awareness. Children with parents who were suddenly out of work, like

Alessia, were helped by the Hotelier Institute of Paola which provided her with a PC for the whole semester of home study.
It has been a journey made of places, faces, stories.
Like that of Halima, who grew up in Casablanca and arrived in Italy only three years ago. She passed the secondary school final exam from the living room of her house in Catanzaro, while her mother Fatima listened to her, understanding perhaps too little of what her daughter was excited about. On the wall the photographs of her brothers and father who were still in Morocco, but that day they were silent witnesses of their little woman's success.
I witnessed a reversal of roles. Teachers struggling with a technology that is often hostile, helped by their native digital pupils. Students were discussing their exams on the professors' desk while the committee sat by their desks, arranged in a horseshoe shape. Signs on the school floors, safety distance, masks, and disinfectants, made the corridors look increasingly similar to hospital lanes.
I saw many teachers give themselves without boundaries of ideas and time. And I saw my daughter Giulia heroically completing primary school after spending hours in front of a monitor, far from her friends and teachers, in a suspended world.

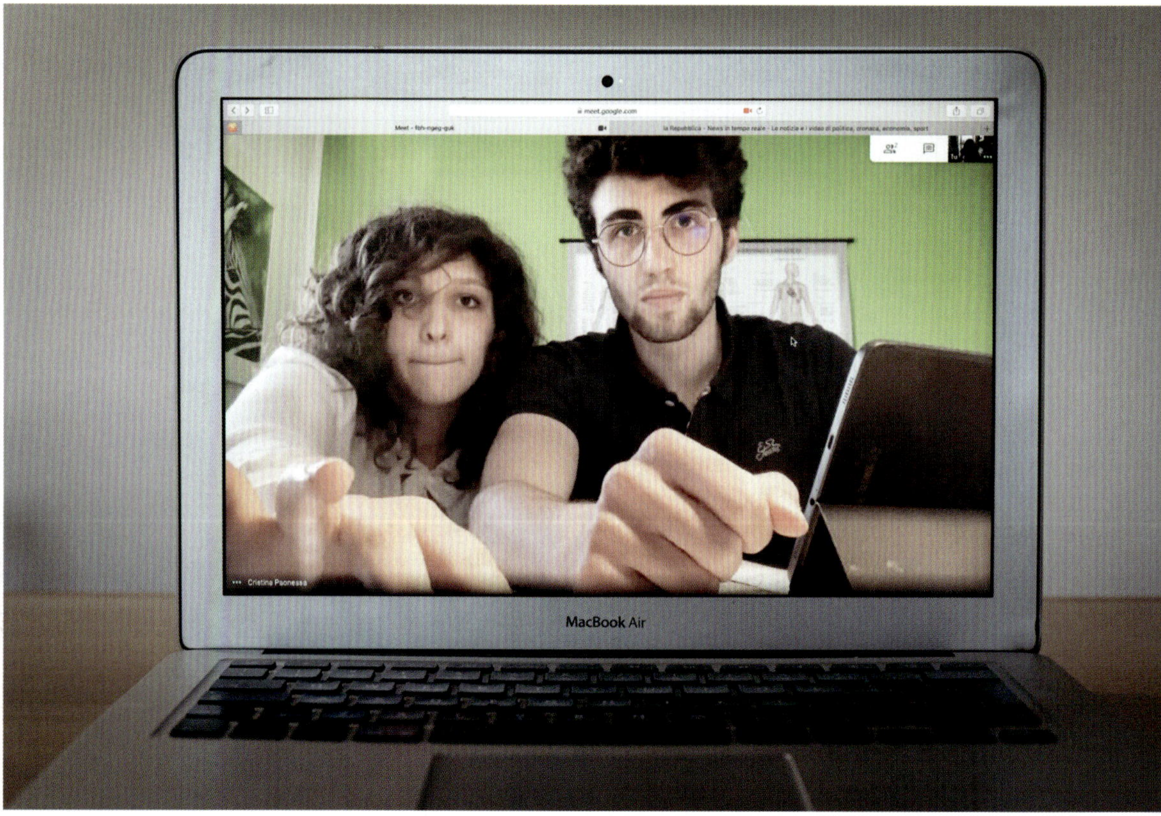
meet.google.com
Cristina Paonessa
MacBook Air

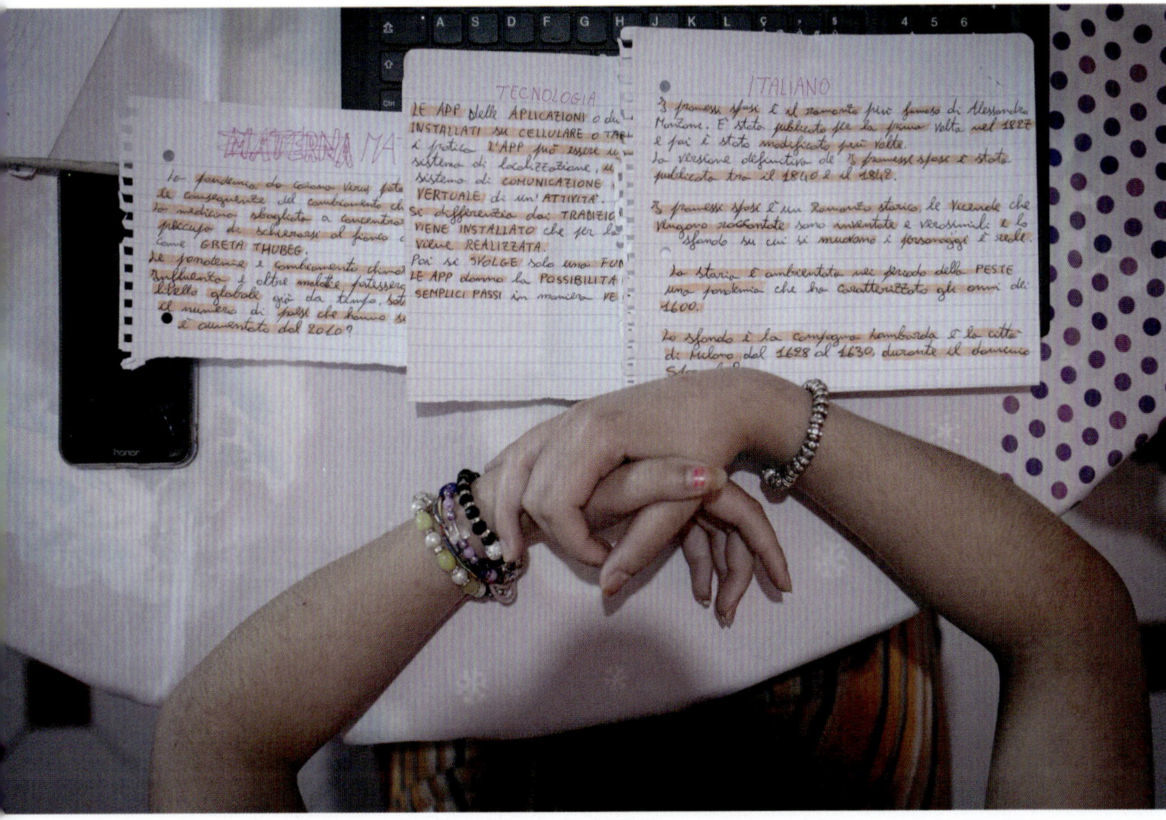
TECNOLOGIA
ITALIANO
GRETA THUBEG
honor

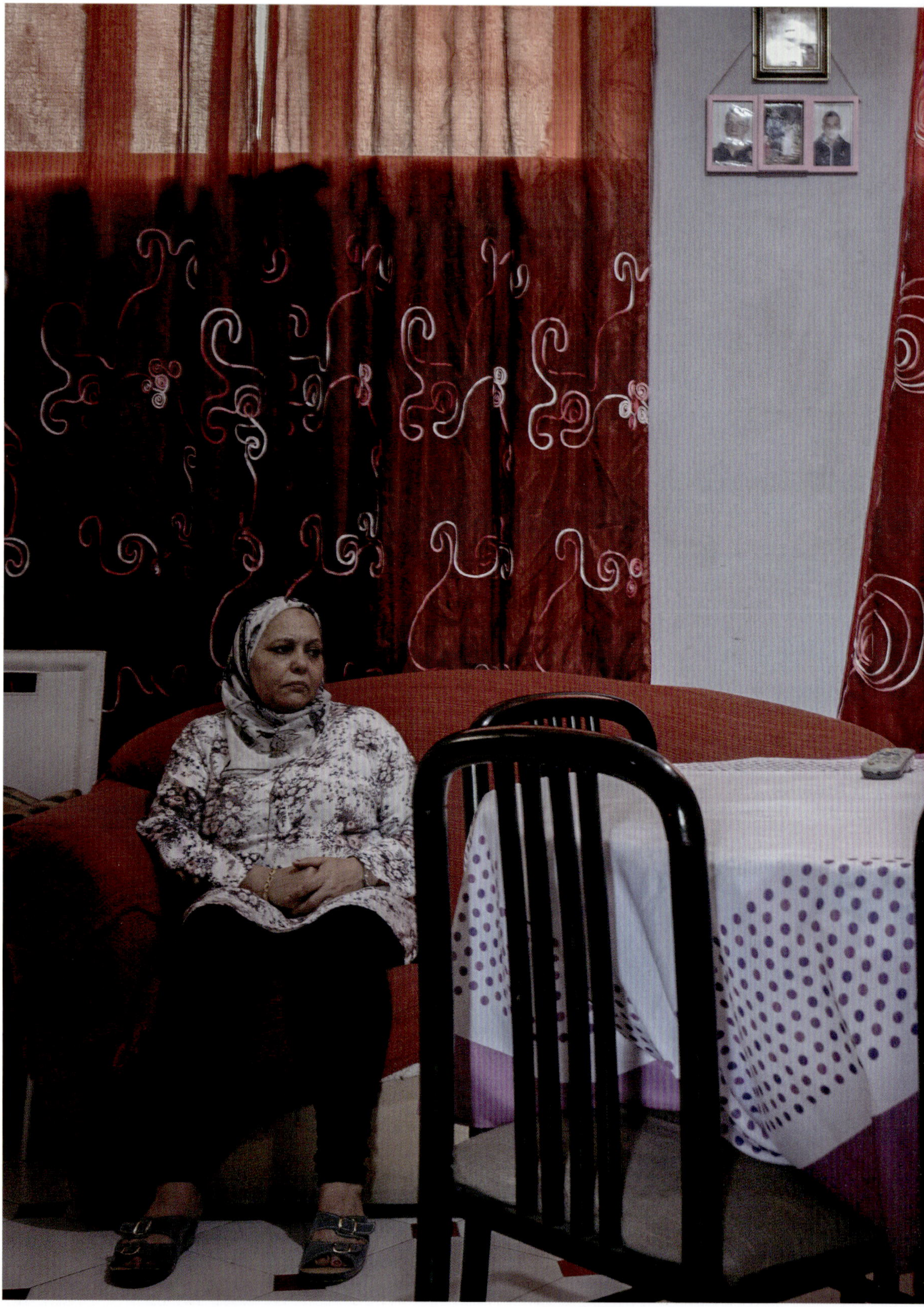

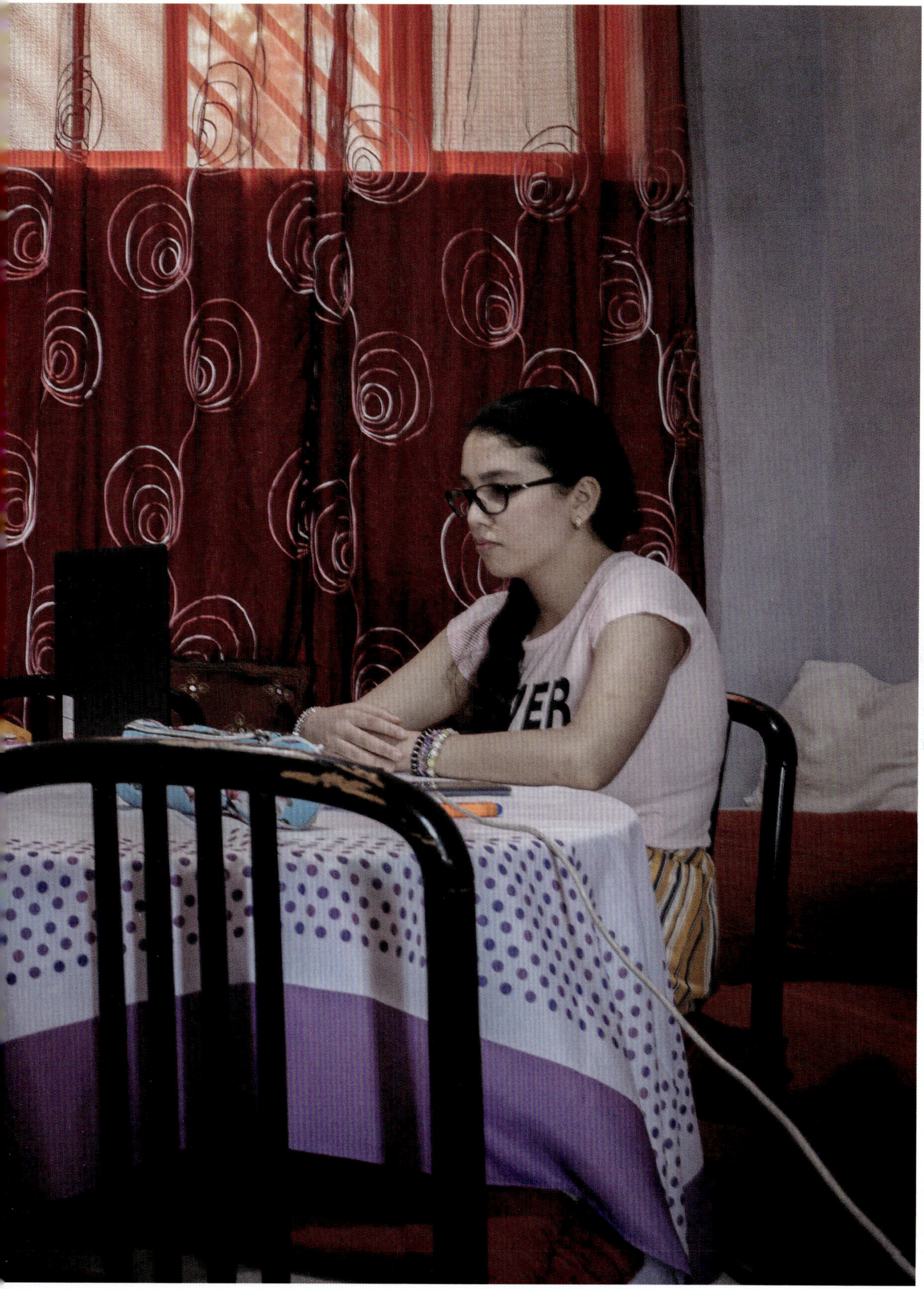

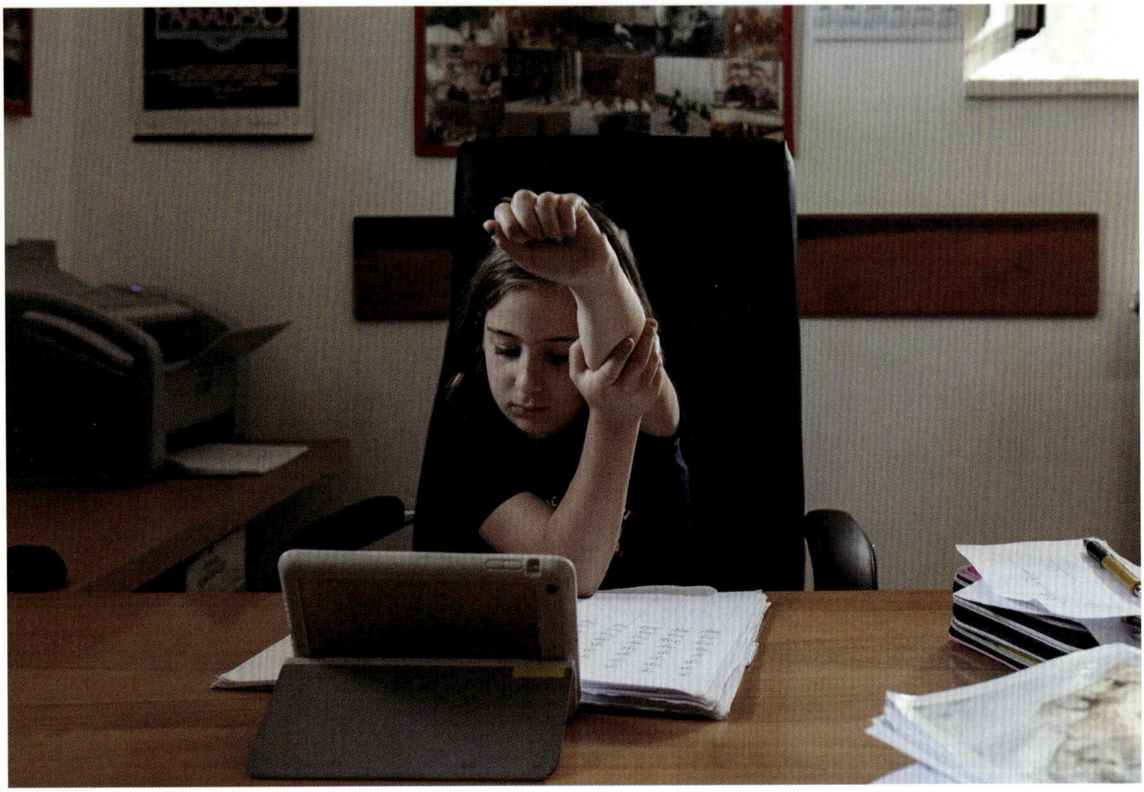

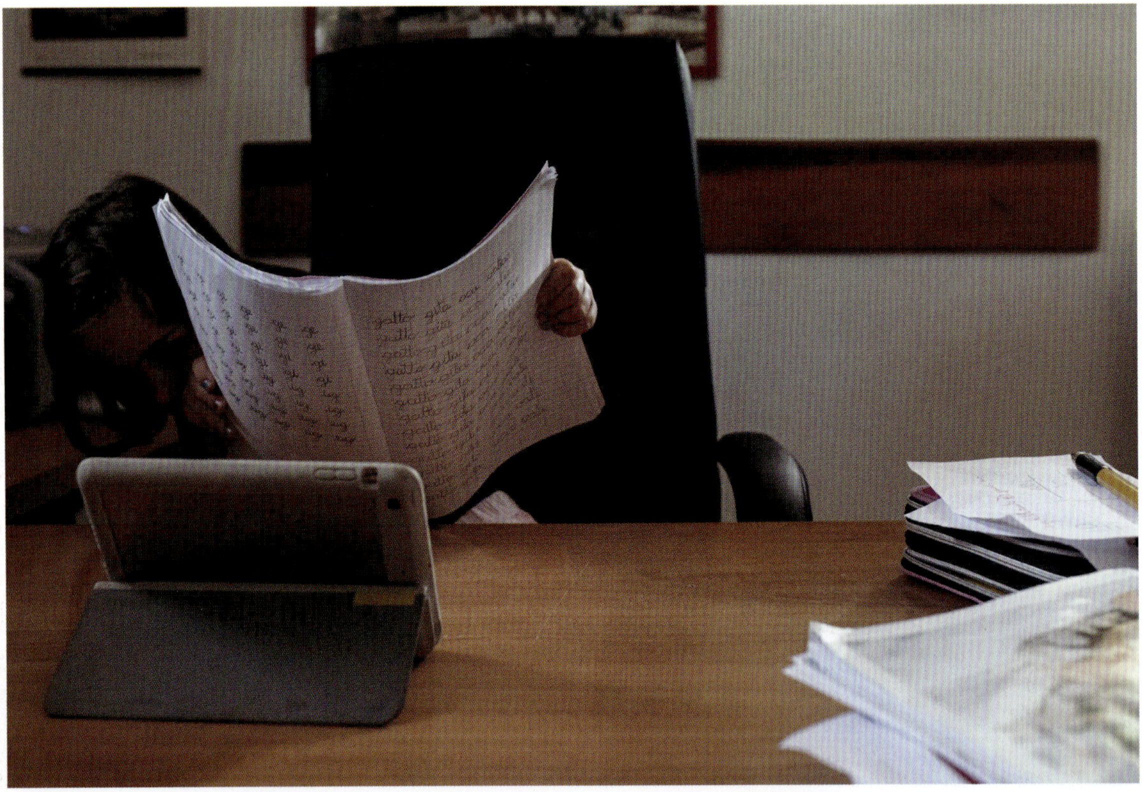

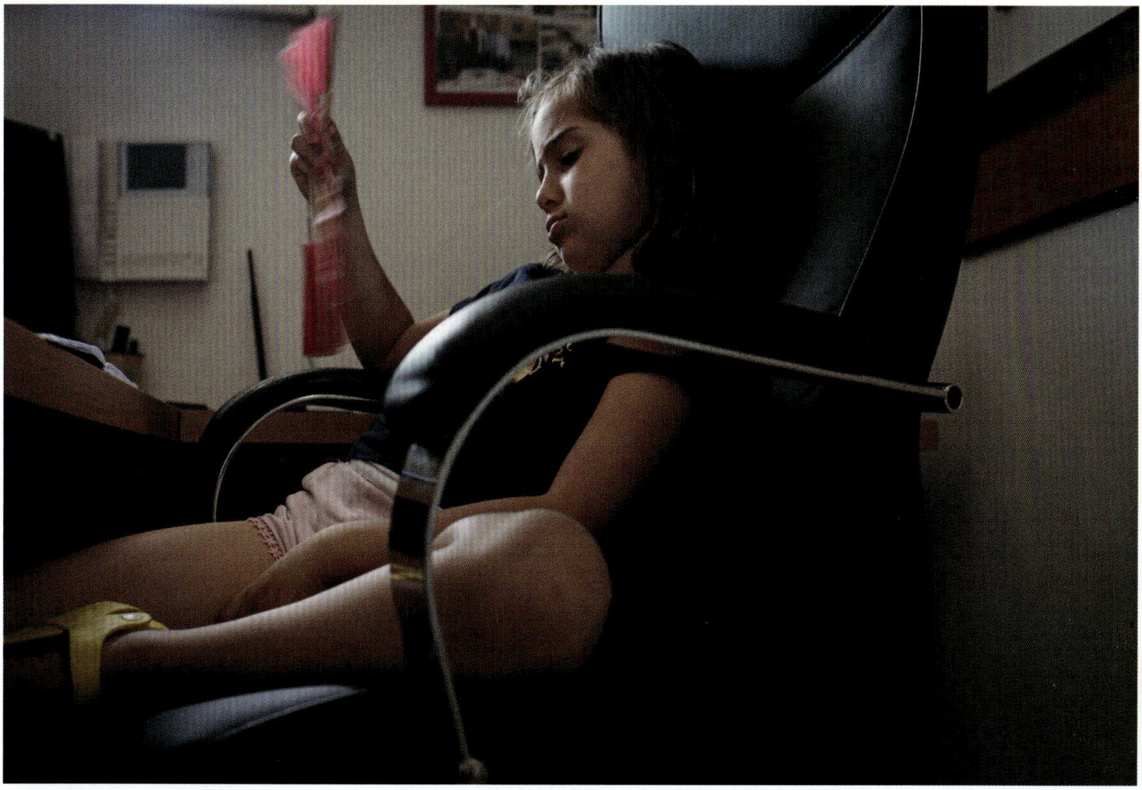

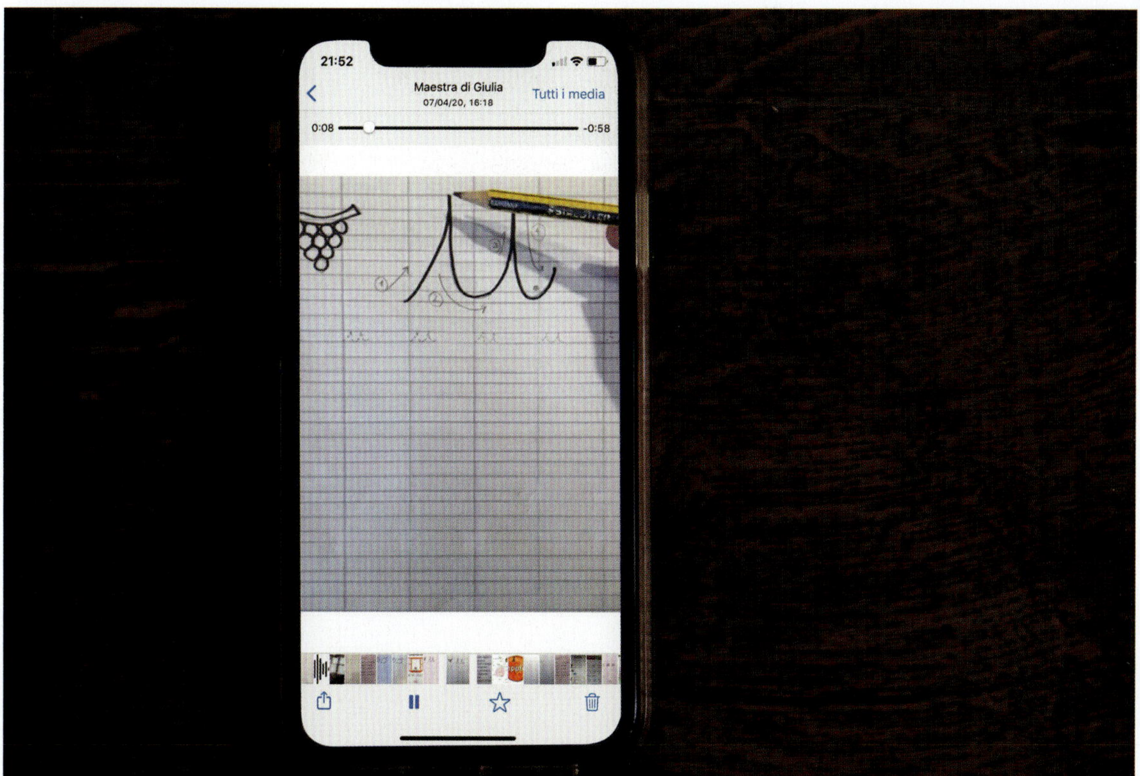
21:52
Maestra di Giulia
07/04/20, 16:18
Tutti i media
0:08
-0:58

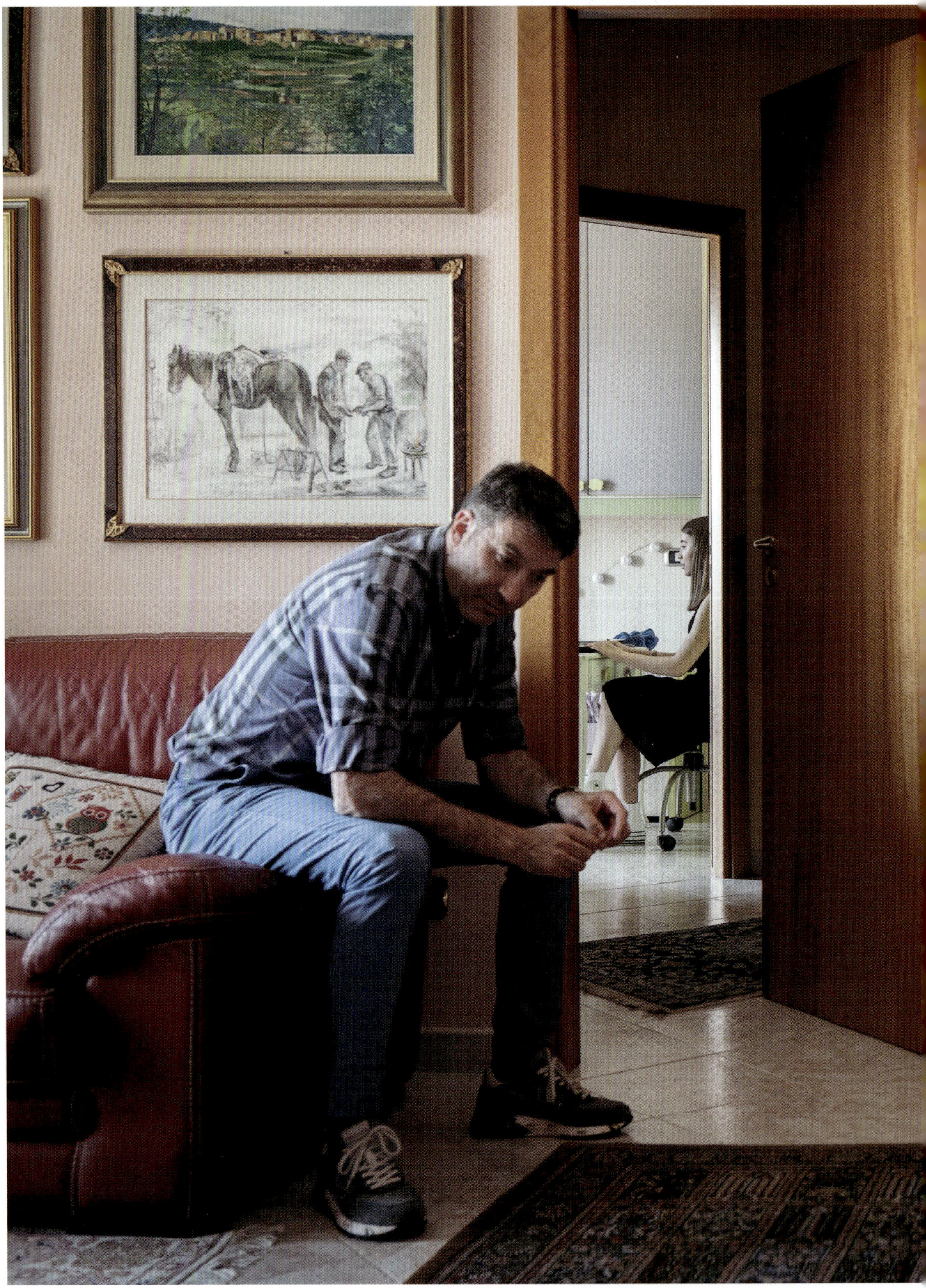

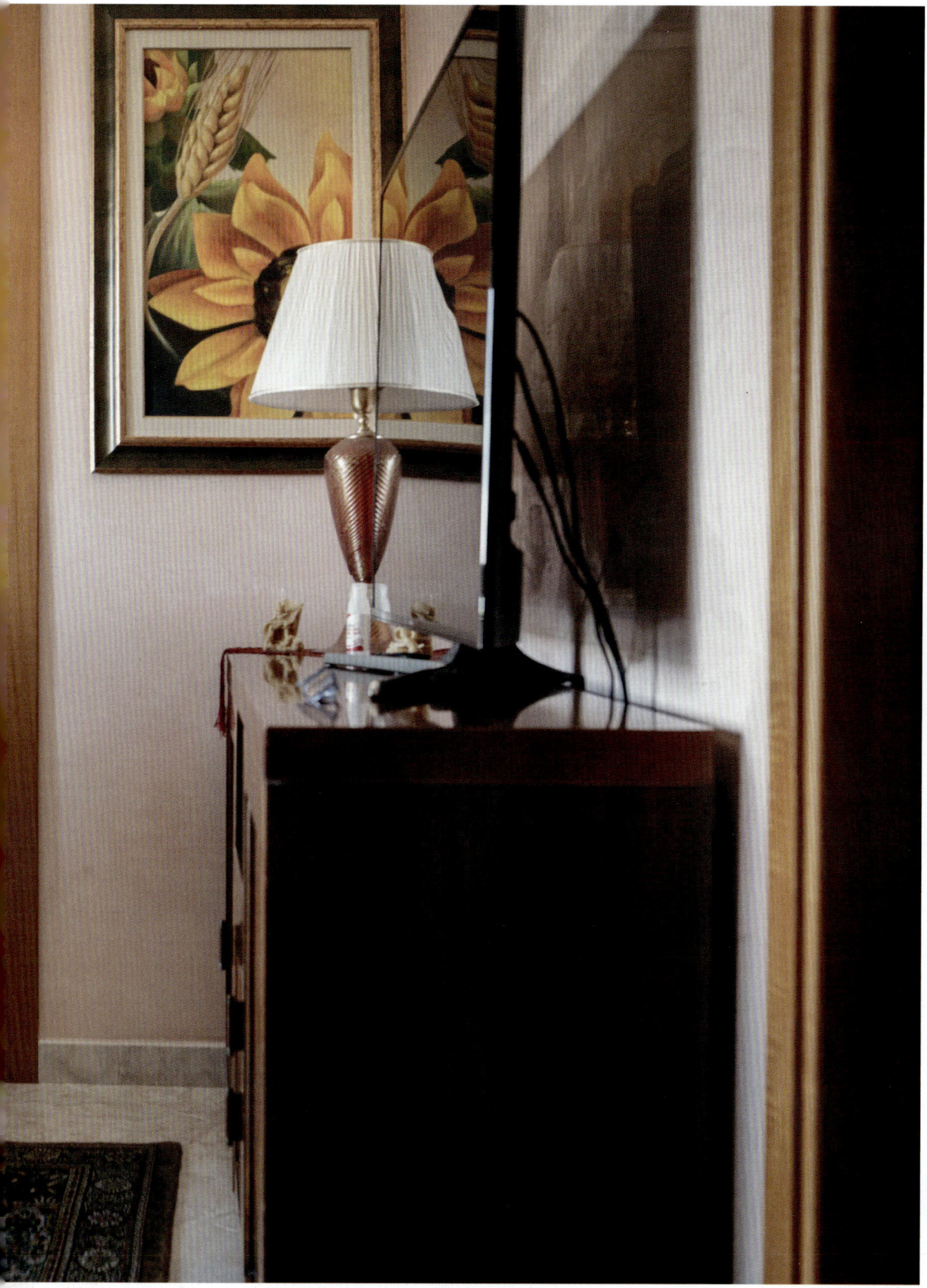

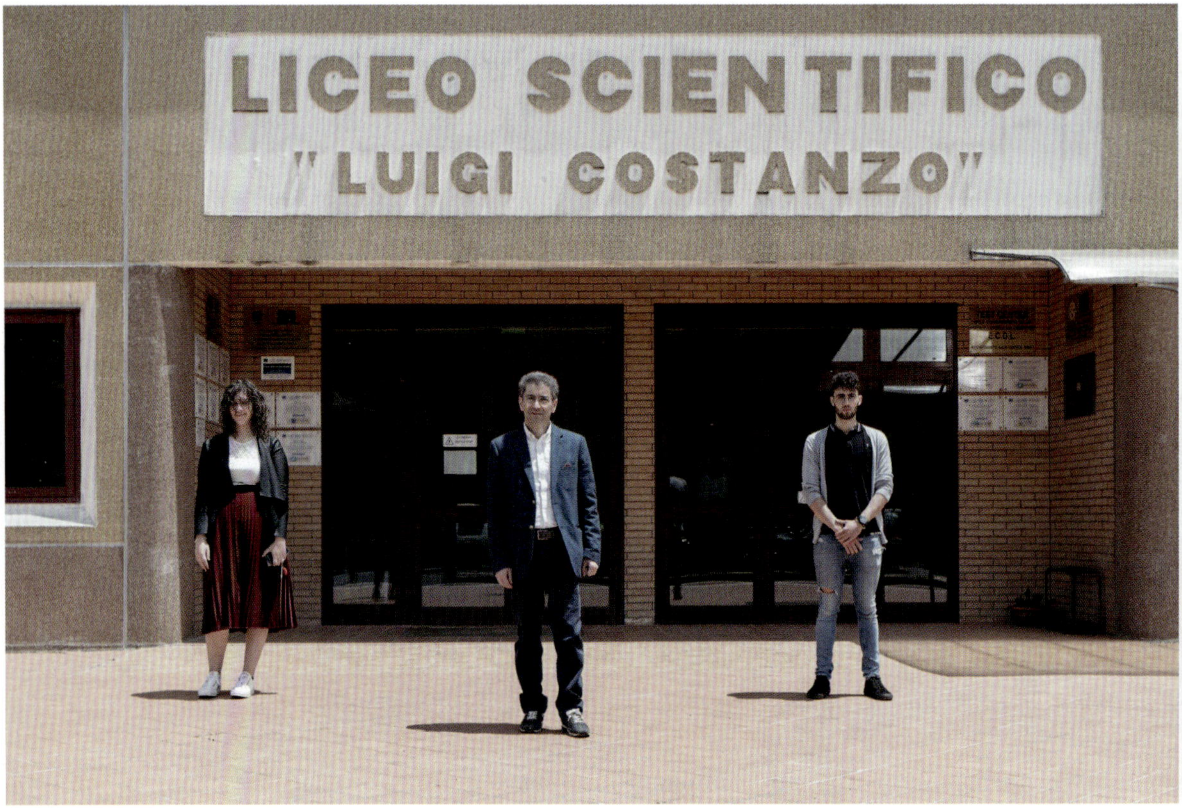
LICEO SCIENTIFICO
"LUIGI COSTANZO"

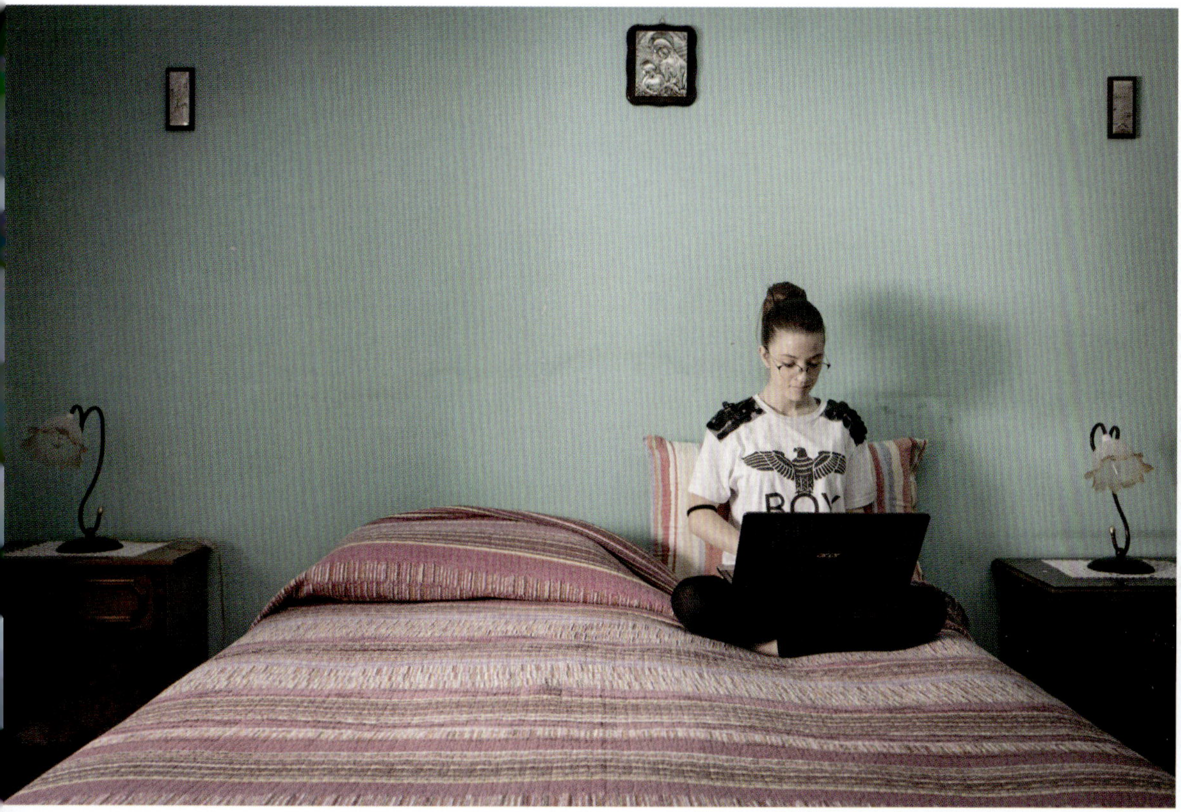

Alberto Bernasconi, Italy
Covid's Long Term Effects

In early spring 2020, Bergamo was a startling warning sign of the virus' fury, a city where sirens rang through the night and military trucks lined up outside the public hospital to ferry away the dead. Bergamo has dramatically curtailed the virus' spread, but it is now offering another kind of warning, this one about the long aftermath, where recoveries are proving incomplete and sometimes excruciating. Those who survived the peak of the outbreak in March and April are now negative. The virus is officially gone from their systems.
The follow-ups with the once-hospitalised patients are the basis for medical research: their health records now fill 17 bankers' boxes, and scientific reports are on the way. Bergamo doctors say the disease clearly has full-body ramifications but leaves wildly differing marks from one patient to the next, and in some cases few marks at all. Among the first 750 patients screened, some 30% still have lung scarring and breathing trouble. The virus has left another 30% with problems linked to inflammation and clotting, such as heart abnormalities and artery blockages. A few are at risk of organ failure. Beyond that, according to interviews with eight doctors from the Papa Giovanni XXIII Hospital involved in the study, many patients months later are dealing with a galaxy of daily conditions and have no clear answer on when it will all subside: leg pain, tingling in the extremities, hair loss, depression, severe fatigue.
Some patients had preexisting conditions, but doctors say survivors are not simply experiencing a version of old problems. Some patients who were self-reliant before contracting the virus remain so weakened that, when they arrive for their follow-up appointments, they're helped to the waiting room by relatives, or in wheelchairs. Four people so far were too frail to make it through the several hours of testing and were rushed instead to the emergency room. Other times, people show up months later, having been through the worst — oxygen support, intubations — and are, improbably, almost fine. Doctors say one of the virus' mysteries is how recoveries can be swift for some and brutal for others.
The Bergamo research is led by the same doctors who worked frantic 14-hour days in March, sometimes falling sick themselves, while watching patients rapidly outnumber the beds. Now, wearing just masks, those same doctors and patients are sitting down together in a way that was impossible months ago. Bergamo, in March, was a place with six-hour waits for ambulances and 16-hour waits in the

ER. At one point, the hospital had 92 people on ventilators and so many who required breathing assistance that it needed to pipe in oxygen from a rush-delivered emergency tank. Subsequent antibody sampling, according to the government, indicated that one-quarter of Bergamo's 1.1 million people were infected with the virus at the time. The hospital was admitting only the worst cases, and to keep pace with the influx, it sometimes had to discharge patients before they were fully ready — something confirmed when the hospital started calling people for the follow-ups. In addition to the 440 people who died while hospitalised, 220 died after being told to go home.

The study in Bergamo is one of multiple efforts around the world to examine aspects of Covid's lingering damage. Other studies are underway to look specifically at "long-haulers" — a subset of people, some never hospitalised, who nonetheless have fatigue and other symptoms months after the illness.

For the patients who have been able to regain a semblance of their lives, the last barrier is the trauma itself — the raw memory of being in a hospital where so many were dying, and wondering if they might be next.

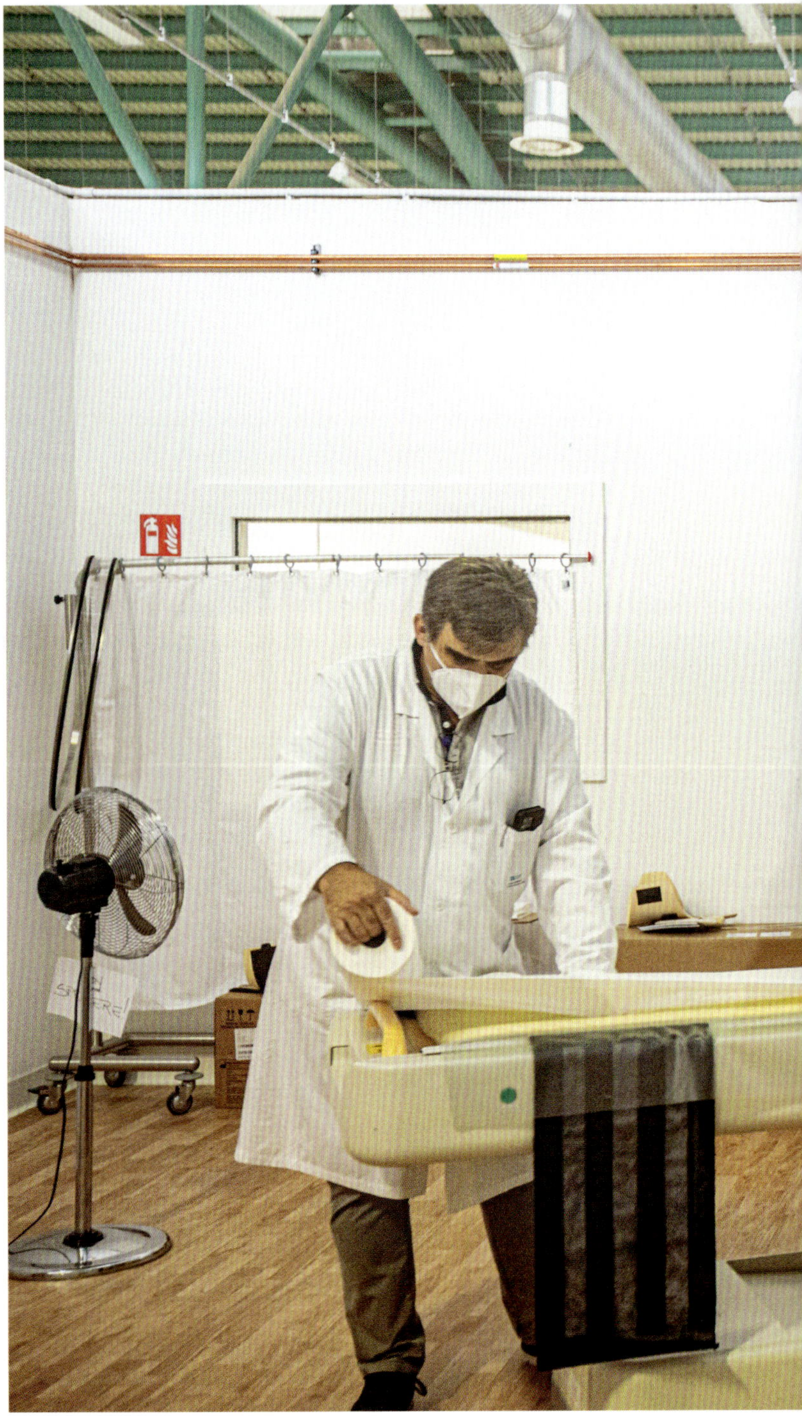

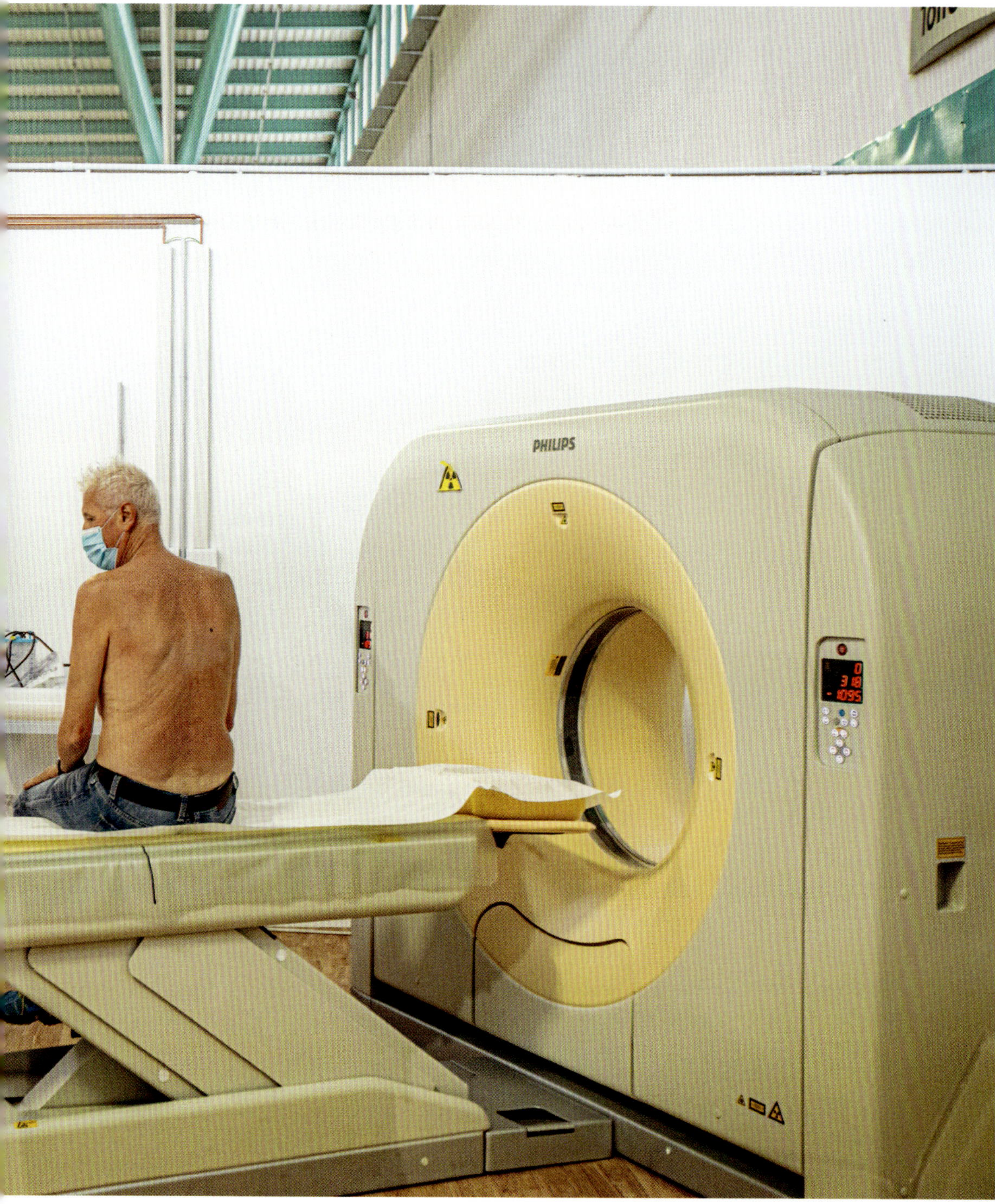
PHILIPS

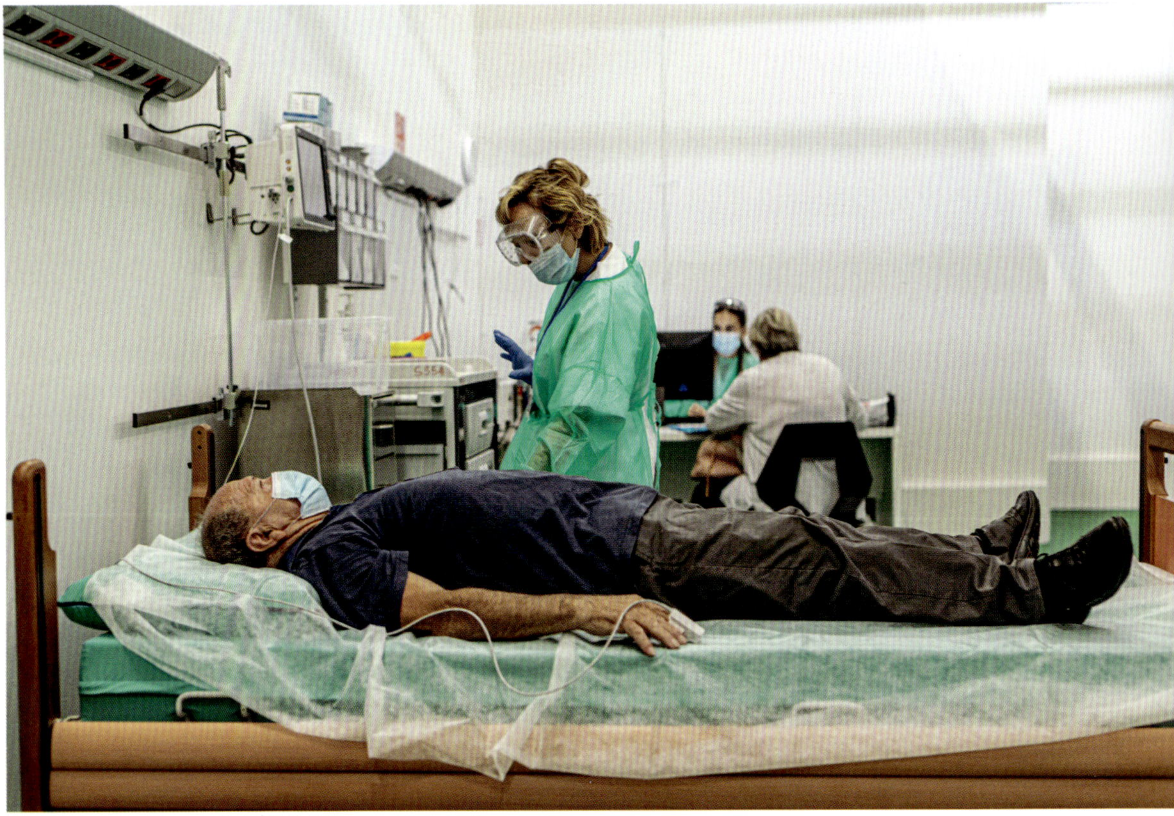

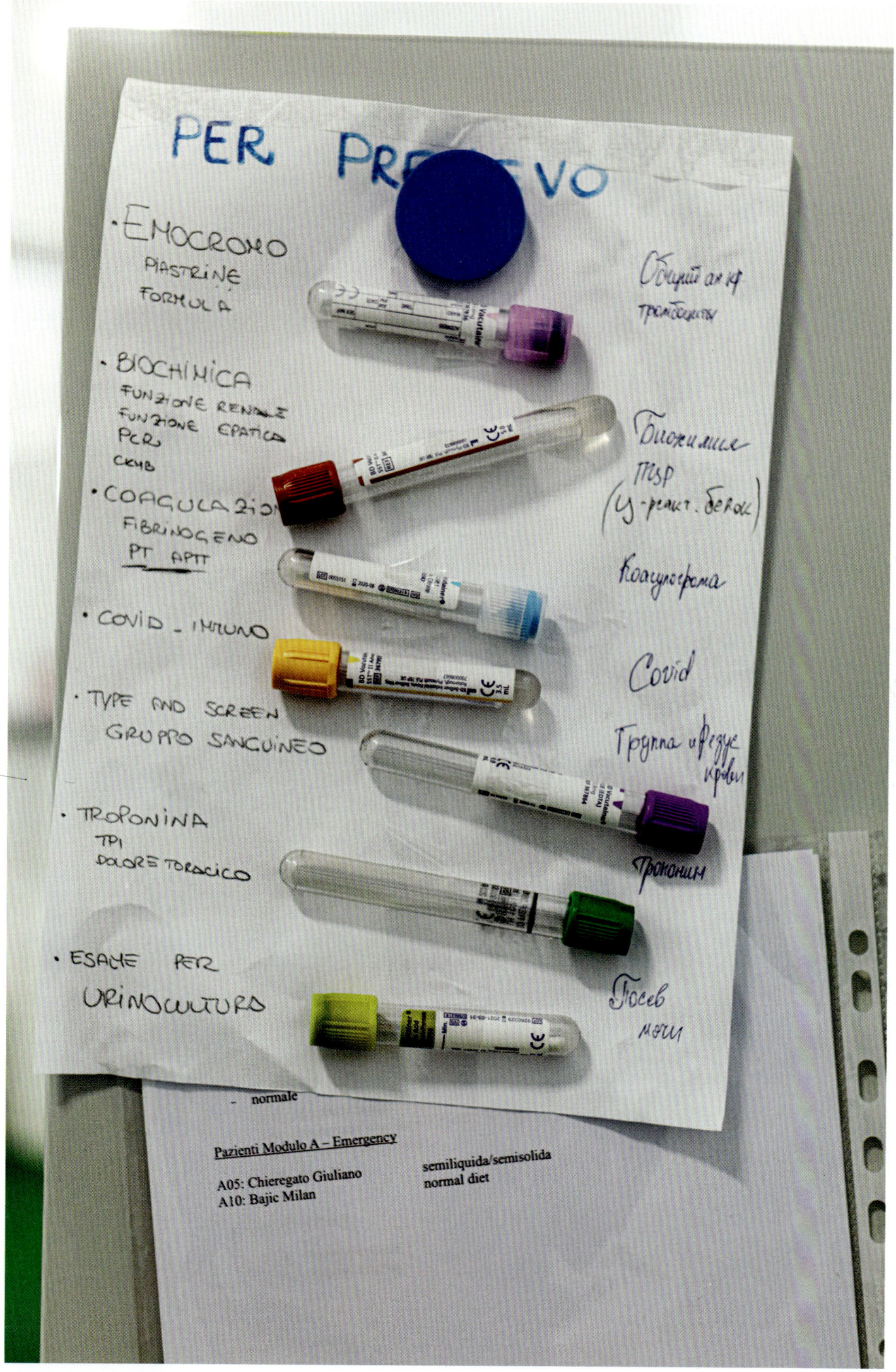
PER
• EMOCROMO
PIASTRINE
FORMULA
• BIOCHIMICA
FUNZIONE RENALE
FUNZIONE EPATICA
PCR
CKMB
• COAGULAZIO
FIBRINOGENO
PT APTT
• COVID - IMMUNO
• TYPE AND SCREEN
GRUPPO SANGUINEO
• TROPONINA
TPI
DOLORE TORACICO
• ESAME PER
URINOCULTURA
тромбоциты
Биохимия
(С-реакт. белок)
Коагулограма
Covid
Группа и резус крови
Тропонин
Посев мочи
- normale
Pazienti Modulo A – Emergency
A05: Chieregato Giuliano
A10: Bajic Milan
semiliquida/semisolida
normal diet

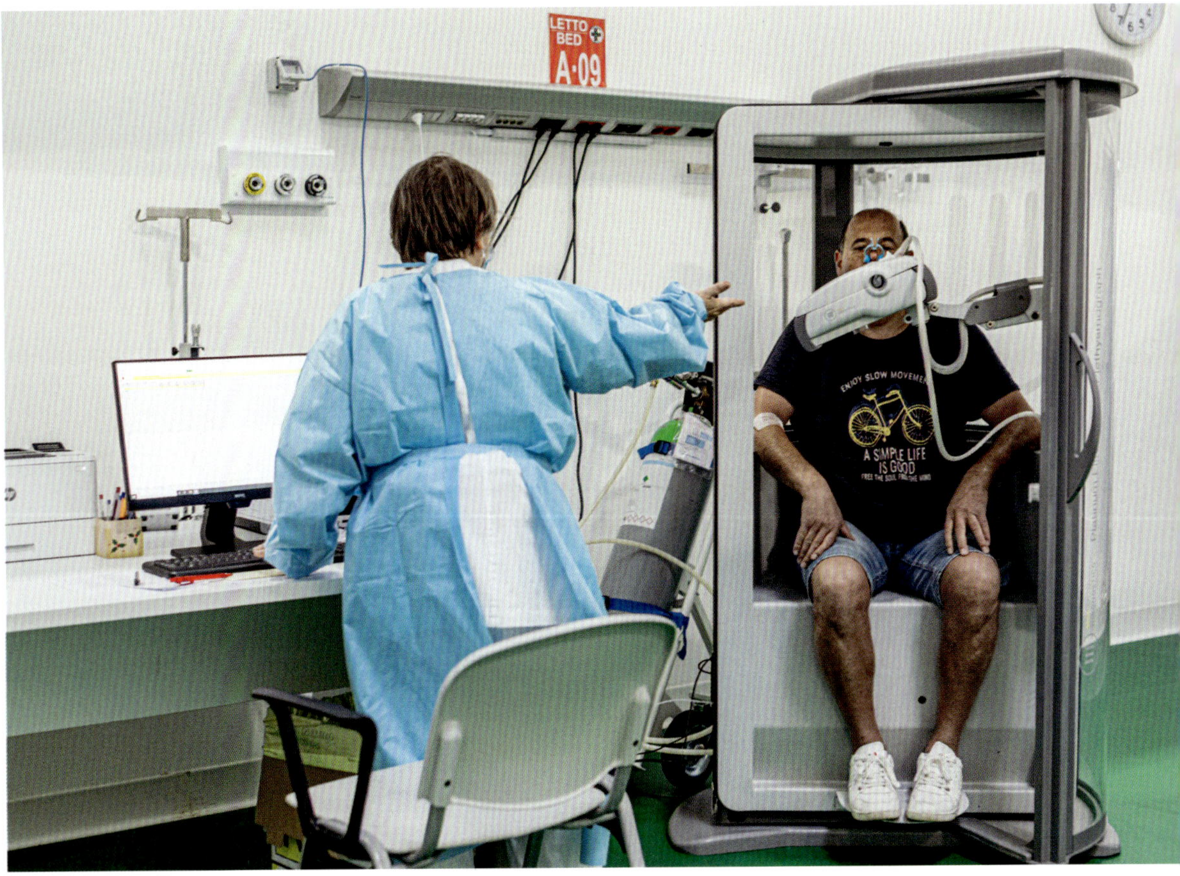
LETTO
BED
A·09
A SIMPLE LIFE
IS GOOD

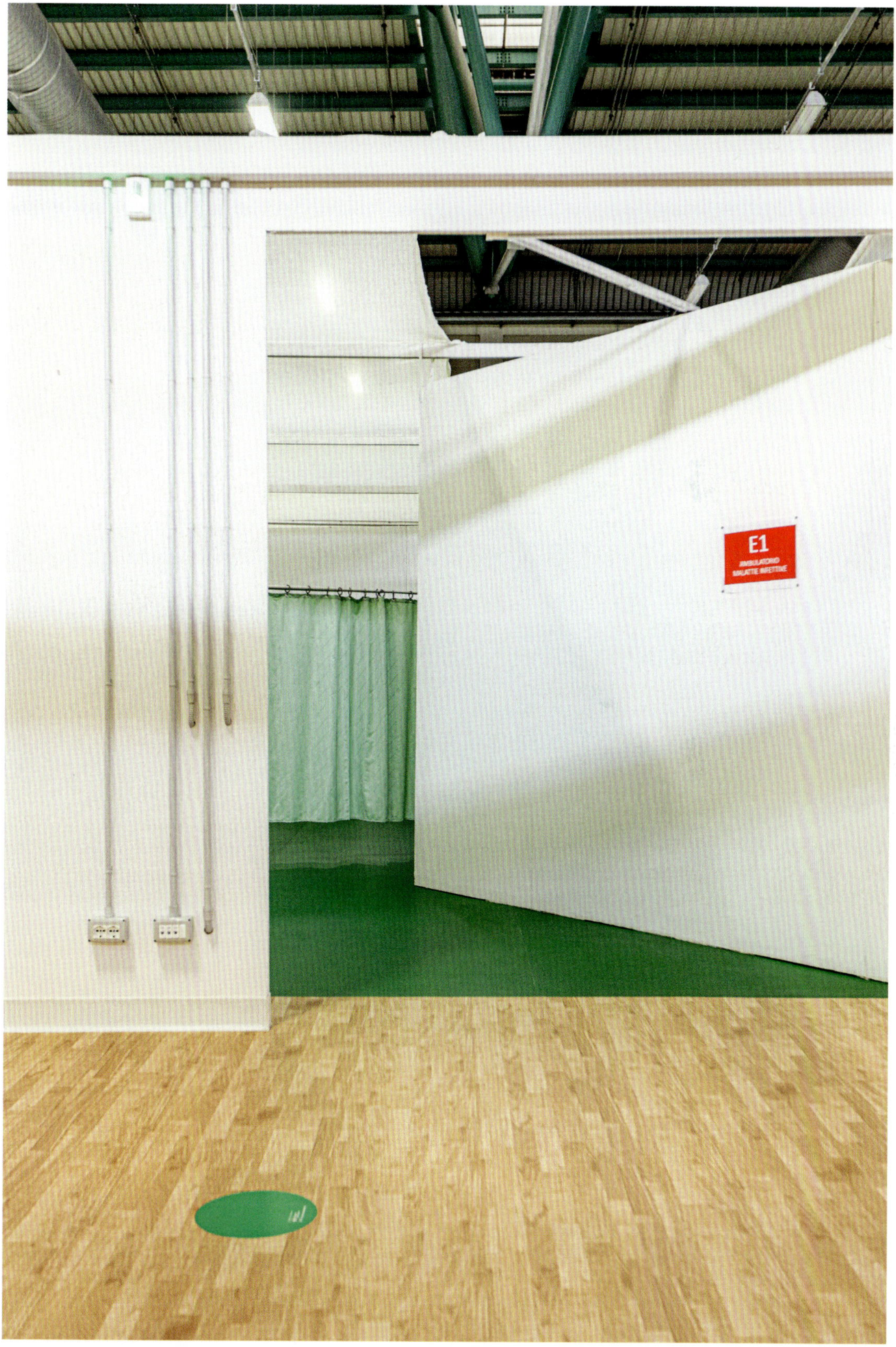
E1

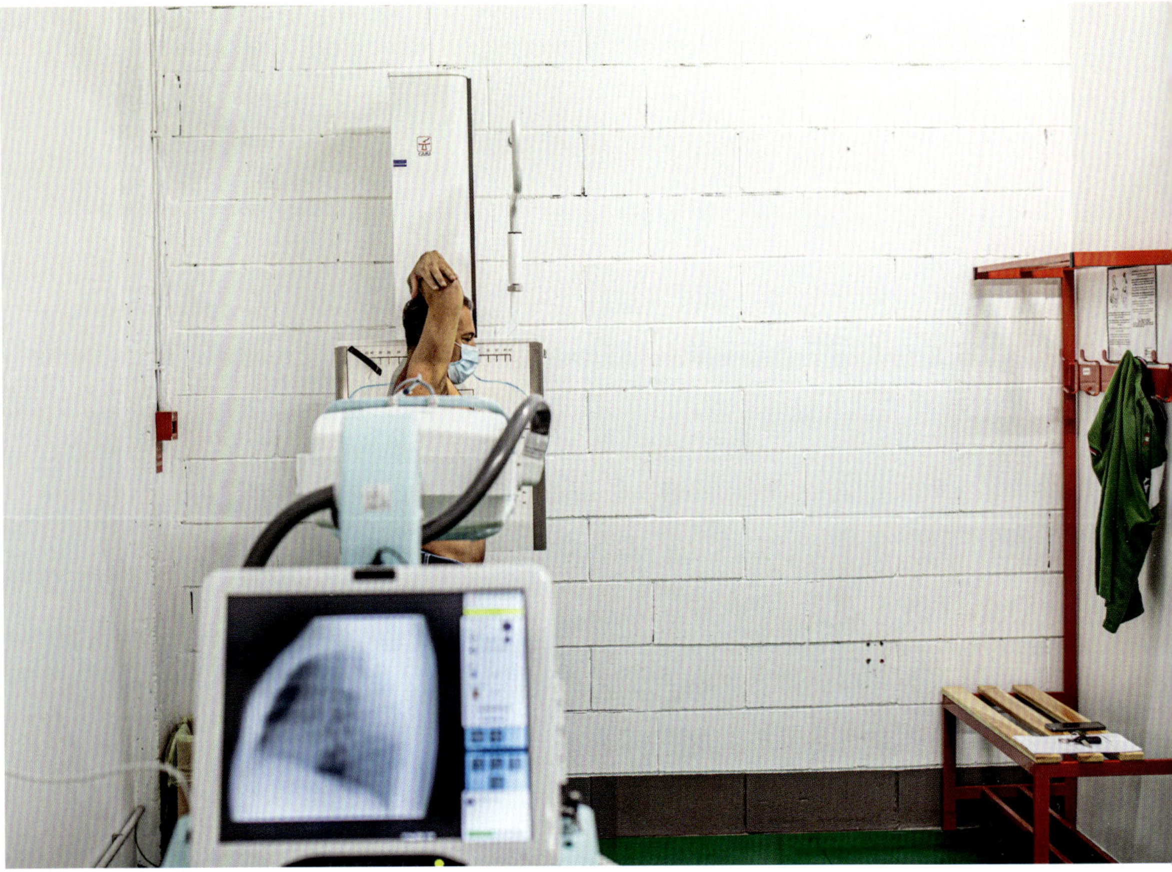

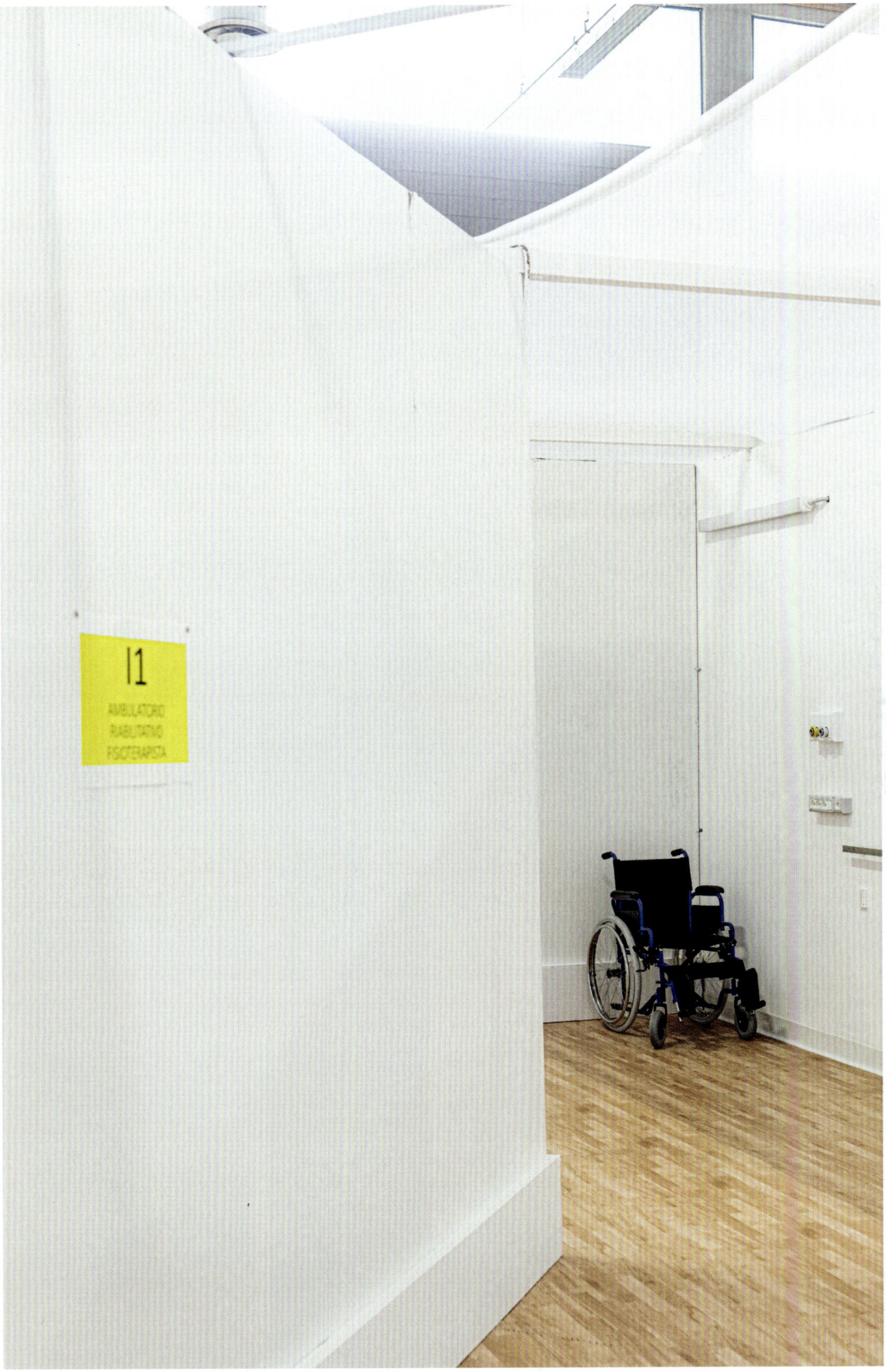
I1
AMBULATORIO
RIABILITATIVO
FISIOTERAPISTA

Niccoló Rastrelli, Italy
COVID-19 Face Wear

"The dress code to participate in the Coronavirus Masked Ball."
Undeniably, we live in a masked world, where the iconic item on the throne is now the face-mask; wearing it to leave our homes as stealthy cats with our self-certification in hand. It appears that during the time of quarantine the imagination of many has thrived. Indeed, numerous alternative proposals of the standard produced face-mask arose, potentially, to create a new cool reputation for the object or just to make it socially more acceptable.
So, while strolling down the street, we see a sea of covered faces with masks of every liking, from the standard surgical ones, ffp2 or ffp3, to more fashionable and sporty ones. Truly today the face-mask is a symbol of protection against diseases and pollution, so instilling a sense of security, however, it is also becoming an accessory intrinsically involved in our sense of identity. While wearing a face-mask half of our facial features disappear however, it most prominently hides the one feature linked to our verbal language and smiling ability. So inevitably nullifying an essential part of our interpersonal communication.
We have been forcibly transformed into interpreters of this new page of history that is "the War against the virus", we prepare, and live our daily lives, as the legendary warriors of the past. Just like knights, tailored in armor, masking and shielding their faces, intimating the enemy with a glance and ready to step into battle.

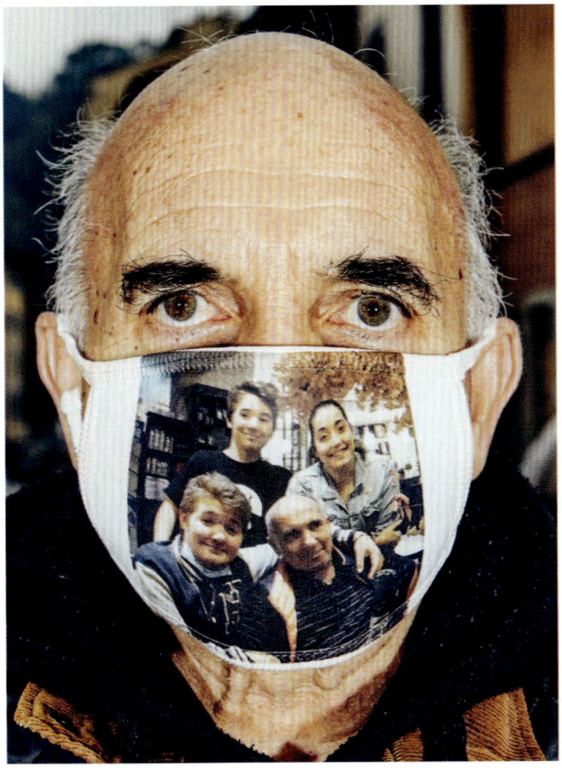

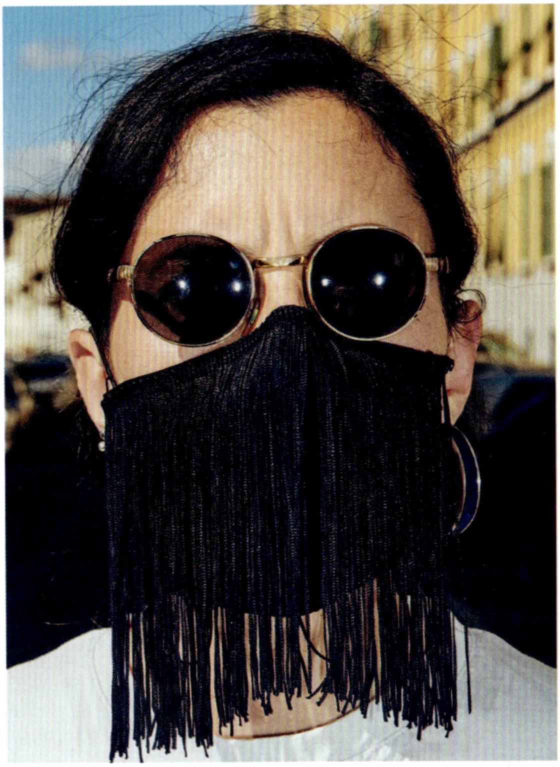

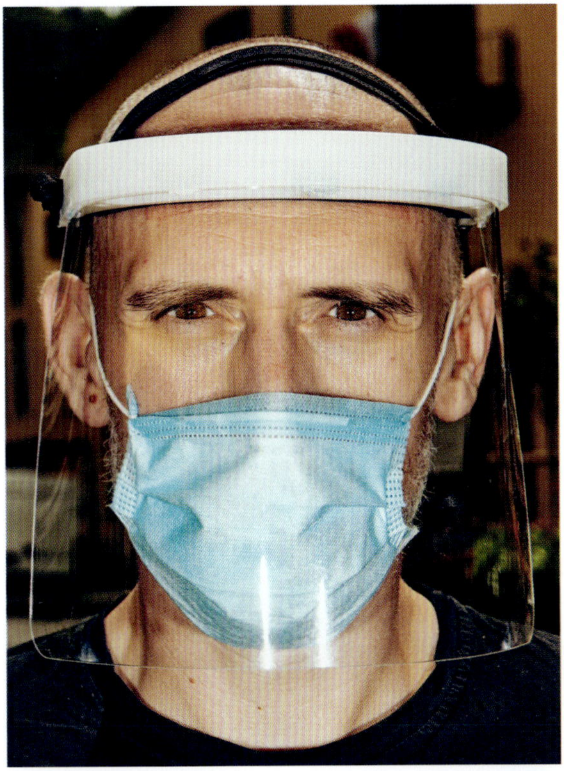

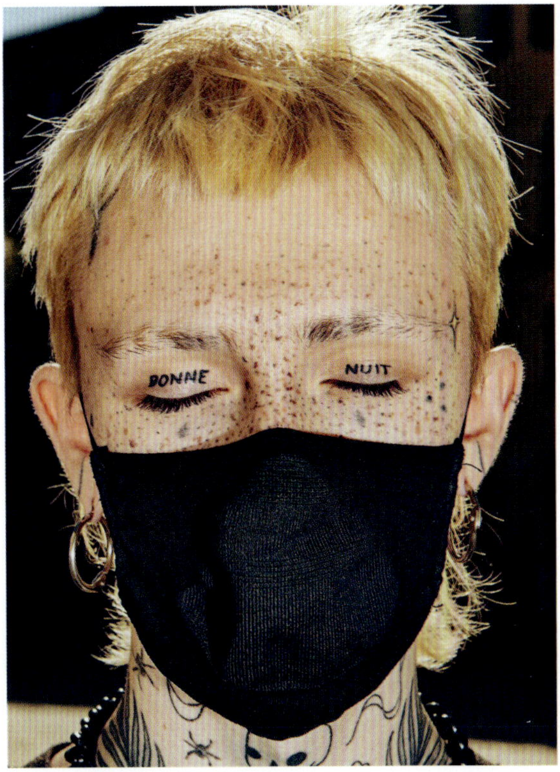
BONNE
NUIT

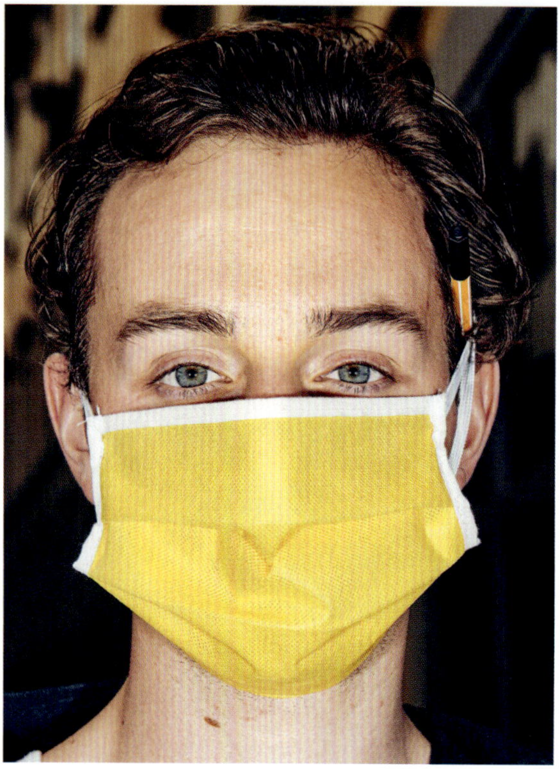

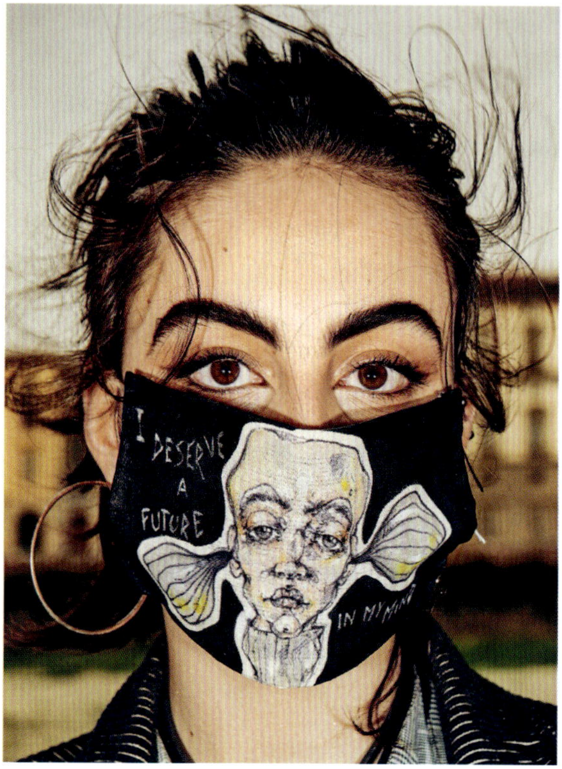
I DESERVE A FUTURE

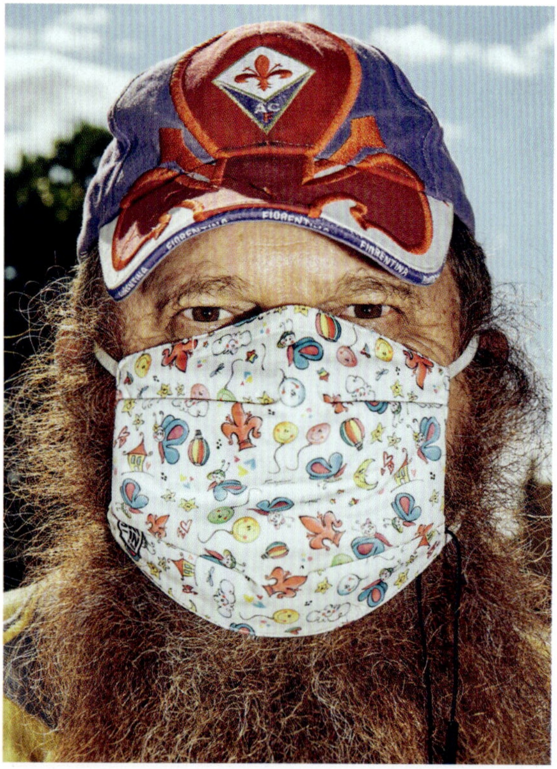
FIORENTINA

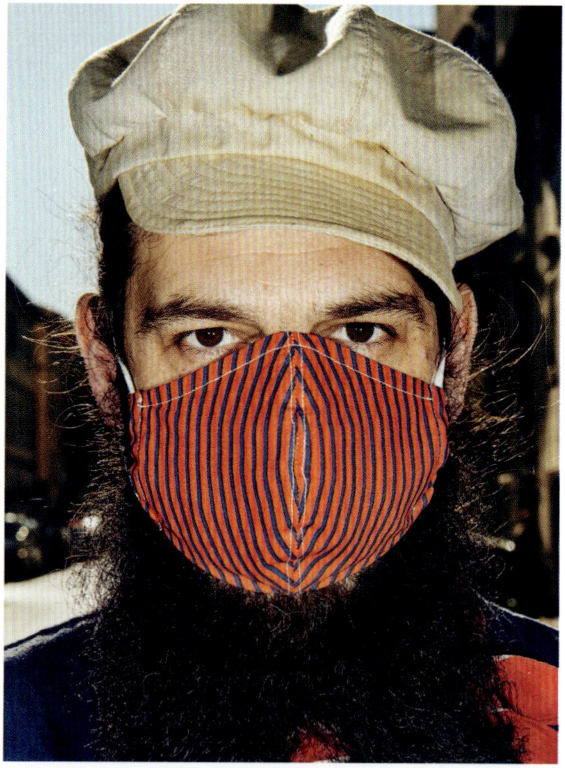

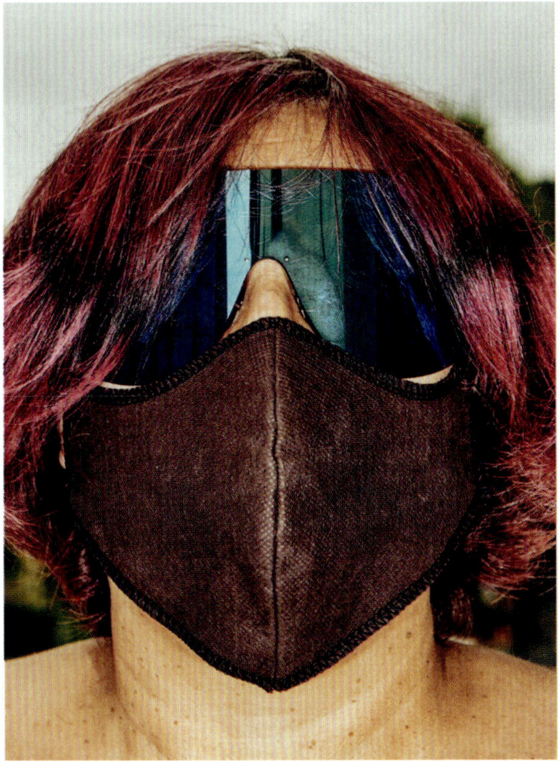
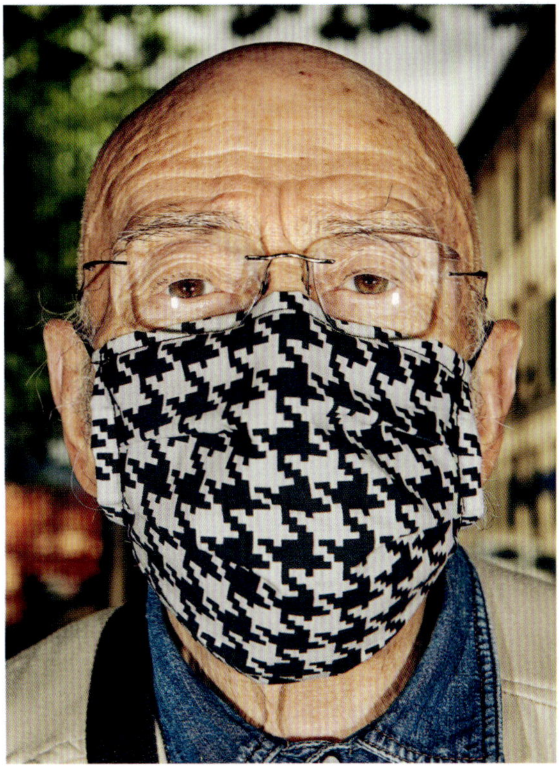
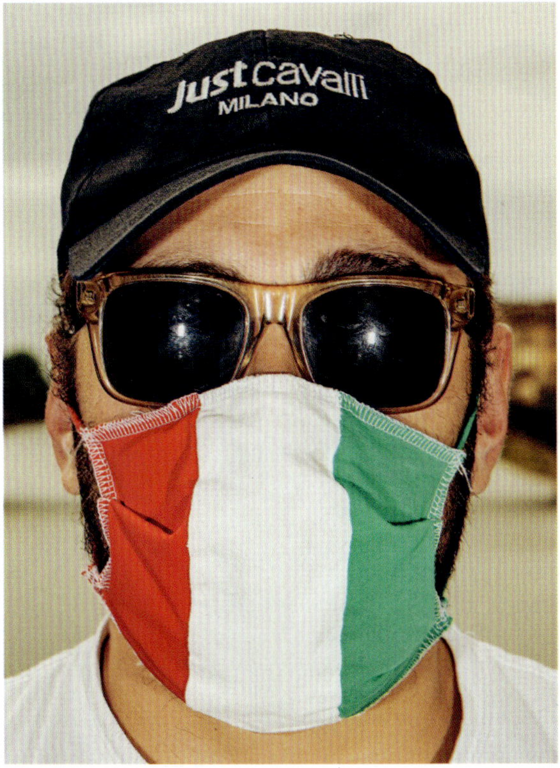
Just cavalli
MILANO
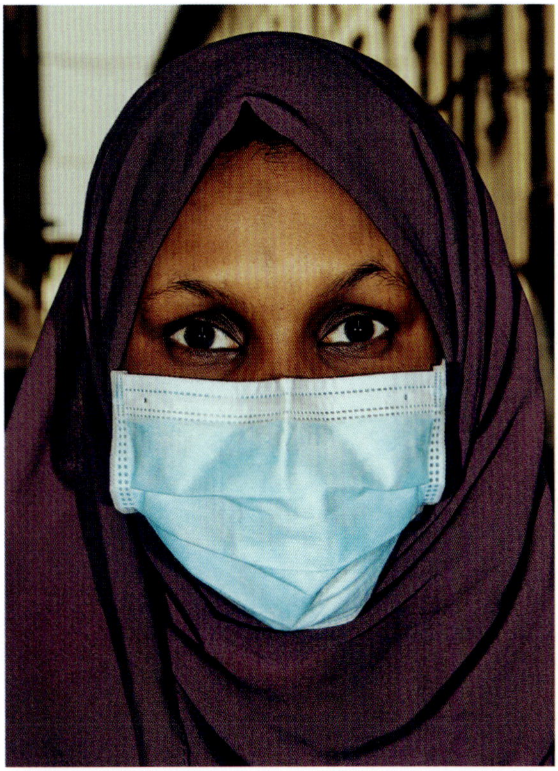

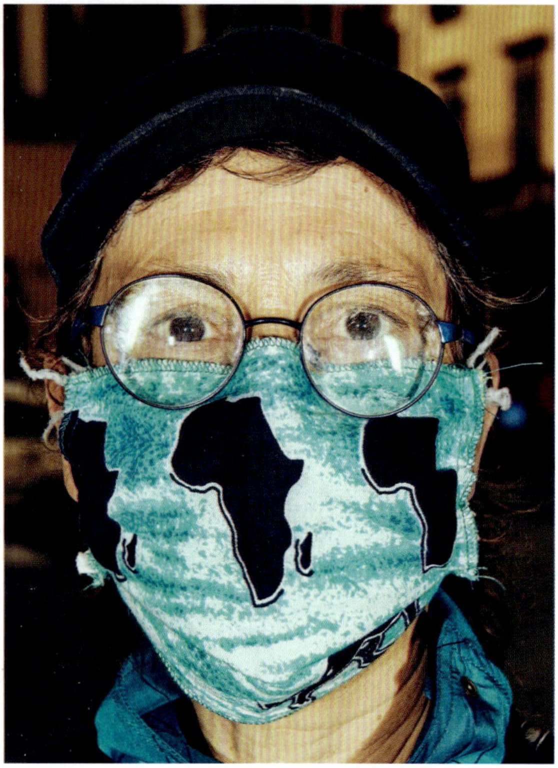

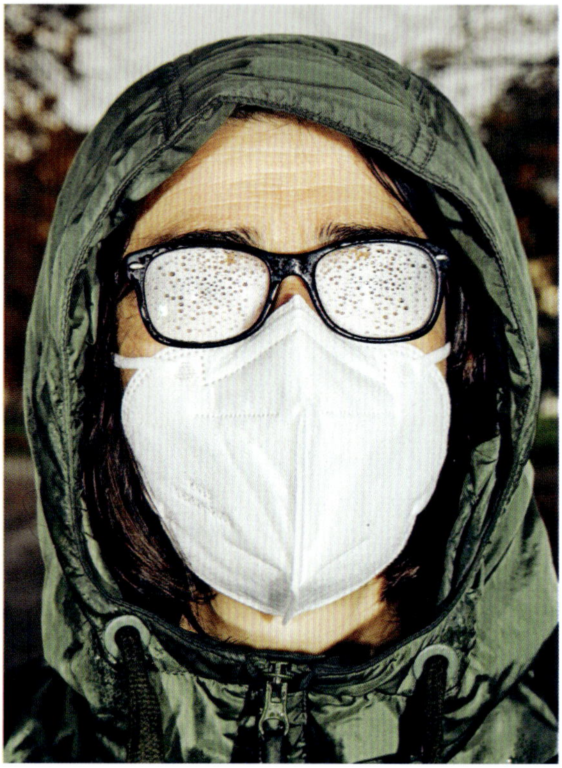

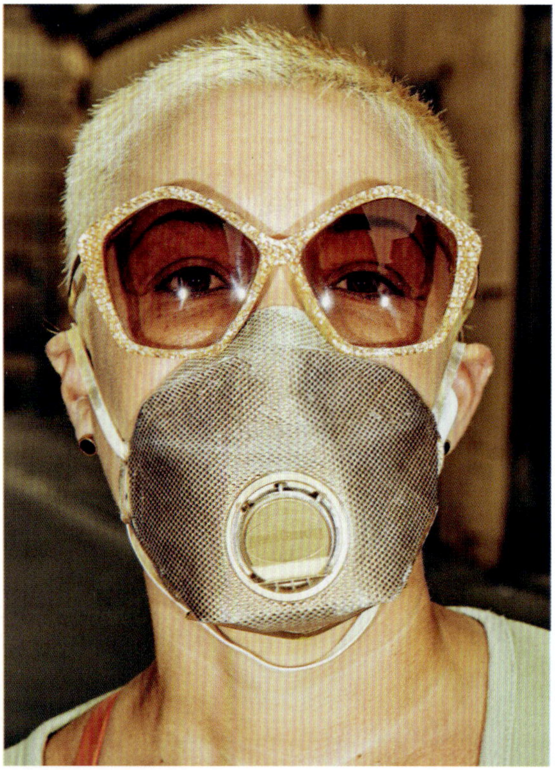

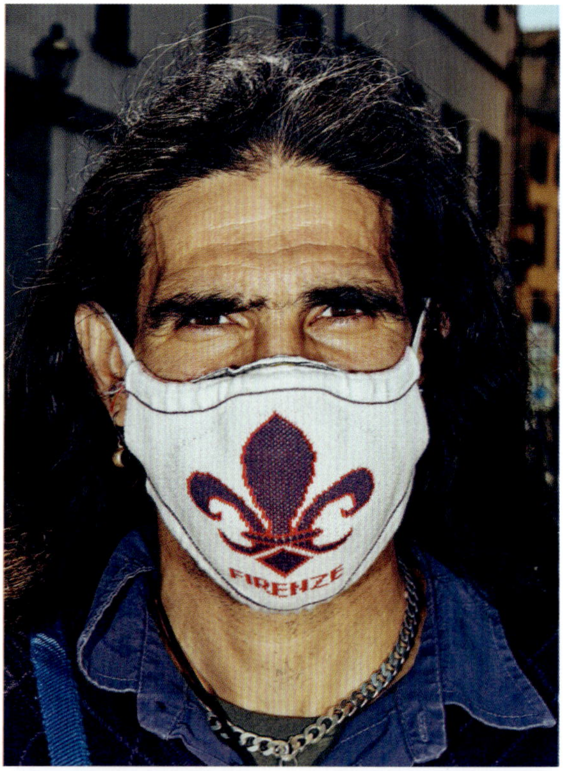
FIRENZE

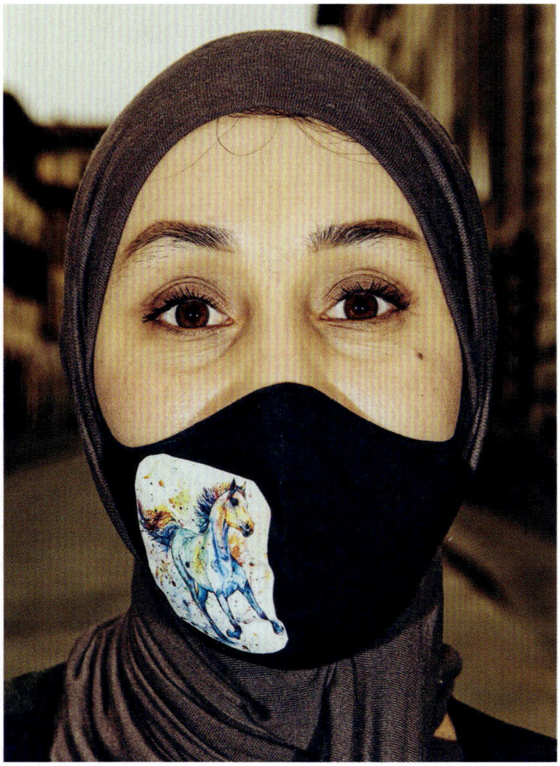

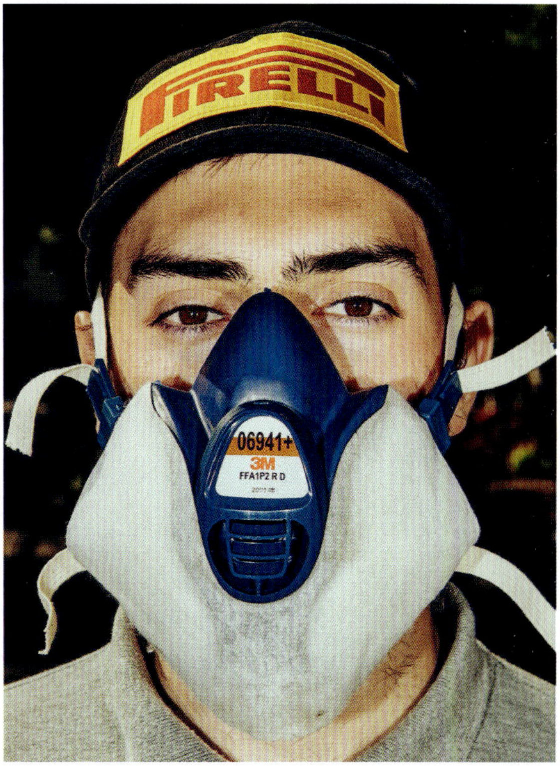
PIRELLI
06941+
3M
FFA1P2 R D

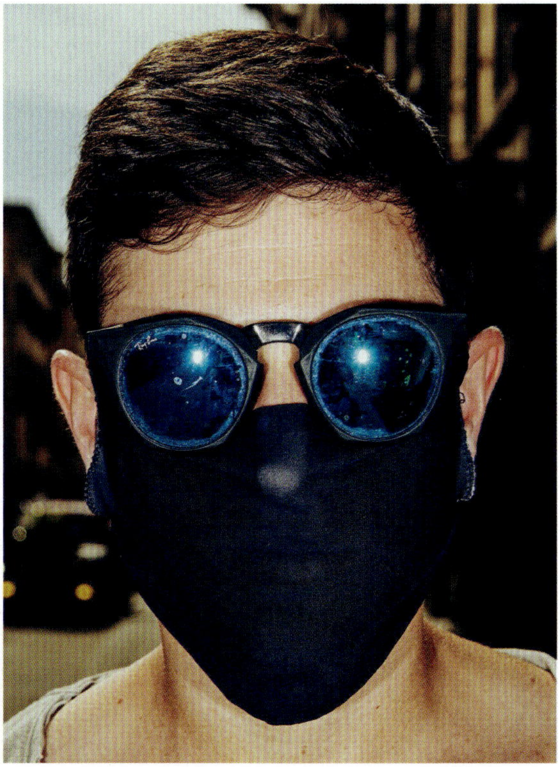

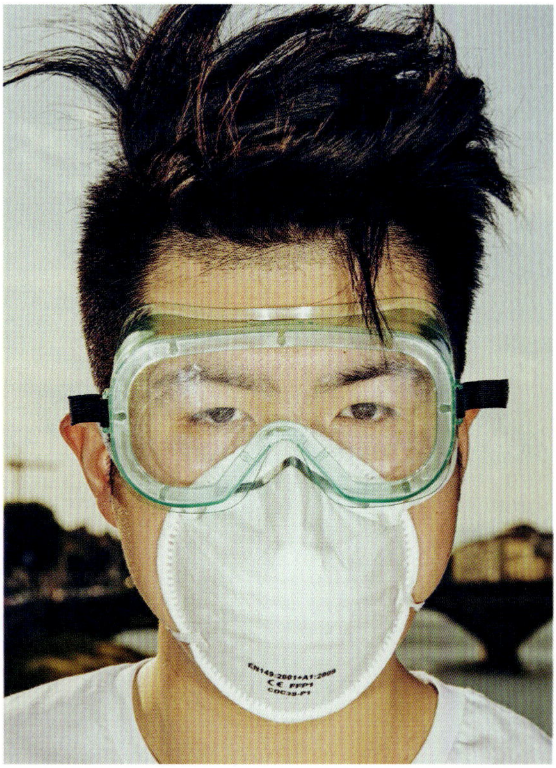

Paolo Pellegrin, Italy
L'Altro

Annalisa D'Angelo
and Alessandro Vitali

"What would happen if a man's face could adequately express his suffering, if his entire inner agony were objectified in his facial expression? Could we still communicate? Wouldn't we then cover our faces with our hands while talking? Life would really be impossible if the infinitude of feelings we harbor within ourselves were fully expressed in the lines of our faces. Nobody would dare look at himself in the mirror, because a grotesque, tragic image would mix in the contours of his face with stains and traces of blood, wounds which cannot be healed, and unstoppable streams of tears."
Emil Cioran

The global pandemic that began in March 2020 has altered our habits and caused us to rethink many aspects of our lives. The way we hug, shake hands, sit next to each other, say hello with a smile, has changed. In dialogue with others and before there is any physical contact, our face is the immediate sign that defines our openness to communication. However, since masks have become part of our daily lives, communication has become more problematic. How do we interpret these new restrictions, what new languages help us to communicate, what happens to our minds?

L'Altro (the other) is a reflection on the effects of COVID-19 and social distancing. It is the culmination of Paolo Pellegrin's urgent need to visually explore this universal unknown. Over the years, Pellegrin has repeatedly questioned the theme of surveillance, opting for a number of techniques used as expedients to suggest an aesthetic of control: the choice of positioning oneself in strategic points from which to mechanically capture places and physical actions, the act of photographing without revealing one's presence, cancelling the physical distance from the subject through his gaze.
The work introduces us to the chaos of disarranged crowds, the blurred lines of the city, the new principles of social organisation. The experience of the individual returns to the centre of the debate, through the faces that emerge from the blackness. Social distancing is emerging as a new concept imposed in the Western, political lexicon, radically transforming each individual's experience of their own body.
L'Altro does not intend to draw conclusions about the effects of the pandemic, this would be impossible in such a short space of time. Instead, photographs are used to question the new paradigms of the society in which we prepare to live.

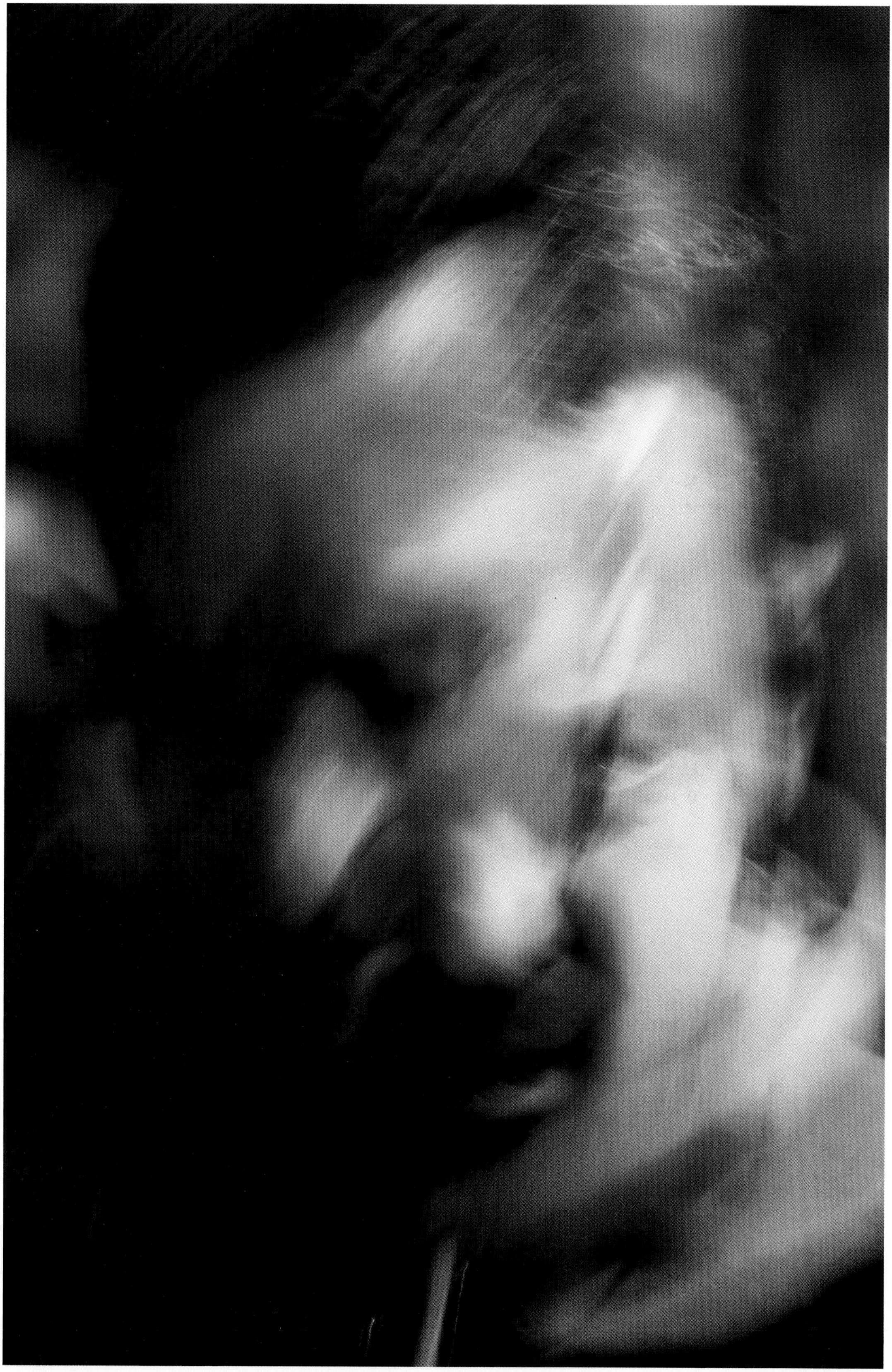

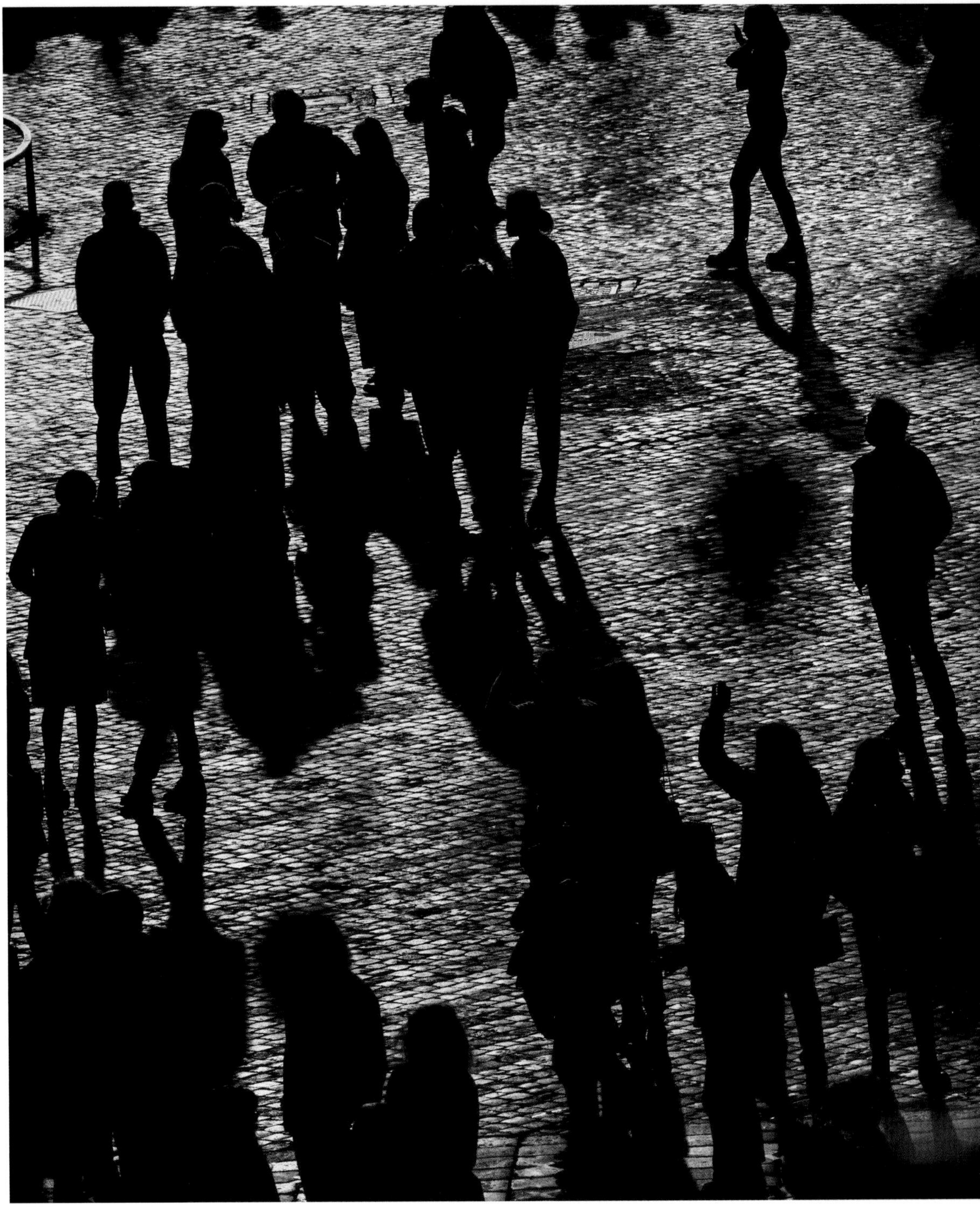

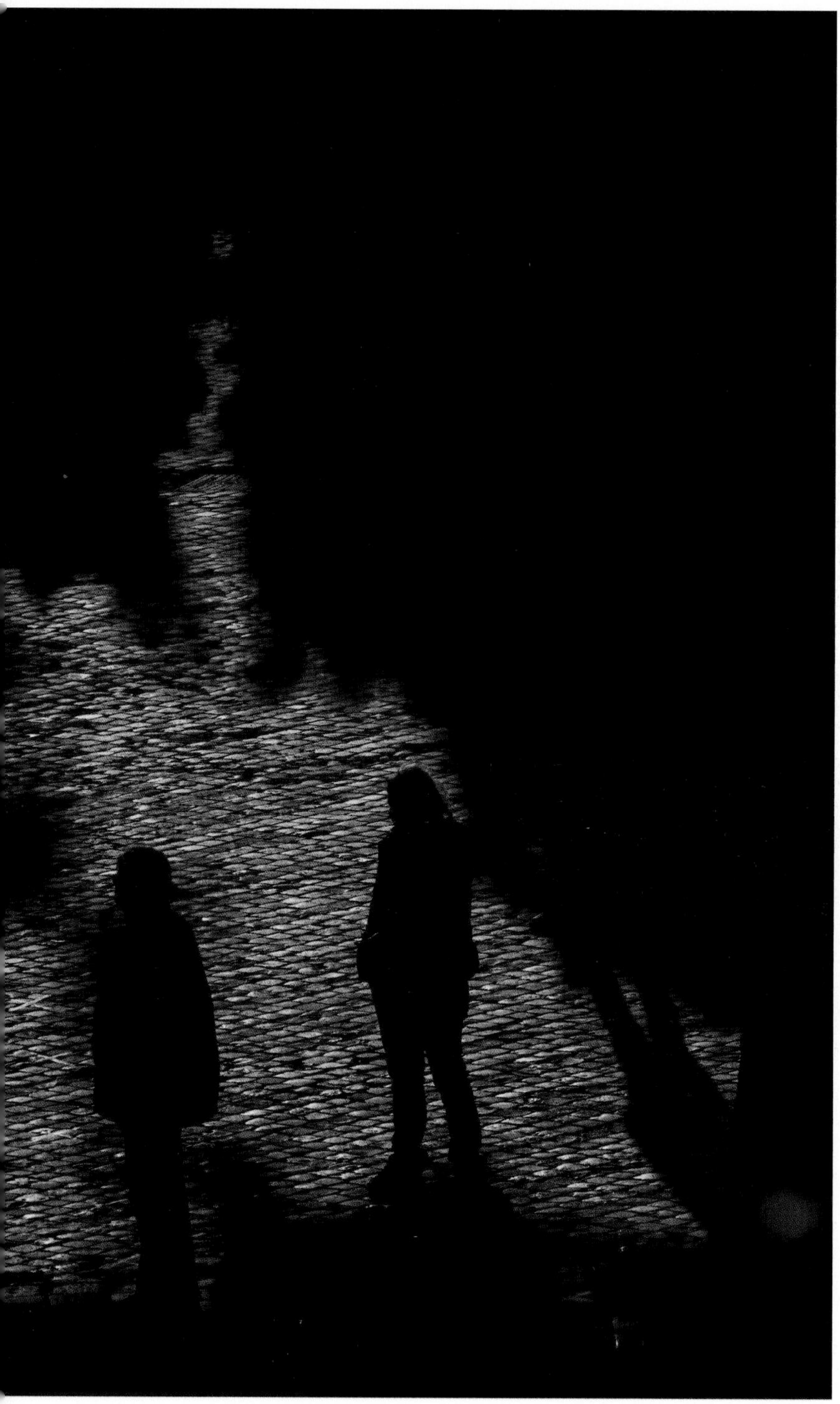

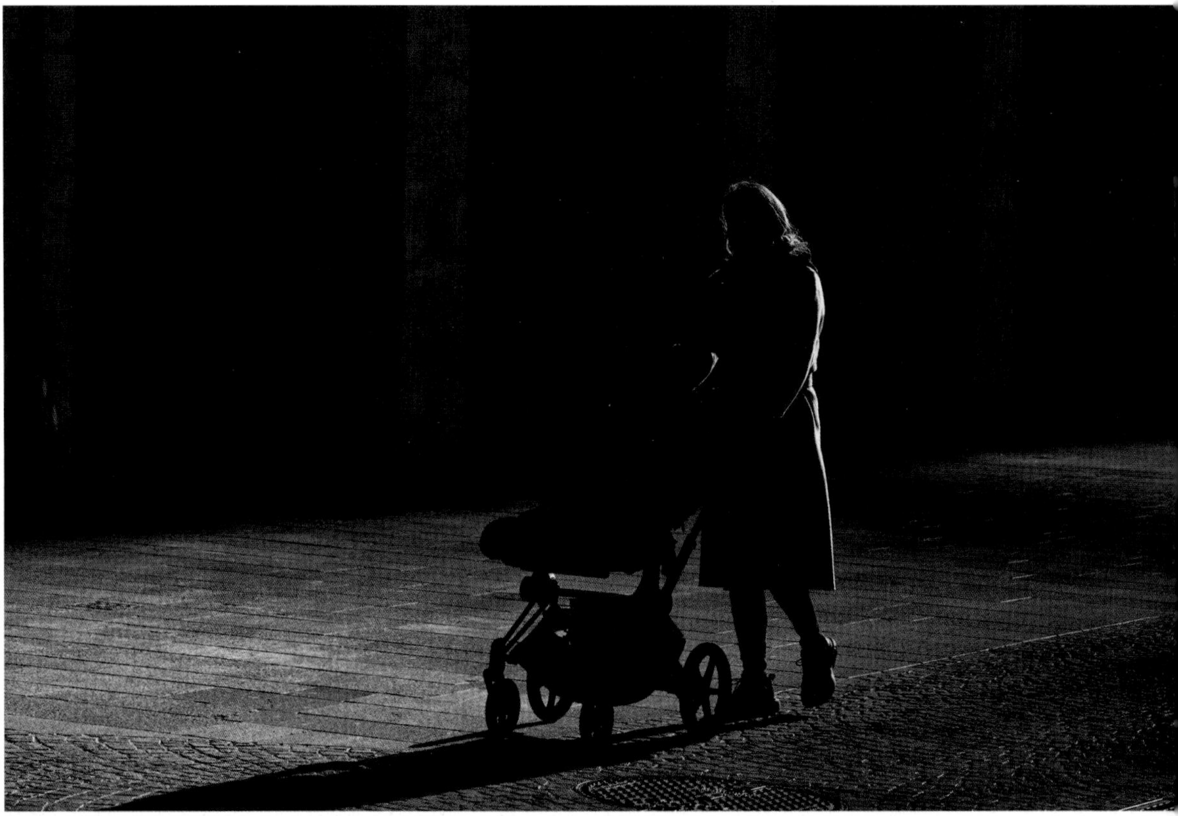

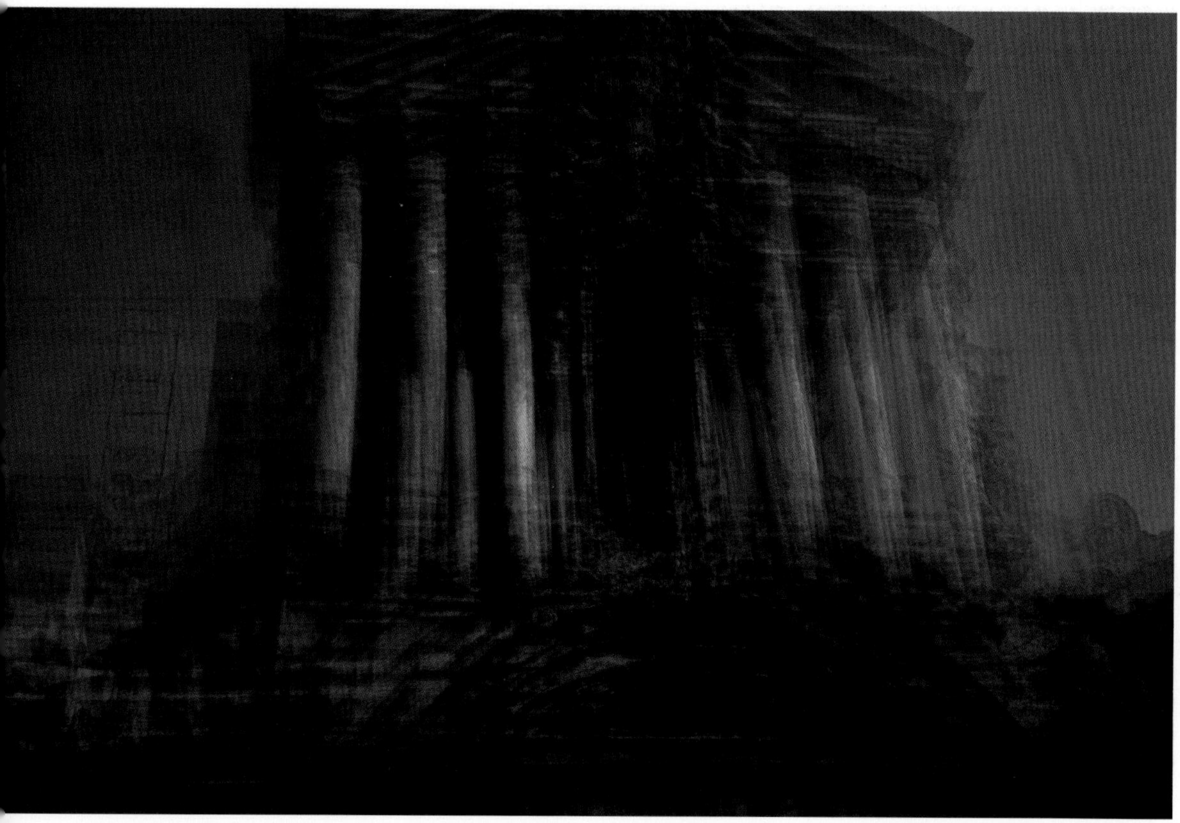

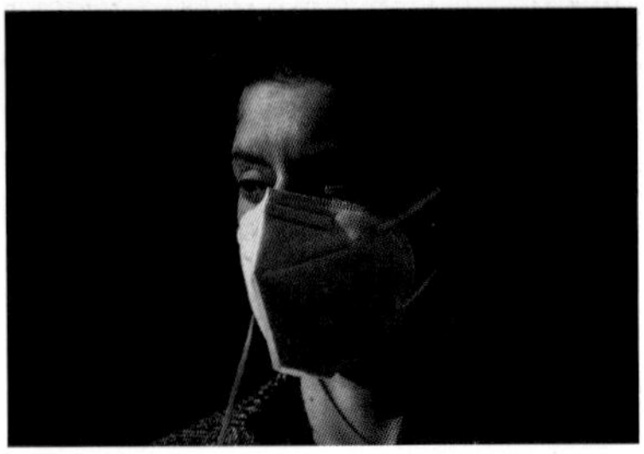
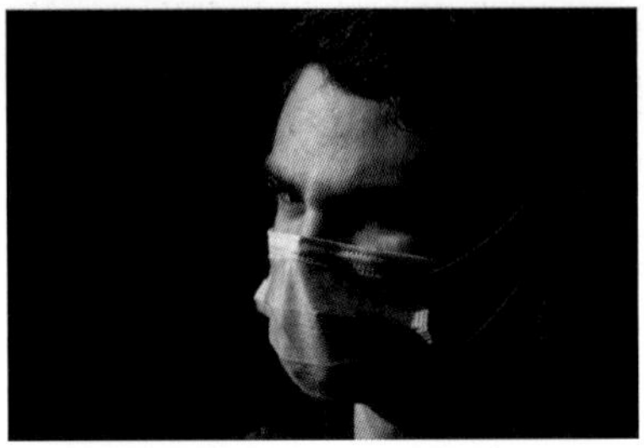
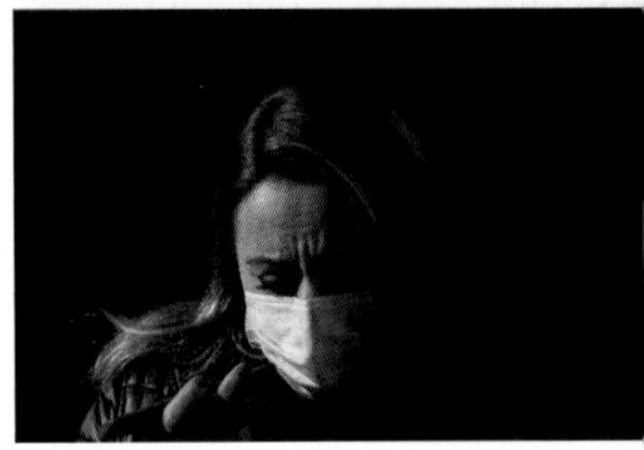
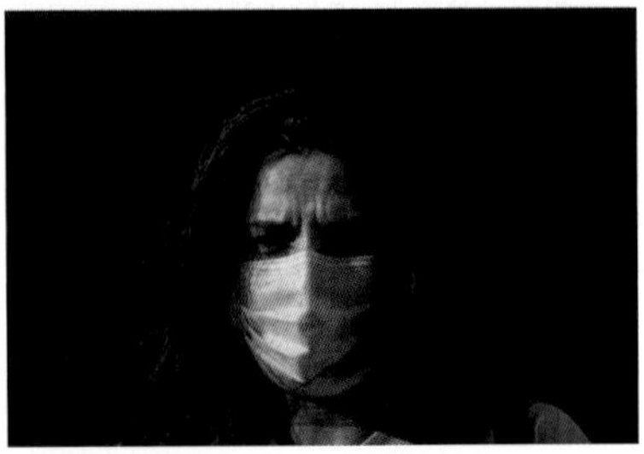
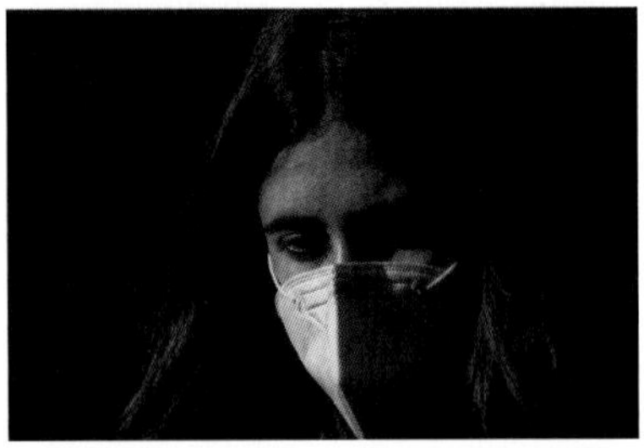
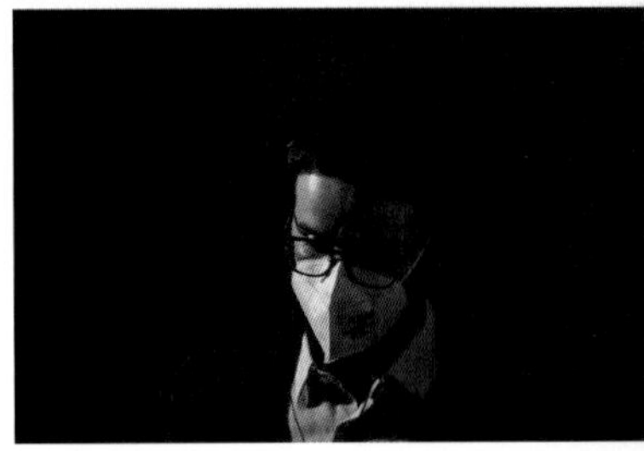
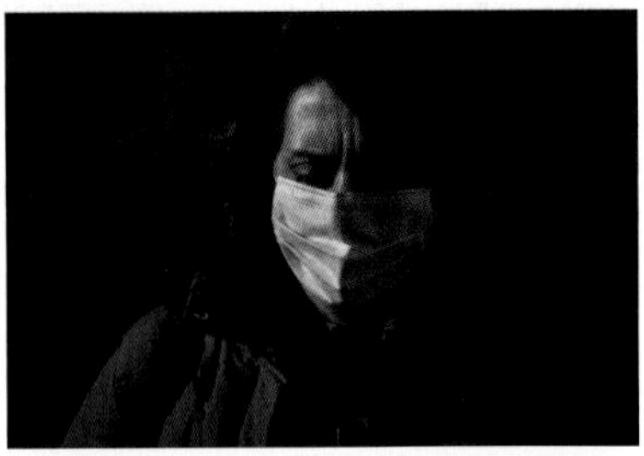
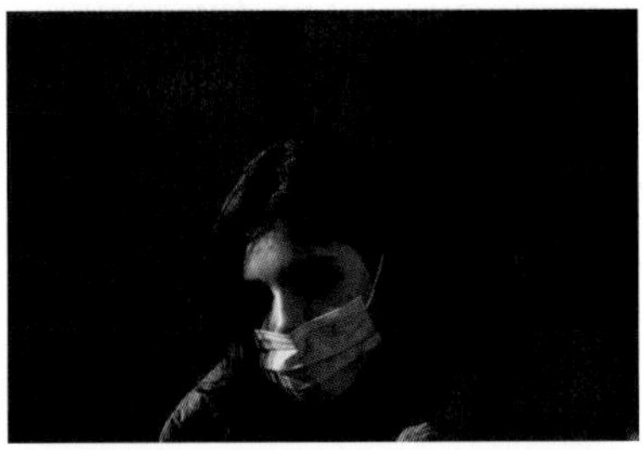
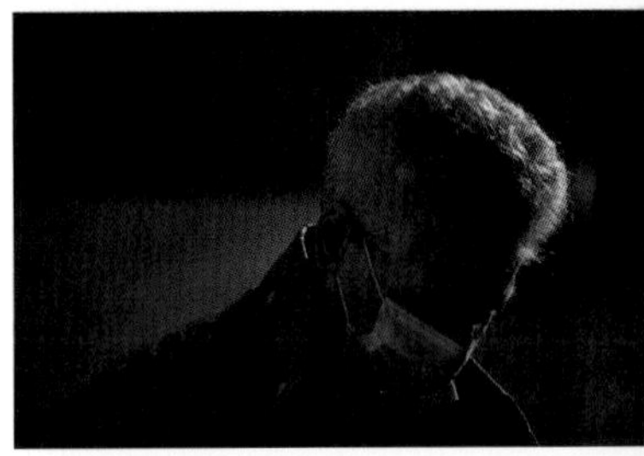
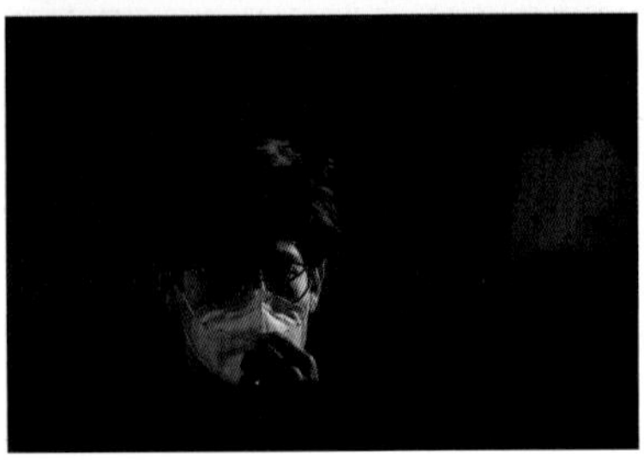
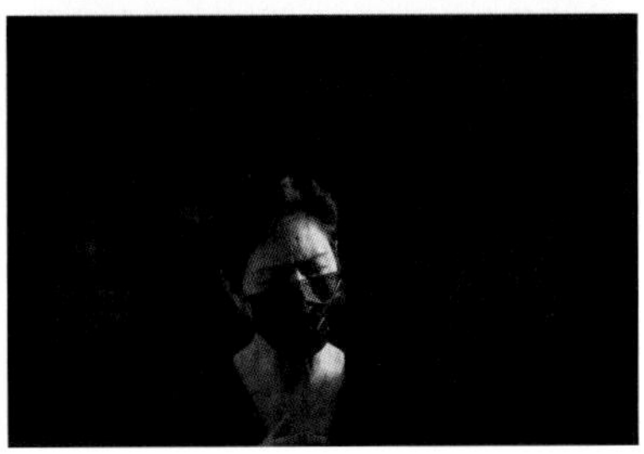
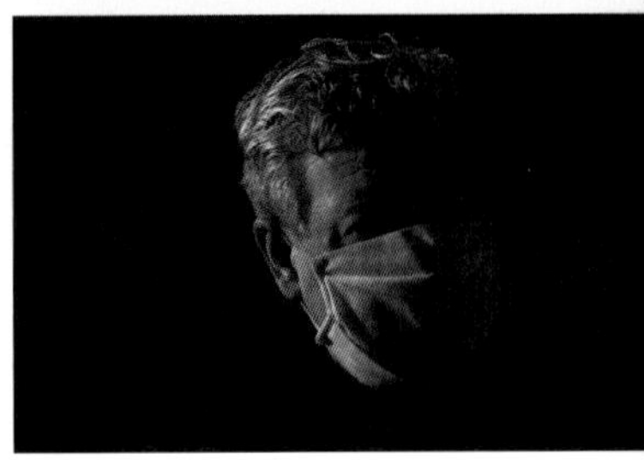

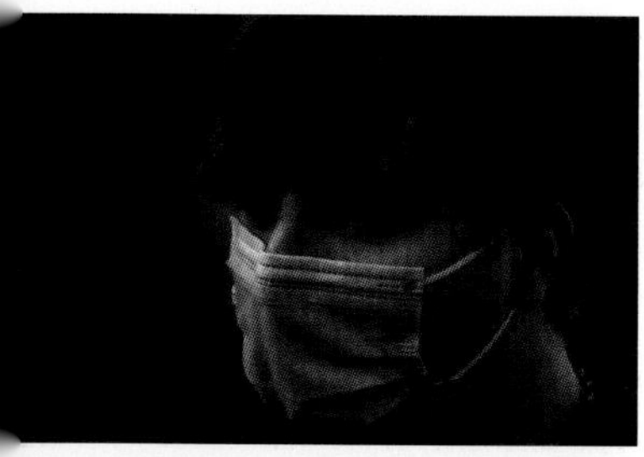
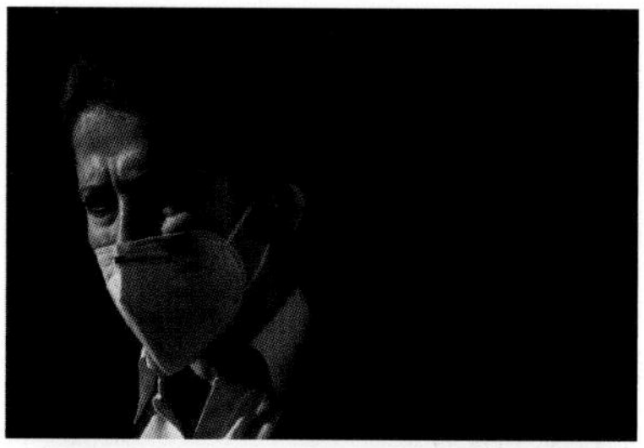
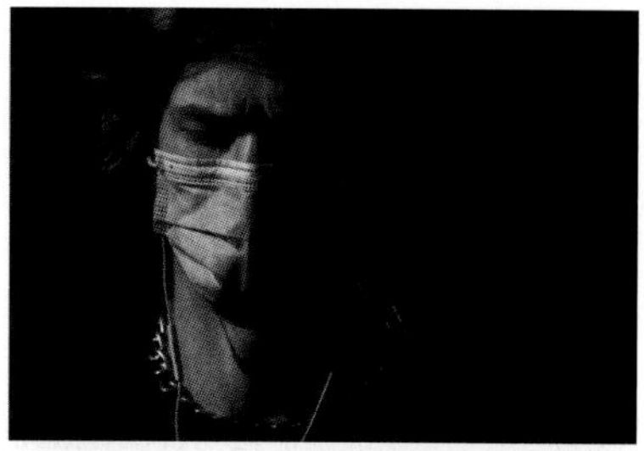
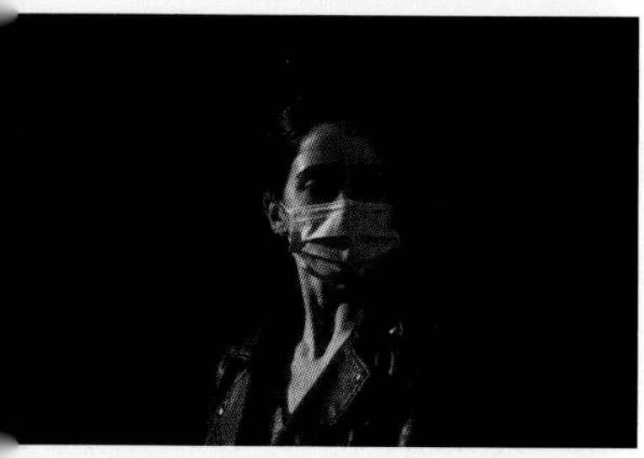
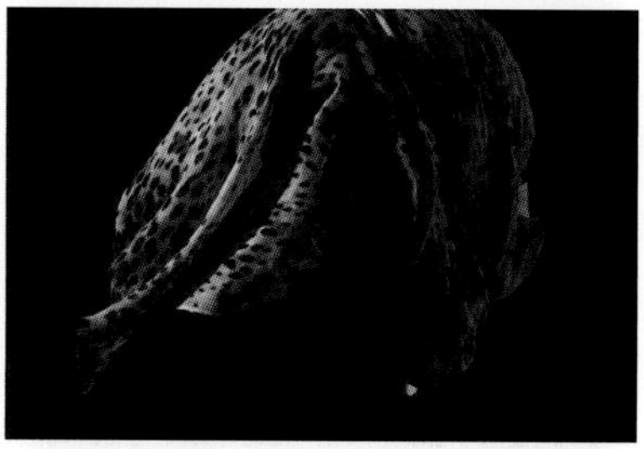
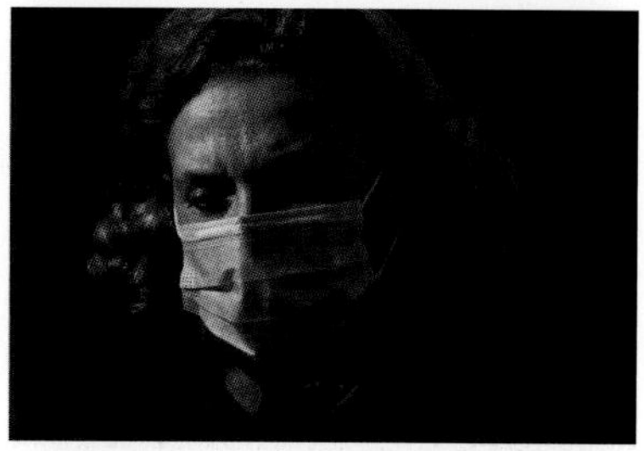
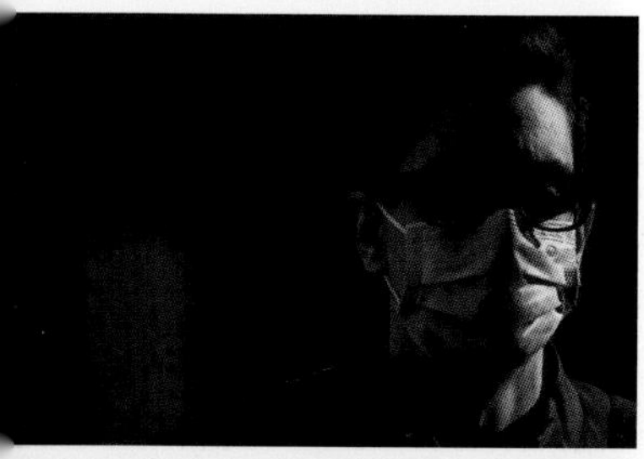
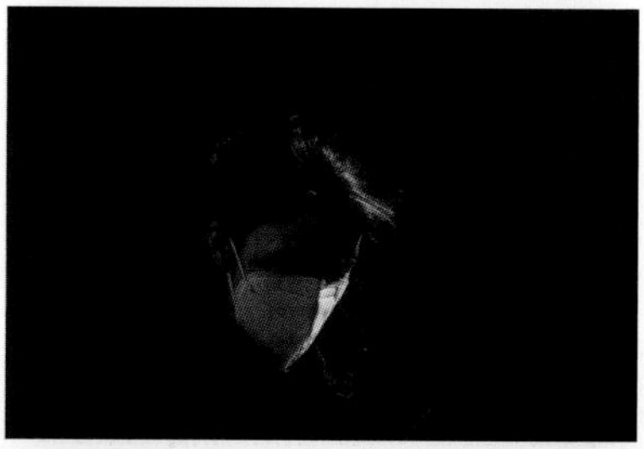
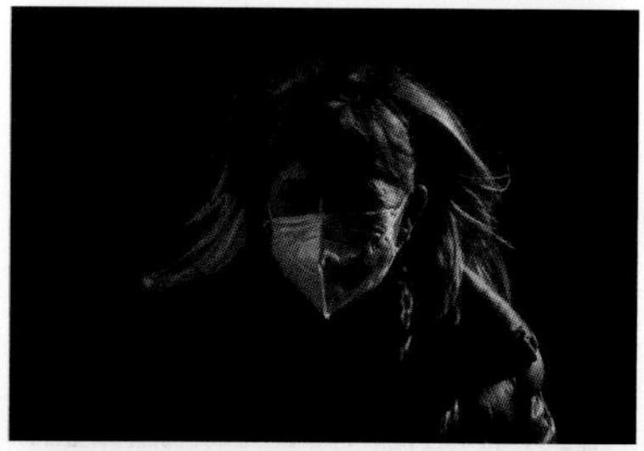
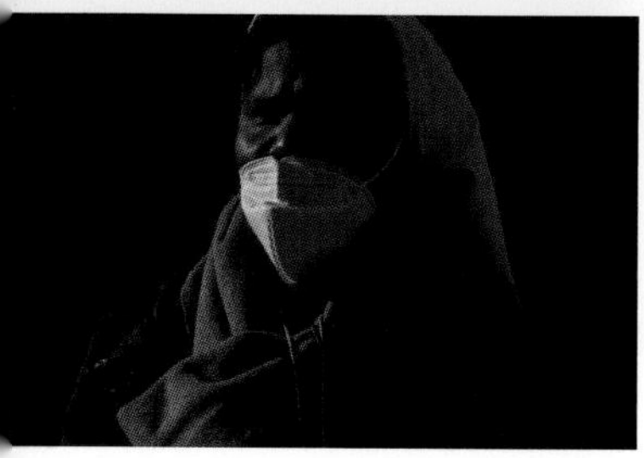
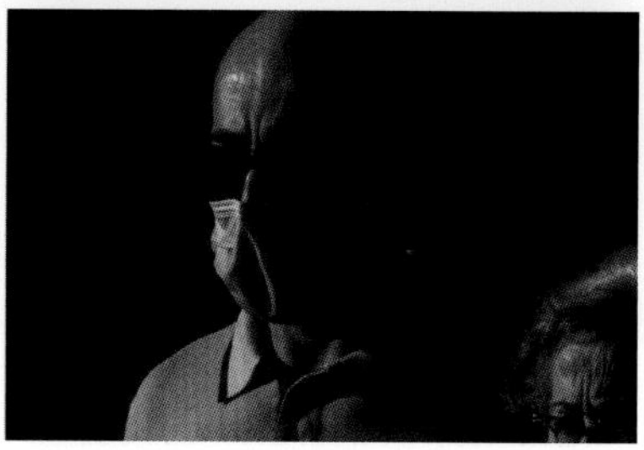
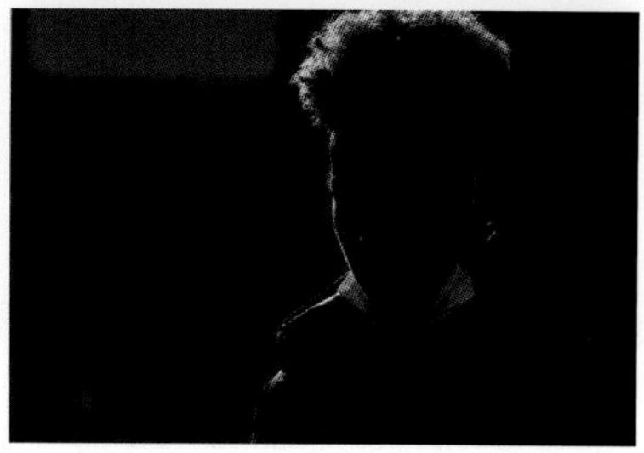

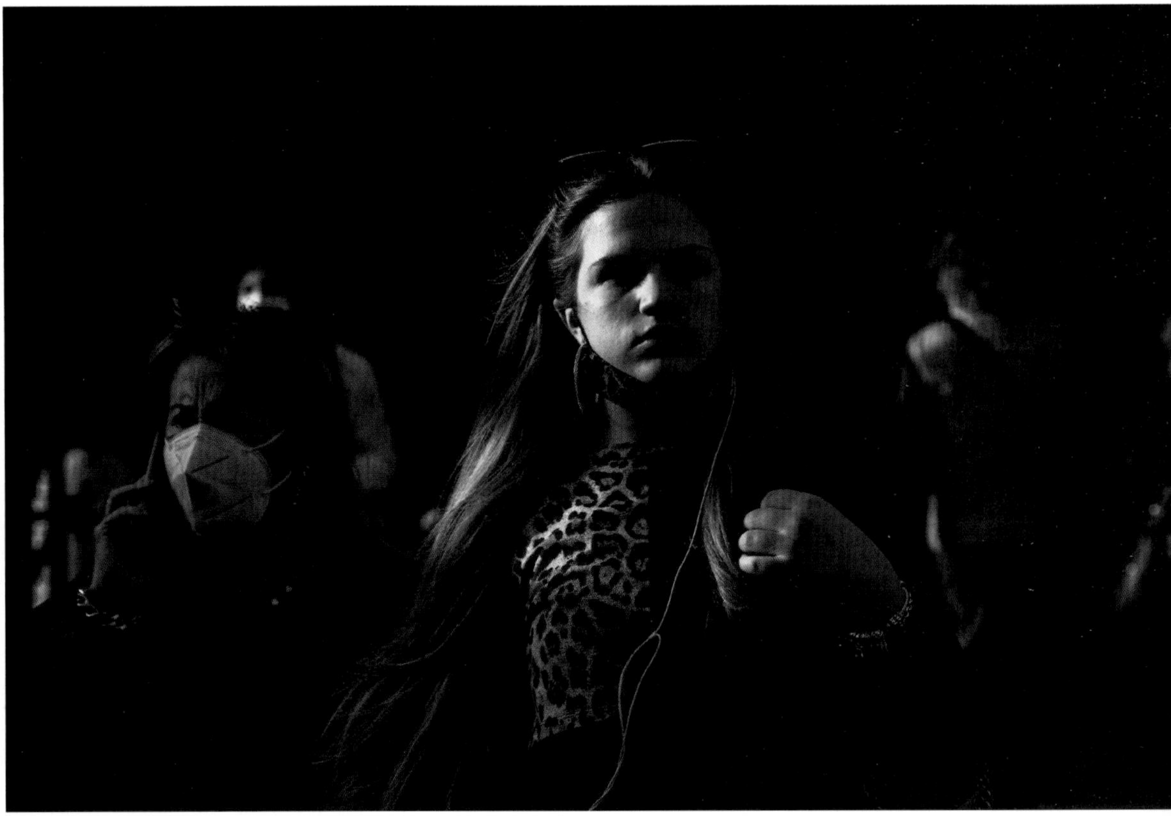

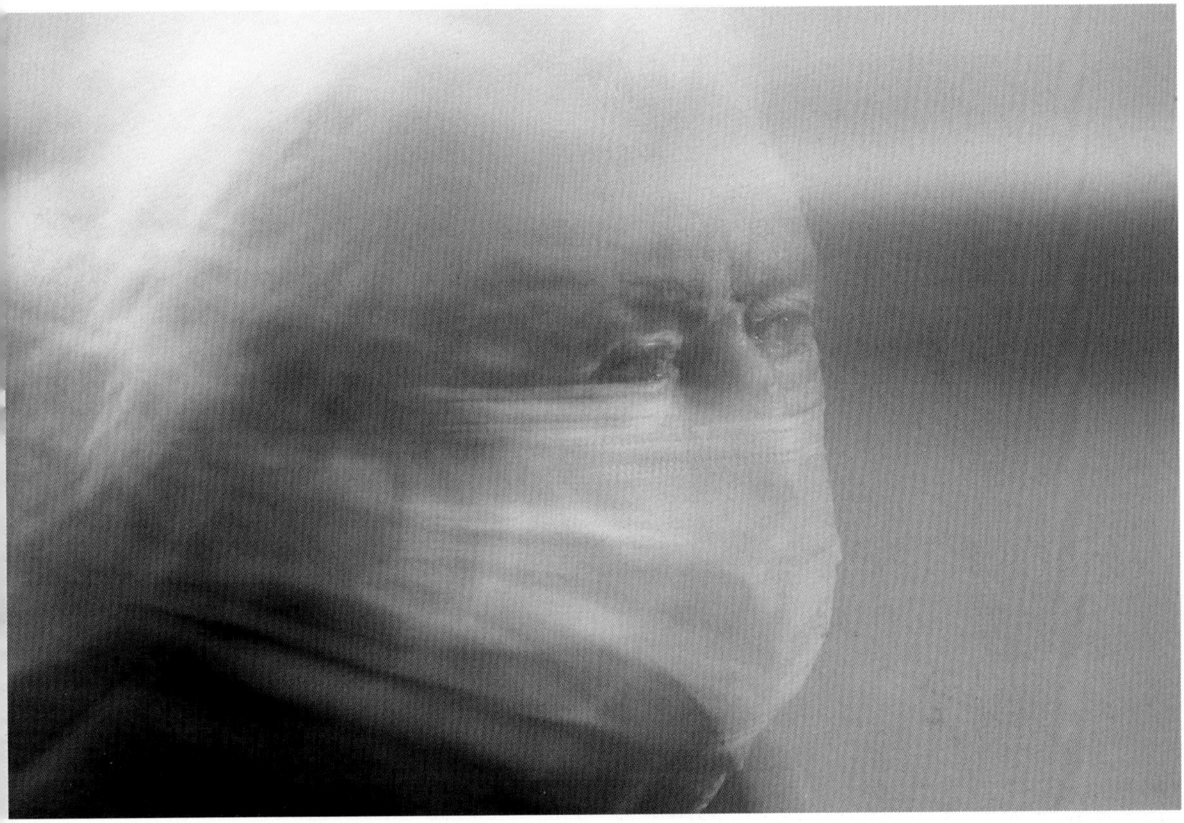

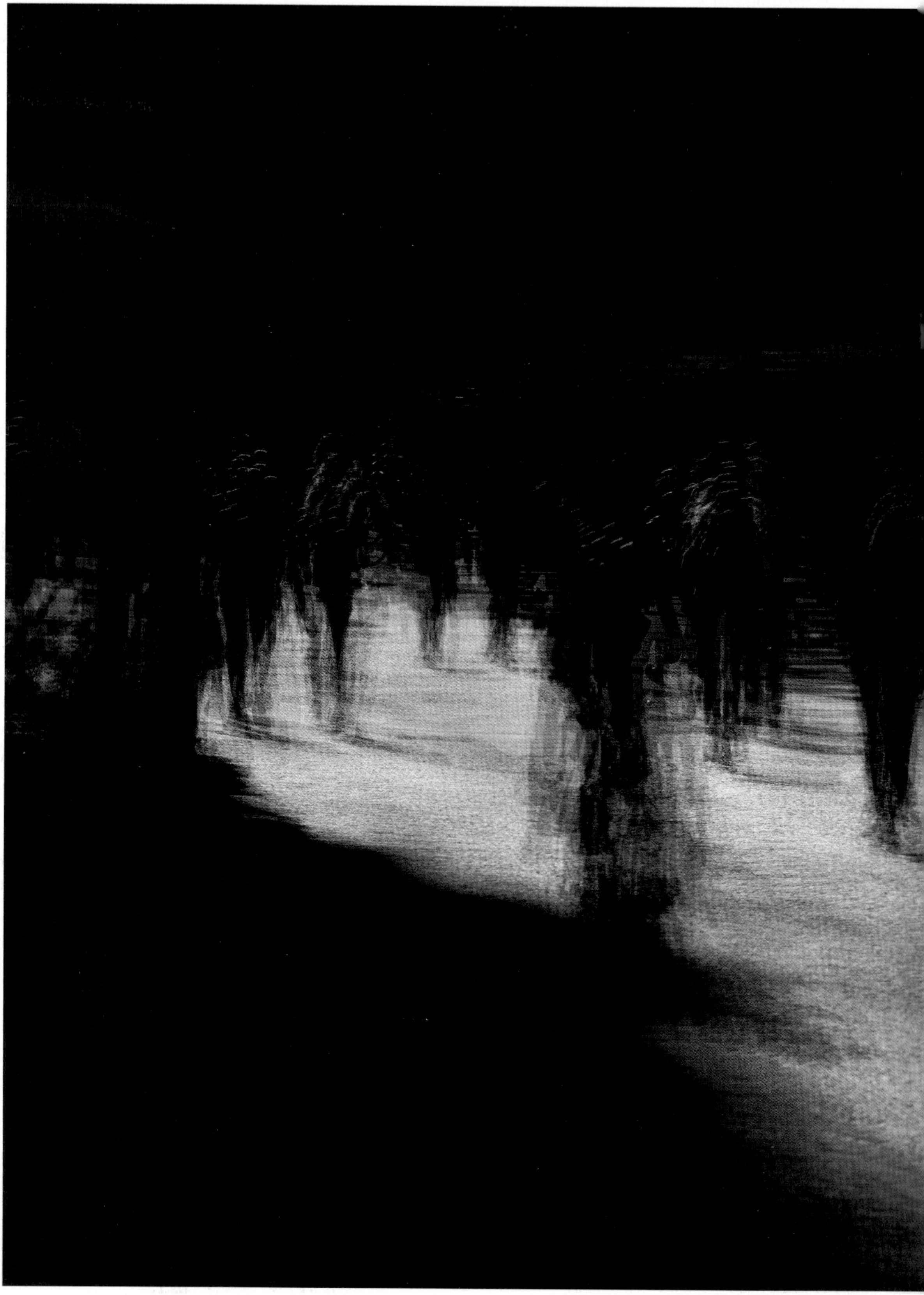

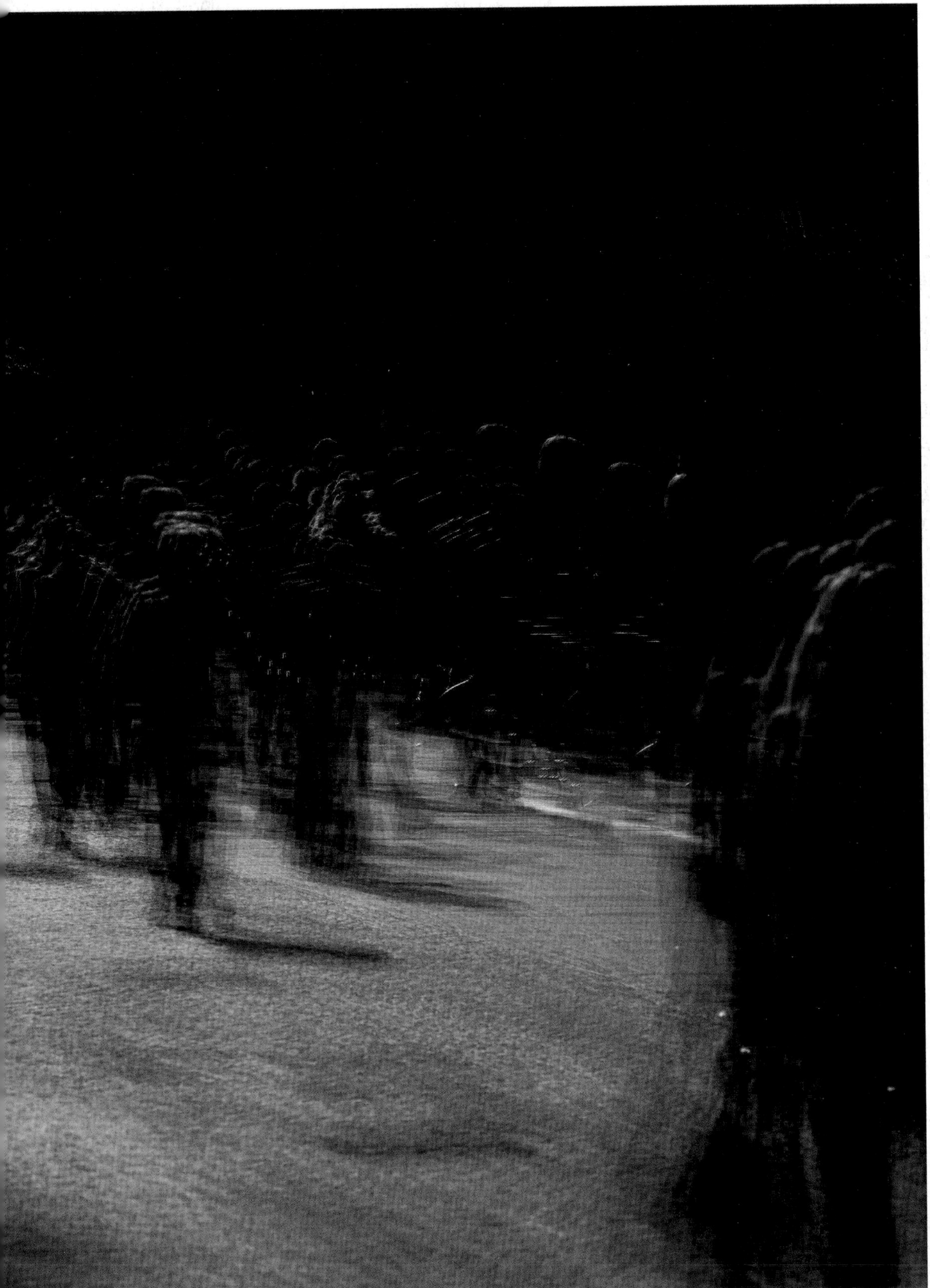

06. A New Normal
Captions

Michele Borzoni, Italy

Mass in the Cathedral of Santa Maria del Fiore, Florence. 31 May 2020.
(Page 391)

Modern history lesson at the University of Florence in the Space Cinema of Novoli, Florence. 12 October 2020.
(Pages 392–393)

Shopping centre of Ponte a Greve, Florence. 20 March 2020.
(Pages 394–395)

Mass at the Parish of Montughi in Florence. 30 May 2020.
(Pages 396–397)

Friday prayer in the garden of Piazza dei Ciompi, Islamic community of Florence. 30 October 2020.
(Pages 398–399)

Headquarter of COVID-19 contact tracers, temporarily set up inside the exhibition fair of the Fortezza da Basso in Florence. 11 November 2020.
(Pages 400–401)

Davide Bertuccio, Italy

The photographs were taken in October 2020.

As before COVID-19, every time a ship departs from a port, visitors stop to admire and photograph the sunset.
(Page 403)

The indoor five-a-side football pitch used as a COVID-19 area. In this area, swabs are carried out directly on board the ship. Those who test positive are either not allowed on board or they are isolated in special areas.
(Page 404)

One of the many dance lessons on board. Like for everything else, regulations must be respected and a limited number of participants is set.
(Page 405)

Miniature golf on board. Places for recreational activities are limited and queuing for participation is regulated by special stickers on the ground, applied specifically to encourage a safe distance.
(Pages 406–407)

Every day, for a few hours, all the sunbeds on the ship are sanitised.
(Page 408)

The gaming area on board the ship is the only area that has changed little from what it was before. Access has always been limited, therefore the only differences are the obligation to wear a mask and the constant sanitisation of every element in the room.
(Page 409)

MSC Grandiosa's main swimming pool, with an image of the sea projected onto the screen.
(Pages 410–411)

Anna Catalano, Italy

The photographs were taken between April and July 2020.

Decollatura (Catanzaro). Cristina and Sergio have prepared together the written test for the high school graduation exam.
(Page 414)

Eighth grade examinations. Catanzaro, Patari-Rodari School. During the exams Halima talked first about Manzoni and then about Covid, topics she had prepared with the help of some classmates.
(Page 415)

Eighth grade exams. Catanzaro, Patari-Rodari School. Halima arrived in Italy when she was three years old, from Morocco. She lives in a flat with her mother, one of her brothers, her sister-in-law and niece. The Institute gave her a PC and activated an internet connection to allow her to study from home during these months, like all the other kids who needed it.
(Pages 416–417)

Giulia learned to write in italics during lockdown with DAD (Distance Learning). At the end of each exercise she showed the exercise book to her teacher, who gave her live feedback on what she had done.
(Page 418, top and bottom)

Distance Learning for several hours a day triggered moments of tiredness and carelessness that were often difficult to manage.
(Page 419, top)

Since the beginning of DAD, every evening, the main teacher sent us parents a preview of the next day's lesson, also acting as an intermediary for the other teachers. These Whatsapp messages were intended to prepare the children for the next day's lesson and we, the parents, had to arrange the necessary material for it.
In this picture, the teacher showed the children a video in which she explained in person how to write the vowel U correctly in italics.
(Page 419, bottom)

Catanzaro, Patari-Rodari Comprehensive Institute. Giovanna's father watches her daughter's examination from the living room. Like all parents, he came from a period when sharing living space and time required a great spirit of sacrifice, but at the same time he was very excited to see his child pass the exam for which they had prepared so carefully.
(Pages 420–421)

Decollatura (Catanzaro), Luigi Costanzo High School. The school manager, Luigi Caligiuri, together with Sergio and Cristina Maturandi. The Luigi Costanzo High School is a 4.0 school, with a strong technological vocation. Being educated to a certain didactic approach, the transition to DAD was immediate and fluid on the part of the students, who often gave their support to the teachers.
(Page 422)

Paola (Cosenza), San Francesco Technical Institute for Tourism. Alessia studies on the bed in her room, as she did almost the whole lockdown period. Her father lost his job.
Her mother is a housewife.
(Page 423)

Alberto Bernasconi, Italy

The photographs were taken at the COVID-19 Follow up Department in Bergamo at the end of August 2020.

CT scan. The CT scan for the lungs can clearly shows the scars due to the coronavirus.
(Pages 426–427)

Routine tests, blood pressure, heart beat etc.
(Page 428)

Different type of samples according to the colours for different blood test.
(Page 429)

Respirometer test. A patient gets his respiration rate checked. Among the first 750 patients screened, about 30% showed breathing trouble and permanent lung scarring.
(Page 430)

Waiting hall.
(Page 431)

Rx-ray. A patient gets an X-ray at a convention centre that was converted for COVID-19 patients in the spring and is now used for follow-up care.
(Page 432)

The convention centre that was converted for COVID-19 patients in the spring is now used for follow-up care.
(Page 433)

Niccoló Rastrelli, Italy

Daniele, 12 November 2020, Florence.
(Page 435, top left)

Eva, 1 June 2020, Florence.
(Page 435, top right)

Francesco, 19 May 2020, Florence.
(Page 435, bottom left)

Manfredi, 21 May 2020, Florence.
(Page 435, bottom right)

Levi, 15 May 2020, Florence.
(Page 436, top left)

Gaia, 14 May 2020, Florence.
(Page 436, top right)

Andrea, 25 May 2020, Florence.
(Page 436, bottom left)

Luigi, 21 May 2020, Florence.
(Page 436, bottom right)

Mariasol, 16 May 2020, Florence.
(Page 437, top left)

Edo, 15 May 2020, Florence.
(Page 437, top right)

Daniele, 13 May 2020, Florence.
(Page 437, bottom left)

Zahira, 13 May 2020, Florence.
(Page 437, bottom right)

Francesca, 10 May 2020, Florence.
(Page 438, top left)

Marcella, 3 November 2020, Florence.
(Page 438, top right)

Faten, 5 May 2020, Florence.
(Page 438, bottom left)

Salvatore, 6 May 2020, Florence.
(Page 438, bottom right)

Rebiha, 13 May 2020, Florence.
(Page 439, top left)

Oliver, 11 May 2020, Florence.
(Page 439, top right)

Matteo, 10 May 2020, Florence.
(Page 439, bottom left)

Lyu, 8 May 2020, Florence.
(Page 439, bottom right)

Cover
Rafael Heygster & Helena Manhartsberger, Germany
Corona Rhapsody

Design
Luigi Fiore

Editorial coordination
Emma Cavazzini

Copy editing
Filomena Moscatelli

Layout
Evelina Laviano

Translations
Valentina Scaramella

First published in Italy in 2022
by Skira editore S.p.A.
Palazzo Casati Stampa
via Torino 61
20123 Milano
Italy
www.skira.net

Printed and bound in Italy.
First edition

ISBN: 978-88-572-4793-9

Distributed in USA, Canada, Central & South America
by ARTBOOK | D.A.P.
75 Broad Street Suite 630,
New York, NY 10004, USA
Distributed elsewhere in the world
by Thames and Hudson Ltd.
181A High Holborn, London
WC1V 7QX, United Kingdom

Credits

pp. 26–35
Alex Majoli/Magnum Photos

p. 96
Andrea Frazzetta
Excerpt from the article by Jason Horowitz published in the *New York Times Magazine*, April 7, 2020. Interviews by Raffaele Panizza.

pp. 120–129
Santi Palacios
This work is part of "Archivo Covid. Una cápsula del tiempo" (Covid Archive: Capsule of Time), a project created by a group of Spanish photojournalists and industry professionals together with the University of Alcalá.
It can be viewed at www.archivocovid.com

pp. 282–291
Loulou D'Aki
This essay on the Greek summer season during the COVID-19 pandemic was produced with the support of a National Geographic Grant from the COVID-19 Emergency Fund and Fujifilm Nordic.

pp. 293–299
Luana Rigolli
This photographic work is part of COVISIONI: a collective project involving 40 photographers from 20 Italian regions for a period of 12 months, in collaboration with Luz photo agency.

pp. 328–339
Nanna Heitmann/Magnum Photos

p. 402
Davide Bertuccio
Excerpt from a text by Davide Bertuccio and Chiara Di Giorgio.

pp. 424–425
Alberto Bernasconi
Excerpt from the article by Chico Harlan and Stefano Pitrelli in the *Washington Post*, September 8, 2020.

pp. 441–451
Paolo Pellegrin/Magnum Photos

The COVID-19 Visual Project was conceived and produced by Cortona On The Move in partnership with Intesa Sanpaolo between 2020 and 2021.
The complete project can be viewed on the online platform covid19visualproject.org